Clinical Ophthalmic Pathology

Principles of Diseases of the Eye and Associated Structures

To our families

Acquisitions editor: Melanie Tait
Development editor: Zoë Youd
Production controller: Chris Jarvis
Desk editor: Jane Campbell
Cover designer: Alan Studholme

Clinical Ophthalmic Pathology

Principles of Diseases of the Eye
and Associated Structures

John Harry BSc MB BCh FRCPath FRCOphth

Honorary Consultant Ophthalmic Pathologist, Birmingham and Midland Eye Centre, City Hospital NHS Trust, Birmingham, UK
Formerly:
Consultant Ophthalmic Pathologist, West Midlands Regional Health Authority, based at the Birmingham and Midland Eye Hospital, UK
Honorary Senior Clinical Lecturer in Pathology, University of Birmingham Medical School, UK
Senior Lecturer in Pathology, Institute of Ophthalmology, University of London, UK
Honorary Consultant Pathologist, Moorfields Eye Hospital, London, UK
Examiner, The Royal College of Ophthalmologists

Gary Misson BSc MB BS DO FRCS FRCOphth

Consultant Ophthalmologist, Warwick Hospital, South Warwickshire NHS Trust, Warwick, UK
Honorary Consultant Ophthalmologist, Walsgrave NHS Trust, Coventry, UK

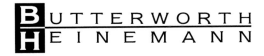

BUTTERWORTH
HEINEMANN

OXFORD   AUCKLAND   BOSTON   JOHANNESBURG   MELBOURNE   NEW DELHI

Butterworth-Heinemann
Linacre House, Jordan Hill, Oxford OX2 8DP
225 Wildwood Avenue, Woburn, MA 01801-2041
A division of Reed Educational and Professional Publishing Ltd

R A member of the Reed Elsevier plc group

First published 2001

British Library Cataloguing in Publication Data
Harry, John
    Clinical ophthalmic pathology: principles of diseases of the eye and associated structures
    1. Eye–Abnormalities   2. Eye–Diseases   3. Ophthalmology
    I. Title   II. Misson, Gary
    617.7′1

Library of Congress Cataloguing in Publication Data
Harry, John.
    Clinical ophthalmic pathology: principles of diseases of the eye and associated structures / John Harry, Gary Misson.
    p. ; cm.
    Includes bibliographical references and index.
    ISBN 0 7506 2171 0
    1. Eye – Pathophysiology.   2. Eye – Diseases.   I. Misson, Gary.   II. Title.
    [DNLM: 1. Eye Diseases – pathology.   2. Optic Nerve Diseases – pathology. WW 100
    H323c 2001]
    RE67.H375 2001
    617.7′1–dc21   2001025847

ISBN 0 7506 2171 0

For information on all Butterworth-Heinemann publications visit our website at www.bh.com

Designed and typeset by Keyword Typesetting Services Ltd, Wallington, Surrey
Printed in India by Ajanta Offset, New Delhi

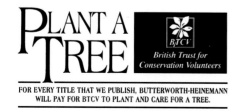

FOR EVERY TITLE THAT WE PUBLISH, BUTTERWORTH-HEINEMANN
WILL PAY FOR BTCV TO PLANT AND CARE FOR A TREE.

Contents

Foreword   vii

Preface   ix

Acknowledgements   xi

1   Injury and repair   1

2   Immunity, inflammation and infection   30

3   Genetics   114

4   Growth, differentiation and development   136

5   Degenerations, dystrophies and deposits   212

6   Vascular, circulatory and blood disorders   265

7   Disorders of nerve and muscle   295

8   The clinician and the laboratory   318

    Glossary   329

    Further reading   333

    Index   335

Foreword

It is a great pleasure to write this Foreword to *Clinical Ophthalmic Pathology*, an important new arrival in the ophthalmic literature. The recipe for the success of this book lies in the partnership of a clinician, with a particular interest in disease processes, and an ophthalmic pathologist of many years experience of diagnosis and teaching. They have generated a natural companion volume for Kanski's *Clinical Ophthalmology*.

In ophthalmology clinical and pathological disciplines are closely integrated and it can surely be no coincidence that many of the key figures in ophthalmology who have made notable contributions to clinical practice have spent some time training in ophthalmic pathology. The eye offers a remarkable ringside seat on pathological processes, biomicroscopy being an important daily activity of ophthalmologists. This allows for a much more indepth appreciation of disease mechanisms and hence options for therapeutic intervention than is immediately accessible in other systems. Well-illustrated, contemporary text that presents pathology in a clinically relevant way should be available to all clinical ophthalmologists, trainees and their more experienced colleagues who might feel in need of an update. This book is also relevant for others including optometrists, histopathologists, microbiologists and ophthalmologists who examine or report on ophthalmic specimens.

Clinical Ophthalmic Pathology provides precisely what is required to foster an understanding of disease processes. By taking a pathogenetic approach as opposed to an anatomical one, the reader is encouraged to crystallize mechanistic concepts in the mind. This is the central power and excitement of pathology that can all too often be lost in cataloguing the huge repertoire of diseases. Indeed, the large and growing base of ophthalmic diseases is only tractable when organized around a coherent framework of the understanding of disease processes as presented in this book.

There is no substitute for teaching on real cases around a microscope, yet current constraints on medical education are in many instances conspiring to limit this. *Clinical Ophthalmic Pathology* will assist both those trying to read microscope slides, and those learning remote from the microscope. Pictures of histology are worth more than a thousand words and the abundance of high quality colour illustrations in this volume hugely enhances its value. I would draw the reader's attention to the care with which definitions have been presented; such clarity is always used as a vehicle for understanding rather than as pedantry.

Finally, with all the excitement of sequencing the human genome and the ever-growing number of diseases caused by defined mutation, it is crucial to be able to integrate this new information into a framework of what goes on in actual disease states. To this end, pathology is about to undergo something of a revolution. That revolution can only rationally be built on a solid basis of morphology. The authors of *Clinical Ophthalmic Pathology* are to be congratulated for presenting us with exactly that.

Professor Philip Luthert BSc MBBS FRCP FRCPath FRCOphth
Department of Pathology
Institute of Ophthalmology, UCL
London, UK

Preface

Our main purpose in writing this book is to give ophthalmologists, optometrists and others in allied professions a knowledge of ophthalmic pathology necessary for the management of their patients. We consider that trainees should familiarize themselves with ophthalmic pathology at the outset of their specialist careers and that this is best done by applying the fundamentals of disease processes. Consequently the book is formulated around pathological mechanisms rather than anatomical structures. We have been precise in terminology throughout and it will be especially noted that 'ocular' is used to relate specifically to the eye and 'ophthalmic' to include the eye and its associated structures. Similarly, the term 'tumour' is also used in its original sense to mean any space-occupying lesion and does not refer exclusively to neoplasms. The book reflects the multidisciplinary aspect of pathology with particular attention being paid to morphology, immunology and microbiology, and to the ever-growing fields of cell biology and molecular genetics. Necessarily there have been omissions, and topics such as ocular toxicology and antibiotic sensitivities are not included. We have also excluded information about infection control because current recommendations are under review, particularly with regard to prions and the use of disposable surgical equipment. While the book is aimed primarily at those preparing for professional examinations, it will be of value to established ophthalmologists and other senior colleagues including pathologists who report on ophthalmic specimens and teach. A glossary of abbreviations is included but we have deliberately restricted references to key textbooks on the assumption that online or other reference databases are readily available. Above all, we hope that we have written a book that is readable, yet comprehensive, and will inspire further and more detailed study.

John Harry
Gary Misson

Acknowledgements

We acknowledge the generous help, advice and support given by many colleagues in the preparation of this book. We are especially grateful to Professor Philip Luthert for making available archival material from the Department of Pathology at the Institute of Ophthalmology, London. Our thanks also to past and present colleagues in the Department, notably the late Professor Norman Ashton FRS, the late Dr René Barry (subsequently also of Birmingham), Professor Alec Garner, Dr Gwyn Morgan, Dr Ross Cox, Dr Amjad Rahi, Dr Ramesh Tripathi, the late Mr George Knight, Mr Victor Elwood, Mr John Peacock, Mr Robert Alexander, Mr Ian Rhodes, Miss Rosalind Hart, Mr Melville Matheson, Mr Robin Howes and Miss Eileen Robins. We also thank colleagues in the Department of Pathology at the Birmingham and Midland Eye Hospital (now closed), in particular Mr Peter Bond, Mr Robert Hickton, Mr Geoffrey Rimmington, Mr Charles Shaikh and Mrs Angela Minto.

For advice and comments on sections of the text we thank Professor Luthert, Mr Peacock, Mr Alexander and Mr Matheson of the Institute of Ophthalmology, Dr Geoffrey Ridgway of University College London Hospitals, Dr Karin Loeffler of University Angenklinik mit Poliklinik, Bonn, Mr John Bertrand of St. Thomas' Hospital, London and Professor Philip Murray, Dr Peter Barber, Miss Lucilla Butler, Dr Paul Dodson, Miss Erna Kritzinger and Miss Saaeha Rauz, all of Birmingham.

The following kindly provided illustrations: Dr R. J. Campbell, Rochester MN, USA (Figs 4.81a, 4.81b), Dr M. P. Carey, Birmingham (Figs 4.57, 7.12), Dr B. J. Clark, London (Figs 2.6, 6.11), Mr J. K. G. Dart, London (Figs 2.59a, 2.59b), Dr P. M. Dodson, Birmingham (Figs 6.14b, 6.16), Electron Microscope Unit, Bristol Public Health Laboratory (Figs 2.37, 2.38), Dr S. I. Egglestone, Bristol (Fig. 2.52), Miss C. E. Gilbert, London (Fig. 2.62), Professor I. Grierson, Liverpool (Figs 7.6, 7.10), Dr P. S. Hiscott, Liverpool (Fig. 5.11), Dr J. W. Ironside, Edinburgh (Figs 3.6, 4.56b, 7.3a, 7.3b), Professor W. R. Lee, Glasgow (Fig. 5.13d), Dr J. H. McCarthy, South Shields, Tyne and Wear (Fig. 5.15a), Mr P. J. McDonnell, Birmingham (Fig. 5.20a), Dr I. F. Moseley, London (Fig. 4.50a), Professor P. I. Murray, Birmingham (Figs 2.27, 2.40a, 2.40b, 2.41a), Mr E. C. O'Neill, Birmingham (Fig. 7.4b), Dr. G. L. Ridgway, London (Figs 2.45a, 2.45c), Dr G.-M. Sarra, London (Fig. 5.7c), Mr S. Scotcher, Birmingham (Fig. 3.8), Mr A. Sharma, Birmingham (Fig. 4.84c), Mr G. A. Sutton, Birmingham (Fig. 4.31a), Miss M. D. Tsaloumas, Birmingham (Fig. 6.17a), Mr D. H. Verity, London (Figs 2.15, 2.16, 2.29a, 2.29b, 2.30, 2.44, 4.5, 4.38a, 4.75a, 5.5a, 5.40, 5.41a, 6.20a) and Professor F. T. Wojnarowska, Oxford (Fig. 2.31). Dr R. E. Bonshek, Manchester, provided the histological section for Fig. 2.13a and Dr McCarthy the material for Fig. 5.15b.

Our thanks to the staff of the Medical Library and the Department of Medical Illustration, City Hospital, Birmingham, and to Carl Stokes and Philip Sidaway of Dunn's Imaging Group plc, Cradley Heath, West Midlands. For secretarial support we are especially grateful to Helen R. Miles of Bromsgrove and, for printing draft copies of the manuscript, we thank Colin Hanson of Solihull. Finally, but not least, our thanks to Caroline Makepeace, Melanie Tait, Zoë Youd and others at Butterworth-Heinemann for their tolerance and forbearance throughout.

Chapter 1

Injury and repair

Cell and tissue injury

Reversible injury
Irreversible injury
Physical injury
  Mechanical injury
    The ophthalmic manifestations of mechanical injury
    Non-accidental injuries in children
    Penetrating and perforating wounds
  Thermal injury
  Ultrasound
  Electrical injuries
    Conduction of electricity
    Electrolysis
    Thermal injury
  The electromagnetic spectrum
    Ocular protective mechanisms
    Effects of electromagnetic radiation
    Non-ionizing electromagnetic radiation
    Ionizing radiation
  Chemical injury
    Alkali burns
    Acid burns
    Organic solvents
    Other chemical irritants
  Hypoxic injury
  Vitamin deficiencies and toxicity
    Vitamin A
    Vitamin B complex
    Vitamin C
    Vitamin D
    Vitamin E family
    Vitamin K family

Wound healing

Growth factors
  Cell types in wound healing
  The healing process
    Regeneration
    Repair
  Modifying influences in wound healing
  Outcome of injuries
    Skin
    Conjunctiva and episclera
    Cornea
    Sclera
    Lens
    Uvea and RPE
    Retina
    Orbit
  Neovascularization
    Ocular neovascularization

Injury resulting from therapeutic intervention

Contact lens wear
  Mechanisms of injury
  Structures damaged
Ophthalmic surgery
  Complications of ophthalmic surgery
    General complications
    Complications following specific procedures

CELL AND TISSUE INJURY

Cell and tissue injury results from a multitude of physical, chemical and biological insults. The changes produced may be reversible or irreversible.

REVERSIBLE INJURY

Sub-lethal injury is manifest as acute cellular oedema, fatty change and disorders of growth. These changes are either completely reversible or herald irreversible damage.

Acute cellular oedema (hydropic change, cloudy swelling)

Hypoxia, metabolic disturbance, fever, chemical injury and other noxious stimuli damage sodium and potassium transport, and other mechanisms controlling cell volume. The resulting osmotic disturbance leads to intracellular accumulation of isotonic fluid, swelling of organelles including the endoplasmic reticulum and mitochondria, and changes in the nucleolus. Affected cells appear swollen and pale on light microscopy.

Fatty change

Noxious stimuli also result in the intracellular accumulation of triglycerides. These are derived from peripheral fat stores and, because of their inability to couple with proteins, accumulate in the cell cytoplasm. Affected cells appear vacuolated in routine histological sections, but the fatty content of the vacuoles is demonstrable on light microscopy of appropriately stained frozen sections.

Disorders of growth

Disorders of growth in response to persistent stress include hypertrophy, hyperplasia, metaplasia and dysplasia.

IRREVERSIBLE INJURY

The irreversible breakdown of function results in cell death due to necrosis or apoptosis. Cell death may follow the reversible changes if the injurious agent is sufficiently great. Less commonly, injury is such that cells remain viable. Hypertrophy, hyperplasia, metaplasia and dysplasia may be irreversible or damaged cells may become neoplastic. The self-digestion of dead cells by lytic enzymes is autolysis, while the digestion of dead and dying cells by enzymes derived from surrounding cells such as neutrophils and macrophages is heterolysis. Cell death leads to atrophy of tissues or organs.

Necrosis

Necrosis is cell death accompanied by inflammation. There are a number of types:

Coagulative necrosis is the commonest type and affects the cytoplasm and organelles, the nucleus and the cell membrane. It is a feature of much acute pathology. Swelling of the cytoplasm and organelles, particularly the mitochondria, is followed by dissolution. Irreversible changes in the nucleus (karyolysis) include swelling and loss of basophilia, shrinkage and increased basophilia (pyknosis) and fragmentation (karyorrhexis). The increased cytoplasmic volume disrupts the cell membrane and the cell disintegrates. The dead tissue is firm and slightly swollen, but the general architectural pattern is retained.

Caseous necrosis is a type of coagulative necrosis in which the dead tissue appears structureless on microscopy. It is characteristic of tuberculosis.

Colliquative (liquefaction) necrosis is total liquefaction due to the effect of hydrolytic lysosomal enzymes and the lack of supporting tissue. It occurs particularly in the CNS, where the outcome is the formation of a cystic cavity surrounded by a glial reaction.

Gangrene is necrosis with putrefaction due to the action of bacteria, especially *Clostridia* spp.

Fibrinoid necrosis is seen in the smooth muscle of arteriolar walls where fibrin is deposited following seepage of plasma into the media. It is characteristic of accelerated hypertension.

Fat necrosis occurs when fat is liberated following trauma or enzymatic lysis. Some of the released fat undergoes lipolysis with the release of fatty acids and glycerol.

Apoptosis

Apoptosis is a programmed cell death not accompanied by inflammation and may be genetically determined. There are two underlying events, priming and triggering. Priming involves the accumulation of endogenous nucleases; the mechanism of this is as yet unknown. Triggering may be physiological or pathological and is the name given to subsequent events which involve an increase in the intracytoplasmic calcium ions, stimulation of mRNA activity and protein synthesis. The cell nucleus and cytoplasm condense and shrink, and membrane-bound fragments (apoptotic bodies) containing structurally intact organelles are formed. Physiological triggering occurs in the remodelling of embryonic tissues, in the deletion of unwanted lymphocyte clones and in the elimination of potentially neoplastic cells. Pathological triggering occurs when injury is insufficient to cause necrosis. This may follow radiation damage, minor ischaemia, viral infections, autoimmunity, and neuro-degenerative and dystrophic disorders of the CNS, including the retina. Apoptotic bodies are phagocytosed by macrophages or adjacent parenchymal cells, but cell surface membrane components are not released and an inflammatory response does not occur.

Atrophy

Atrophy is the decrease in the size of an organ or cell by a reduction of cell numbers and/or a reduction in cell size. It must be distinguished from hypoplasia (failure to grow to normal size) and aplasia (failure of normal forma-tion). Atrophy is a consequence of cell death, and may be physiological or pathological. Physiological atrophy occurs throughout life from embryogenesis to old age, and results from apoptosis. Pathological atrophy results from disease; diminished functional activity, denerva-tion, hypoxia, anoxia and disordered nutrition are among the many causes.

PHYSICAL INJURY

Physical injury results from mechanical forces, extremes of temperature, ultrasound, electricity, and electromag-netic or ionizing radiation.

Mechanical injury

The effects of mechanical injury depend on the amount of force, its rate of transfer, the surface area over which it is applied and the area affected. Tissues are disrupted and cells die. Concussion injuries are soft tissue injuries in which overlying structures remain intact. They result from direct or indirect compressive force. A contusion is a concussion injury of sufficient force to disrupt blood vessels and cause focal haemorrhage, producing discrete collections of blood known as haematomas. Soon after the formation of a haematoma, the blood becomes deoxygenated. This results in blue or blue-black discol-oration, which turns yellow as erythrocytes are ingested by macrophages and haemolysis results in the produc-tion of bilirubin. The yellow fades to yellow-green as bile pigments are further metabolized and removed. Abrasions are disruptions of an epithelial surface and result from direct or tangential impact. Lacerations are torn or ragged wounds, usually due to unidirectional tangential force. Incisions are clearly defined wounds made by sharp objects or cutting instruments.

The ophthalmic manifestations of mechanical injury

The various tissues are best considered individually because they respond differently to mechanical trauma. The response may also depend on the presence of foreign material introduced at the time of injury.

Lids and conjunctiva

Abrasions, minor lacerations, vasodilatation, oedema and haemorrhage result from blunt trauma. Foreign material frequently causes non-specific inflammation or granulomatous reactions. Non-specific inflammation is produced by particles of grit, wood, metal, glass, lime, cement and coal dust, by insect stings, by the lipid base of drops and ointments, and by the injudicious use of cosmetics. Psychologically disturbed individuals can introduce irritant materials that cause 'conjunctivitis artefacta'. In response to trauma, particularly if self-induced, active fibroblastic proliferation may result in a lesion that mimics a sarcomatous neoplasm. Granulomatous reactions include stitch or synthetic fibre granulomas, granulomas caused by caterpillar hairs, and chronic inflammation due to a diversity of foreign bodies.

Orbit

Orbital injury is manifest as oedema, haemorrhage, frac-tures of the bony walls, avulsion of the optic nerve, dis-insertion or rupture of extraocular muscles, and peripheral nerve damage.

Corneoscleral coat

Mechanical trauma can result in loss of corneal epithe-lium (abrasion), disruption of Bowman's layer and Descemet's membrane (this may rupture following birth trauma), and tears in the corneal and scleral lamel-lae. Foreign particles may damage the corneal surface or penetrate into stromal tissue (Fig. 1.1); invariably there is associated conjunctival irritation. Foreign bodies con-taining iron can result in corneal siderosis. Melanin deposition on the posterior corneal surface may result from accidental trauma; the melanin is contained within corneal endothelial cells or macrophages as phagocy-tosed granules, or is present within stromal melanocytes or epithelial cells that have migrated from the iris. The eye may rupture at the point of impact, on the opposite side (contre coup) or at a site of structural weakness such as the limbus, the equator (where the sclera is thinnest) or the lamina cribrosa. The sites of staphylomas or old scars are particularly liable to rupture.

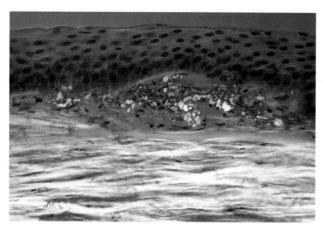

Figure 1.1 Multiple refractile foreign bodies in the superficial cornea. Partially polarized light.

Iris and ciliary body

Blunt injury may result in mild uveitis. Stromal lacerations, in addition, result in specific damage which includes:

Iridodialysis: detachment of the iris root from the ciliary body.

Anterior chamber angle recession: separation of the longitudinal outer fibres of the ciliary muscle from the circular and radial inner fibres; the ciliary processes become posteriorly displaced.

Cyclodialysis: detachment of the ciliary muscle from the scleral spur.

Hyphaema: blood released from damaged vessels is diluted by the aqueous and either rapidly dissolves by fibrinolysis or organizes with granulation and scar tissue formation, and resultant adhesions. Cholesterol crystals and macrophages may be present, and blood staining of the cornea can develop if the intraocular pressure is raised.

Pupillary disorders and iris stromal damage: physical injury can damage iris muscles and nerve fibres. This may be manifest as sphincter rupture and transient miosis followed by mydriasis, iridoplegia and cycloplegia.

Melanin dispersion: damage to the pigment epithelium releases melanin pigment granules.

Zonule and lens

Concussion injuries may rupture the zonular fibres and the lens may subluxate or completely dislocate into the anterior chamber or vitreous. If the iris impacts on the anterior lens surface, a pigmented ring (Vossius' ring) remains. Cataract can develop in undislocated and dislocated lenses; most commonly the opacity is at the pos-

terior pole and takes the form of a rosette due to forcible separation of the suture lines. Rupture of the capsule can result in cataract, anterior subcapsular fibrosis (due to metaplasia of the lens epithelium), phacolytic glaucoma and lens-induced endophthalmitis (both due to the release of lens material).

Vitreous

Vitreous detachment and subhyaloid haemorrhage can result from blunt injuries. There may only be a macrophage response but organization leads to fibroglial membranes and tractional retinal detachment.

Retina

Oedema, haemorrhage and tearing of retinal tissue can all occur. Commotio retinae and retinal dialysis are specific entities.

Commotio retinae (Berlin's oedema) is a contre-coup injury seen as transient grey-white opacification of the retina, most prominent at the macula. It is probably due to direct neuroretinal cell trauma. The affected retina exhibits intracellular oedema with fragmentation of the photoreceptor outer segments. Commotio retinae can lead to macular cysts and holes, focal scotomas and RPE changes, particularly hyperplasia.

Retinal dialysis is disruption of the peripheral retina from the ora serrata. It is most likely to occur in the inferotemporal and superonasal quadrants, and probably results from avulsion of the vitreous base.

Choroid

Bruch's membrane is relatively inelastic compared with the retina and sclera and, together with the RPE and choriocapillaris, may rupture when the retina and/or sclera are deformed by compressive force. Oedema and haemorrhage lead to choroidal detachment and, if Bruch's membrane is ruptured, fluid and blood exude into the sub-RPE and/or subretinal space and cause RPE and/or retinal detachment.

Optic nerve

The optic nerve can be damaged by direct mechanical injury (shock wave) or compression by sheath oedema and/or haemorrhage. Avulsion of the optic nerve is a severe injury usually accompanied by damage to other ophthalmic tissues.

Non-accidental injuries in children

Non-accidental injuries in children are considered under two headings:

The battered child

Intraocular manifestations of blunt injuries include subluxated, dislocated and cataractous lenses, anterior chamber angle recession, iridodialysis, cyclodialysis, retinal disinsertion or detachment and haemorrhages (anterior chamber, vitreous, subhyaloid, retinal, subretinal). There may also be periorbital, optic nerve sheath and intracranial haemorrhage. Recent or previous injury to the trunk and limbs is often evident.

The shaken baby

Intraocular injury produced by shaking takes the form of haemorrhages in the posterior segment. Initially haemorrhages are subhyaloid and subretinal, but later there are retinal and optic nerve sheath haemorrhages. The intraocular haemorrhages are probably due to shearing forces caused by vitreous traction, and are likely indicators of the coexistence of intracranial subdural haemorrhage. The intraocular haemorrhages, so characteristic of shaking, are not pathognomonic of trauma, and a similar picture may result from other causes such as blood dyscrasias, asphyxia and cardiopulmonary resuscitation.

Penetrating and perforating wounds

A penetrating wound is one that causes entry into a structure without traversing its entire substance, whereas a perforating wound extends through the entire structure. A perforating wound of the corneoscleral envelope only penetrates the globe, which is described as perforated if there is an exit wound in addition to an entry wound ('through and through' perforation is possibly more explicit but inaccurate terminology for this type of wound).

Perforation of the corneoscleral coat

Perforation of the corneoscleral coat may result in intraocular pathology similar to that following concussion and contusion injuries. It may also result in severe inflammatory disorders and extensive structural changes that often have serious consequences. Complications may arise from the presence of an intraocular foreign body.

Inflammatory disorders

Inflammatory disorders following corneoscleral perforation are either infective or immune-mediated. Endophthalmitis and panophthalmitis result from infection due to bacteria or fungi. Immune-mediated inflammations include sympathetic ophthalmitis and lens-induced endophthalmitis.

Structural changes

Structural changes following corneoscleral perforation include displacement of epithelium into the globe, lens damage, and disorganization of the ocular architecture.

Epithelial displacement: surface epithelial cells from the conjunctiva or cornea can be implanted into the globe at the time of perforation or grow down a wound track, particularly if the wound edges are malaligned. The displaced epithelial cells can form cysts (epithelial implantation cysts) or proliferate to cover intraocular structures in the anterior segment (epithelialization of anterior segment – Fig. 1.2).

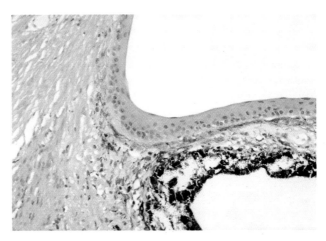

Figure 1.2 Epithelial displacement. Stratified squamous epithelium lining the anterior iris surface and the filtration angle.

Lens damage: lens material may escape into the ocular cavities and changes that occur include Soemmering's ring cataract (a doughnut-shaped structure formed from peripheral lens material – Fig. 1.3), Elschnig's pearls (large globular cells formed from the proliferation of lens epithelium), phacolytic glaucoma and lens-induced endophthalmitis.

Disorganization of the intraocular architecture varies in proportion to the severity of the cause. It includes incarceration of iris tissue into the wound (Fig. 1.4), adhesion of intraocular contents to a full-thickness corneal scar (adherent leukoma – Fig. 1.5), and, in severe injury, may lead to phthisis bulbi.

Intraocular foreign bodies

Most intraocular foreign bodies (IOFBs) gain access to the eye through a perforating corneal wound; a lesser number enter via a scleral perforation. The kinetic energy of foreign bodies on entry is determined by their weight and velocity. Small IOFBs are retained anteriorly, while large IOFBs are usually found in the posterior segment. Some IOFBs become walled off by a connective tissue

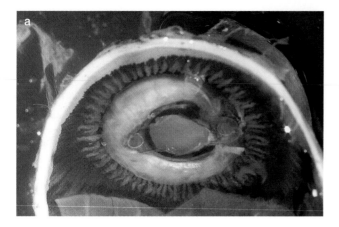

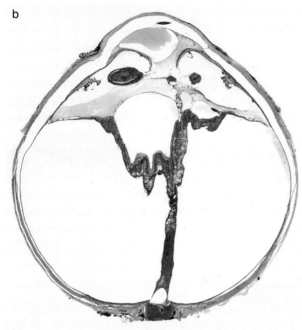

Figure 1.3 Soemmering's ring cataract. (a) Doughnut-shaped lens remnants. (b) The central lens substance is lost but cortical material remains at the periphery. The retina is totally detached in this specimen.

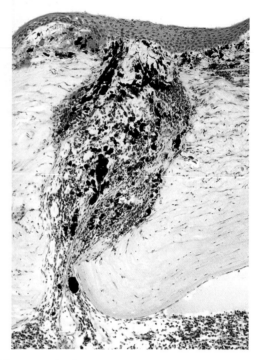

Figure 1.4 Iris tissue incarcerated in a limbal perforation.

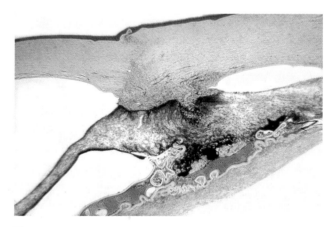

Figure 1.5 Adherent leukoma. Damaged iris and lens tissue adhere to the posterior corneal surface.

capsule and, although there may be degenerative and atrophic changes in the ocular tissues, if no harmful breakdown substances are produced can remain in the eye without damaging sequelae. Small particles are often phagocytosed without any clinical complications. IOFBs are either organic or inorganic. Organic IOFBs include suture material, wood, plant and vegetable matter, and eyelashes; they often provoke a granulomatous inflammatory reaction (Fig. 1.6a). Inorganic IOFBs include iron (or steel), copper, glass, plastics, lead (Fig. 1.6b), gold and silver, and compounds of carbon and calcium; most are relatively innocuous, but iron (or steel) can result in siderosis and copper in chalcosis.

Thermal injury

Extremes of temperature may result in tissue injury. Where the effect is widespread and associated with a change in body temperature, the effects of cold or heat are referred to as hypo- or hyperthermia respectively. Greater extremes of temperature may be concentrated in particular areas and this focal hypo- or hyperthermia results in characteristic lesions depending on the tissue affected, the temperature and the duration of exposure. Very rapid heating to high temperature in small areas

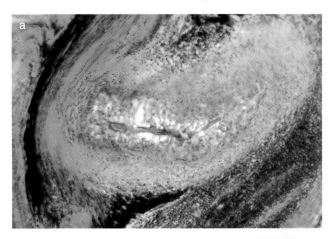

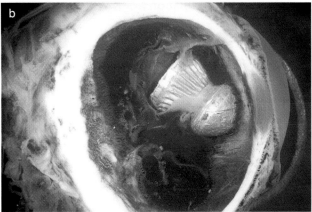

Figure 1.6 Intraocular foreign bodies. (a) Plant fibre and granulomatous inflammatory reaction in ciliary body region. (b) Airgun pellet.

causes vaporization of water or plasma (superheated ions and electrons) formation, and this has an explosive effect that mechanically disrupts tissues.

Focal hypothermia

Focal reduction in tissue temperature causes local vaso-constriction. If the temperature is sufficiently low, freezing occurs and the effects depend on the rate of cooling. Small vessel endothelial cells are those most significantly affected by cold injury, and this results in changes in vascular permeability. Transudation of plasma results in local oedema and blisters, and the cell injury causes acute inflammation. Freezing of the extremities results in frostbite, but serious cellular injury may also result from prolonged cooling short of freezing, with endothelial cell damage, thrombosis, vascular occlusion and gangrene (as occurs in trenchfoot).

Slow freezing

If freezing is relatively slow, ice crystals form within cells and in the extracellular spaces. This increases the electro-

lyte concentration in the surrounding fluid. Injury to cells and organelles is due to mechanical disruption from the ice crystals and the marked changes in ionic concentration in that part of the intracellular and extracellular fluid that remains liquid.

Fast freezing

Ice crystals are unable to form in rapid freezing, and an amorphous water-solid forms within cells and in the extracellular space. This causes much less cell damage during the freezing phase, but the most significant damage occurs during thawing when the water-solid may crystallize.

Focal hyperthermia

Focal hyperthermia sufficient to cause injury (burns) mainly involves the skin of the lids. The degree of damage depends on the temperature and the length of exposure. Heat coagulates protein, thus disrupting the structure and function of cells, and appears histologically as coagulative necrosis. Cutaneous burns are classified as first degree (erythema only), second degree (epidermal necrosis and blistering) or third degree (epidermal and dermal necrosis). Associated conjunctival reactions include hyperaemia, oedema and an inflammatory cell infiltrate. The major complication of thermal burns is scarring of the lids, which can result in cicatricial entropion and lagophthalmos.

Ocular thermal injury

Both heating and freezing damage ocular tissues, and the scarring that occurs may be used therapeutically to bring about retinochoroidal adhesion. Diathermy can result in necrosis of all the ocular coats and associated extensive inflammatory reactions. Cryotherapy is much less destructive, but the sensory retina undergoes coagulative necrosis, the RPE becomes vacuolated with dispersion of its melanin granules, and the inflammation induced results in retinal and choroidal scarring. Heat damage may be caused by light (thermocoagulation) and this is the basis for the therapeutic effect of lasers.

Ultrasound

Ultrasound is used in ophthalmology for diagnostic imaging and biometric measurements at energies and frequencies well within the tolerance of ocular tissues. Focused high-energy ultrasound is used during phaco-emulsification cataract surgery, and causes injury as a result of mechanical and thermal effects.

Electrical injuries

Electrical injury may be due to the passage of an electric current, to electrolysis or to thermal injury.

Conduction of electricity

The effects of conduction of electricity through the body are seen in injuries due to high voltage electricity and lightning. Systemic effects include tetany and disturbances in the electrical activity of the heart and brain, leading to cardiac arrest and seizures respectively. In the eye, high voltages (including lightning) damage the anterior epithelium and the posterior subcapsular fibres of the lens to produce cataract. Lightning cataracts are nearly always bilateral, whereas those produced by other electrical injuries are usually unilateral although not always on the side of injury. Younger individuals are more susceptible to electric lens damage, which, after a variable latent period, begins as vacuoles and punctate linear opacities. These changes may remain stationary or progress over a number of months to a mature cataract.

Electrolysis

Electrolysis is the process by which a chemical change is induced in a substance by the passage of a direct electrical current. Electrolysis results in localized tissue damage from the production of heat and hydroxyl ions at the negative electrode. This is used therapeutically in the focal destruction of small areas of tissue such as hair follicles.

Thermal injury

Electric current passed through a resistor produces heat in a quantity related to the current and resistance. The passage of a sufficiently large current through tissues causes heating that can result in injury. With high current densities disseminating from a small area, such as from the tip of a diathermy probe, arcing occurs with the generation of very high local temperatures that result in vaporization of water and explosive destruction of cells. Further from the source of the current, where temperatures are lower, coagulative tissue damage results from protein denaturation and dehydration.

The electromagnetic spectrum

The electromagnetic spectrum is arbitrarily subdivided according to wavelength. The longest (10^5 m; long-wave radio) and the shortest (10^{-13} m; γ-rays) are transmitted through the eye, but many radiations of inter-mediate wavelength are partially or wholly absorbed. The eye has evolved to transmit and absorb visible light (400–760 nm) which, together with infrared (> 760 nm) and ultraviolet (200–400 nm), may cause injury. Microwaves, infrared and ultraviolet light, and electromagnetic ionizing radiation (X-rays, γ-rays) are all capable of damaging ocular tissue. Ionizing events may also result from the interaction of charged particles (α and β particles) with tissues and, although not forming part of the electromagnetic spectrum, may have similar effects. The damage produced by radiation depends on the properties of the radiation, the ability of tissues to transmit/absorb it, and the susceptibility of the tissue.

Properties of the radiation

These include the intensity, duration of exposure and energy (this is inversely proportional to the wavelength). Tissue injury is more likely to result from focused radiation that is of high intensity, long duration and short wavelength.

The ability of tissues to transmit/absorb the radiation

The eye is unique in its ability to transmit light of visible wavelengths, but light-induced damage can occur. The eye can also transmit radiation of non-visible wavelengths such as microwaves, X-rays and γ-rays, but others such as ultraviolet radiation are selectively absorbed by the cornea and lens.

The susceptibility of tissue to radiation injury

Tissues containing rapidly dividing cells, such as corneal epithelium, intestine and bone marrow, are particularly susceptible.

Ocular protective mechanisms

Mechanisms have evolved to protect the eye from electromagnetic radiation in the visible and near-visible wavelengths. These mechanisms include behavioural responses such as aversion responses and the blink reflex, together with anatomical and other physiological factors such as the eyebrow ridge and pupillary miosis. The cornea reflects up to 60 per cent of light not perpendicular to its surface, and absorbs most short wavelength ultraviolet (UV-B, 280–315 nm; UV-C, < 280 nm) and some infrared. The lens absorbs longer wavelength ultraviolet (UV-A, 315–400 nm) and, depending on age, visible blue light. Within the retina and choroid, macular xanthophyll absorbs blue light and near ultraviolet, melanin absorbs a wide spectrum of electromagnetic radiation, the choroidal circulation controls temperature, and free radicals are scavenged by intracellular molecular mechanisms.

Effects of electromagnetic radiation

The effects of electromagnetic radiation are molecular, thermal or mechanical, and more than one process may occur simultaneously.

Molecular

Short-wavelength electromagnetic and ionizing radiation cause damage at the molecular level by free radical production, genetic damage or molecular fragmentation.

Free radical production
The radiolysis of water, whereby free oxygen radicals are produced, causes cell membrane injury, lipid peroxidation and interaction with vital cellular macromolecules, and cell death results. While this is an acute effect of exposure to ionizing radiation, it may also explain the photochemical damage of ultraviolet and visible blue wavelengths.

Genetic damage
Ionizing radiation and ultraviolet light damage DNA either directly by the absorption of energy or indirectly through the production of free radicals. This may lead to failure of cell replication or to mutation, the latter being associated with neoplastic transformation.

Molecular fragmentation
Radiation of appropriate wavelength (typically UV) and intensity causes resonance and breakage of intermolecular bonds, resulting in molecular fragmentation and evaporation of tissues (photoablation). This is the mode of action of excimer lasers that operate in the UV wavelengths.

Thermal

Electromagnetic radiation energy when absorbed is converted into heat. Damage is therefore most severe at the site of maximal absorption. For visible light, melanin-containing tissues have a great absorptive capacity and play a major role in converting electromagnetic waves into thermal energy. A retinal temperature rise of 10–20°C causes protein denaturation and enzyme inactivation, resulting in coagulation, necrosis and haemostasis. This occurs with moderate irradiance and exposure durations $> 1\,\mu$s, particularly with the longer visible and infrared wavelengths.

Mechanical

The energy of very high intensity, very short duration (10^9–10^{12} s) electromagnetic radiation may strip electrons from molecules to create superheated (15 000°C) ions and electrons (plasma). The intense energy produced results in an acoustic shock wave that causes local tissue disruption (photodisruption). This is the mode of action of the Nd:YAG (neodymium:yttrium aluminium garnet) laser, which operates at the IR wavelength of 1064 nm.

Non-ionizing electromagnetic radiation

Most of the electromagnetic spectrum is non-ionizing and may be derived from many different sources. All wavelengths occur naturally, but some are generated artificially for commercial, domestic and medical use. An artificial source of particular ophthalmic importance is the laser.

Laser (light amplification by stimulated emission of radiation)

Lasers emit monochromatic electromagnetic radiation that is coherent, collimated and can be very precisely controlled with respect to intensity, duration and focus. Lasers emitting infrared, visible and ultraviolet light differ in their effects on tissues, and are widely used in the treatment of ocular conditions. The effect of infrared and visible light lasers is predominantly thermal (photocoagulation), the Nd:YAG is a pulsed infrared photodisruptive laser, and excimer lasers are pulsed ultraviolet lasers that cause photoablation.

Microwaves (30 cm–1 mm)

Prolonged exposure to microwaves damages the lens and cataract develops, particularly in the anterior and posterior cortex. There is no evidence that microwave ovens produce cataract in the human eye.

Infrared (760 nm–1 mm)

The cornea absorbs the longer wavelengths within the infrared spectrum, but the shorter wavelengths penetrate the eye and inflict damage mainly on the lens and retina.

Lens
Although the lens itself absorbs very little infrared light, it is damaged by the heat energy resulting from the absorption of infrared rays by the melanin pigment in the adjacent iris. The damage is manifest as true exfoliation of the capsule, which curls into the anterior chamber, and as anterior and posterior subcapsular opacities – changes which are the basis of glassblowers' cataract.

Retina
Infrared rays absorbed by the melanin of the RPE are converted, as in the iris, into thermal energy and result in

a macular burn. Initial oedema with loss of the foveal reflex resolves to leave a cyst or hole. Retinochoroidal atrophy and a fibroglial scar eventually develop; the RPE is lost at the centre of the lesion but is hyperplastic at the margins. This type of lesion is produced by certain lasers, such as infrared diode lasers. Infrared absorption, together with the photochemical effects of visible light, is responsible for the lesions induced by direct solar observation without adequate protection (solar retinopathy, eclipse blindness).

Nd:YAG (neodymium:yttrium aluminium garnet) laser
The Nd:YAG laser is a solid-state laser that operates at the infrared wavelength of 1064 nm. The two modes of operation are continuous wave and pulsed. The continuous wave mode produces an output of continuous intensity and relatively low power, and causes photocoagulation. The Nd:YAG laser is more frequently used in the pulsed mode, when it delivers energy packed into a very small time (40 mJ in 50 ns). This causes plasma formation and an acoustic shock wave that disrupts and vaporizes tissue.

Visible light (400–760 nm)

The ocular media transmit up to 90 per cent of visible light, which is absorbed by melanin in the RPE and choroid, and by macular pigments. Visible blue wavelengths and ultraviolet light at intensities below the coagulation threshold can cause photochemical reactions that result in tissue damage. Sources include sunlight, welding arcs, lasers and the light from ophthalmic instruments, including operating microscopes. Functional deficits occur at or soon after exposure, and visible lesions develop 24–48 hours later. Damage is predominantly at the level of the photoreceptor outer segments and RPE, and is thought to be due to the production of free radicals. The effect is enhanced by increased temperature and an increased blood oxygen tension. The role of visible light in the pathogenesis of retinopathy of prematurity, age-related macular degeneration and other conditions is unclear.

Photocoagulation
The therapeutic effect of laser light applied to the posterior segment results from the absorption of light energy and its conversion to heat. The major sites of absorption are the RPE and uveal melanocytes, but the green light of the argon laser is also absorbed by haemoglobin within the retinal and choroidal vasculature. The maximal effects are exerted on the RPE, choriocapillaris and outer layers of the retina. Minimal to moderate doses spare the inner retinal layers but more intense energies destroy them, including the retinal vasculature. Burns produced by lasers appear clinically as white areas. Microscopy shows retinochoroidal atrophy, fibrogliosis

and RPE changes similar to those produced by infrared rays. Therapeutic burns in the posterior segment are made by the argon laser (green light of 457, 488, 514 and 610 nm wavelength), the krypton laser (red light of 641 nm wavelength) or the diode laser (infrared). Laser burns are used to destroy hypoxic retinal tissue, to seal peripheral holes and tears, and to destroy blood vessels.

Ultraviolet (200–400 nm)

Ultraviolet (UV) light is classified as UV-A (315–400 nm), UV-B (280–315 nm) and UV-C (< 280 nm). The epidermis, cornea and conjunctiva absorb UV-B and UV-C and the lens most UV-A, but are damaged when exposure is excessive. The main effect of ultraviolet light damage is on the corneal epithelial cells, in which mitosis is inhibited in the early prophase; nuclei fragment and the cytoplasm is denatured. The result is an acute painful superficial punctate keratopathy with small epithelial erosions that stain with fluorescein. Longer wavelengths are transmitted to the lens, where they produce lesions in the anterior cortical and subcapsular regions. Ultraviolet light damage is caused by sunlight, especially when reflected from water, snowfields (snow blindness) and deserts, circumstances in which the amount of energy delivered to the eye is virtually doubled. Other sources of ultraviolet light include sunlamps and welding arcs (arc eye), when there is usually a latent period of several hours between exposure and the onset of symptoms. Chronic exposure to ultraviolet light induces melanin pigmentation (suntan), and may also result in the formation of cutaneous basal and squamous cell carcinomas and cutaneous melanomas. Ultraviolet light exposure plays a role in the development of pingueculae, pterygia and spheroidal corneal degeneration.

The excimer laser
The excimer laser delivers high energy levels of short ultraviolet wavelengths (e.g. 193 nm for the argon fluoride laser) in very short pulses (10 ns) and, in conjunction with computerization, is used to remove corneal scars and other lesions from the anterior third of the cornea. It is also used in the treatment of corneal dystrophies and to reshape the anterior corneal surface to correct errors of refraction. Ultraviolet photons break intermolecular bonds and volatilize molecular fragments from the tissue surface. Damage is limited to the immediate vicinity of the target, small amounts of tissue can be excised, and the smooth surface remaining allows for re-epithelialization without significant collagen formation.

Ionizing radiation

Ionizing radiation is either electromagnetic or particulate. Only the short wavelengths of the electromagnetic spectrum have photons of sufficiently high energy to produce ionizing events, and X-rays and γ-rays are the cause of most damage. Certain subatomic particles, including α- and β-particles, produce ionization but their penetration of tissues is limited. Their effect may be enhanced if their source is ingested.

Radiation damage

The effects of ionizing radiation are predominantly at the molecular level, where DNA is damaged and free radicals are produced. Injury to cells or blood vessels underlies most pathological changes. With widespread irradiation, tissues may also be affected by the breakdown products of cellular metabolism. Single-dose irradiation causes earlier and more severe damage than comparable doses given on multiple occasions (fractionated doses). The major ophthalmic consequences of exposure to ionizing radiation are dry eye, cataract, vasculopathy and retinopathy.

Dry eye is due to loss of tears because the lacrimal glands become atrophic.

Radiation cataract follows damage to equatorial lens epithelial cells (i.e. cells that are actively proliferating). Months or years following exposure, these cells degenerate and become atypical, and the subcapsular regions opacify. The lens fibres become vacuolated due to the intracellular accumulation of fluid, and the whole lens becomes opaque. The lens is the ocular structure most susceptible to radiation, and those of the young are particularly vulnerable.

Radiation vasculopathy is essentially an endarteritis. The vessel wall exhibits an inflammatory cell infiltrate and spindle cell proliferation. The consequent narrowing of the lumen results in ischaemic necrosis of the affected tissue. This is the basis of radiotherapy.

Radiation retinopathy is a variation of radiation vasculopathy and usually occurs within 3 years of exposure. All retinal neural cells are radioresistant, but the dividing retinal vascular cells are particularly sensitive to radiation damage. Radiation exposure leads to the death and loss of vascular endothelial cells although vascular pericytes are relatively well preserved (cf. diabetic retinopathy). Endothelial cell loss activates the clotting cascade, resulting in localized capillary occlusion. Small dilated telangiectatic collateral vessels bypass these ischaemic areas. Other vascular abnormalities include microaneurysms, IRMAs, exudates and cotton-wool spots. Rarely, if the ischaemia is particularly severe, neovascularization may occur. The appearance is very similar to diabetic retinopathy, although the macular telangiectatic vessels and relative lack both of microaneurysms and of neovascularization are distinctive features.

Radiation and neoplasms

Ionizing radiation has therapeutic and harmful effects in relation to malignant neoplasms.

Radiotherapy
Radiotherapy can be used for malignant neoplasms of the lid, orbit and eye. Fractionation allows for a higher dose to be given without increasing the side effects. Each treatment fraction induces tissue damage, and attempts at repair follow. Neoplastic cells replicate more rapidly and repair less effectively than normal cells and are, therefore, more radiosensitive.

Neoplasia
Malignant neoplasms, particularly of the bone marrow and skin, are induced by ionizing radiation. Examples include leukaemia, basal and squamous cell carcinomas, and sebaceous carcinomas.

Chemical injury

Many chemicals damage ophthalmic tissues. The effects depend on the nature and concentration of the chemicals, and the duration of exposure. Limited exposure results in hyperaemia and oedema of the lids and conjunctiva, and lacrimation. Prolonged exposure, especially to more toxic substances, leads to necrosis and sloughing of tissues with subsequent fibrosis and scarring. Injury can be produced by a wide range of substances including alkalis, acids, organic solvents and other chemical irritants.

Alkali burns

Alkalis are especially destructive because of their ability to saponify fats. They react with the lipid component of cell membranes to form soluble compounds (soaps) that allow for rapid penetration, further dissolution and denaturation of proteins. Of the common alkalis, the least penetrative is calcium hydroxide; potassium hydroxide, sodium hydroxide and ammonium hydroxide are increasingly penetrative, the latter being particularly damaging because of its fat solubility and ability to diffuse rapidly through tissues. In moderate to severe injury the effect on the eye is almost immediate, with destruction of epithelium and corneoscleral penetration. Keratocytes coagulate, the glycosaminoglycan ground substance of the cornea is destroyed and collagen fibres swell. Dissolution of collagen follows due to the action of collagenases. Further penetration of the alkali leads to necrosis of intraocular tissue. Damaged tissues appear on microscopy as acellular, oedematous and necrotic. The main consequence of alkali burns is extensive scarring. Lid and conjunctival scarring results in ectropion, entropion and symblepharon, and the loss of mucus-secreting goblet cells leads to dry eye. The scarred cornea is vascularized and possibly epidermidalized (the formation of surface keratin and rete ridges). Intraocular changes possibly lead to iridocorneal and iridolenticular adhesions, cataract and secondary glaucoma.

Acid burns

Although acids coagulate tissue proteins in the lids, conjunctiva and cornea, diffusion into the eye is limited. Severe burns, however, particularly by organic acids, can cause corneal, scleral and intraocular damage.

Organic solvents

Organic solvents and petroleum substances used in industry do not usually penetrate the conjunctival and corneal epithelium and do not cause serious ophthalmic problems, but if the epithelial basement membrane is damaged recurrent erosions may develop.

Other chemical irritants

Tear gas damages the epithelium of the conjunctiva and cornea and causes profuse lacrimation but no permanent damage. Agents used in chemical warfare, such as mustard gas, cause severe conjunctivitis and corneal damage that leads to stromal scarring and vascularization and, in many instances, blindness.

Hypoxic injury

Hypoxia is a state in which tissue dysfunction and injury occur as a consequence of starvation of oxygen. This results from interruption of the blood supply of vascularized tissues (ischaemia) or reduced oxygenation of avascular structures such as the cornea in contact lens wearers. If the hypoxia is of short duration and not severe its effects are reversible, but if it persists above certain levels damage is irreversible and may continue despite reoxygenation to physiological levels. With decreasing oxygen tension, reduced mitochondrial phosphorylation results in a decline in the synthesis of ATP, lack of which leads to partial failure of the sodium pump and intracellular oedema. The rate of anaerobic glycolysis increases, and lactate and inorganic phosphate accumulate; both these substances lower the intracellular pH. Protein synthesis declines and changes occur in the cytoskeleton. All these changes are reversible, but if hypoxia persists mitochondria swell, flocculent intracellular

material accumulates and intracellular membranes fragment as a result of hydrolysis of their phospholipids. Cell nuclei disintegrate (karyolysis), cell membranes become freely permeable and the cell finally dies and disintegrates. The continuation of irreversible damage following the restoration of blood flow and reperfusion of previously ischaemic tissues results from the excessive synthesis of toxic oxygen species (O_2^-, H_2O_2, OH^-) from sources including neutrophils and metabolic processes involving xanthene oxidase.

Vitamin deficiencies and toxicity

Vitamin deficiencies (and occasionally excesses) are responsible for several ophthalmic disorders. Deficiencies are usually associated with an inadequate diet, and are rarely related to a single vitamin.

Vitamin A

Vitamin A refers to the group of fat-soluble unsaturated 20-carbon cyclic colourless compounds exhibiting the biological activity of retinoids. Vitamin A is mainly derived from preformed vitamin A in animal foods or from β-carotene in green plants. Vitamin A is necessary for the maintenance of normal epithelial architecture, particularly of mucous membranes, and is an integral part of retinal photopigments. Deficiency leads to night blindness and xerophthalmia including keratomalacia, which in developing countries is a leading cause of blindness in children, especially those between the ages of 6 months and 3 years. It is estimated that vitamin A-induced ophthalmic disease affects 5 million children annually, at least one-quarter of whom become blind from keratomalacia. Vitamin A deficiency also contributes to measles-associated blindness in developing countries, particularly in Africa and Asia.

Night blindness

Vitamin A forms part of the rhodopsin molecule, and is necessary for normal retinal function. In deficiency states, rod function is preferentially affected and night blindness is an early manifestation, with cone function becoming affected in more advanced disease. Loss of rhodopsin is accompanied by degenerative changes in the photoreceptor outer and inner segments and cell nuclei.

Xerophthalmia

Xerophthalmia refers to the external ocular manifestations of vitamin A deficiency and progresses through a number of stages:

Stage 1 Conjunctival xerosis: the conjunctiva becomes dry, thickened, wrinkled and opaque (stage 1A). Small refractile plaques (stage 1B – Bitot's spots) with bubble-like structures embedded in their surface later form on the limbal interpalpebral bulbar conjunctiva, particularly on the temporal side.

Stage 2 Corneal xerosis: the corneal surface loses its normal lustre and develops a fine pebbly appearance before becoming cloudy. There is a predisposition to ulceration.

Stage 3 Corneal ulceration and keratomalacia: corneal ulceration (stage 3A) follows stage 2. Early ulcers are small sharply punched-out partial- or full-thickness defects located on the nasal side. Full-thickness defects are usually plugged by iris tissue and the anterior chamber remains formed. Ulcers heal rapidly following vitamin A therapy but, if allowed to progress, extend on to the visual axis. Secondary infection may ensue. Keratomalacia (stage 3B) is full-thickness necrosis of the cornea with or without an acute inflammatory cell infiltrate, and occurs only in children. It is characterized by corneal sloughing, which is often bilateral and appears as a sharply demarcated cloudy gelatinous greyish-yellow lesion. A descemetocele may form or perforation may lead to loss of the anterior chamber and possibly infective endophthalmitis.

Vitamin A deficiency causes loss of conjunctival goblet cells. The conjunctival and corneal epithelia become keratinized and rete ridges form (epidermidalization), and saprophytic organisms (especially *Corynebacterium xerosis*, a Gram-positive diphtheroid) invade the abnormal surface. Bitot's spots are localized areas of the conjunctival epithelium where the surface keratinization is particularly marked. Chronic inflammatory cells may infiltrate the substantia propria of the conjunctiva and anterior corneal stroma. Keratomalacia is liquefactive corneal necrosis with fragmentation and dissolution of stromal collagen and loss of keratocytes. Its pathogenesis is unclear, but may result from activation of collagenolytic enzymes derived from polymorphonuclear leukocytes.

Vitamin B complex

The vitamin B complex comprises several independent water-soluble substances.

Vitamin B₁ (thiamine)

Thiamine in its phosphorylated form acts as a coenzyme for the decarboxylation of pyruvate. Thiamine deficiency leads to Wernicke's syndrome (ophthalmoplegia, ataxia and mental confusion) and beri beri, in which there may be peripheral neuritis and optic neuritis.

Vitamin B₂ (riboflavin)

Riboflavin is a precursor of coenzymes for several oxidation–reduction reactions involved in the transfer of electrons to oxygen. Riboflavin deficiency is manifest clinically in parts of the body exposed to ambient light, i.e. the skin and eye, and the lesions produced include seborrhoeic dermatitis, corneal vascularization and photophobia.

Vitamin B₁₂ (cyanocobalamin)

The commonest cause of cyanocobalamin deficiency is pernicious anaemia. The retinal haemorrhages and cotton-wool spots that may be seen probably result from the anaemia rather than from vitamin B₁₂ deficiency. Optic neuropathy is a rare complication.

Nutritional amblyopia occurs in those maintained on deficient diets. It is reversible in the early stages, but may become permanent. The cause remains unknown, although a deficiency of one or more members of the vitamin B complex is thought to be important. Degenerative changes in the papillomacular bundle result in central or paracentral scotomas.

Vitamin C (ascorbic acid)

Vitamin C is necessary for the hydroxylation of procollagen, and plays an important role in maintaining connective tissues. It is present in high concentration in the corneal epithelium and lens. Deficiency causes scurvy, in which haemorrhages result from increased capillary fragility. Petechiae or larger haemorrhages may occur in the lids, conjunctiva, orbit and intraocular tissues.

Vitamin D (calciferol)

The principal function of vitamin D is the control of calcium metabolism through the mediation of polar hydroxylated metabolites. Excess ingestion of vitamin D causes hypercalcaemia, which may result in band keratopathy.

Vitamin E family (tocopherols)

Vitamin E (alpha-tocopherol) is a powerful antioxidant for unsaturated lipids, and protects lipid membranes from attack by free radicals. Vitamin E is concentrated in the photoreceptor outer segments and, together with vitamin A, may protect against light-induced damage. It may also play a prophylactic role in the pathogenesis of retinopathy of prematurity and age-related macular degeneration.

Vitamin K family

Several related substances form the vitamin K family, which is chemically related to vitamin E. Vitamin K plays an important role in blood coagulation, and haemorrhages occur in deficiency states.

WOUND HEALING

All living organisms are constantly subject to destructive agents that can result in cell death and tissue injury. Wound healing is a complicated sequence of events, the purpose of which is to restore integrity to the damaged tissues. Wound healing involves chemotaxis, the division of cells, the synthesis of extracellular matrix proteins, neovascularization and scar tissue formation. Growth factors and particular cell types are important in the mechanisms.

GROWTH FACTORS

Growth factors are peptides that initiate mitosis. They may act on the producer cell (autocrine stimulation), on adjacent cells (paracrine stimulation) or on distant cells (endocrine stimulation); membrane-bound growth factors interact with adjacent cells (juxtacrine stimulation). Growth factors initiate their effects by binding to and activating specific high-affinity receptor proteins located in the cell membrane of target cells. The following are of particular importance:

Epidermal growth factors

Epidermal growth factors include epidermal growth factor (EGF) and transforming growth factor-alpha (TGF-α).

EGF is synthesized in most cells as a large transmembrane glycoprotein precursor molecule which, when proteolytically cleaved, releases a small biologically active fragment. EGF is found in substantial amounts in platelets, from where it is released during the early phase of wound healing. It is also synthesized by several tissues including the lacrimal gland and is found in tears. It stimulates the migration and division of cells and promotes epithelial cell regeneration in corneal injuries.

TGF-α is initially synthesized as a transmembrane glycoprotein and is produced by a large variety of cells, including activated macrophages, eosinophils and keratinocytes, and functions by autocrine and paracrine mechanisms. It is an important factor in angiogenesis, and other effects are similar to those of EGF.

Transforming growth factors

Transforming growth factors (TGFs) include TGF-β (TGF-β1, TGF-β2, TGF-β3) and are characterized by the ability to reversibly inhibit the growth of a number of cell types, particularly keratinocytes and leukocytes. Each TGF-β subunit is initially synthesized as an inactive precursor molecule, which is then proteolytically processed to generate a smaller fragment. TGF-βs are produced by platelets and by a wide variety of cells including activated macrophages, T cells, fibroblasts and bone cells. In the eye it is synthesized by the ciliary epithelium and RPE. Two of the most important actions in the context of tissue repair are the ability to stimulate the chemotaxis of inflammatory cells and the synthesis of extracellular matrix.

Insulin-like growth factors

Insulin-like growth factors (IGFs) include IGF-I and IGF-II. IGF-I synthesis is influenced by pituitary-derived growth hormone. Sites of synthesis are mature tissues including the liver, heart, lung, kidney, pancreas, cartilage, brain and muscle. It is found in substantial levels in platelets and, together with other growth factors in platelets, is released during clotting. It is a potent chemotactic agent for vascular endothelial cells. IGF-II synthesis is prominent during fetal development.

Platelet-derived growth factors

Platelet-derived growth factor (PDGF) and vascular endothelial growth factor (VEGF) are important platelet-derived growth factors (PDGFs). They have similar structures, but bind different receptors and stimulate different actions.

PDGF is secreted by platelets, and cells including placental cells, fibroblasts, vascular smooth muscle cells and vascular endothelial cells. PDGF is primarily a mitogen for cells of mesenchymal origin.

VEGF is a heparin-binding protein, and is found in astrocytes and Müller cells in the developing retina where blood vessels are forming and also in hypoxic retinal tissue. It plays a major role in ocular angiogenesis.

Fibroblast growth factors

Fibroblast growth factors (FGFs) are important regulators of wound healing; the group comprises acidic FGF (aFGF), basic FGF (bFGF) and keratinocyte growth factor (KGF).

aFGF and bFGF are single chain proteins derived from precursor molecules synthesized by a variety of cells, including fibroblasts, astrocytes and smooth muscle cells. They are potent mitogens for cells derived from mesoderm and neuroectoderm, and stimulate proliferation of most of the major cell types involved in wound healing, such as keratinocytes, fibroblasts and vascular endothelial cells. An important characteristic of FGFs is their ability to bind to heparin and heparan sulphate. bFGF is often found in basement membranes and extracellular matrix.

KGF is a single chain polypeptide synthesized only by fibroblasts and is probably a paracrine effector of epithelial cell growth.

Endothelial cell angiogenesis factor

Endothelial cell angiogenesis factor (ECAF) is a small molecule of unknown structure that releases enzymes required for basement membrane lysis and potentiates the mitogenic activity of FGFs.

Cell types in wound healing

The capability of cells to replace those that are lost is foremost among the many factors that determine the outcome of injury. In this respect there are three types of cells: labile, stable and permanent.

Labile cells continually divide and proliferate. They have a short lifespan and a rapid turnover time. Lost cells are soon replaced, but their high turnover renders them highly susceptible to the toxic effects of radiation or drugs that interfere with cell division. Examples of labile cells include epithelial cells and haemopoietic cells.

Stable cells divide infrequently and have less capacity than labile cells to regenerate. Most cells fall into this category, but those principally involved in repair are mesenchymal stem cells and fibroblasts.

Permanent cells normally divide only during fetal life. They are highly specialized, do not undergo mitotic activity and are not replaced following injury. They include neurons and cardiac and skeletal muscle cells, although the latter have a limited capacity for regeneration.

The healing process

Healing essentially comprises regeneration and repair. The specific processes depend on the characteristics of the involved tissues, but there are some general principles:

Regeneration

Regeneration is the replacement of lost cells. The term is applicable only to the labile cell population. An example of regeneration is the healing of a minor surface abrasion by the multiplication of epithelial cells which migrate from the margin of the lesion to cover the defect. When a confluent layer is formed, the stimulus to proliferate is switched off due to contact inhibition.

Repair

If tissue damage is such that reconstitution necessitates more than regeneration, then restructuring takes place through the formation of granulation tissue that matures into a fibrous scar.

Granulation tissue

Granulation tissue (Fig. 1.7) is a loosely-formed arrangement of capillary loops and specialized fibroblasts (myofibroblasts). Solid buds of capillary endothelial cells flow into the damaged area and fibroblasts are stimulated to divide and secrete collagen; in addition, they acquire bundles of muscle filaments (myofibroblasts) and attach themselves to adjacent cells and the underlying stroma. Myofibroblasts play an important role in wound contraction.

Organization, wound contraction and scarring

Organization is the formation of mature scar tissue following the contraction of granulation tissue. Extracellular matrix proteins are produced by fibroblasts and are laid down initially as Type III collagen, which is subsequently replaced by Type I collagen. Contraction takes place as the collagen accumulates, and a fibrous

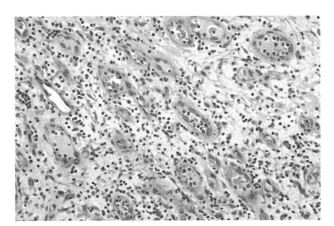

Figure 1.7 Granulation tissue. Inflamed vascularized connective tissue.

scar is formed. At the same time, dead tissue is removed by neutrophils and macrophages. Remodelling of a fibrous scar continues for many years.

Modifying influences in wound healing

Wound healing is affected by age, disorders of nutrition, vascular disturbance, denervation and the use of drugs.

Age

In children, wounds usually heal rapidly. The ability to repair damaged tissue diminishes with age, particularly in the presence of vascular or malignant neoplastic disease.

Disorders of nutrition

Protein malnutrition due to dietary deficiency or gastro-intestinal disease impairs wound healing. Vitamin C is necessary for the hydroxylation of protein in collagen synthesis, and its deficiency has an adverse effect on heal-ing mechanisms.

Vascular disturbance

Normal cellular function depends upon an adequate blood supply, but if this is impaired by ischaemia further tissue damage ensues.

Denervation

Denervated tissues may be unresponsive to repeated minor trauma, intercurrent inflammation or infection. Moreover, nerves play a part in mediating the inflamma-tory response that limits the effects of injury.

Drugs

Corticosteroids, antimetabolites and other drugs impair healing by interfering with the formation of granulation tissue.

Outcome of injuries

The general principles of wound healing apply in all ophthalmic tissues.

Skin

Minor abrasions of the skin heal by complete restitution. In larger wounds, healing occurs in three phases: the inflammatory phase occurs soon after the initial injury and is followed by the cellular phase, which merges with the phase of contracture and remodelling. Incisional wounds, the edges of which are brought together by apposition, are associated with little damage to adjacent

tissues and heal by first (primary) intention. During the inflammatory phase, fibrin is precipitated locally and holds the wound edges together, granulation tissue for-mation is minimal and epidermal cells proliferate super-ficially. Fibroblast activity and collagen deposition during the cellular phase increase the stability and tensile strength of the wound. Wound contracture starts at about 1 week and may continue for many months. The strength of the final wound is usually 70–80 per cent that of the original tissue. Epidermal cells occasionally become incorporated into a healing wound or along a suture tract, and their continued growth can lead to the formation of an inclusion cyst.

If for some reason the wound edges are not apposed at an early stage or if there is tissue loss, local haemorrhage or infection, healing occurs by second intention; macro-phages phagocytose debris, granulation tissue fills the gaping defect, and epidermal cells eventually grow inwards to cover the surface. The wound contraction and scarring that follow can, in the lids, lead to cicatricial entropion, madarosis and lagophthalmos. Excessive pro-liferation of fibroblasts with increased collagen produc-tion can result in the formation of a keloid nodule, a genetically determined phenomenon more common among black people. Differentiated structures such as hair follicles, and sebaceous and sudoriferous glands are not reformed.

Conjunctiva and episclera

Conjunctival wounds heal by the migration of epithelial cells from adjacent areas. There is little stroma to be affected but, as in the skin, inclusion cysts may form. Fibroblast proliferation is not a significant problem other than in association with glaucoma filtration sur-gery, where episcleral fibrosis can result in failure of the procedure. Antimetabolites, such as 5-fluorouracil and mitomycin C, are agents that limit fibroblast prolifera-tion when applied to the filtration site at or immediately following surgery.

Cornea

The commonest corneal injury is an epithelial abrasion, where there can be considerable epithelial loss without underlying involvement. If the cornea is perforated and the wound edges accurately apposed, then healing takes place by first intention. Corneal wounds complicated by substantial loss of tissue, infection, haemorrhage, retained foreign material or material which cannot be dealt with at an early stage heal by second intention, with resultant severe scarring and vascularization. Consequent developments include surface epithelial ingrowth, adhesion between the wound and the iris, lens or vitreous, with endothelial cell proliferation and possibly a Descemet-like membrane being laid down over affected intraocular tissue.

Corneal epithelial healing

This depends on the extent of injury, but regeneration from the limbus is the basic underlying feature in the healing of areas of epithelial cell loss. Small defects are rapidly covered due to amoeboid movement and extension of epithelial cells across the denuded area until they touch other migrating cells. At this stage, contact inhibition stops further migration. If epithelial injury is widespread, healing occurs in three phases.

1. Latent phase: within several hours of epithelial cell loss, polymorphonuclear leukocytes migrate from the tear film to the wound margin and remove necrotic cells and debris. Epithelial cells at the wound margin become rounded and lose their microvilli; cells of the basal epithelial layer lose their hemidesmosomal attachments to the basement membrane, flatten, slide over each other and form cellular projections (filopodia and lamellipodia) in the direction of the tissue loss.

2. Cell migration and adhesion: lateral migration of epithelial cells across the wound depends on the functioning of cytoskeletal elements and precedes mitosis and cell proliferation. Extracellular matrix proteins such as fibronectin, laminin and tenascin are also necessary. Fibronectin appears within hours of injury, and forms a transient subepithelial matrix to which migrating epithelial cells adhere. It has numerous functions including the stimulation of cells to synthesize plasminogen activator, which converts plasminogen into plasmin. Plasmin breaks down adhesions between cells to allow migration. When migration of the epithelial monolayer is complete, the cells become more firmly anchored to the basement membrane and Bowman's layer by the formation of hemidesmosomes and anchoring filaments containing Type VII collagen. Damage to the basement membrane will delay the formation of permanent hemidesmosomal attachments.

3. Cell proliferation: epithelial proliferation results from stem cell activity at the limbus, and produces a layer of normal thickness. Stem cells initially produce rapidly dividing transient amplifying cells, which form part of the basal cell population and migrate in a whorl-like centripetal pattern that gives rise to the characteristic vortex keratopathy seen in conditions such as Fabry's disease and amiodarone use. Epithelial wound healing is completed by further differentiation from postmitotic cells to mature corneal epithelial cells and the formation of additional hemidesmosomes to firmly anchor the cells to underlying structures.

Recurrent erosions

Failure of normal adhesion may result from abnormalities in the basement membrane and the formation and function of molecules necessary for normal adhesion and migration. This may occur as a result of trauma, damage caused by infections (e.g. herpetic disease), metabolic disorders (e.g. diabetes mellitus), or corneal dystrophies.

Bowman's layer

This never regenerates, and defects are filled by surface epithelial cells (corneal facet) or scar tissue formed from the stroma.

Stromal wound healing

Stromal wound healing is avascular, and the process is one of fibrous rather than fibrovascular proliferation that occurs in other tissues. It takes place at a much slower rate than the healing of epithelium and other connective tissues, and requires interaction between epithelial cells and keratocytes; growth factors play an important role. Following stromal injury, epithelial integrity must be regained before keratocytes become active. When epithelial defects are covered, epithelial cells and extracellular components form a plug in the deep aspect of the wound; this may persist for many months. Neutrophils are brought to the site by tears, and proteolytic enzymes initiate healing. Two to three days following injury, keratocytes form fibroblasts which proliferate and synthesize collagen, glycoproteins and proteoglycans to form new extracellular matrix. For several months the new collagen fibrils are larger than normal because of the higher concentrations of chondroitin/dermatan sulphate; collagen types I, III, V and VI are the predominant determinants of tensile strength. Stromal remodelling, under the influences of metalloproteinases, takes months, but leads to essentially normal structure and transparency, although tensile strength is seldom fully regained. Extensive stromal destruction prevents this type of healing, and the disorganized collagen found following such injury leads to an opaque scar.

Descemet's membrane

This does not regenerate but a new membrane is laid down, often in a multilaminar fashion, by endothelial cells. A retrocorneal fibrous membrane containing fibroblast-like cells, collagen and basement membrane proteins is an additional layer that may form posterior to the new membrane.

Endothelial cells

Endothelial cells do not regenerate, but cells migrate towards a defect in an amoeboid-like manner over the exposed Descemet's membrane/stroma or fibronectin submatrix.

Sclera

Scleral tissue is avascular and acellular, and does not heal itself. In the healing of scleral wounds, whether by first or second intention, scar tissue develops from episcleral fibroblasts. Contraction of the fully formed scar produces a pinched-in appearance.

Lens

A very small defect in the lens capsule may close as the result of fibrin deposition and the proliferation and migration of subcapsular epithelial cells; new capsular material is synthesized and fills the defect. Larger capsular defects permit fluid entry into the lens and consequent cataract formation. Some injuries stimulate the lens epithelium to undergo fibrous metaplasia. Escape of lens material into the ocular cavities can result in phacolytic glaucoma or lens-induced endophthalmitis.

Uvea and RPE

The aqueous contains fibrinolysins that inhibit fibrin clot formation and prevent scar tissue developing in the iris stroma. Uveal melanocytes do not regenerate. The collagenous scar tissue that forms in traumatized ciliary body and choroid results from scleral fibroblasts. Iris and ciliary epithelium and the RPE proliferate in response to trauma. The RPE can also undergo fibrous and osseous metaplasia to eventually produce bone.

Retina

Damaged photoreceptor outer segment lamellae can possibly regenerate but, as with all nerve fibres of the CNS, any interruption of axons within the nerve fibre layer leads to irreversible damage. Ascending optic atrophy develops, and perivascular astrocytes and Müller cells replace damaged nerve cells in the process of gliosis.

Orbit

Adipose tissue, bone, muscle, peripheral nerves and the optic nerve may all be involved.

Adipose tissue

Fibrosis follows fat necrosis, which occurs when fat is liberated from lipocytes.

Bone

Devitalized fragments of bone are removed by macrophages, and osteoblasts accompany the capillaries and myofibroblasts in granulation tissue. New bone (callus) is laid down and is later remodelled with more orderly bone formation.

Muscle

Skeletal muscle cells are mostly permanent, and their destruction usually leads to the formation of fibrous scar tissue. Vascular smooth muscle cells proliferate as new vessels are formed.

Peripheral nerves

Damage to peripheral nerves affects the axons and supporting structures. If a nerve is severed, axons degenerate proximally over a distance of one or two nodes; distally, axonal (Wallerian) degeneration is followed by proliferation of Schwann cells, which form channels down which the axons flow if the cut ends of the nerve are realigned. If the nerve is malaligned or amputated, axons proliferate as a tangled mass referred to as an amputation neuroma.

Optic nerve

Loss of axons, demyelination and astrocytic proliferation are the responses to optic nerve damage.

Neovascularization

In the physiological state, vascular endothelial cells are continually lost through haemodynamic damage and apoptosis, and are in constant need of renewal. Under pathological conditions the formation of new vessels (angiogenesis) is an extension of this physiological response. Its control is finely tuned by the release or activation of stimulatory and inhibitory factors. The three key events required for angiogenesis are basement membrane lysis, endothelial cell proliferation and endothelial cell migration.

Basement membrane lysis

An intact basement membrane prevents anchorage of proliferating endothelium to extracellular matrix and binds angiogenic growth factors in an inactive state. Membrane dissolution and the release of these factors are essential for angiogenesis. Basement membrane lysis appears to involve metalloproteinases.

Endothelial cell proliferation

In pathological states, endothelial cell proliferation results from an imbalance between stimulatory and inhibitory factors. Substances capable of supporting the growth of vascular endothelium include growth factors (particularly TGF-α, IGF-I, VEGF, FGFs), low molecular weight angiogenic factors (e.g. lactate, nucleotides and their derivatives), minerals (e.g. copper ions, selenium) and inflammatory mediators (e.g. IL-1). Antiproliferative agents (e.g. heparin, platelet factor IV, corticosteroids) inhibit stimulatory growth factors.

Endothelial cell migration

Activated endothelial cells, free from the constraints of the basement membrane, move away from the parent vessel. It appears that growing vessels provide their own source of stimulation.

Ocular neovascularization

Neovascular tissue within the eye originates from the retinal or uveal circulation. Corneal neovascularization is derived from limbal vessels. Angiogenic growth factors stimulate vascular endothelial cell proliferation. Inhibitory influences include the vitreous and RPE.

Retinal vasoproliferation

The three prerequisites for retinal vasoproliferation are:

1. The presence of living tissue.
2. Low oxygen tension in the tissue – hypoxic retinal tissue releases a number of angiogenic growth factors including VEGF.
3. Poor venous drainage – this ensures that angiogenic growth factors are maintained at effective levels.

Proliferating retinal blood vessels give rise to preretinal or intraretinal neovascularization.

Preretinal neovascularization: this is a well-recognized feature of diabetic retinopathy, branch retinal vein occlusion, retinopathy of prematurity and sickle cell disease. The new vessels arise from the venous side of the capillary bed at the margins of ischaemic areas, the neovascularization being preceded by an increase in the calibre of the parent vein. Two patterns of proliferation are identified by the extent of fibrosis: rete mirabile and fibrotic vasoproliferation.

Rete mirabile (Fig. 1.8a) is the type of growth frequently seen in diabetic and sickle cell retinopathies, the proliferating plexuses in the latter condition also being described as seafans. Rete mirabile are budding solid cords of endothelium that canalize and, although initi-

ally flat, develop into delicate fronds, which account for the characteristic clinical appearance. Associated fibrosis is sparse.

Fibrotic vasoproliferation (Fig. 1.8b) is similar to embryonic vasogenesis, and occurs in the neonatal period as retinopathy of prematurity. Undifferentiated cells appear to be the source of both the definitive endothelium and the fibroblasts. The endothelial cells form intercommunicating strands, which acquire a lumen and become recognizable as capillaries. These eventually secrete a basement membrane and acquire an outer layer of pericytes, the origin of which is not entirely clear. The fibroblasts give rise to extensive fibrosis.

In preretinal neovascularization, new vessels may regress to leave a flat vitreoretinal scar. Regression is most marked where there is least collagen, and rete mirabile are more likely to regress than fibrotic vasoproliferations. The untoward effects of preretinal neovascularization relate to the fragility of immature vessels and cicatrization of the accompanying fibrous

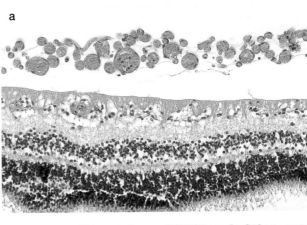
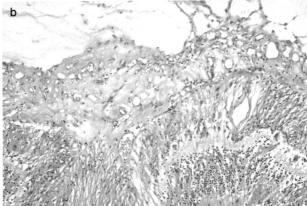

Figure 1.8 Preretinal neovascularization. (a) Rete mirabile; new vessels on the inner retinal surface with minimal fibrosis. (b) Fibrotic vasoproliferation; new vessels on the inner retinal surface with marked fibrosis.

tissue, and are manifest as haemorrhage, and retinal tearing and detachment.

Intraretinal neovascularization: the term intraretinal microvascular abnormality (IRMA) is non-committal and reflects the uncertainty surrounding the presence of vascular channels within the retina. It is not known if IRMAs represent remodelling of pre-existing defunct vessels or completely new formations, but their presence in relation to areas of capillary closure is undoubted.

Uveal vasoproliferation

Uveal vasoproliferation occurs in the choroid and iris.

Choroidal vasoproliferation: vasoproliferation from the choriocapillaris is an essential component of the exudative form of age-related macular degeneration, where new vessels grow through gaps in Bruch's membrane. Proliferation initially occurs between Bruch's membrane and the RPE, but eventually spreads into the space between the RPE and neurosensory retina. Macrophages are important in the pathogenesis.

Iris vasoproliferation: vasoproliferation on the anterior iris surface (rubeosis iridis – Fig. 1.9a) originates from venules at the pupillary margin or near the iris root. Dilatation and increased permeability of the parent vessels is followed by neovascularization and a variable degree of accompanying fibrosis. The resultant fibrovascular membrane leads to peripheral iridocorneal adhesion and possibly neovascular glaucoma, and ectropion uveae (Fig. 1.9b). Predisposing causes include retinal ischaemia, retinal neoplasia and anterior intraocular inflammation. It is thought that angiogenic growth factors released from hypoxic retinal tissue drain anteriorly into the aqueous and stimulate new vessels to grow, and that stimuli derived from retinoblastomas and inflammatory mediators in anterior intraocular inflammation have a similar effect.

Corneal vasoproliferation

The causes of vasoproliferation within the cornea are many and varied. Essentially they are infective, traumatic, allergic, toxic or metabolic. Oedema, hypoxia and inflammation are all important in the pathogenesis. The new vessels originate from the perilimbal plexus of venules and capillaries and may invade the cornea at any level.

Pannus: this is a fibrovascular proliferation between the epithelium and Bowman's layer (Fig. 1.10a), and is either inflammatory or degenerative.

Inflammatory pannus is associated with a conspicuous inflammatory cell infiltrate and Bowman's layer is often focally destroyed.

Degenerative pannus has far fewer inflammatory cells and less prominent vascularity. Regression leaves a fibrous scar. Degenerative pannus may be associated with glaucoma and chronic epithelial oedema.

Stromal neovascularization: this commonly follows inflammatory disorders (Fig. 1.10b) that are associated with stromal oedema. The vessels are straight and follow the divisions of the corneal lamellae. They branch in a brush-like manner and, being relatively free of surrounding collagen, there is little stromal opacification. Their presence erodes much of the cornea's immune privilege and increases the risk of lipid keratopathy.

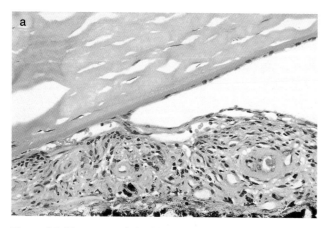

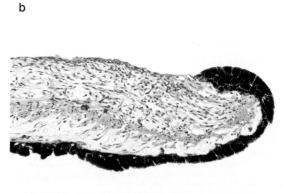

Figure 1.9 Iris neovascularization. (a) Rubeosis iridis; neovascularization on the anterior iris surface and closure of the filtration angle by peripheral iridocorneal adhesion. (b) Ectropion uveae; eversion of the iris pigment epithelium on to the anterior iris surface in association with a fine neovascular membrane.

a
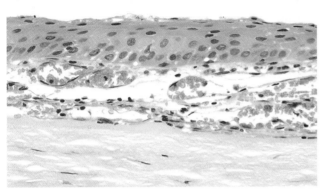

b
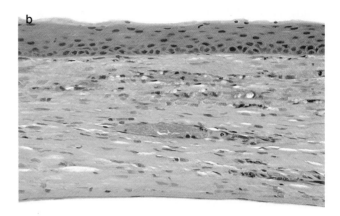

Figure 1.10 Corneal neovascularization. (a) Pannus. (b) Stromal blood vessels in a chronically inflamed cornea.

INJURY RESULTING FROM THERAPEUTIC INTERVENTION

Many therapeutic interventions lead intentionally or unintentionally to pathological processes. Such interventions are wide ranging and include contact lens wear, ophthalmic surgery and medications.

CONTACT LENS WEAR

Contact lenses are associated with significant ocular morbidity, particularly if the lenses are abused or poorly fitting or if there is pre-existing local pathology.

Mechanisms of injury

Ocular injury from contact lens wear results from four possible mechanisms: hypoxia/hypercapnia, allergy/toxicity, mechanical, and osmotic. Hypoxia/hypercapnia and allergy/toxicity are the most important.

Hypoxia/hypercapnia

Normal corneal aerobic metabolism depends on oxygen/carbon dioxide exchange at the tear/air interface. When a contact lens is worn, this gaseous exchange is diminished and the oxygen tension in the cornea is dependent on the permeability of the lens and the flow of tears between it and the corneal epithelium. Hypoxia/hypercapnia leads to the suppression of aerobic metabolism and decreased production of ATP. Anaerobic glycolysis is thus stimulated and lactate production is increased; the decrease in stromal pH (acid shift) and changes in the ionic composition of the extracellular matrix lead to oedema and predispose to neovascularization. The deep stroma and endothelium are at less risk of hypoxia/hypercapnia than the epithelium and superficial stroma because of gaseous exchange with the aqueous.

Allergy/toxicity

Allergic/toxic responses in susceptible individuals may be directed at any of a number of potential substances present on or in the contact lens or contact lens solutions.

Mechanical effects

Mechanical injury may damage the surface epithelium, particularly if it is already hypoxic. Diffuse widespread mechanical forces may alter the shape of the cornea. Steep-fitting rigid lenses induce corneal distortion or can leave a surface imprint, possibly leading to warping.

Osmotic effects

The volume and composition of tears is affected by contact lens wear. Following adaptation to the use of contact lenses, aqueous tear flow is reduced and its osmolarity raised due to increased evaporation as a consequence of disturbance in the lipid component of the tear film. These changes in the tears increase the risk of epithelial damage.

Structures damaged

The cornea, conjunctiva, tear film and lids are the structures primarily affected.

Cornea

The cornea is the structure most commonly injured, and any or all of the layers can be involved. The major predisposing cause to damage is hypoxia/hypercapnia.

Epithelium

Mechanical and non-mechanical trauma damage the epithelium. Mechanical injury may follow the incompetent insertion or removal of a lens, or may result from a scratched or cracked lens or debris trapped in the tear film. Tight-fitting soft lenses may cause wrinkling of the epithelial surface. Hypoxia/hypercapnia and, to a lesser extent, lens disinfecting solutions are the primary causes of non-mechanical damage and lead to cell swelling, reduced mitotic activity, reduced cellular adhesion and desquamation. The manifestations of damage include mild epithelial oedema (Sattler's veil), punctate epithelial keratopathy, abrasions, epithelial erosions and microcysts, severe ocular surface disorders with indolent ulceration, anterior stromal scarring and superficial vascularization. Epithelial injury also predisposes to infective keratitis.

Stroma

Stromal oedema is due to hypoxia/hypercapnia and presents as corneal thickening with striae and folds, corneal distortion and increased light back scatter secondary to disruption of the regular pattern of collagen lamellae. Other stromal lesions include neovascularization, sterile infiltrates, infective keratitis and corneal deformation.

Neovascularization in the deep stroma is due to hypoxia/hypercapnia, and occurs in both rigid and soft contact lens wearers. Although the progression of the neovascularization may be limited by cessation of lens wear, the vessels persist but shrink to form non-perfused ghost vessels. Lipid keratopathy (see Fig. 5.41) is a complication.

Sterile infiltrates are aggregates of inflammatory cells. They are a relatively common complication of soft contact lens wear, are usually small and multiple, and are most often seen at the limbus, although clusters may involve the central region. Their pathogenesis is not fully understood, but possible causes include hypersensitivity to the various chemicals associated with contact lens use, exposure to environmental toxins, staphylococcal lid disease, bacterial contaminants of contact lens solutions and chronic exposure of the corneal surface to debris adherent to the lens.

Infective keratitis is the most serious complication of contact lens wear, and is usually associated with failure to adhere to appropriate lens-care protocols. The users of extended wear soft lenses are 10–15 times more likely to be affected than those wearing daily contact lenses. Most cases of infective keratitis are bacterial, and *Pseudomonas aeruginosa* is the most frequent isolate. Less common pathogens include fungi and *Acanthamoeba* spp., which are seen particularly in soft lens wearers.

Corneal deformation (warpage) is due to a combination of diffuse widespread mechanical forces and hypoxic injury. It occurs in both hard and soft lens wearers, and usually resolves within 3–4 weeks following cessation of lens wear.

Endothelium

Endothelial cells are susceptible to stromal acidosis, and the changes that may occur include reversible blebs and irreversible polymegathism (variation in size) and pleomorphism (variation in shape). Reversible endothelial cell blebs are focal collections of oedematous cells disrupting the normal mosaic that resolve within 30 minutes of removal of the lens and are not associated with any long-term sequelae. Polymegathism and pleomorphism are frequently associated with long-term polymethylmethacrylate (PMMA) lenses and extended wear lenses and, to a lesser extent, day-wear soft lenses.

Conjunctiva

The number of conjunctival goblet cells increases in contact lens wearers. Inflammation is often associated with contact lens abuse, trauma, toxicity and immune reactions. Specific conditions include toxic conjunctivitis, allergic conjunctivitis, giant papillary conjunctivitis and superior limbic keratoconjunctivitis.

Toxic conjunctivitis is due to contact lens-related chemicals, but does not depend on the dose of irritant or the susceptibility of the individual. Presentation is with a papillary conjunctivitis, particularly pronounced in the inferior fornix.

Allergic conjunctivitis also presents as a papillary response, but is distinguished from toxic conjunctivitis by the presence of intense itching and chemosis. The allergen may be a contact lens-related chemical or an external substance, exposure to which is increased because of the presence of a contact lens.

Giant papillary conjunctivitis presents with itching, excess mucus and giant papillae of the upper tarsal conjunctiva. It is thought to be a Type IV hypersensitivity reaction to proteinaceous material accumulating on the surface of the lens, and is more frequent in those who use extended wear soft lenses.

Superior limbic keratoconjunctivitis is usually bilateral and symmetrical, and is characterized by superior bulbar conjunctival inflammation with thickening and redundancy of the conjunctiva, which exhibits epithelial irregularity. The cornea shows punctate epithelial erosions. The pathogenesis is not clear, but preservative toxicity and mechanical irritation may be significant.

Tear film

Contact lenses are associated with meibomian gland dysfunction and an increase in the number of conjunctival goblet cells. Disruption of the lipid component of tears leads to dry eye syndrome. Ocular surface drying is exacerbated by reduced tear secretion and by the wearing of high-water-content, extended wear hydrogel lenses, which absorb water from the tear lake.

Lids

Inflammation of the lids as a result of contact lens wear is usually subclinical but may underlie complications such as dry eye. Chronic low-grade inflammation leads to meibomian gland dysfunction, which interferes with normal tear film composition and dynamics and causes accumulation of irritant contact lens deposits. Blepharoptosis is associated with the long-term wearing of rigid contact lenses. It is due to levator aponeurosis disinsertion, although the pathogenesis is unclear.

OPHTHALMIC SURGERY

Surgery is the deliberate and controlled manipulation and/or wounding of tissue in order to produce a beneficial result. As in any form of trauma, the response depends on the site, nature and extent of the injury. Ophthalmic surgical procedures mostly involve cutting, coagulation by heat, electrical current or freezing, or exposure to ultrasound, light or ionizing radiation. Drugs, irrigating fluids and disinfecting solutions are often used, as are sutures, orbital implants, extraocular plombs, intraocular lenses, viscoelastic materials and gases.

The basic manoeuvres of surgery involve the creation and closure of wounds, procedures that are carried out in such a way as to minimize complications and maximize the therapeutic aim. Wounds are created by incision or the use of a diathermy or laser. Wounds may then be closed with sutures, tape or other surgical devices that bring the cut edges together. Healing of closed wounds is said to occur by primary intention (i.e. this being the 'primary intention' of the surgeon). Alternatively, wounds may be left open to allow granulation tissue formation and re-epithelialization, and heal by second intention. Although wound healing is tissue specific and is different for skin and ocular tissues such as cornea, sclera and RPE, there are important similarities.

Healing by primary (first) intention

In closed wounds there is no tissue deficit, and healing results in the adhesion and reintegration of the apposed surfaces with the formation of a relatively small scar. The tensile strength of the wound increases with time, although for skin it may be as low as 5 per cent of normal at 5 days. Corneal tensile strength may not return to normal values for many months. As the wound edges are apposed, re-epithelialization is rapid and, if sutures remain *in situ* for a protracted period (e.g. > 1 week for skin), the suture tracts may become lined with epithelium. Suturing is associated with a greater inflammatory response than that occurring in non-sutured wounds, but the degree of inflammation depends on the number of sutures, the suture technique and the suture material (e.g. silk, nylon, polyester, catgut, polyglycan). Silk and catgut cause much greater inflammatory responses than synthetic materials such as nylon, polyester or polyglycan; polyglycan rapidly biodegrades and is removed by phagocytes; nylon is slowly hydrolysed by lysosomal enzymes; both silk and nylon (but not polyester) biodegrade.

Healing by second intention

Healing by second intention occurs in wounds that have unopposed edges or where tissue is lost between the wound edges. Partial thickness skin wounds and conjunctival and corneal epithelial defects heal without scarring. Re-epithelialization of partial thickness cutaneous wounds originates from both the wound edges and remnants of epidermal/epithelial tissues left in the bed of the wound, such as those originating from transected epidermal-associated structures. In full thickness skin wounds, following a time lag corresponding to the inflammatory phase, granulation tissue forms in the base of the wound and scarring is usual. Re-epithelialization occurs only from the wound edges, as epidermal-associated structures have been lost. Retraction of connective tissue causes gaping, which delays the healing of underlying structures. Collagen orientation is relatively random, but remodelling occurs later and depends on contact guidance, chemotaxis and the distribution of mechanical stresses. Corneal wounds may gape as a result of the retraction of lamellar collagen fibres, and this is influenced by intraocular pressure, gravity and the mechanical effects of the lids. Random orientation of collagen in the cornea results in opacification, and elsewhere is evident as a scar that differs in consistency from the surrounding tissue.

Complications of ophthalmic surgery

Surgical intervention occasionally deviates from the predicted course, with resulting harmful effects. Complications are best classified as non-specific and common to many procedures, or procedure-specific.

General complications

General complications include those due to faulty incisions and suturing, haemorrhage and thrombosis, intraocular pressure variations, intraocular manipulation and inflammation.

Faulty incisions and suturing

Faulty incisions may create the wound in an inappropriate location or extend it into adjacent structures. Inaccurate suturing may cause persistent deformity, and the consequences depend on the tissues involved. Malalignment and distortion of the lid, corneal astigmatism and iris prolapse with incarceration all result from inaccurate suturing. A malaligned wound of the eye may leak and act as a route for intraocular infection or epithelial ingrowth.

Haemorrhage and thrombosis

Haemorrhage is classified as primary (at the time of surgery), reactionary (within 24 hours of surgery due to reperfusion of cut blood vessels) or secondary (7–14 days after surgery and usually due to infection). Thrombosis is an unusual complication of ophthalmic surgery other than in the retinal vasculature as a consequence of elevated intraocular pressure.

Intraocular pressure variations

Fluctuations in intraocular pressure commonly follow intraocular surgery and, if not prolonged or extreme, are of little consequence. Pressure variations include hypotony and secondary glaucoma.

Hypotony: opening the eye lowers the intraocular pressure and may result in expulsive haemorrhage. The hypotony following filtration procedures or inadequate wound closure is associated with serous choroidal detachment, which in turn reduces aqueous secretion, thereby further lowering the intraocular pressure. Hypotony may result in a shallow anterior chamber and lenticuloiridocorneal adhesion, cataract and corneal endothelial damage.

Secondary glaucoma: persistent elevation of the intraocular pressure can lead to retinal arteriolar or venous occlusion, the former being a particular complication of vitreoretinal surgery where encircling bands or internal tamponade are used. Elevation of the intraocular pressure is common during the first few post-operative days of intraocular surgery, and relates to the use of viscoelastic materials and the presence of particulate matter and cells in the trabecular meshwork. Post-operative corticosteroid medication is another cause of a more persistent and potentially serious elevation of intraocular pressure.

Intraocular manipulation

Complications arising from intraocular manipulation include those due to corneal endothelial and lens damage.

Corneal endothelial cell damage leads to stromal and epithelial oedema. Predisposing factors include a reduced cell count and polygmegathism. Immediately following focal endothelial damage, the cells in the region of injury lose their hexagonal shape and uniform size as they try to cover the defect. Stromal oedema rapidly resolves as the endothelial pump mechanism is restored to normality, but structural changes may persist for months. Severe endothelial damage results in chronic stromal and epithelial oedema.

Lens damage may lead to subluxation, dislocation, cataract, phacolytic glaucoma or lens-induced endophthalmitis.

Inflammation

Inflammatory complications include cystoid macular oedema, post-operative infective endophthalmitis, lens-induced endophthalmitis and sympathetic ophthalmitis.

Cystoid macular oedema (CMO) is macular oedema characterized by the presence of cyst-like fluid accumulations in the outer plexiform layer (Fig. 1.11). It is uncertain whether the fluid accumulations are extra- or intracellu-

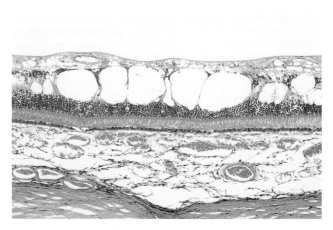

Figure 1.11 Cystoid macular oedema. Cyst-like spaces in the outer plexiform layer of the retina.

lar, although the first ultrastructural change is the appearance of fluid within Müller cells. In some instances, chronic inflammatory cells infiltrate in relation to the perifoveal capillaries and other intraocular vessels. In the later stages, serous exudate separates the central photoreceptors from the RPE. The cause of CMO is unknown, but a putative role for prostaglandins is the rationale behind the use of cyclo-oxygenase inhibitors in its treatment.

Complications following specific procedures

Complications may follow corneal and corneolimbal incisions, keratoplasty, corneorefractive procedures, cataract, glaucoma and vitreoretinal surgery, eviscerations, enucleations and exenterations, and extraocular surgery.

Corneal and corneolimbal incisions

Epithelial injury is commonly caused by surgical manipulation and the use of topical medications, but healing is usually quick and uneventful.

Descemet's membrane detachment and/or rupture initially leads to stromal and epithelial oedema, but most cases resolve if the corneal endothelium remains viable. A detached Descemet's membrane may fall back into place, but rupture is usually followed by the formation of a new Descemet's membrane that covers exposed stroma.

Endothelial cell loss leads to stromal and epithelial oedema which, in the presence of an intraocular lens, is referred to as pseudophakic keratopathy.

Retrocorneal membranes appear clinically as fine grey lines on the posterior corneal surface. They may be part of an epithelialized anterior segment or follow fibrous ingrowth (Fig. 1.12).

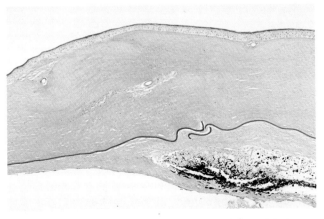

Figure 1.12 Retrocorneal fibrous membrane with associated disruption of Descemet's membrane and of the underlying adherent iris.

Epithelialization of the anterior segment (Fig. 1.2) follows the implantation or ingrowth of epithelial cells. Epithelial implantation occurs when conjunctival or corneal epithelial cells are implanted into the aqueous at the time of surgical incision. Epithelial ingrowth is the proliferation of conjunctival or corneal epithelium into the anterior chamber, either through a non-healed wound or as a consequence of the incarceration of epithelial cells in a wound track. If the epithelial cells proliferate into the trabecular meshwork, intractable secondary glaucoma is a possible consequence.

Fibrous ingrowth is similar to epithelial ingrowth, although the offending tissue is thought to be the subconjunctival connective tissue. Fibroblasts proliferate through poorly healing wounds and invade the anterior chamber. Retrocorneal fibrous membranes may also arise from malaligned corneal wounds, from the organization of inflammatory or haemorrhagic exudates in the anterior chamber, and from fibrous metaplasia of the corneal endothelium.

Endothelialization of the anterior segment is rare. Endothelial cells migrate throughout the anterior segment and deposit a Descemet-like membrane and, as with epithelialization, secondary glaucoma may result from trabecular involvement.

Keratoplasty

The healing processes involved in penetrating keratoplasty are those of normal corneal wound healing. The antigenic difference between the graft and the host makes the possibility of rejection a considerable threat, predominating over other potential general complications following procedures that breach the corneoscleral coat. The latter include retrocorneal fibrous membrane formation consequent upon malalignment of the wound edges, fibrous metaplasia of the corneal endothelium, epithelialization of the anterior segment, and infection. Lamellar keratoplasty and epikeratophakia create a large interface between host and graft tissue in the plane parallel to the surface; this remains structurally weak and is the potential site for the ingrowth of epithelium and the formation of intrastromal cysts.

Normal healing of keratoplasty wounds

Following keratoplasty, the anterior aspect of the wound tends to gape because of the elasticity of Bowman's layer. Deeper within the cornea, the exposed stroma of host and graft becomes oedematous and helps to bring the wound edges into apposition. Migrating and proliferating epithelial cells fill the gap to the level of apposed stroma. Activated keratocytes later migrate into the area and lay down collagen and extracellular matrix, which lacks the structural regularity of normal stroma and tends to be opaque. Endothelial cells migrate over the posterior surface of the wound and lay down a new Descemet's membrane in deficient areas. With time, the wound remodels with reorientation of corneal lamellae. Stromal healing is less efficient in the plane parallel to the corneal surface.

Complications and abnormal healing

Faulty wound alignment and tissue incarceration interfere with normal healing, encourage astigmatism and neovascularization, and predispose to immune rejection, which accounts for at least 35 per cent of graft failures. Structures likely to become incarcerated include Bowman's layer, Descemet's membrane and intraocular tissues. Endothelial cells may undergo fibrous metaplasia to produce collagen and a retrocorneal fibrous membrane. Graft endothelial cells may be damaged at the time of surgery, and surviving cells may be lost at a greater than normal rate, possibly becoming so depleted as to produce endothelial failure.

Corneorefractive procedures

Keratotomy

Keratotomy wounds are similar to other unsutured corneal wounds. The location and size of incisions allow for the correction of spherical (radial keratotomy) and astigmatic (arcuate and transverse keratotomy) errors. The location, depth and type of incision influence healing, deep or radial incisions taking longer to heal than shallow or tangential incisions. Normal healing proceeds with regression of the epithelial plug by 2 weeks. Fibroblasts migrate into the wound, and cells and collagen are orientated parallel to the wound margin such that closure is complete by 2 weeks and stable by 6 months. Complete healing, however, may take 5 or more years. Keratotomy sites remain relatively weak, and may rupture following blunt trauma. The persistence of an epithelial facet and gaping of the wound are common, and epithelial inclusion cysts may form at the site of incision. Delayed healing is a cause of refractive instability and may lead to epithelial defects that have the potential to become infected.

Photorefractive/phototherapeutic keratectomy

Wound healing following excimer laser photorefractive keratectomy (PRK) or phototherapeutic keratectomy is similar to that of simple superficial keratectomy. The initial injury in excimer laser keratectomy involves complete loss of the epithelium and Bowman's layer and partial loss of the superficial stroma. A thin, amorphous pseudomembrane of coagulated material initially covers the base of the wound and forms a smooth surface that facilitates re-epithelialization. Epithelial cell mitosis occurs within hours and is soon followed by migration across the exposed stroma, so that re-epithelialization is complete within 3–5 days. Thereafter the epithelium becomes hyperplastic and, over the next 6 months, continues to thicken in proportion to the depth of the ablation. Epithelial hyperplasia may contribute to myopic regression. Normal epithelial attachment complexes regenerate within weeks, and recurrent erosions are rare. Bowman's layer never regenerates, and scarring occurs when it is removed (Fig. 1.13). Destruction of Bowman's layer and the associated stromal changes are major determinants of the refractive results of PRK. These changes are minimized with laser-assisted *in situ* keratomileusis (LASIK), where Bowman's layer is left intact. Within 24 hours of treatment inflammatory cells invade the stroma from the tear film, but dissipate within several days. Keratocytes become fibroblastic and migrate into the zone of ablation, where they persist for many months. These activated keratocytes synthesize collagen and extracellular matrix, excessive production of which probably accounts for the corneal haze of the post-operative period. Stromal changes continue for months or years. Changes in Descemet's membrane include a fibrillar response in its anterior portion. Endothelial changes are minimal unless ablation approaches Descemet's membrane, where acoustic and shock wave damage results in endothelial cell loss.

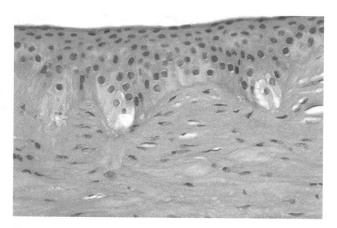

Figure 1.13 Superficial corneal scarring with loss of Bowman's layer following excimer laser photorefractive keratectomy.

Cataract surgery

In cataract surgery, extracapsular extraction is performed through a small sutureless incision using phacoemulsification. The changes produced relate to the creation of a corneal, limbal or scleral wound, and include perforation and decompression of the eye, manipulation within the anterior chamber, manipulation and response of the lens capsule and lens substance, implantation of an intraocular lens and closure of the wound with subsequent healing. General complications include those associated with corneolimbal incisions and opening the eye, while specific complications relate to manipulation of the lens and its capsule and to the implantation of an intraocular lens. Damage to the corneal endothelium is reduced by the use of viscoelastic materials, but remains a potential complication.

Manipulation of the lens and its capsule

The creation of an accurate anterior capsulotomy by continuous curvilinear capsulorrhexis is critical. A tear can extend posteriorly to threaten the integrity of the posterior capsule, and an irregular capsulorrhexis and zonular dehiscence may compromise the centration and stability of an intraocular lens. Inadequate removal of lens material can result in late post-operative complications, including Soemmering's ring cataract (Fig. 1.3), Elschnig's pearls, and contraction and opacification of the remaining capsule.

Intraocular lenses

Capsule bag-fixated posterior chamber intraocular lens implantation is used to correct the aphakia of uncomplicated extracapsular cataract extraction. Intraocular lenses (IOLs) comprise a central optic with a surrounding support (haptic) which is either of a plate-like configuration or consists of loops that maintain placement within the capsular bag or ciliary sulcus. The materials of which the optic and haptic are composed vary depending on the type of implant, but all are biologically inert. Polymethylmethacrylate (PMMA) is rigid and not ideal for small-incision phacoemulsification surgery, and foldable IOLs made of silicone, hydrogel and acrylic are used. Their surface properties may cause different responses, particularly in the posterior capsule. Silicone IOLs lead to thickening of the posterior capsule and tend to discolour with time, and silicone oils adhere to their surface. Acrylic is less likely to be associated with posterior capsular thickening. PMMA and polypropylene are currently used for loop haptics. Plate haptics are of the same material as the optic, the whole IOL being manufactured from one piece of material. Complications of posterior chamber implants include decentration and dislocation into the vitreous due to posterior capsular rupture and zonular dehiscence, pigment dispersion due to rubbing of the iris pigment epithelium on the lens surface, and post-operative infective endophthalmitis (it is thought that the electrostatic charge on the surface of some lenses attracts pathogens at the time of implantation).

Glaucoma surgery

The aim of glaucoma surgery is to reduce the intraocular pressure. In open-angle glaucoma this is achieved by reducing the secretion of aqueous by altering the structure and/or function of the ciliary body, or increasing the outflow of aqueous by modifying the drainage apparatus. The commonest procedure is filtration surgery. Laser energy may be applied to the trabecular meshwork in argon laser trabeculoplasty (ALT), and to the ciliary body in cyclophotocoagulation. In closed angle glaucoma, peripheral laser iridotomy or surgical iridectomy overcomes pupil block.

Procedures on the ciliary body (cyclodialysis and cyclodestruction)

Cyclodialysis is an obsolete surgical technique in which the longitudinal muscle of the ciliary body is separated from the scleral spur. It may profoundly disrupt aqueous dynamics, and can result in hypotony. Cyclodestructive procedures, particularly those using controlled laser energy, are used when other methods fail.

Cyclodestruction

Destruction of part of the ciliary body reduces intraocular pressure by decreasing aqueous production. Laser cyclophotocoagulation has largely superseded destruction of the ciliary body by freezing (cyclocryotherapy).

The effect of trans-scleral cyclocryotherapy is due to the production of intracellular ice crystals that cause cell death. There is a direct effect on ciliary epithelial cells, and an indirect effect of infarction resulting from the destruction of the ciliary microcirculation. A fibrotic scar replaces necrotic tissue, and the location of lesions depends on accurate placement by the surgeon. Various lasers have been used in trans-scleral photocoagulation of the ciliary body (cyclophotocoagulation), including Nd:YAG, argon, krypton and diode lasers. Argon and diode lasers have also been used in transpupillary and endo-cyclophotocoagulation. Laser energy is selectively absorbed by melanin in the ciliary body epithelium and results in focal coagulative lesions.

Procedures involving the trabecular meshwork

Procedures involving the trabecular meshwork reduce intraocular pressure by increasing the aqueous outflow. This is achieved by enlarging pre-existing apertures or creating new outflow pathways.

Argon laser trabeculoplasty

Focal photocoagulation of the trabecular meshwork can significantly reduce intraocular pressure. The mechanism of action is unclear, but it is postulated that focal photocoagulation of the trabecular meshwork causes shrinkage of collagen and dilatation of trabecular pores between laser scars. Physiological changes in the extracellular matrix and trabecular cells following treatment may contribute to the increased outflow facility resulting from this procedure.

Filtering procedures

Filtration (fistulizing) procedures are currently the principal methods of surgical control of intraocular pressure in the open-angle glaucomas. Their aim is to lower intraocular pressure by creating a passage between the anterior chamber and subconjunctival space to allow direct flow of aqueous. Full thickness surgical sclerostomies have the disadvantage of profound hypotony with its subsequent complications. Laser sclerostomies have had limited success because of closure of the fistula. Trabeculectomy is currently the treatment of choice, and overcomes the problems of sclerostomy by placing a partial thickness scleral flap over the fistula (guarded sclerostomy).

Trabeculectomy

In most successful trabeculectomies, aqueous filters through and/or around the partial thickness scleral flap to produce a cystic elevation of the overlying conjunctiva (filtration bleb). Thereafter aqueous diffuses through the conjunctiva to the tear film or enters vascular or perivascular spaces, lymphatics and aqueous veins. Trabeculectomy involves manipulation and cautery of the sclera and of the highly reactive, fibroblast-rich episcleral tissues. Traumatic inflammation and subsequent healing processes cause a significant number of procedures to fail because of scarring of the filtration bleb. This is seen histologically as a marked inflammatory response associated with proliferation of fibroblasts and the production of collagen and glycosaminoglycans in the subconjunctival space. Filtration blebs may also become encapsulated by a fibrovascular response of the episclera, and such blebs usually present within the first post-operative month as smooth, vascularized elevations. The frequency of failure has led to the development of techniques for modulating wound healing of the conjunctival and episcleral tissues in the region of the drainage site. Corticosteroids are undoubtedly beneficial in maintaining the function of the filtration site by reducing the inflammatory responses and inhibiting cellular migration into the wound area. Fibroblast proliferation and collagen production may be inhibited by the use of antimetabolites that interfere with DNA replication. The fluorinated pyrimidine analogue 5-fluorouracil (5-FU) is such a compound, but is only effective on actively dividing cells and so must be applied in the post-operative period when fibroblast activity is greatest. Mitomycin C has a similar effect, but is 100 times more potent than 5-FU and its action does not depend on the presence of actively dividing cells. Both are used in trabeculectomy where there is a known risk of failure, although their use is associated with an increased risk of complications, including hypotony, scleral ulceration (mitomy-cin C), conjunctival wound leaks and corneal epithelial defects.

Implant devices

Numerous implant devices including tubes and valves have been devised to facilitate drainage of filtration procedures. Most fail due to fibrosis but some, such as the Molteno implant, remain of use in treating eyes with complicated glaucoma. Failure may result from tissue responses that almost invariably include formation of a thick collagenous wall around the implant and the presence of metaplastic myoblasts. Hypotony is the main post-operative complication, and may be caused by valve or ligature failure, leakage around the tube or reduced aqueous production following ciliary body malfunction after surgery. Other complications include vitreous haemorrhage, retinal detachment, malignant glaucoma, hyphaema, choroidal effusion, endothelial cell loss and endophthalmitis.

Eviscerations, enucleations and exenterations

Eviscerations, enucleations and exenterations may be complicated by haemorrhage and infection. Eviscerations must be meticulously performed, as leaving behind any uveal tissue can lead to sympathetic ophthalmitis. Orbital implants can be extruded.

Extraocular surgery

Manipulation of the conjunctiva, episclera and extraocular muscles is necessary in squint and extraocular retinal detachment surgery. Episcleral tissue contains abundant fibroblasts and reacts swiftly to trauma and, while this is a disadvantage in glaucoma surgery, it is beneficial in squint and retinal detachment surgery, where it allows for rapid reattachment of muscles and attachment of explants. Complications relating to manipulation of extraocular tissues include epithelial inclusion cysts and granulomatous responses to foreign bodies such as sutures and explants. Any procedure in which an extraocular muscle is detached necessitates cutting the anterior ciliary vessels and can lead to anterior segment ischaemic necrosis. In most instances, this only occurs after detachment of more than two rectus muscles. Features include pain, lid and conjunctival oedema, anterior uveitis and hypotony.

Vitreoretinal surgery

The clinicopathological features of uncomplicated vitreoretinal surgery include those of the general response to extraocular manipulation, cryotherapy, laser photocoagulation and the processes that occur during reapposition of a previously detached retina to the RPE. In addition to the general complications of intraocular surgery, proliferative vitreoretinopathy is relatively common, particularly following complex or multiple procedures. Other complications (e.g. secondary glaucoma, retinal vascular occlusion) are associated with intraocular injections of materials such as gases and fluids including silicones and halogenated hydrocarbons.

Chapter 2

Immunity, inflammation and infection

Immunity

The immune system
  Cellular constituents of the immune system
    The myeloid system
    The lymphoid system
  Molecular constituents of the immune system
    Major histocompatibility complex
    Adhesion molecules
    Cytokines
    The complement system
The adaptive immune response
  Afferent limb
  Central processing
  Efferent limb
  Regulation of the immune system and tolerance
Immunity of the eye and associated structures
  Innate immunity
  Adaptive immunity

Inflammation

Acute inflammation
  The acute early response
    The release of chemical mediators
    Vascular changes
    Leukocyte activation
  The delayed cellular response and phagocytosis
  The outcome of acute inflammation
    Resolution
    Organization
    Chronicity
  The systemic response to acute inflammation
Chronic inflammation
  Non-granulomatous chronic inflammation
  Granulomatous chronic inflammation
    Chalazion

Sarcoidosis
Clinicopathological features of inflammation of the eye
  and associated structures
  Extraocular inflammation and inflammation of the
    corneoscleral coat
    Blepharitis
    Conjunctivitis
    Orbital cellulitis
    Keratitis
    Scleritis
  Intraocular inflammation
    Anterior intraocular inflammation
    Posterior intraocular inflammation
    Sequelae of intraocular inflammation

Disorders of immunity

Immunodeficiency
  Primary immunodeficiencies
    Non-specific primary immunodeficiencies
    Specific primary immunodeficiencies
  Secondary immunodeficiencies
    HIV infection and AIDS
Hypersensitivity
  Ophthalmic hypersensitivity
    Allergic disease of the conjunctiva and other
      mucous membranes
    Allergic disease of the lids, conjunctiva and
      cornea
    Allergic disease with cutaneous and/or systemic
      involvement
Autoimmunity
  Autoimmunity and the conjunctiva
  Autoimmunity and the corneoscleral coat
  Autoimmunity and the uvea
    Acute anterior uveitis
    Chronic anterior uveitis

Posterior/panuveitis
Autoimmunity and the lens
Autoimmunity and the orbit
Immunology of tissue transplantation
Corneal allograft reactions
Tolerance of corneal allografts
Rejection of corneal allografts
Graft-versus-host reactions

Infection

Prions
Viruses
DNA viruses
Papovaviruses
Adenoviruses
Herpesviruses
Poxviruses
RNA viruses
Picornaviruses
Paramyxoviruses
Togaviruses
Orthomyxoviruses
Retroviruses
Bacteria
Rickettsiae
Chlamydiae
Mycoplasmas
Cocci and bacilli
Cocci
Bacilli
Cocci, bacilli and ophthalmic infection

Gram-negative bacilli, autoimmune uveitis and
arthritis
Mycobacteria
Tuberculosis
Leprosy
Spiral bacteria (spirochaetes)
Syphilis
Lyme disease
Fungi
Fungal infection in ophthalmology
Classification
Protozoa
Toxoplasma gondii
Toxoplasmosis
Acanthamoeba spp.
Helminths
Nematodes
Toxocara spp.
Trichinella spiralis
Onchocerca volvulus
Loa loa
Wuchereria bancrofti
Trematodes
Schistosoma mansoni, S. haematobium and
S. japonicum
Cestodes
Taenia solium
Echinococcus granulosus
Arthropods
Insecta
Arachnida

IMMUNITY

Immunity is the ability of the host to protect itself against antigens such as those of pathogenic organisms. Antigens are usually high molecular weight proteins, but low molecular weight substances (haptens), including drugs and the polysaccharide component of pathogenic organisms, can initiate an immune response if bound to a carrier protein before introduction to the body. An effective immune response necessitates the presence of a functioning immune system.

THE IMMUNE SYSTEM

The immune system is an intricate interdependent network of cells, tissues, molecules and compounds, and has two functional divisions, the innate and adaptive systems; the response of each results in inflammation. The innate (natural or native) immune system is the first line of defence. It provides immediate protection but is non-specific, lacks memory and does not necessitate central processing. The substrates of the system include skin and mucous membranes and their associated secretions, and cells with phagocytic and cytotoxic activity. The adaptive (acquired) immune system provides a defensive response to specific pathogenic organisms and antigens. Two key features of adaptive immunity are memory of previous antigenic encounters and the ability to recognize self from non-self. An adaptive immune response takes several days to develop because of the complex series of events following antigen recognition. Antigen initially binds to specific antigen-presenting cells, which migrate to a central processing station of lymphoid tissue wherein it is presented to other cells of the immune system. These cells then mature into immunocompetent antigen specific effector cells or cells that ultimately secrete antibodies (immunoglobulins). Clonal proliferation follows, and a cell-mediated or antibody (humoral) response is mounted against the antigen.

Cellular constituents of the immune system

The cellular constituents of the immune system include leukocytes and the tissue macrophage system. Granulocytes (neutrophils, eosinophils, basophils, mast cells), mononuclear phagocytic cells (monocytes, macrophages) and dendritic cells comprise the myeloid system and are derived from precursors in bone marrow; apart from dendritic cells they are the cellular basis of innate immunity. Cells of the lymphoid system (lymphocytes, plasma cells) also originate in bone marrow, but their development is more complex and involves the thymus and secondary lymphoid organs (lymph nodes, spleen, mucosa-associated lymphoid tissue). The lymphoid system is essential to adaptive immunity. The different functions of immune cells are reflected in protein molecules on their surfaces, which are identifiable by monoclonal antibodies and form the basis of the CD (cluster designation/cluster of differentiation) classification. CD numbers enable pathologists to categorize morphologically similar cells such as lymphocytes in blood and in inflammatory and neoplastic lesions.

The myeloid system

Granulocytes and mononuclear phagocytic cells are directly involved in the non-specific killing of micro-organisms and the removal of damaged host tissue. All have surface receptors that bind to the material they ingest.

Granulocytes

Granulocytes, so called because of their granule-rich cytoplasm, comprise neutrophils, eosinophils, basophils and mast cells. Neutrophils, eosinophils and basophils circulate in the blood stream (polymorphonuclear leukocytes); mast cells reside in extravascular tissue. Granulocytes are approximately $15\,\mu m$ in diameter, express CD45 protein on their surface and constitute 60–70 per cent of the total blood leukocytes.

Neutrophils (Fig. 2.1) constitute 40–75 per cent of circulating leukocytes. Their nuclei are segmented into three or four lobes and have densely staining chromatin. Their cytoplasm contains primary and secondary granules. Primary (azurophilic) granules are lysosomes containing microbiocidal proteins such as myeloperoxidase and lysozyme, and enzymes that can degrade proteins, carbohydrates and lipids. Secondary (specific) granules are more numerous than primary granules and contain lysozyme and lactoferrin, an iron-binding protein that has bacteriostatic and bactericidal properties. Lactoferrin can also interact with lipopolysaccharide and thereby alter the cell wall of Gram-negative bacteria, allowing subsequent lysis by lysozyme. Specific granules also contain other enzymes, including C5-cleaving enzyme, which splits the fifth component of complement.

Neutrophils circulate in the blood for 6–7 hours before entering tissues, where they die after 1–4 days. Neutrophils are not only produced in bone marrow but are also stored therein, and can be mobilized in response to cytokines and complement fragments produced during inflammation and infection.

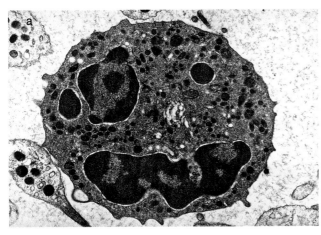

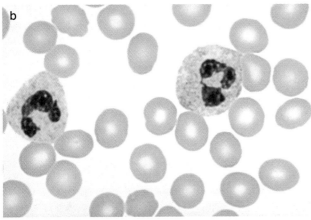

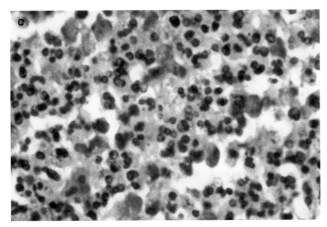

Figure 2.1 Neutrophils. (a) Irregular segmented nucleus and cytoplasmic granules. TEM. (b) Multilobed nuclei and granular cytoplasm. Blood film. (c) Inflammatory exudate.

Neutrophils function as scavengers and provide an early defence against bacterial infection. At sites of injury or bacterial invasion, locally released factors chemotactically promote their migration from the blood into tissues. Neutrophils express receptors for complement fragments and the Fc (fragment crystallizable) portion of immunoglobulin G, thus facilitating binding to micro-

organisms and subsequent phagocytosis. The phagosomes so formed contain engulfed material and fuse with lysosomes to form phagolysosomes, into which numerous digestive enzymes are released. Neutrophils are important in Type III hypersensitivity reactions in which immune complexes bind to Fc receptors. The resultant degranulation releases enzymes that injure surrounding tissue.

Eosinophils constitute 2–5 per cent of circulating leukocytes. They have a bilobed nucleus and large eosinophilic cytoplasmic granules (Fig. 2.2). They are chemotactic to various factors including platelet-activating factor (PAF) and eosinophilic chemotactic factor of anaphylaxis (ECF-A) produced by mast cells. Degranulation of eosinophils is induced by the stimulation of cell membrane receptors for complement fragments and the Fc portion of immunoglobulins A, E and G. Eosinophilic granules contain cytotoxic proteins, including eosinophilic cationic protein, eosinophilic peroxidase and eosinophilic major basic protein (EMBP). Each is toxic to helminths,

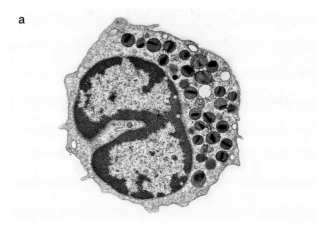

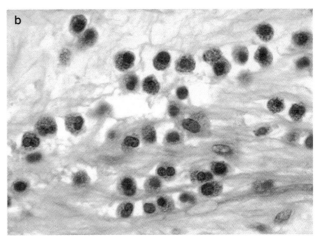

Figure 2.2 Eosinophils. (a) Bilobed nucleus and large cytoplasmic granules. TEM. (b) Bilobed nuclei and eosinophilic granular cytoplasm; inflammatory exudate.

and EMBP stimulates mast cell degranulation. Eosinophils are thus conspicuous in helminth infections and Type I hypersensitivity reactions. Paradoxically, eosinophils inactivate mast cell mediators released during allergic reactions.

Basophils constitute < 0.2 per cent of circulating leukocytes. They are the circulating equivalent of mast cells. Large basophilic cytoplasmic granules (Fig. 2.3) obscure their indented or partially lobulated nucleus. The granules contain histamine, serotonin and heparin, and are released as a consequence of lysosomal activity following the stimulation of surface membrane receptors for complement factors and immunoglobulin E.

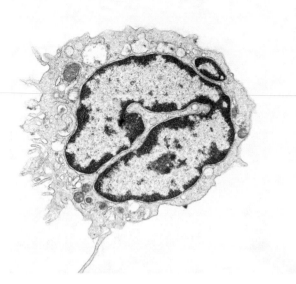

Figure 2.4 Monocyte. TEM.

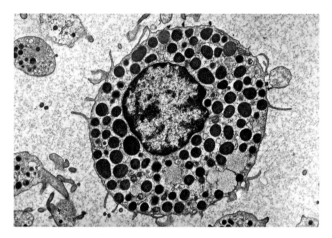

Figure 2.3 Basophil. Large cytoplasmic granules. TEM.

Mast cells have round to oval nuclei and slightly basophilic granular cytoplasm. They have high affinity immunoglobulin E receptors on their cell membranes and, together with basophils, function as the effector cells of Type I hypersensitivity. The Fc portion of the immunoglobulin E molecule binds to these receptors, degranulation occurs, and chemical mediators including histamine, serotonin, proteolytic enzymes and chemotactic factors are released. As a result, the arachidonic pathway is stimulated and prostaglandins and leukotrienes are synthesized.

Mononuclear phagocytic cells

Mononuclear phagocytic cells are either circulating monocytes or tissue macrophages.

Monocytes comprise 3–8 per cent of circulating leukocytes. They measure about 20 μm in diameter, and have oval or reniform nuclei and abundant granular cytoplasm (Fig. 2.4). Monocytes are the immature precursors of macrophages.

Macrophages (histiocytes – Fig. 2.5) develop from circulating monocytes that migrate into tissues. They are widespread throughout the body, being present in skin, connective tissue, pleura, peritoneum, synovium, lung, lymph nodes, liver (Kupffer cells), spleen, bone (osteoclasts) and CNS (microglia). Macrophages are relatively large, long-lived cells and express CD68 protein on their surface. Their nuclei are oval, indented or irregular, and their abundant cytoplasm is rich in lysosomes and may contain phagocytic granules. Macrophages are essential to innate and adaptive immunity, and to the inflammatory response. They secrete enzymes such as lysozyme, and their principal function is microbiocidal phagocytosis. Additionally, macrophages act as antigen-presenting

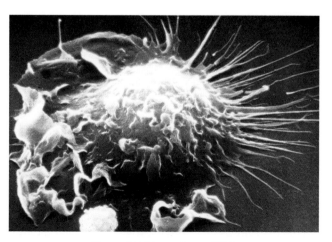

Figure 2.5 Macrophage. SEM.

cells and are also important in wound healing, tissue remodelling and the removal of senescent cells.

Dendritic cells

Dendritic cells are leukocytes with a characteristic arborizing morphology that partake in the adaptive immune response, in which they act as professional antigen-presenting cells. They originate from myeloid precursors in the bone marrow, and are classified as either interdigitating or follicular.

Interdigitating dendritic cells act as an antigen surveillance system at sites of high antigen exposure. These include the skin, conjunctiva and peripheral cornea, where they lie within the epithelium as Langerhans cells, which are identified by the characteristic Birbeck granules in their cytoplasm (Fig. 2.6). They are rich in major histocompatibility complex class II molecules and migrate as veiled cells to lymphoid tissue, where they present antigen to T cells.

Follicular dendritic cells are found in the B cell areas of lymph nodes and spleen. They lack major histocompatibility complex class II molecules, and present antigen to B cells.

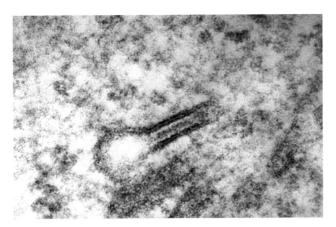

Figure 2.6 Langerhans cell. Birbeck granule. TEM.

The lymphoid system

The lymphoid system consists of primary and secondary lymphoid organs and lymphocytes.

Primary lymphoid organs

The primary lymphoid organs are the bone marrow and thymus. Lymphocytes originate from bone marrow, but during embryonic life some precursors migrate to the thymus where they differentiate and mature into T (thymus-dependent) lymphocytes, while others remain in the bone marrow and differentiate into B lymphocytes. After birth, lymphocytes emanate from both the bone marrow (B cells and T cell precursors) and the thymus (T cells). Many lymphocytes die by clonal deletion and/or apoptosis during the maturation process.

Secondary lymphoid organs

The secondary lymphoid organs are the lymph nodes, the spleen and mucosa-associated lymphoid tissue. They are populated by T and B cells and antigen-presenting cells. The secondary lymphoid organs act as traps and processing stations for antigen, and are the centres from which an adaptive immune response is initiated and sustained.

Lymph nodes comprise follicles of B cells and diffuse paracortical areas of T cells (T cell zones), and receive antigen from professional antigen-presenting cells via lymphatics. Lymphatics from the lids and conjunctiva carry such cells to the preauricular and submandibular nodes.

The spleen is composed of red pulp (the site of red blood cell disposal) and white pulp (areas of lymphocytes surrounding the arterioles entering the organ). The inner region of the white pulp is divided into a periarteriolar lymphoid sheath containing mainly T cells and a flanking corona of B cells. The spleen receives and processes antigen-presenting cells from all regions of the body, and traps those that may have bypassed regional lymph nodes and those originating from structures devoid of lymphatics, such as the eye, orbit and brain. The white pulp is a major site of antibody production.

Mucosa-associated lymphoid tissue (MALT) consists of focal aggregates of lymphoid tissue in relation to mucous membranes. It traps antigen from local sites. MALT in the gut is probably primary and developmental and is evident as Peyer's patches, while in the conjunctiva it is possibly acquired secondary to prolonged low-grade local antigenic stimulation. MALT consists of B cell follicles in the subepithelial tissue and T cells within the epithelium. Conjunctival MALT is more specifically referred to as CALT (conjunctiva-associated lymphoid tissue).

Lymphocytes

Lymphocytes comprise 20 per cent of circulating leukocytes. They are approximately $10\,\mu$m in diameter and circulate in the blood, where they appear as cells with a round or slightly indented darkly staining nucleus and very little cytoplasm (Fig. 2.7). They recognize antigens via antigen-specific cell surface receptors. Most lymphocytes express multiple copies of a single receptor specific for one antigenic determinant and are only able to

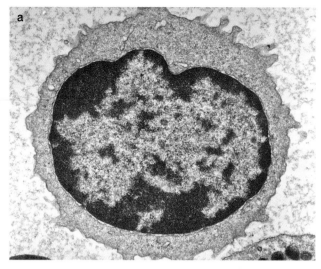

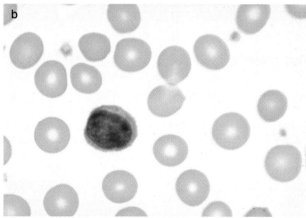

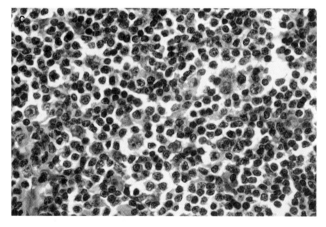

Figure 2.7 Lymphocytes. (a) Slightly indented nucleus and little cytoplasm. TEM. (b) Darkly staining nucleus and little cytoplasm. Blood film. (c) Inflammatory exudate.

respond to that antigen, but as the total lymphocyte population is approximately 2×10^{12}, a large number of different antigens can be recognized. Lymphocytes have distinct characteristics and functions, and are classified as T cells (including NK cells), B cells or null cells.

T cells

T cells are fundamental to cell-mediated immunity. All express CD3 antigen on their surface. T cell precursors arise from bone marrow and migrate to the thymus, where they mature before passing into the blood. They constitute 70–80 per cent of circulating lymphocytes, and pass into the lymph nodes, spleen and MALT. T cells recognize antigen by T cell receptors.

T cell receptors (TCRs) fall into one of two categories. Both consist of two polypeptide chains linked to form a heterodimer. The commonest form has chains designated α and β ($\alpha\beta$ receptor – TCR2) and constitutes 90 per cent of all TCRs. The rarer form consists of γ and δ peptides ($\gamma\delta$ receptor – TCR1) and is expressed on primitive types of T cells. TCR2 in association with CD3 forms the TCR/CD3 signalling complex, a group of transmembrane proteins expressed on all mature T cells. The complex is central to T cell activation following the binding of antigenic peptide to major histocompatibility complex molecules on the surface of antigen-presenting cells.

Functional subsets of T cells

T cells exhibit two main functional subsets that relate to the major histocompatibility complex: helper (T_H/CD4+) and cytotoxic/suppressor ($T_{C/S}$/CD8+) cells.

Helper T (T_H/CD4+) cells recognize specific antigens in association with major histocompatibility complex class II molecules. When stimulated, they proliferate and release cytokines that facilitate B cell activity. Helper T cells express CD4 protein on their surface and constitute 45 per cent of circulating lymphocytes. Naïve T_H cells clonally expand towards T_{H1} and T_{H2} subsets in the adaptive immune response. T_{H1} cells secrete interferon gamma, tumour necrosis factors alpha and beta, and interleukin 2, which drives their growth. T_{H2} cells secrete interleukins 4, 5, 6 and 10, all of which activate B cells. Growth of T_{H2} cells is driven by interleukin 4.

Cytotoxic/suppressor T ($T_{C/S}$/CD8+) cells recognize antigen presented in association with major histocompatibility complex class I molecules, and kill host cells infected by viruses or other intracellular pathogens. They express CD8 protein on their surface and constitute 25 per cent of circulating lymphocytes.

B cells

B cells are responsible for humoral immunity. In birds they originate from the bursa of Fabricius (hence 'B' cell), but in mammals, where no such organ exists, they arise from bone marrow. B cells either circulate, where they constitute 10–15 per cent of blood-borne lymphocytes, or remain within the lymph nodes or spleen. They express CD20 and CD79a proteins on their surface. Appropriate presentation of antigen to unprimed B cells leads to their transformation into plasma cells. Each B cell has specificity for only one antigen and produces only one type of immunoglobulin, but a particular cell may switch from producing one type of immunoglobulin to another (isotype switching). B cells can also act as antigen-presenting cells.

Plasma cells are confined to tissues and are ovoid in shape, with eccentrically placed nuclei in which the peripherally situated chromatin gives rise to a clock-face or cartwheel appearance (Fig. 2.8a, 2.8b). Their cytoplasm is slightly basophilic and large amounts of RNA are present in the rough endoplasmic reticulum, which is actively involved in antibody synthesis. Each plasma cell produces only one class of immunoglobulin specific for a particular antigen. Plasma cells containing eosinophilic granules (Russell bodies) within their cytoplasm are known as plasmacytoid cells. Russell bodies are composed of immunoglobulin and enlarge before being extruded to lie freely as globules within inflamed tissue (Fig. 2.8c). Plasma cells express CD79a on their surface.

Null cells and natural killer (NK) cells

Null cells are neither T cells nor B cells. Natural killer (NK) cells are a type of T cell and constitute 5–10 per cent of peripheral blood lymphocytes. Their cytoplasm is granular, and they are otherwise known as large granular lymphocytes (LGLs). NK cells kill IgG antibody-coated target cells in the process known as antibody-dependent cell-mediated cytotoxicity (ADCC).

Molecular constituents of the immune system

Major histocompatibility complex

Major histocompatibility complex (MHC) molecules are cell surface proteins expressed by a wide variety of cells. When bound to antigenic peptides they allow that cell to be recognized by T cells. The MHC gene complex is located on chromosome 6 (6p21). MHC molecules are also known as human leukocyte antigens (HLAs), and their genetic loci by letters (A, B, C, DP, DQ, DR, E, F and G). Over 100 individual alleles are identified by numbers following the letters, and those tentatively identified have the letter 'w' ('workshop') inserted. HLAs are divided into two main classes, class I and class II molecules.

MHC class I molecules

MHC class I molecules (HLA-A, -B, -C, -E, -F) are expressed on the surface of all nucleated cells and blood platelets, but not on mature red cells. They

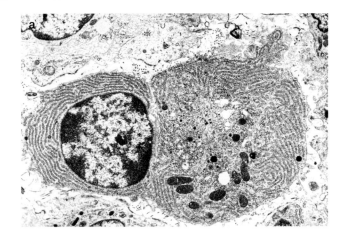

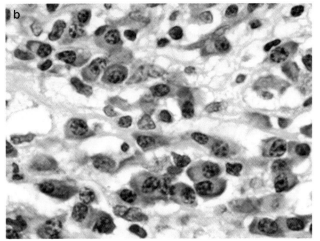

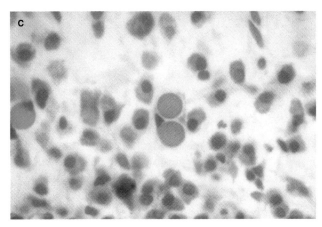

Figure 2.8 Plasma cells. (a) Ovoid eccentrically placed nucleus with peripheral chromatin. TEM. (b) Ovoid cells having eccentric nuclei with peripheral chromatin (clock-face or cartwheel appearance) in an inflammatory exudate. (c) Russell bodies; eosinophilic globules of immunoglobulin.

bind peptides originating from within cells, and are recognized by T cells expressing CD8 molecules (class I restriction).

MHC class II molecules

MHC class II molecules (HLA-DP, -DQ, -DR) have a limited distribution but are expressed on antigen-presenting cells, although during an immune response their expression may be induced on other cell types. They bind peptides originating from outside cells, and are recognized by T cells expressing CD4 molecules (class II restriction).

Adhesion molecules

Adhesion molecules, like MHC molecules, are cell surface proteins expressed by a wide variety of cells. They are of particular importance in the binding of T cells, and the four main groups are selectins, mucin-like vascular addressins, integrins and the immunoglobulin superfamily.

Selectins

Selectins are important for leukocyte homing to specific tissues, and can be expressed on either leukocytes (L-selectin) or vascular endothelium (P-selectin and E-selectin). They have a common core structure and are distinguished from each other by different lectin-like domains in their extracellular portion.

Mucin-like vascular addressins

Mucin-like vascular addressins are mucin-like cell adhesion molecules (MAd CAMs) expressed on vascular endothelium, including that of specialized venules (known as high endothelial venules) in lymph nodes. MAd CAM-1 is expressed on the vascular endothelium of mucosal surfaces, and guides lymphocyte entry into MALT.

Integrins

Integrins are a large family of cell surface proteins that mediate intercellular and cell-matrix adhesion in immune and inflammatory responses, and are important in tissue organization and cell migration during development. An integrin molecule consists of a large α-chain that pairs non-covalently with a smaller β-chain. All T cells express a leukocyte integrin known as lymphocyte function-associated antigen-1 (LFA-1), which is the most important adhesion molecule for lymphocyte activation.

Immunoglobulin superfamily

Immunoglobulin superfamily members include T cell receptors, CD4, CD8, CD19 and intercellular adhesion molecules (ICAM), which are especially important in T cell activation. ICAM-1, ICAM-2 and ICAM-3 all bind to T cell LFA-1. ICAM-1 and ICAM-2 are expressed on vascular endothelium and APCs, and binding to these molecules enables lymphocytes to migrate through vessel walls. ICAM-3 is expressed only on leukocytes, but is thought to play an important part in adhesion between APCs and T cells.

Cytokines

Cytokines are a heterogeneous group of soluble molecules that are short-lived mediators of cellular interactions involved in the immune response. Some act locally, but others are released into the blood stream and act at a distant site. They are secreted in response to a specific stimulus, and are effective at very low concentrations. Cells that release them include lymphocytes (lymphokines), neutrophils, mast cells, monocytes, macrophages (monokines) and fibroblasts, and the many known groups include interleukins, interferons, tumour necrosis factors, transforming growth factors, colony stimulating factors and chemokines. The function of specific cytokines may change depending on their target, while their interaction with other mediators results in additive, synergistic or antagonistic effects.

Interleukins

The name interleukins (ILs) refers to the role of these molecules in mediating interaction between leukocytes. They are produced by and interact with a wide range of cells, and at least 15 different types (IL-1 to IL-15) have been described. They have wide-ranging effects and act particularly on T cells, B cells and eosinophils. Functions for which they are responsible include chemotaxis, isotype switching and haemopoiesis. IL-1, IL-2 and IL-6 are particularly noteworthy for their role in intraocular inflammation. IL-1 is produced by macrophages. It acts on T cells, promoting CD4 + (T_H) cell activation, and is essential in the inflammatory response, where it promotes leukocyte and macrophage chemotaxis and cytotoxic activity. It acts together with prostaglandins to induce fever and muscle proteolysis. IL-1 also activates the RPE and retinal vascular endothelium. IL-2 is produced by T cells. It is the principal cytokine in T cell mediated responses, and plays a key role in T and B cell proliferation and maturation. IL-2 receptors have been demonstrated on both intraocular and freely circulating lymphocytes in active endogenous uveitis. IL-6 is produced by many cells, including CD4 + (T_H) cells, mast cells, macrophages, fibroblasts and RPE cells, and its wide-ranging effects include the limitation of tissue damage. It has been detected in the aqueous in active intraocular inflammation.

Interferons

The interferons (IFNs) are a group of proteins that inhibit viral replication and promote MHC class I induction.

Three major classes (α, β, γ) are identified. IFN-α is produced by macrophages and IFN-β by fibroblasts. IFN-γ is released from antigen-stimulated T_{H1} cells, and is an activator of macrophages.

Tumour necrosis factors

Tumour necrosis factors (TNF-α and -β) exist in soluble and membrane-bound forms. TNF-α, like IFN-γ, is produced by T_{H1} cells and is a macrophage activating factor. TNF-β is also produced by T_{H1} cells, and is cytotoxic.

Transforming growth factors

Transforming growth factors (TGFs) are secreted as inactive precursors. There are at least six types, of which TGF-β is the most important. It is produced by platelets, activated macrophages, T cells, fibroblasts and bone cells. In the eye it is produced by the ciliary epithelium and RPE. TGF-β is an inflammatory mediator, has potent immunosuppressive activity and is also important in wound healing.

Colony stimulating factors

Colony stimulating factors (CSFs) are produced by monocytes, macrophages and T cells, and act on bone marrow to control the growth and maturation of cells. The granulocyte/macrophage factor (GM-CSF) commits precursors to the myeloid cell line, while G-CSF and M-CSF later determine whether these cells become granulocytes or mononuclear phagocytic cells.

Chemokines

Chemokines are small polypeptides synthesized by phagocytes, vascular endothelial cells, keratinocytes, fibroblasts and smooth muscle cells. They recruit phagocytic cells to local sites of infection.

The complement system

The complement system is considered as part of the innate immune system, but also participates in adaptive immunity. It comprises a cascade of about 25 soluble serum proteins synthesized in the liver and mononuclear phagocytes. The components normally exist as inactive precursors, but once activated each acts as a substrate for the preceding protein in the cascade and then as an enzyme for the next protein in the sequence. The enzymatic action of a precursor releases at least two fragments. A large fragment, usually designated 'b', binds to membranes of the triggering complex and becomes the next active enzyme in the sequence. Small fragments, designated 'a', are important in chemotaxis and the mediation of inflammation. The proteins are identified by the designation C1–C9. Confusingly, the numbers correspond to their order of discovery, not to their sequential order of activation. C1 is a complex of three proteins, two molecules each of C1r and C1s being bound to a molecule of C1q.

Complement activation occurs in two phases: activation of the C3 component by the classical, alternative or lectin pathways, and the lytic sequence, which involves the sequential activation of C5, C6, C7, C8 and C9 that leads to cell death. The classical pathway is activated by immune complexes, notably those of IgM or IgG. The complexes bind to C1q and activate a cascade in the order C4, C2, C3. In the alternative pathway, C3 is usually activated by microbial products such as endotoxins. The alternative pathway is slow and less efficient than the classical pathway, and requires high concentrations of the components. The lectin pathway is initiated by the binding of a serum mannan-binding lectin to mannose-containing proteins or carbohydrates on bacteria and viruses.

Complement provides a mechanism for removing and destroying antigen that does not depend exclusively on antibodies. The principal actions of the complement system are opsonization, chemotaxis, mediation of inflammation, and cytotoxicity. C3b is necessary for opsonization, and C5a promotes the chemotaxis of neutrophils. C3a, C4a and C5a are potent inflammatory mediators which, when bound to receptors on mast cells, promote degranulation and the release of histamine and other inflammatory agents. The cytotoxic function of complement is due to the formation of polymers of C9, which form tubular structures that perforate cell membranes and result in non-specific transmembrane ion transfer and osmotic cell lysis.

THE ADAPTIVE IMMUNE RESPONSE

The presence of a foreign antigen results in a complex and co-ordinated response, the adaptive immune response, that ultimately leads to its neutralization and removal. In a primary response, where antigen is presented for the first time, activation of naïve lymphocytes leads to their proliferation and differentiation into either effector cells (CD4+/T_H and CD8+/$T_{C/S}$ cells from T cells; plasma cells from B cells) or memory cells (memory T cells; memory B cells). Memory cells are long-lived and, on re-exposure to antigen, generate a secondary response in which effector and memory cells are produced in greater numbers. Antibody production in a secondary response is more rapid than in a primary response and consists predominantly of IgG at higher concentrations and with greater antigen affinity. In the adaptive immune response, an afferent limb and central processing precede an effector limb.

Afferent limb

The processing of antigen by specific cells termed antigen-presenting cells (APCs) is the first stage in the adaptive immune response. Antigen is transported by APCs to lymphoid tissue (lymph nodes, spleen, MALT), where the immune response is initiated. The professional APCs are dendritic cells, macrophages and B cells. Interdigitating dendritic cells present antigen to T cells, macrophages internalize and present particulate antigen, and B cells present antigen to T cells via receptors that allow them to internalize large amounts of specific antigen.

Central processing

Central processing involves the processing of antigen and the activation of lymphocytes.

Antigen processing

Antigen processing is a complex mechanism in which antigens are altered in such a way that they can be recognized by T cells. It involves the conversion of proteinaceous material into smaller peptides which then bind to MHC class I or class II molecules on APC surfaces, the preference for one or other class being termed restriction. Those with class I restriction are recognized by $CD8+$ ($T_{C/S}$) cells, and those with class II restriction by $CD4+$ (T_H) cells.

Lymphocyte activation

Lymphocyte activation in a primary immune response involves naïve $CD4+$ (T_H) cells which leave the blood by crossing high endothelial venules that deliver them to the cortical region of lymph nodes. T cell activation involves complex intracellular biochemical changes that influence their clonal proliferation, differentiation and functional maturation. Previously sensitized $CD4+$ (T_H) cells either sustain the primary response or initiate a secondary response by activating memory cells that have persisted within the immune system following previous exposure.

Efferent limb

Specific mechanisms in the efferent limb are either cell-mediated or antibody-mediated. Non-specific mechanisms include the activation of complement.

Cell-mediated immunity

Cell-mediated immunity (CMI) involves mechanisms in which cellular interactions predominate, and although antibodies are present they do not have a prominent role. The principal cellular component of CMI is the antigen-activated $CD4+$ (T_H) cell, which modulates the activity of other cells including $CD8+$ ($T_{C/S}$) cells, NK cells and macrophages. Cytokines are the key intercellular messengers that co-ordinate the responses of participating cells.

Antibody-mediated immunity

Antibody-mediated (humoral) immunity necessitates the production and appropriate functioning of antibodies, which are soluble or membrane-bound immunoglobulins produced by B cells/plasma cells in response to a specific antigen. Antibodies bind to antigen and cross-link it to leukocytes or complement, and thereby start a chain of events leading to elimination of the antigen. Immunoglobulins are proteins consisting of an identical pair of long polypeptide chains (heavy – H chains) linked by disulphide bonds to an identical pair of short polypeptide chains (light – L chains). Five types of heavy chain (α, δ, γ, μ, ε) determine the isotype or class (IgA, IgD, IgG, IgM, IgE). Light chains are of two types (κ and λ), and an immunoglobulin has only one or other type. The H and L chains are folded into a number of domains which are the basic building blocks for many molecules of importance in the immune system, such as TCRs, HLAs, CD4 and CD8.

The basic immunoglobulin molecule can be split into three fragments by digestion with the enzyme papain. Two identical fragments bind antigen (Fab – fragment antigen binding) and consist of a complete L chain and a section of an H chain; the third fragment consists of the remainder of the H chain and may be crystallized (Fc – fragment crystallizable). The immunoglobulin molecule binds antigen at a site (paratope) on its Fab portion, while its Fc portion attaches to cell membranes or fixes complement.

Each heavy and light chain is made up of domains in which the amino acid sequence for immunoglobulin molecules of the same isotype or subclass is constant (constant – C regions). Conversely, other regions of both H and L chains show considerable variation in amino acid sequence (variable – V regions) in different immunoglobulins. Depending on the isotype, heavy chains have three or four constant (C_H) regions and one variable (V_H) region; light chains have one constant (C_L) and one variable (V_L) region. The C_H regions are within the Fc portion and the variable regions (V_H and V_L) are within the Fab portion. Hypervariable regions within V_H and V_L constitute the antigen-binding site. The amino acid sequence of the hypervariable regions is unique to that immunoglobulin molecule and specific for a particular antigen (idiotype).

IgM (molecular weight 900 kDA) is the first major immunoglobulin produced in primary immune responses. It is a star-shaped pentamer consisting of five monomers joined by a molecule known as the J chain. With 10 antigen-binding and 5 complement-binding sites per molecule, it is an effective agglutinator of particulate antigens and a potent activator of complement. IgM comprises 6 per cent of the total serum immunoglobulin, and is important in the defence against bacterial infections and in the aetiology of autoimmune disease.

IgG (molecular weight 150 kDA) is the major antibody produced during secondary immune responses. It has a higher binding capacity for antibody than IgM, and is able to activate a wider range of effector mechanisms. IgG is a monomer distributed equally between the intravascular and extravascular compartments of the body, and constitutes 80 per cent of the total serum immunoglobulin. It binds to the Fc receptors of neutrophils, eosinophils, macrophages, B cells and null cells, and can act as an opsonin. There are four subclasses, IgG_1, IgG_2, IgG_3 and IgG_4. IgG_1, IgG_2 and IgG_3, but not IgG_4, are able to activate complement via the classical pathway. IgG, because of its small size, can cross the placenta, and is the only immunoglobulin to do so.

IgA (molecular weight 320 kDA) can be either monomeric or dimeric, and comprises 13 per cent of the total serum immunoglobulin. The monomeric form is present in serum and the dimeric form in the secretions of various mucosal surfaces. In the dimeric form, two molecules are connected by a J chain. The secretory form of dimeric IgA has an additional glycoprotein called the secretory piece that facilitates its transport through mucosal surfaces and makes it more resistant to degradation. Secretory IgA is the principal immunoglobulin formed by plasma cells in the lacrimal gland and conjunctiva, and is present in tears. It is also present in saliva and milk, and in the secretions of the respiratory and gastrointestinal tracts. IgA prevents the binding of viruses to epithelial cells, and is found in the superficial conjunctival epithelium in some types of conjunctivitis. IgA can also activate complement via the classical pathway.

IgD and IgE are both monomers and present only in small amounts in normal serum and body fluids, where they act mainly as cell regulators. IgD (molecular weight 185 kDA) acts on the surface of B cells, and IgE (molecular weight 200 kDA) binds to receptors on the surface of mast cells. The cross-linking of surface IgE by antigen, which results in the release of inflammatory mediators from mast cells, is the basis of Type I hypersensitivity. IgE is also important in the immune response to helminths.

Antibody production

Efficient antibody production necessitates APC and B cell function and regulatory T cell activity. Each B cell produces an antibody with a unique V_H–V_L combination that is both expressed on its surface and secreted. CD4 + (T_H) cell cytokines stimulate clonal proliferation of B cells and their subsequent differentiation into plasma cells that are sensitive to and produce identical specific antibody against the target antigen. On first exposure to antigen, individual B cells initially produce IgM or IgD. The same B cell/plasma cell later switches to secreting IgG, IgA or IgE, and although the isotype is different the affinity for the antigen is maintained. This phenomenon, known as isotype switching, is under T cell control, and occurs in an antibody response where the predominant circulating immunoglobulin of the primary response is IgM and that of the secondary response, where memory cells are activated, is IgG.

The basic function of antibody is to bind antigen to form antigen–antibody (immune) complexes. Antibody activity is manifest in neutralization, opsonization, complement activation and antibody-dependent cell-mediated cytotoxicity (ADCC). In neutralization, antibody binds directly to soluble toxins and many viruses, and renders them safe by preventing them binding to tissue receptors; the resulting immune complexes are removed from the circulation and destroyed by macrophages. Opsonization is the coating of insoluble antigens by antibodies and/or complement; this is recognized by phagocytic cells and results in phagocytosis. Fc and C3 receptors are present on neutrophils and macrophages, and both types of cell can phagocytose IgG-coated antigens. Fc-related phagocytosis is relatively inefficient but is greatly facilitated by the involvement of complement (C3b) activated by either antibody (the classical pathway) or bacterial cell walls (the alternative pathway). ADCC requires NK cell activity.

Regulation of the immune system and tolerance

The immune system is regulated by complex interactions and feedback mechanisms, and many cytokine pathways play an important role. Tolerance is an antigen-induced inhibition of the development, growth or differentiation of antigen-specific lymphocytes. It is acquired during lymphocyte development and accounts for the immune system being able to distinguish self from non-self antigens, there being no response to self antigens. The mechanisms by which tolerance develops are clonal deletion, in which the thymus destroys autoreactive T cell clones during development; clonal inactivation, whereby antigen-specific lymphocytes are rendered unresponsive;

and possibly the suppression of an immune response by specific down-regulatory suppressor T cells. In clonal deletion and inactivation the immune system does not respond to self antigen, while in suppression, although self antigen is recognized, there is no inflammatory response. Other mechanisms of tolerance include the absence of presentation and processing of self antigen, antigen receptor blockade and the synthesis of anti-idiotype autoantibodies.

IMMUNITY OF THE EYE AND ASSOCIATED STRUCTURES

Ocular defences comprise the lids, tears and conjunctiva, the bones and soft tissues of the orbit, the coats of the eye, and innate and acquired immune mechanisms.

Innate immunity

The substrates of innate immunity include the lids and blinking, tears, normal conjunctival/lid flora, and the mechanical barrier of an intact mucous membrane.

Lids and blinking

The lashes are accurate sensors in the blink reflex, and trap micro-organisms. Lid closure cleans the ocular surface and augments the lacrimal pump mechanism, thus increasing tear flow and flushing.

Tears

Antibacterial defence results from components within tears, including lactic acid and fatty acids produced by the meibomian glands and glands of Zeiss, and lysozyme and lactoferrin contained within the aqueous component produced by the lacrimal and accessory lacrimal glands. Tears also have specific anti-adhesive properties for bacteria. Leukocytes are present in the tear film, and their numbers increase when the lids are closed.

Normal flora

The normal bacterial flora (commensals) of the skin, lids and conjunctiva are acquired early in life and consist largely of aerobes, principally *Staphylococcus epidermidis* and diphtheroids; the principal anaerobe is *Propionibacterium acnes*. Commensals help to prevent colonization with more virulent organisms. This occurs particularly at the lid margins, where *Staphylococcus epidermidis* helps to prevent infection by *Staphylococcus aureus*.

Mechanical barrier of an intact mucous membrane

The tightly adherent non-keratinized stratified epithelium of the conjunctiva and cornea is a strong barrier against invasion by pathogenic organisms, and a break is usually required for their entry. *Corynebacterium diphtheriae*, *Neisseria gonorrhoeae*, *Haemophilus aegyptius* and *Listeria monocytogenes* are organisms that can break an intact corneal epithelium.

Adaptive immunity

The substrates for adaptive immunity in the eye and associated structures include MALT, Langerhans cells, immunoglobulin A, the choroidal circulation, the vitreous, and immune privilege.

MALT is the system through which environmental antigen is processed.

Langerhans cells are dendritic APCs in the epithelium of the conjunctiva and corneal periphery.

Immunoglobulin A is present in the aqueous component of tears produced by the lacrimal and accessory lacrimal glands.

The choroidal circulation is rapidly affected by systemic influences and acts as a trap for many blood-borne antigens. It is a repository for immunoreactive cells, and in extreme circumstances assumes the histological appearance of a lymph node.

The vitreous may act as a long-term storage depot for foreign antigens.

Immune privilege is the special relationship that the eye has with the immune system, whereby the adaptive immune response is modulated in such a way as to preserve and maintain the delicate highly specialized ocular structures. A potential danger of this special status is the possibility of an inadequate response to a foreign antigen. Many factors contribute to ocular immune privilege:

Corneal avascularity: the avascularity of the cornea and its lack of APCs (other than at the periphery) and effector cells are the reasons for the excellent survival of corneal transplants. This component of immune privilege is lost when the cornea is vascularized.

Blood–ocular barriers: the interior of the eye is isolated from the cellular and humoral components of the immune system by the relative impermeability of the blood–ocular barriers. The increased permeability that occurs in ocular inflammation may facilitate chronicity and recurrence.

Absence of lymphatic drainage: the absence of lymphatic drainage for the eye and orbit profoundly affects immune mechanisms. Antigens from intraocular and orbital tissues are presented to the spleen, whereas those from the lids and conjunctiva are presented to MALT and regional lymph nodes.

MHC class II expression: the adaptive immune response is modified by the absence of MHC class II expression in the endothelium of the cornea and trabecular meshwork, and in the ocular vascular endothelium, RPE and neurosensory retinal cells.

Immunosuppressive ocular fluids: factors in the aqueous that modify the adaptive immune response include TGF-β, α-melanocyte-stimulating hormone (α-MSH), vasoactive intestinal peptide (VIP), calcitonin gene-related peptide (CGRP), anti-complement activity, and low levels of cortisol-binding globulin.

Fas ligand (Fas L)-mediated apoptosis: Fas is a transmembrane protein of the tumour necrosis factor receptor (TNFR) family expressed on many cells, including those of the myeloid and lymphoid systems. Fas ligand (Fas L) is another transmembrane protein also present on many cell types. Cells expressing Fas are induced into apoptosis on binding with Fas L. Ocular Fas L expression occurs in the cornea (epithelium and endothelium), iris, ciliary body and retina. Fas L expression causes apoptosis of Fas + T cells, thereby destroying invading activated immune cells with the potential to damage ocular structures.

Uveitogenic antigens: uveitogenic antigens sequestered within the eye are normally isolated from the immune system, and their exposure results in intraocular inflammation. Such antigens include retinal S-antigen, interphotoreceptor retinoid binding protein (IRBP), rhodopsin and possibly others.

Anterior chamber associated immune deviation (ACAID): this is an unusual adaptive immune response to antigen in the anterior chamber, requiring an intact eye–spleen axis. It is characterized by a selective and transient depression of cell-mediated immunity, but preservation of the humoral response that produces complement-fixing antibodies. ACAID has evolved as a way of limiting potentially dangerous delayed-type hypersensitivity, and may in part account for the rarity of corneal allograft rejection, lens-induced endophthalmitis and sympathetic ophthalmitis. The absence of ocular lymphatics and the slow drainage of antigen through the trabecular meshwork into the venous system are important factors in the mechanism. ACAID is in part mediated by cytokines, which induce ACAID behaviour in intraocular APCs. Antigens captured by these APCs are transported to the spleen, a humoral response ensues and cytotoxic cells are directed against the inciting antigens. Phenomena similar to ACAID occur within the vitreous and subretinal space.

INFLAMMATION

Inflammation is the vascular and cellular response of the host to tissue injury. Causes include physical and chemical agents, invading pathogenic organisms, ischaemia, and the excessive or inappropriate operation of immune mechanisms as in hypersensitivity and autoimmunity respectively. It is characterized by a reaction of the microcirculation in which increased vascular permeability leads to the migration of cells of the innate and acquired immune systems. Inflammation facilitates the immune response and the subsequent removal of antigenic material and damaged tissue. At the outset, the recognition of tissue injury initiates mechanisms that localize and clear foreign substances and damaged tissues. Following this, the response is amplified by the activation of inflammatory cells and the production of soluble mediators. Finally, after the elimination of foreign agents and damaged tissue, specific inhibitory factors terminate the response. Inflammation is classified as acute or chronic, depending on the persistence of injury, the cellular response and the clinicopathological features.

ACUTE INFLAMMATION

The essential features of acute inflammation are vasodilatation, increased vascular permeability, the intravascular stimulation of platelets, and the accumulation of polymorphonuclear leukocytes. Vasodilatation and the increased vascular permeability that lead to the accumulation of fluid and plasma give rise to the four cardinal clinical signs of redness (rubor), heat (calor), pain (dolor) and swelling (tumor).

The acute early response

The acute early response begins immediately and relates to changes within the microvasculature, particularly at the level of the capillary and post-capillary venule. The vascular network contains all the components necessary for acute inflammation, and the acute early response involves the release of mediators, vascular changes and leukocyte activity.

The release of chemical mediators

Mediators released from platelets, cells and tissues include vasoactive amines, acidic lipids, leukocyte-derived mediators, cytokines, neuropeptides, endothelium-derived mediators, platelet-activating factor and reactive oxygen metabolites. Enzymatic cascade systems within plasma that facilitate inflammation include the complement system, the kinin system, and the clotting cascade and fibrinolytic sequence.

Vasoactive amines include histamine and serotonin, which are released from mast cells and basophils. Histamine causes vasodilatation and increases vascular permeability. Serotonin is a vasoconstrictor.

Acidic lipids comprise prostaglandins, thromboxane and leukotrienes. They are all derived from the arachidonic acid component of cell membranes. Prostaglandins cause vasodilatation, thromboxane is a vasoconstrictor, and leukotrienes are chemotactic for neutrophils.

Leukocyte-derived mediators emanate from cytoplasmic granules. They are numerous and include enzymes that degrade basement membranes, increase vascular permeability and generate chemotactic fragments from C5.

Cytokines include interleukins, interferons, tumour necrosis factors, transforming growth factors, colony stimulating factors and chemokines. They are released from a variety of cells, particularly lymphocytes, granulocytes, monocytes and macrophages.

Neuropeptides are found in nerves and include substance P, calcitonin gene-related peptide (CGRP) and vasoactive intestinal peptide (VIP). Among their many functions, substance P is a vasodilator and increases vascular permeability, CGRP is a slow-onset long-lasting vasodilator, and VIP inhibits lymphocytic proliferation and the synthesis of leukotrienes.

Endothelium-derived mediators are derived from vascular endothelium and include endothelins, nitric oxide and prostacyclin. Endothelins are potent vasoconstrictors, and nitric oxide and prostacyclin are vasodilators.

Nitric oxide also inhibits and reverses platelet aggregation, acting synergistically with prostacyclin.

Platelet-activating factor (PAF) comprises a group of phospholipids produced by platelets and a variety of cells including neutrophils, eosinophils, basophils and macrophages. Pro-inflammatory properties of PAF include platelet aggregation, vasoconstriction, enhanced release of histamine and serotonin, increased arachidonic acid metabolism and increased neutrophil activity.

Reactive oxygen metabolites include superoxide anion (O_2^-), hydrogen peroxide (H_2O_2), hydroxyl radical (OH^-) and hypochlorous acid $(HClO_3^-)$. All are produced during the increased oxidative metabolic activity (respiratory burst) of neutrophils and are prime mediators of tissue injury.

The complement system includes the small 'a' fragments that are important in the mediation of inflammation; C3a, C4a and C5a are particularly potent.

The kinin system comprises kinins, small inflammatory peptide mediators, produced from plasma precursors (kininogens) by specific cleaving enzymes (kallikreins) or cellular proteases released from neutrophils and mast cells.

The clotting cascade and fibrinolytic sequence manifests itself in converting fibrinogen to fibrin and subsequent fibrinolysis, as a consequence of which chemotactic and vasoactive fibrinopeptides are liberated.

Vascular changes

Vascular changes result from the release of inflammatory mediators. The major response is vasodilatation, although initial retraction of vascular endothelium is accompanied by transient vasoconstriction. Blood flow increases, capillary channels open, and cells (particularly neutrophils) and plasma leak into the extravascular tissues with consequent oedema. An increase in lymphatic drainage helps to reduce oedema and results in the transport of antigen to lymphoid tissue. At the same time, the normally flat endothelial cells enlarge and protrude into the vascular lumen, cytoplasmic granules increase in number, and adhesion molecules are expressed.

Leukocyte activation

Leukocytes marginate to the periphery of the blood stream and come to lie in contact with the vascular endothelium. They appear to roll along the inner surface of the vessel in the direction of the blood flow before adhering to the endothelium and migrating into extravascular tissue.

The delayed cellular response and phagocytosis

In addition to polymorphonuclear leukocytes, other components activated include mast cells, mononuclear phagocytes and platelets. Lymphocytes enter the site of acute inflammation at about the same time as monocytes, but await activation by antigen-primed APCs. Lytic enzymes released from neutrophils and macrophages damage tissue, as does complement, which has a direct effect (non-antibody-dependent complement-mediated cell lysis) and promotes NK cell activity (ADCC). Phagocytosis is a key mechanism in the removal of pathogens and necrotic tissue and, while it may occur spontaneously, it is facilitated by opsonization.

The outcome of acute inflammation

Acute inflammation resolves, organizes or becomes chronic.

Resolution

Elimination of the cause of the inflammation and subsidence of the acute response, followed by the restoration of normal tissue architecture and function, is the ideal outcome. The return to normality depends on the ability of the tissue to replace lost cells with cells of identical type, and on the preservation of the vascular framework and connective tissue in which the cells are arranged.

Organization

If the damaged cells are unable to regenerate or if the vascular framework and connective tissue are significantly disturbed, organization results in the formation of a scar, the morphology and consistency of which depend on the tissue involved. Epithelial surfaces are restored by cell migration and proliferation. In connective tissue, vascularization occurs and the extracellular matrix is remodelled by the deposition of glycosaminoglycans, fibroblast activity and the production of collagen. Abscess formation is a possible consequence of local organization, an abscess being a walled-off localized collection of pus, a protein-rich liquid containing acute inflammatory cells and cellular debris (Fig. 2.9) and, if the cause was infection, micro-organisms. Pus formation results from the activity of enzymes released by neutrophils during acute inflammation.

Chronicity

If the acute inflammatory response does not eliminate the cause of the inflammation, the reaction becomes chronic.

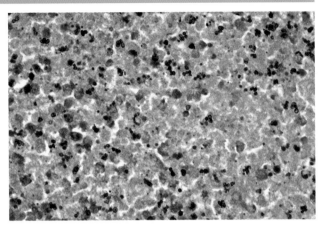

Figure 2.9 Abscess. Cellular and necrotic debris.

The systemic response to acute inflammation

Severe acute inflammation is associated with fever, malaise and hypotension, effects that are known as the acute phase response. This response is produced by inflammatory mediators, particularly cytokines, released at the site of tissue injury. IL-1 and IL-6 act on the hypothalamic temperature control system to induce fever and cause transcription of acute phase reactants by hepatocytes. Acute phase reactants such as C-reactive protein and serum amyloid components A and P enhance innate defence mechanisms, inhibit the effect of cytokines, elevate plasma viscosity (PV) and increase the erythrocyte sedimentation rate (ESR).

CHRONIC INFLAMMATION

Persistent inflammation is designated as chronic, but the term 'chronic inflammation' has come to mean a specific type of response characterized by the presence of mononuclear inflammatory cells (lymphocytes, plasma cells, macrophages) and, in certain circumstances, eosinophils. Acute and chronic inflammation represent the opposite ends of a spectrum of responses, and the histological features of both types may be present at the site of inflammatory activity. Chronic inflammation may develop as a continuation of the acute response, but in viral, protozoal, helminth and some bacterial infections a chronic inflammatory cell infiltrate may represent the primary response. Chronic inflammation can also occur as an immune response to self and non-self antigens and, as with acute inflammation, serves to eliminate the cause. Immune and non-immune mechanisms are involved, and granulation tissue formation and fibrosis frequently develop. Chronic inflammation is histologically of two types, non-granulomatous and granulomatous.

Non-granulomatous chronic inflammation

The characteristic cells of non-granulomatous chronic inflammation are lymphocytes, plasma cells and macrophages, but other cells are sometimes seen.

Lymphocytes modulate both cell-mediated and antibody-mediated (humoral) immunity. T lymphocytes are the effector cells in cell-mediated immunity. B lymphocytes are plasma cell precursors and predominate in antibody-mediated immunity.

Plasma cells are the source of antibodies.

Macrophages are phagocytic and also function as a source of immune and inflammatory mediators. They play a key role in chronic inflammation by regulating the response of lymphocytes and releasing mediators that control the proliferation and function of vascular endothelial cells and fibroblasts.

Other cells seen in non-granulomatous chronic inflammation include eosinophils, particularly in Type 1 hypersensitivity responses and helminth infections.

Granulomatous chronic inflammation

Granulomatous chronic inflammation exhibits the features of non-granulomatous reactions but the characteristic additional feature is the presence of aggregates of epithelioid histiocytes (granulomas) and sometimes histiocytic giant cells, two specialized forms of macrophages. Granulomatous inflammation can only be diagnosed histologically, although its presence is inferred if the cause of the inflammation is otherwise established as being due to a specific granulomatous disorder.

Epithelioid histiocytes (epithelioid cells) are modified macrophages that morphologically resemble epithelial cells by having large pale vesicular nuclei, prominent nucleoli and pale-staining eosinophilic cytoplasm (Fig. 2.10). They have limited phagocytic activity, but appear to be adapted to a secretory function (they secrete angiotensin converting enzyme – ACE) and may fuse to form histiocytic giant cells.

Histiocytic giant cells (giant cells) are multinucleate, and form when two or more epithelioid cells fuse while simultaneously attempting to engulf the same particle. They are commonly seen in granulomatous inflammation, but are not a defining feature; nor do solitary giant cells in the absence of epithelioid cells constitute a granuloma. Giant cells have little phagocytic activity and no other known function. Three types are identified: Langhans', Touton and foreign body (Fig. 2.11).

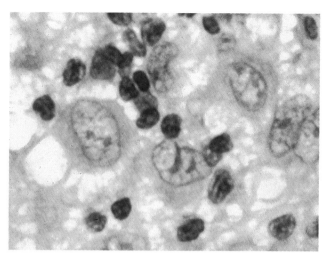

Figure 2.10 Epithelioid histiocytes. Large pale vesicular nuclei, prominent nucleoli and pale eosinophilic cytoplasm.

Langhans' giant cells have a horseshoe arrangement of nuclei at the periphery (Fig. 2.11a) and are seen in the non-caseating granulomatous inflammation of sarcoidosis and the caseating granulomatous inflammation of tuberculosis.

Touton giant cells have a ring of nuclei in the mid-periphery (Fig. 2.11b), outside which is a vacuolated cytoplasm. They occur in xanthomatous lesions such as juvenile xanthogranuloma.

Foreign body giant cells have randomly distributed nuclei and are present in relation to exogenous or endogenous foreign material (Fig. 2.11c). Exogenous foreign bodies include talc and sutures, and examples of endogenous substances include the haematogenous residues of a cholesterol granuloma (Fig. 2.12), keratin leaking from a keratinous cyst and the sebaceous material present in a chalazion.

Granulomatous inflammation is characteristic of tuberculosis, leprosy and syphilis, certain fungal infections, ocular toxocariasis, sarcoidosis, immune-mediated reactions when Type 3 and sometimes Type 4 mechanisms are involved, and foreign body reactions. The commonest granulomatous reaction in the lids is a chalazion.

Chalazion ('meibomian cyst')

In spite of the commonly used name, 'meibomian cyst', a chalazion is not a cyst and is not exclusively derived from the meibomian glands. It is a granulomatous inflammatory reaction in the lid caused by retained sebaceous secretion leaking from the meibomian glands, the glands of Zeiss or other sebaceous glands into the stromal tissues to produce a focal (Fig. 2.13a) or diffuse reaction

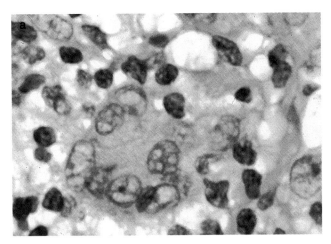

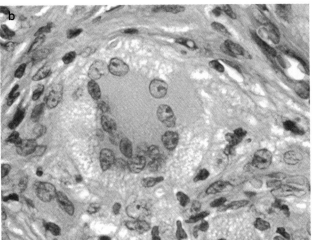

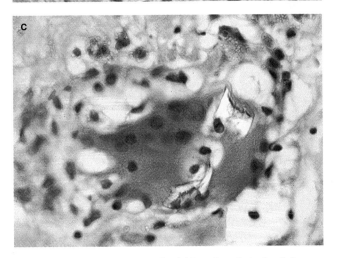

Figure 2.11 Histiocytic giant cells. (a) Langhans' giant cell; horse-shoe configuration of peripheral nuclei. (b) Touton giant cell; mid-peripheral ring of nuclei and vacuolated peripheral cytoplasm. (c) Foreign body giant cell; the nuclei are randomly distributed. Note particles of birefringent foreign material. Partially polarized light.

that may involve the whole lid (Fig. 2.13b). Chalazions occur more commonly in the upper lids, and may be solitary or multiple. A chalazion may resolve and disap-

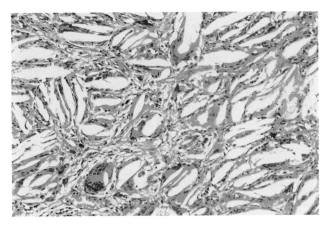

Figure 2.12 Cholesterol granuloma. Cholesterol clefts, epithelioid histiocytes and foreign body giant cells.

pear or remain stationary, but frequently increases in size and presents as a lid mass. Chalazions may be associated with blepharitis (which may be infective), but the chronic inflammation of chalazions is not primarily infective although secondary infection may later lead to the development of an abscess. It is sometimes difficult clinically to distinguish a chalazion from a neoplasm. The histological features are those of a lipogranuloma (Fig. 2.13c, 2.13d) in which a granulomatous inflammatory reaction occurs in response to lipid. The lipid is leached out during the processing of excised material, and appears in routine histological sections as well-demarcated empty spaces. In addition to the epithelioid histiocytes of a granuloma, giant cells, lymphocytes and plasma cells and, on occasions, neutrophils and eosinophils are seen.

Sarcoidosis

Sarcoidosis is an idiopathic granulomatous inflammatory condition that can affect almost every part of the body, but particularly the mediastinal and peripheral lymph nodes, the lungs, liver, spleen, kidneys and heart, the phalangeal bones, the parotid and lacrimal glands, the skin and the eyes. It occurs more usually in young adults. Males and females are equally affected, and the condition is more common in Afro-Caribbeans than in Caucasians. Approximately 30 per cent of cases exhibit ophthalmic involvement, which may develop without evidence of active systemic disease. The uvea, retina and lacrimal gland are the structures principally affected, and the commonest ocular manifestation is anterior uveitis, which may be acute but is more usually chronic, with mutton-fat keratic precipitates, and Busacca and Koeppe nodules. In posterior segment involvement the eye is not clinically inflamed, but there may be intermediate uveitis with snowball opacities in the vitreous. Vascular sheathing and perivascular exuda-

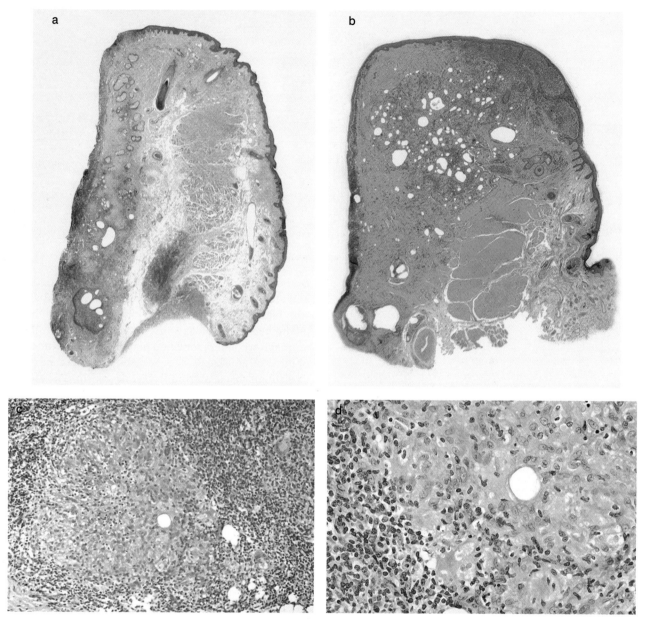

Figure 2.13 Chalazion: lipogranuloma. (a) Localized lesion in lid. (b) Diffuse lesion in lid. (c) Curetted material. Low magnification. (d) Curetted material. High magnification.

tion (candle-wax drippings) are evidence of retinal periphlebitis, and there may be venous occlusion, macular and optic disc oedema, and retinal neovascularization. Unilateral or bilateral involvement of the orbit usually affects the lacrimal glands, which become enlarged. Tear production is possibly reduced, and keratoconjunctivitis sicca may develop. Other ophthalmic manifestations of sarcoidosis include band keratopathy, follicular conjunctivitis and sarcoid nodules of the conjunctiva and lids.

All the involved tissues show discrete non-necrotizing granulomas, usually with a surrounding rim of lymphocytes (Fig. 2.14). The granulomas either resolve or

become fibrosed. Blood eosinophilia may be accompanied by raised serum levels of calcium, lysozyme and angiotensin converting enzyme (ACE). In sarcoid uveitis, the aqueous ACE may be raised despite a normal level in the serum.

The Kveim test is now obsolete, but was formerly used in the investigation of sarcoidosis. The subject under investigation had an intracutaneous injection of a sterile particulate suspension of human spleen affected with sarcoidosis. A positive response was the formation of a nodule 2–6 weeks following injection; biopsy revealed non-necrotizing granulomatous inflammation. The

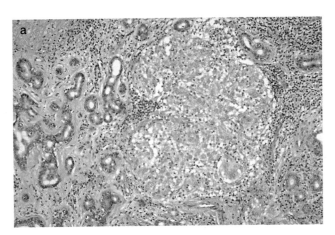

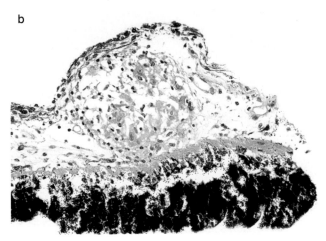

Figure 2.14 Sarcoidosis. (a) Sarcoid granuloma in lacrimal gland. (b) Sarcoid granuloma in iris.

mechanism of the positive reaction is unknown. The test was positive in about 80 per cent of those affected, with only a small number of false positives. The test is now obsolete because of the risks of transmission of infection, but other disadvantages include unavailability of antigen, lack of standardization, delay in the time to diagnosis and the interference of systemic medication with the results of the test.

The cause of sarcoidosis remains unknown, but T cell function is defective whereas B cell responses remain normal. An increased ratio of CD4+ to CD8+ cells occurs in the aqueous of those with sarcoid uveitis and in the conjunctiva of those with sarcoid follicles. One of the major genetic factors contributing to the development of sarcoidosis is located within the DRB1 locus of the HLA class II region.

CLINICOPATHOLOGICAL FEATURES OF INFLAMMATION OF THE EYE AND ASSOCIATED STRUCTURES

Inflammation has a number of causes, the most important of which are immune-mediated or infective. Extra- and intraocular tissues can be affected; the reactions are either acute or chronic, and their sequelae may have a profound effect on vision.

Extraocular inflammation and inflammation of the corneoscleral coat

Extraocular inflammation includes inflammation of the lid margins (blepharitis), the conjunctiva (conjunctivitis) and orbital connective tissues (orbital cellulitis). The sequelae of chronic severe blepharitis and conjunctivitis are similar, and include distortion of the lids, ectropion,

entropion, trichiasis, madarosis and symblepharon (Fig. 2.15). The consequence of orbital inflammation is tissue scarring, possibly with diminished ocular movement (frozen orbit). Involvement of the lacrimal gland can result in diminished tear secretion and dry eye.

Inflammation of the corneoscleral coat comprises keratitis and scleritis. The possible sequelae of keratitis include epithelial oedema, destruction of Bowman's layer, thickening or thinning and vascularization of the scarred stroma, lipid keratopathy, loss of endothelial cells and staphyloma formation. Sequelae of scleritis are scarring, thickening or thinning, and possibly staphyloma formation (Fig. 2.16).

Blepharitis

The clinicopathological features of blepharitis include scaling, crusting, vascularization, telangiectasis and thickening. There is often accompanying inflammation of the conjunctiva and cornea. Blepharitis is classified as

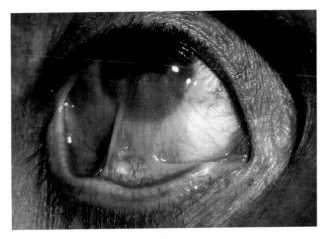

Figure 2.15 Symblepharon.

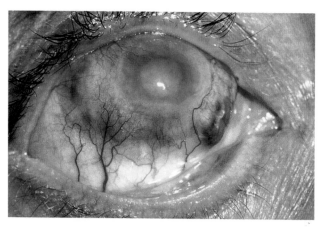

Figure 2.16 Ciliary body staphyloma.

anterior or posterior, and diffuse or focal. Anterior ble-pharitis is essentially due to staphylococcal infection, while posterior blepharitis results from meibomian gland dysfunction.

Anterior blepharitis (staphylococcal blepharitis)

This is characterized by lid margin ulceration and pust-ular folliculitis with a positive culture for *Staphylococcus aureus*. Lid bacteria contribute to blepharitis directly by infection and the release of toxins, or indirectly through their action on lipids and the production of irritant fatty acids. Acute focal infection is manifest as an external hordeolum (stye), which is an infection (usually staphy-lococcal) of a lash follicle and its associated glands of Zeiss and Moll. It presents as a tender inflamed swelling at the lid margin, often with a protruding lash, that later develops into an abscess from which the causative organ-ism may be cultured.

Posterior blepharitis

Posterior blepharitis is due to meibomian gland dysfunc-tion and is the principal manifestation of acne rosacea, a chronic oculodermal disorder primarily affecting the sebaceous glands of the face and the meibomian glands of the lids. In acne rosacea there also appears to be enhanced cell-mediated immunity to *S. aureus*. There may at times be an association with seborrhoeic derma-titis. The clinicopathological features result from meibo-mian gland blockage, possibly due to keratinization of the ducts, inflammation (meibomitis), and the altered pH and lipid content of tears, and the effect on the lids and ocular surface. In posterior blepharitis the tarsus of the lids is often thickened, and the meibomian glands are enlarged and appear to push above the surface. In pos-terior blepharitis conjunctival injection is common, and

there may be a papillary reaction. Abnormalities of the tear film account for the symptoms of meibomian gland dysfunction (burning sensation on waking and blurred vision) and for the inconsistent ocular surface wetting that leads to punctate epithelial erosions, subepithelial infiltrates and vascularization of the peripheral cornea. The degree of inflammation is variable, but there may be internal hordeolum and chalazion formation. An inter-nal hordeolum is a localized infection (usually staphylo-coccal) of a meibomian gland. Inflammatory signs are localized around the orifice of the involved gland, and a yellowish tender inflamed nodule is produced in the palpebral conjunctiva; as with an external hordeolum, there is abscess formation from which the causative organism can be cultured.

Conjunctivitis

Conjunctivitis is manifest as vasodilatation, oedema, dis-charge, membranes and pseudomembranes, follicles, papillae and lymphadenopathy.

Vasodilatation is most conspicuous in the fornices.

Oedema (chemosis) may be widespread, and is due to increased vascular permeability.

Discharge is watery (viral infections), mucoid (vernal keratoconjunctivitis, keratoconjunctivitis sicca), muco-purulent (mild bacterial infections) or purulent (severe bacterial infections).

Membranes and pseudomembranes represent different degrees of the same process in which inflammatory exudate, fibrin and other constituents of serum form a coagulum in relation to the conjunctival surface. In true membrane formation this coagulum permeates the sur-face, and attempts at removal result in tearing of the epithelium and bleeding from the underlying stroma. Pseudomembranes are not entirely dissimilar, but the inflammatory process is less intense and the membrane can usually be peeled off the epithelium. *Corynebacter-ium diphtheriae* and *Streptococcus pyogenes* are the usual bacterial pathogens. Other causes include ocular cicatri-cial pemphigoid, the Stevens–Johnson syndrome and ligneous conjunctivitis, an idiopathic chronic inflamma-tion characterized by the presence of a coagulum of fibrin on the conjunctiva (Fig. 2.17). In ligneous conjunctivitis the lids feel woody on palpation (hence ligneous), the cornea may be involved and other mucous membranes (larynx, tracheobronchial tree, vulva, vagina) can be affected.

Follicles are smooth yellowish-white elevations seen par-ticularly in the palpebral conjunctiva and in relation to the limbus. Histologically, they are subepithelial lym-

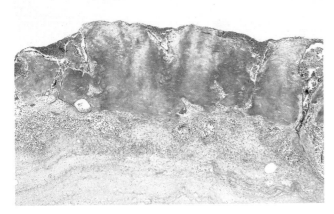

Figure 2.17 Ligneous conjunctivitis. Eosinophilic fibrinous coagulum on conjunctival surface.

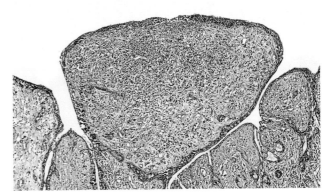

Figure 2.19 Conjunctival papilla. Fibrovascular core and an inflammatory cell infiltrate.

phoproliferative lesions consisting of germinal follicles of lymphocytes with immature cells centrally and mature cells peripherally (Fig. 2.18). They represent reaction to an inflammatory stimulus and occur most often in viral and chlamydial infections, in hypersensitivity to topical medication, and in Parinaud's oculoglandular conjunctivitis (follicular conjunctivitis with preauricular and submandibular lymphadenopathy). Follicles in children are usually of no significance.

Papillae are polygonal elevations, larger than follicles, usually affecting the palpebral conjunctiva, to which they give a red velvety appearance. They comprise a fibrovascular core infiltrated by inflammatory cells and covered by surface epithelium. Large papillae (Fig. 2.19) occur in vernal keratoconjunctivitis and giant papillary conjunctivitis, while small papillae are a non-specific finding in conjunctival inflammation due to any cause.

Lymphadenopathy (preauricular and submandibular) is a feature of viral and bacterial infections.

Orbital cellulitis

The pathological characteristics of inflammation of orbital connective tissue are vasocongestion, oedema and an inflammatory cell infiltrate.

Keratitis

Keratitis is manifest as punctate epitheliopathy, epithelial oedema, corneal filaments, punctate epithelial keratitis, ulceration, stromal infiltrates and oedema, and folds in Descemet's membrane.

Punctate epitheliopathy (punctate epithelial erosions – PEE) are non-specific tiny slightly depressed grey-white spots that stain well with fluorescein (fluorescein stains areas of epithelial cell loss). PEE are located superiorly in vernal keratoconjunctivitis and superior limbic keratoconjunctivitis, inferiorly in keratoconjunctivitis sicca and staphylococcal blepharitis, and in the interpalpebral area in seborrhoeic blepharitis.

Epithelial oedema is manifest as vesicles and bullae, and is indicative of endothelial cell dysfunction.

Corneal filaments are comma-shaped mucus threads that move with each blink. They stain well with rose Bengal. Causes of corneal filaments include keratoconjunctivitis sicca and herpes zoster ophthalmicus.

Punctate epithelial keratitis (PEK) is the hallmark of viral infections, and is revealed as opalescent epithelial cells that stain well with rose Bengal (rose Bengal stains degenerate and dying cells, and mucus).

Ulceration is the loss of epithelium and possibly Bowman's layer and a variable amount of stroma (Fig. 2.20).

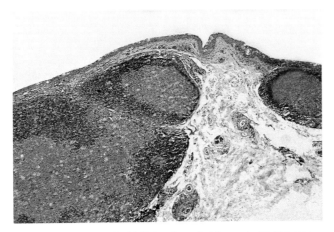

Figure 2.18 Conjunctival follicles. Lymphoid germinal follicles in subepithelial stroma; immature cells centrally and mature cells peripherally.

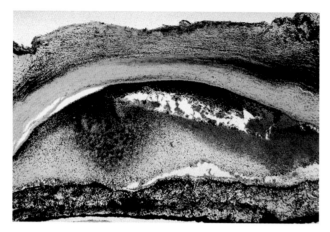

Figure 2.20 Ulcerative keratitis. Corneal ulceration and stromal infiltration with hypopyon and hyphaema.

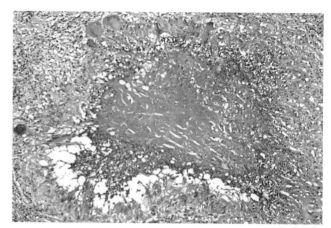

Figure 2.21 Scleritis. Necrotizing granulomatous inflammation with giant cells.

Stromal infiltrates are aggregates of inflammatory cells, and indicate active inflammation.

Stromal oedema usually coexists with infiltrates. On clinical examination, the cornea is opalescent and thickened. Oedematous stroma appears as pale and frothy in histological preparations.

Folds in Descemet's membrane may result from stromal inflammation.

Scleritis

The features of scleritis are vasocongestion and oedema, with histological evidence typically of necrotizing granulomatous inflammation (Fig. 2.21).

Intraocular inflammation

Intraocular inflammation (IOI) includes uveitis, endophthalmitis and panophthalmitis. Uveitis is inflammation of the iris and/or the ciliary body (anterior uveitis – iritis, iridocyclitis and cyclitis) and the choroid (posterior uveitis – choroiditis), and the cellular and vascular reactions that accompany inflammation targeted to adjacent sites, particularly the retina. Endophthalmitis is inflammation of the vitreous, retina and uvea. Panophthalmitis, in addition, involves the corneoscleral coat. IOI may be classified as anterior or posterior.

Anterior intraocular inflammation

Anterior IOI occurs anterior to the iris–lens diaphragm, and includes iritis, iridocyclitis and cyclitis. In acute inflammation, circumcorneal vasocongestion is associated with increased permeability of the blood–aqueous barrier, resulting in iris oedema, aqueous cells and flare.

Chronic inflammation exhibits the features of acute inflammation apart from vasocongestion.

Aqueous cells: inflammatory cells circulating in the thermal convection currents of the aqueous reflect and scatter light from the slit-beam of a biomicroscope and are visible on clinical examination. Inflammatory cells may be deposited on the posterior corneal surface (keratic precipitates, KPs – Fig. 2.22), and range in morphology from the fine diffuse aggregates of acute anterior uveitis to nodular aggregates (mutton-fat KPs) that are assumed to be a clinical characteristic of chronic granulomatous inflammation. Nodular cellular aggregates may also be present at the pupillary margin (Koeppe nodules) or on the anterior iris surface (Busacca nodules). A sediment of inflammatory cells in the anterior chamber is termed a hypopyon.

Aqueous flare: this is the visibility of a beam of light as it passes through the aqueous. It is due to the Tyndall effect (the scattering of light by large protein molecules).

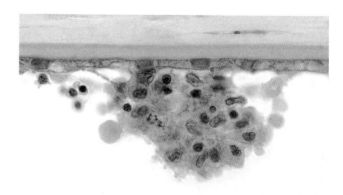

Figure 2.22 Keratic precipitate. An aggregate of inflammatory cells on the posterior corneal surface.

Posterior intraocular inflammation

Posterior IOI refers to intraocular inflammatory conditions posterior to the iris–lens diaphragm, and includes intermediate uveitis (inflammation of the pars plana), posterior uveitis, choroidoretinitis, retinitis, retinal vasculitis and vitritis. The clinicopathological features result from increased permeability of the blood–retinal barrier. The eye does not usually appear inflamed, but floaters and impaired vision are characteristic. There are specific effects in the choroid, retina and vitreous.

Choroid

Extracellular accumulation of fluid results in choroidal and suprachoroidal oedema. Choroidal oedema may result in localized detachment of the RPE and, if the junctional complexes between the RPE cells are broken down, serous detachment of the neurosensory retina. Suprachoroidal oedema can extend anteriorly to produce supraciliary oedema.

Retina

Exudation of fluid into the retina is clinically manifest as an elevation and loss of transparency. The macula is particularly susceptible to inflammatory changes, and cystoid macular oedema (see Fig. 1.11) and retinoschisis may develop. Lymphocytic cuffing of the retinal venules is often seen histologically.

Vitreous

The physical and mechanical properties of the vitreous form a barrier to the inward and outward spread of inflammation. Inflammatory cells lodged in the vitreous may persist after the acute inflammation has subsided, and aggregate and come to lie inferiorly, giving rise to the characteristic vitreous snowballs seen in intermediate and posterior uveitis. Persistent inflammation causes posterior vitreous detachment. Inflammatory infiltrates may settle behind the posterior vitreous face in a way analogous to hypopyon formation in the anterior chamber.

Sequelae of intraocular inflammation

If resolution does not occur, the permanent sequelae of IOI involve all the intraocular structures and can affect the intraocular pressure.

Iris

Neovascularization on the anterior surface (rubeosis iridis – see Fig. 1.9) may be a feature of previous inflammation. Organization of inflammatory exudate in the anterior ocular compartments leads to iridocorneal and iridolenticular adhesions (anterior and posterior synechiae – Fig. 2.23). Peripheral iridocorneal adhesions (peripheral anterior synechiae) can result in the extension of corneal endothelial cells and the development of a Descemet-like membrane on the anterior iris surface.

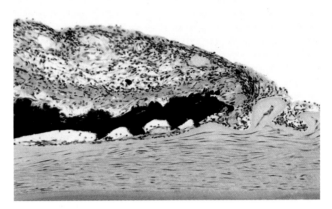

Figure 2.23 Iridolenticular adhesion. A degree of active chronic inflammation is evident and the lens exhibits anterior subcapsular fibrosis.

Ciliary body

Organization of inflammatory exudate posterior to the lens results in the formation of a retrolental membrane. The membrane may become attached peripherally to the ciliary body, and detachment of both the ciliary body and retina can ensue. The ciliary epithelium becomes hyperplastic and the proliferating cells may extend into the cyclitic membrane and assume a pseudoadenomatous appearance (see Fig. 4.61). The ciliary processes can become hyalinized.

Secondary glaucoma and hypotony

Increased viscosity of the aqueous, due to its cellular and proteinaceous content, may reduce the efficacy of drainage and result in elevation of the intraocular pressure. Ciliary body inflammation can lead to a diminished output of aqueous, which may compensate for the hypertensive effect of increased aqueous viscosity. Iridocorneal and iridolenticular adhesions may result in secondary glaucoma, whereas damage to the ciliary epithelium may result in hypotony.

Lens

Cataract, particularly posterior subcapsular, may develop.

Posterior segment

Neovascularization, fibrosis and gliosis (fibrogliosis) underlie choroidoretinal scarring and adhesions (Fig. 2.24). Massive retinal glial proliferation may clinically resemble a neoplasm in the posterior segment. The RPE may become atrophic or hyperplastic and pigment may migrate into the neurosensory retina, particularly in relation to blood vessels. Organized membranes may form in the vitreous.

Phthisis bulbi and atrophia bulbi

Phthisis bulbi (Fig. 2.25) follows severe diffuse IOI. The globe becomes shrunken, the corneoscleral coat thickened and the intraocular structures grossly disorganized

with widespread fibrosis, gliosis and sometimes bone formation. The bone is largely but not exclusively derived from the RPE, which initially undergoes metaplasia to form fibroblasts prior to the subsequent ossification (Fig. 2.26). Choroidal fibroblasts may also undergo osseous metaplasia. Fat is almost always present in relation to the bone, but haemopoiesis is very rare. Atrophia bulbi is similar to phthisis bulbi, but disorganization is less and the choroidal and retinal architecture are preserved.

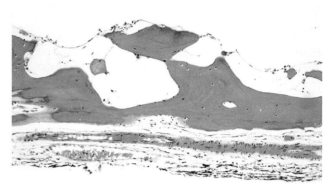

Figure 2.26 Intraocular ossification. The RPE has undergone metaplasia to form bone.

DISORDERS OF IMMUNITY

Immune inflammatory reactions protect the host from antigens and the potentially harmful effects of these responses. Disorders of immunity can affect both the innate and adaptive systems. The three types of immune disorder are: immunodeficiency, hypersensitivity and autoimmunity. Immunodeficiency is a congenital or acquired deficiency of immunity that renders the host incapable of mounting a defence against exogenous antigens. In hypersensitivity, the immune response of the host to exogenous antigens is so exaggerated as to produce collateral tissue damage. In autoimmunity, tolerance is lost and the immune system fails to distinguish self from non-self; the consequence is a response directed against host tissue antigens.

IMMUNODEFICIENCY

Immunodeficiency is either primary or secondary, and arises from abnormalities of non-specific or specific effector mechanisms. The four main clinicopathological manifestations are infections, neoplasms, disorders related to the primary disease, and complications of therapy.

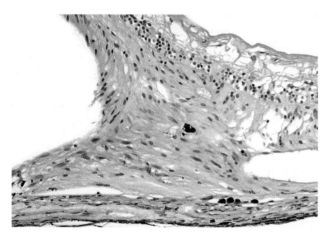

Figure 2.24 Choroidoretinal adhesion. Fibrogliosis with loss of RPE.

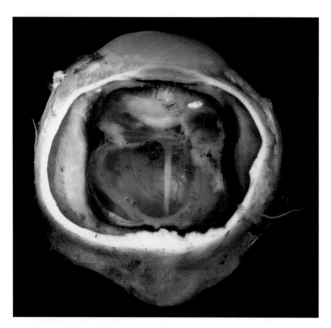

Figure 2.25 Phthisis bulbi. The intraocular contents are disorganized.

Infections

Infections occur as a consequence of disordered innate and adaptive immunity. Disorders of innate defence mechanisms include abnormalities of the lids, tear film, and the ocular surface and its innervation. These predispose to neuroparalytic, exposure and neurotrophic keratopathy and subsequent infection. Disorders of adaptive immunity predispose to exaggerated or opportunistic infections, which are among the most serious and frequent complications.

Neoplasms

Neoplasms, especially high-grade B cell lymphomas, are associated with immunodeficiency. In primary immunodeficiencies, the neoplasms may be due to chromosomal instability related to an underlying genetic defect. In other immunodeficiency states they may relate to defective immune surveillance, to defective immune responses to oncogenic viruses or to the chronic over-stimulation and proliferation of immune cells.

Disorders related to the primary disease

These include the vascular changes and neuro-ophthalmic abnormalities of ataxia telangiectasia and the oculocutaneous albinism of the Chédiak–Higashi syndrome.

Complications of therapy

Complications of therapy are usually infective or metabolic, and include the consequences of corticosteroids or long-term broad-spectrum antibiotics.

Primary immunodeficiencies

Primary immunodeficiencies result from an intrinsic defect in one or more components of the immune system. Most are the manifestations of congenital abnormalities localized at particular points in the system. Non-specific or specific mechanisms may be affected.

Non-specific primary immunodeficiencies

Non-specific primary immunodeficiencies are due to phagocytic or complement deficiencies.

Phagocytic deficiencies

The defensive activity of phagocytes requires a sequence of functions including chemotaxis, adhesion, opsonization, ingestion and intracellular microbial lysis. Disruption of any of these processes leads to phagocytic deficiencies characterized by a susceptibility to chronic and recurrent infection, particularly by bacteria and fungi. Two important disorders of phagocytic deficiency are chronic granulomatous disease and the Chédiak–Higashi syndrome.

Chronic granulomatous disease (CGD) includes a group of disorders characterized by Mendelian inheritance and the inability of phagocytic cells to use molecular oxygen for the generation of bactericidal oxygen radicals during the respiratory burst of phagocyte activation. CGD usually presents in early life with recurrent and chronic infections involving the lungs, skin, gastrointestinal tract, soft tissues, bone and brain. The main ophthalmic manifestations are recurrent blepharoconjunctivitis, marginal or punctate keratitis and progressive atrophic choroidoretinal lesions.

The Chédiak–Higashi syndrome is a rare autosomal recessive disorder comprising partial oculocutaneous albinism, increased susceptibility to viral and bacterial infections, and neurological manifestations including cerebral atrophy. There is pancytopenia, and abnormal granules are present in neutrophils, eosinophils, melanocytes (hence the albinism), renal tubular cells, hepatocytes, thyroid cells and Schwann cells. The ultrastructural abnormalities of melanosomes distinguish the condition from true albinism.

Complement deficiencies

Complement deficiencies lead to specific infections relating to the position of the deficient component in the sequential cascade. Although complement is present in the eye, ocular infections are not a prominent feature; however, those with complement deficiencies may have more severe infections than the immunocompetent.

Specific primary immunodeficiencies

Specific primary immunodeficiencies affect T cells, B cells or both.

T cell deficiencies

Failure of development of the thymus may occur in isolation (Nezelof's syndrome), in association with absence of the parathyroid glands (derived, like the thymus, from the third and fourth pharyngeal pouches), or in association with congenital cardiac defects (Di George's syndrome). If the thymus is absent, T cells cannot be produced and the T cell zones of lymph nodes are not colonized. In the presence of the thymus, cellular immunodeficiency may be a consequence of metabolic abnormalities such as purine nucleotide phosphorylase deficiency. A specific T cell defect against the *Candida* spp. of fungi occurs in chronic mucocutaneous candidiasis (CMC), a condition characterized by severe skin and mucous membrane infections including ulcerative ble-pharitis and keratoconjunctivitis. CMC is also part of a syndrome that includes keratitis, ichthyosis and deafness (KID syndrome).

B cell deficiencies

B cell deficiencies result from absence of B cells, failure of B cells to differentiate into plasma cells, or defective synthesis of antibody. All classes of immunoglobulin may be involved (panhypogammaglobulinaemia). Alternatively, only one class or subclass may be involved (selective deficiency). Most primary antibody deficiencies are rare, but selective IgA deficiency is relatively common and affects 1 : 700 individuals. In all instances there is a risk of opportunistic infection, but despite the fact that IgA is the main immunoglobulin in the tears and conjunctiva, ocular surface infection is more common when other immunoglobulins are deficient.

Combined T and B cell deficiencies

Stem cell deficiency leads to a lack or absence of T and B cell precursors. At its worst the bone marrow fails completely (reticular dysgenesis), and affected infants die of overwhelming sepsis within the first week of life. A defect at the pre-thymus/pre-bursa stage of lymphocyte ontogeny is more common and results in severe combined immunodeficiency (SCID), in which those affected can neither mount an effective cell-mediated immune response nor produce antibodies against viruses or bacteria. The rapidly fatal outcome of combined immunodeficiencies probably explains the lack of ophthalmic findings. Two important types of combined immunodeficiency that are difficult to explain in terms of the development and maturation of the immune system are the Wiskott–Aldrich syndrome and ataxia telangiectasia.

The Wiskott–Aldrich syndrome is an X-linked disorder usually presenting within the first year of life with recurrent infections, haemorrhages secondary to thrombocytopenia, and eczema. Ophthalmic manifestations include lid and ocular surface disease comprising eczema, mollusca contagiosum and herpes simplex virus keratitis. The Wiskott–Aldrich syndrome is characterized by a deficiency in the production of antibodies to polysaccharide antigen (predominantly IgM) and partial T cell immunodeficiency.

Ataxia telangiectasia is a rare autosomal recessive disorder of DNA repair. Clinical features are progressive, and include cerebellar degeneration, spinocerebellar atrophy leading to movement disorders including abnormal ocular motility, telangiectasis involving particularly the conjunctiva and the flexor surfaces of the forearms, and reduced resistance to infections due to abnormalities of both cellular and humoral immunity. Other features include abnormalities of the thymus and reduced plasma levels of IgA and IgE. Affected individuals are predisposed to lymphoma, and death occurs before the age of 20 years.

Secondary immunodeficiencies

Secondary immunodeficiencies result from acquired systemic disease and are more common than their primary counterparts. Reduced synthesis, increased loss or interference with the function of the cellular or humoral components of the immune system results in immunodeficiency. Reduced synthesis of immune components occurs in malnutrition, infection and lymphoma, and as a result of immunosuppressive therapy including drugs and radiotherapy. Immune components are lost in the nephrotic syndrome, protein losing enteropathy and following burns. Disordered function of immune components is evident in abnormal metabolic states such as diabetes mellitus and uraemia, and with corticosteroid medication. The acquired immunodeficiency syndrome (AIDS) is a secondary immunodeficiency that follows infection with the human immunodeficiency virus (HIV) and is invariably fatal.

HIV infection and AIDS

HIV is an RNA virus belonging to the retrovirus group. Retroviruses are unique in that they express reverse transcriptase, an enzyme that synthesizes virus-specific double-stranded DNA from the viral RNA genome. There are two serological types, HIV-1 and HIV-2, which are morphologically similar and produce clinically indistinguishable diseases. HIV-1 is found world-wide, while HIV-2 is more or less confined to West Africa and Portugal. There are two types of HIV-1, type M (consisting of subtypes A–H) and type O; there are five subtypes of HIV-2 (A–E). HIV is present in blood, semen, vaginal secretions, saliva, tears, breast milk and urine, and cerebrospinal, synovial and amniotic fluids. The efficacy of transmission is higher for HIV-1 than HIV-2, as is the incidence of AIDS in those infected with HIV-1. Fifty per cent of infected individuals develop AIDS within 8–10 years.

The specific target cell for HIV is the CD4 + (T_H) lymphocyte, although other cells in the immune system such as B cells and macrophages including microglia are also infected. Free HIV or HIV-infected cells express a surface glycoprotein (gp120) that binds to the CD4 molecule of T_H cells. When an uninfected host cell comes into contact with free virus or an infected cell, its cell membrane fuses with the viral envelope or the surface membrane of the infected cell. Virus particles are internalized into the host cytoplasm, where their RNA is translated into DNA by reverse transcriptase. The DNA so produced is integrated through the action of viral integrase into the genome of infected cells, where it remains latent. When reactivated, the viral DNA acts as a template for the synthesis of viral RNA and the production of virus particles. Release of virus takes place at the surface of infected cells by a process of budding, in which the virus envelope is formed from the host cell membrane to which the surface glycoproteins are added. Cell death, although not inevitable, results from membrane disruption caused by fusion of gp120 and CD4 molecules expressed together on the surface cell membrane of infected lymphocytes. CD4+(T$_H$) cells are critical for cellular and antibody-mediated immunity, and their destruction results in profound immunodeficiency.

Transmission of HIV necessitates direct inoculation and is sexual, parenteral or perinatal. Sexual transmission can be homosexual or heterosexual. In heterosexual transmission, entry of the virus is facilitated by genital trauma and the coexistence of other sexually transmitted diseases. In homosexual men the receptive partner of anal intercourse is at particularly high risk due to the transmission of virus from semen through damaged rectal mucosa. Parenteral transmission includes direct inoculation with infected blood-contaminated needles or syringes, and transfusion of infected blood products. Perinatal transmission can occur in utero, during delivery or postpartum.

There are two patterns of spread of HIV infection. The first affects homosexual or bisexual men, intravenous drug users, transfusion recipients and the heterosexual partners and children of these groups, and occurs in developed countries such as those of Western Europe, Australasia and North America. The second pattern of spread occurs in Africa and the Caribbean, where HIV infection appears in the young heterosexually active population, in transfusion recipients and in the children of affected women. An estimated 5–10 million people are infected with HIV, and 70 per cent of these reside in developing countries. HIV-associated disease is now world-wide, and there have been over 2.5 million cases of AIDS reported since its recognition in 1981.

The clinicopathological features of HIV infection cover a wide range of disease. An asymptomatic infection or acute self-limiting illness in the early stage is followed by a latent period that may last months or years, but infected individuals eventually succumb to the profound immunodeficiency of AIDS. In the early stage HIV infection may be clinically silent, or 2–3 weeks following exposure infected individuals develop an acute febrile illness resembling infectious mononucleosis, with fever, myalgia, lymphadenopathy, sore throat and a macular rash. Most symptoms and signs resolve over a

3-week period, but the myalgia and lymphadenopathy may persist for some months. Persistent generalized lymphadenopathy (PGL) is defined as the presence of enlarged palpable nodes at least 10 mm in diameter at two or more non-contiguous sites persisting for at least 3 months in those infected with HIV and in the absence of any coexistent illness known to cause lymph node enlargement. PGL does not have any prognostic significance with respect to the progression of HIV infection to AIDS. A latent period follows, and during this time those infected with HIV remain asymptomatic. Virus replication eventually resumes and the number of CD4+(T$_H$) cells declines. Viral antigens and antibodies are usually detectable within 6 months of infection, although viral replication can remain minimal for 10 years or more.

HIV-infected individuals usually remain asymptomatic until the total number of CD4+ lymphocytes falls below 500/μl. At this stage there are constitutional symptoms such as weight loss, fever and diarrhoea, and immunodeficiency becomes manifest with the onset of opportunistic infections or neoplasms. A person is designated as having AIDS when the CD4+ lymphocyte count falls below 200/μl or when, in the presence of known HIV infection, one or more AIDS-indicator conditions (Table 2.1) are diagnosed. When the number of CD4+ cells falls below 150/μl progress is rapid, with multiple pathology including widespread opportunistic infections and neoplasms, and death may ensue.

Opportunistic infections

HIV infection leads to widespread opportunistic infections which include *Pneumocystis carinii* pneumonitis, severe mucosal candidiasis, ulcerative herpes simplex, typical and less common mycobacterial infections, cryptococcal infection of the CNS, toxoplasma cerebral abscess and disseminated cytomegalovirus infection.

Neoplasms

HIV is not oncogenic, but neoplasms may develop amongst those infected. These include Kaposi sarcoma, lymphoma, and anogenital and conjunctival carcinoma.

Kaposi sarcoma: this was one of the earliest diseases that defined AIDS. Whether it is a genuine neoplasm or a reactive hyperplasia of vascular endothelium is a matter of dispute. Kaposi sarcoma (see Fig. 4.46) is very much more common in those with sexually transmitted AIDS and appears to be associated with the Kaposi sarcoma virus (KSV), which is also sexually transmitted and possibly oncogenic.

Lymphoma: individuals with HIV infection have an increased incidence of high-grade B cell lymphoma, par-

Table 2.1 AIDS-indicator conditions (based on the 1993 CDC AIDS case definition for surveillance amongst persons over 13 years old)

Opportunistic infections	Viral	Persisting or disseminated HSV, VZV, CMV or EBV infection Progressive multifocal leukoencephalopathy HIV encephalopathy HIV wasting syndrome
	Bacterial	Multiple or recurrent pyogenic bacterial infections Persistent or recurrent *Salmonella* spp., *Shigella* spp. or *Campylobacter* spp. infections Any atypical mycobacterial disease Extrapulmonary tuberculosis
	Fungal	*Pneumocystis carinii* pneumonitis Disseminated histoplasmosis Candidiasis of the oesophagus, trachea and lungs Extrapulmonary cryptococcosis Disseminated coccidioidomycosis
	Protozoal	Cerebral toxoplasmosis Cryptosporidiosis with diarrhoea Isosporiasis with diarrhoea
Neoplasms		Kaposi sarcoma Non-Hodgkin lymphoma, particularly of the CNS EBV-related lymphoma Anogenital carcinoma

ticularly in the CNS, and lymphoma associated with the Epstein–Barr virus (Burkitt's lymphoma).

Anogenital and conjunctival carcinoma: HIV-infected homosexual men have a thousand-fold increased risk of developing anal carcinoma compared with the uninfected. An increased prevalence of cervical intraepithelial neoplasia (CIN) and cervical squamous cell carcinoma occurs in HIV-infected women. Squamous cell carcinoma of the conjunctiva (see Fig. 4.42) occurs in HIV-infected adults. All these anogenital and conjunctival carcinomas are associated with the human papilloma virus (HPV).

Classification of HIV infection

The 1993 revision of the Centres for Disease Control (CDC) classification of all stages of HIV infection allow for three clinical categories (A, B and C) and relate them to the CD4+ cell count (Table 2.2).

Category A: a history, or the presence, of asymptomatic HIV infection, PGL and/or acute (primary) infection with accompanying illness.

Category B: clinical conditions not in categories A or C attributable to HIV infection or complicated by HIV infection due to defective cell-mediated immunity. Examples include candidiasis, herpes zoster, listeriosis, pelvic inflammatory disease and cervical intraepithelial neoplasia (CIN).

Category C: the presence of any AIDS-indicator condition (Table 2.1).

Ophthalmic manifestations of HIV infection

Ophthalmic manifestations of HIV infection are common and occur in up to 75 per cent of those with AIDS. They include retinal microangiopathy, opportunistic infections, Kaposi sarcoma, conjunctival carcinoma and neuro-ophthalmic lesions.

Retinal microangiopathy (HIV retinopathy – Fig. 2.27) is characterized by cotton-wool spots and develops in 50 per cent of those with asymptomatic HIV infection or AIDS. The capillary basement membrane is thickened, pericytes are lost, endothelial cells are swollen and there is microaneurysm formation. The features

Table 2.2 1993 CDC classification of HIV infection

	CD4+ T cell		Clinical manifestations		
Category	Cell count per μl		Category A – asymptomatic, acute HIV or PGL	Category B – symptomatic, not A or C conditions	Category C – AIDS-indicator conditions
1	>500		A1	B1	C1
2	200–500		A2	B2	C2
3	<200		A3	B3	C3

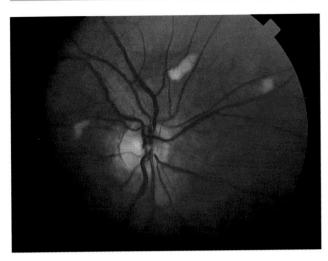

Figure 2.27 HIV retinopathy.

are similar to those of diabetic microangiopathy, but the cotton-wool spots are smaller and longer lasting than those of diabetes mellitus and haemorrhages are relatively uncommon. The incidence of retinal microangiopathy is related to the level of immunodeficiency, and is thought to be due to either the deposition of immune complex in the walls of the arterioles or HIV infection of the vascular endothelium.

Opportunistic infections with molluscum contagiosum virus, herpes simplex virus and varicella zoster virus, atypical mycobacteria, *Pneumocystis carinii*, *Candida albicans*, *Cryptococcus neoformans*, *Histoplasma capsulatum* and *Toxoplasma gondii* may develop. Retinal infections are infrequent, but cytomegalovirus retinitis eventually occurs in up to 40 per cent of those with AIDS.

Kaposi sarcoma (see Fig. 4.46) involves the lids, conjunctiva and orbit in at least 2 per cent of individuals with AIDS.

Squamous cell carcinoma of the conjunctiva (see Fig. 4.42) occurs in AIDS, particularly in equatorial Africa.

Neuro-ophthalmic lesions occur in up to 40 per cent of those with AIDS, and may be demonstrated postmortem in more than 75 per cent of those dying from AIDS. Cranial neuropathy and damage to the visual pathways result from opportunistic CNS infections, most commonly cryptococcal meningitis. Direct infection of the CNS by HIV causes subacute encephalopathy, demyelination and neuronal atrophy, resulting in ocular motility disorders, cranial nerve palsies and visual dysfunction in addition to more generalized neurological features such as dementia (AIDS dementia complex). Other causes of neuro-ophthalmic manifestations include CNS lymphoma.

Investigation for HIV infection and AIDS

The diagnosis of HIV infection is based on the detection of antibodies in the serum by immunological and molecular biological methods. The CD4 + lymphocyte count is important in the classification of HIV infection and in monitoring disease progression. A falling count may precede the clinical manifestations by up to 12–18 months.

HYPERSENSITIVITY

Hypersensitivity reactions are immune responses so exaggerated as to cause collateral tissue damage. Gell and Coombs described four mechanisms: Types I, II, III and IV. Most hypersensitivity disorders involve a combination of these mechanisms, although one type may predominate. The causes of hypersensitivity are those of any immune response, and include allergens (extraneous antigens), infections and autoimmune disorders.

Type I hypersensitivity (anaphylaxis) is manifest as a local or systemic reaction. The bridging by antigen of the Fab portion of two adjacent IgE molecules leads to a complex series of events resulting in the degranulation of mast cells and basophils. Histamine and serotonin, platelet-activating factor (PAF) and the eosinophilic chemotactic factor of anaphylaxis (ECF-A) are released, and prostaglandins, thromboxane and leukotrienes are formed from arachidonic acid. The effects of mediator release include initial vasoconstriction followed by vasodilatation, increased vascular permeability, the chemotactic attraction of granulocytes, particularly eosinophils, and platelet activation.

Type I hypersensitivity mechanisms account for the anaphylactic reactions to penicillin and insect bites, and for the allergic reactions of hay fever and asthma. In addition to other hypersensitivity mechanisms, Type I mechanisms play a role in more complex disorders such as eczema, vernal keratoconjunctivitis and giant papillary conjunctivitis. The histological features of Type I hypersensitivity are those of acute or subacute non-purulent inflammation. Dilatation and congestion of the microvasculature is associated with exudation, tissue oedema and eosinophil infiltration, and mast cells can be identified in various stages of degranulation. Atopy is a state in which individuals are predisposed to Type I hypersensitivity reactions, there being a genetic basis whereby IgE is synthesized more readily and in greater amounts to irrelevant antigens.

Type II hypersensitivity (cytotoxic) results in tissue damage due to the presence of circulating complement-fixing antibodies directed against specific antigens on the surface of particular cells or within tissue components.

Binding of antibody to antigen leads to destruction of target cells and tissue damage by lysis of the cell membrane through activation of the complement system, phagocytosis of the target cell by macrophages mediated through C3b or the Fc portion of immunoglobulin (opsonization), or direct damage to the target cell through the mechanism of antibody-dependent cell-mediated cytotoxicity (ADCC).

Type II hypersensitivity is the underlying mechanism of haemolytic blood transfusion reactions and is involved in disorders such as ocular cicatricial pemphigoid, pemphigus and possibly Mooren's ulcer. Bullous changes and ulceration of mucous membranes are characteristic. Microscopy reveals non-specific features including infiltration by neutrophils, monocytes and macrophages together with cell necrosis. Immunofluorescence techniques demonstrate the presence of bound antibodies and complement in involved tissues, and are important in establishing diagnoses.

Type II hypersensitivity may be directed against a connective tissue component rather than a particular cell type. In both ocular cicatricial pemphigoid, where epithelial basement membrane is involved, and in Goodpasture's syndrome, in which the RPE and Bruch's membrane are involved, antibody is directed against different basement membrane proteins. In pemphigus, a bullous disorder primarily of the skin but which may also affect the eye, antibody is directed against proteins involved in intercellular adhesion.

In some Type II reactions antibody binding leads to functional changes rather than cell and tissue destruction (this is sometimes classified as Type V hypersensitivity). In myasthenia gravis autoantibody inhibits synaptic transmission by competing against acetylcholine for cholinergic receptors at the neuromuscular end plate. By contrast, in Graves' disease autoantibodies directed against thyroid stimulating hormone (TSH) receptors stimulate thyroid acinar cells by mimicking its effects. In both myasthenia gravis and Graves' disease, activation of complement and other immune mechanisms lead to additional destructive structural changes.

Type III hypersensitivity (immune complex-mediated) results when antibodies bind to circulating antigens to form immune complexes which become deposited in tissues. Physicochemical features such as molecular size, immunoglobulin class and haemodynamic turbulence are factors in determining the location of deposition, which includes vascular walls and renal glomeruli. If the complexes contain immunoglobulin, activation of the complement cascade results in an inflammatory response and local tissue damage.

Type III mechanisms are implicated in the pathogenesis of many diseases including serum sickness and autoimmune disorders such as systemic lupus erythematosus and rheumatoid arthritis where vasculitis is a prominent feature. Most types of glomerulonephritis are mediated by Type III hypersensitivity, which is also the mechanism of the Arthus reaction and the vasculitis of the Stevens–Johnson syndrome. The Arthus reaction is an inflammatory reaction characterized by oedema, haemorrhage and necrosis following the administration of an antigen to an animal that already possesses precipitating antibody to that antigen. In the eye, the retinal vasculitis of Behçet's disease is at least in part mediated by Type III hypersensitivity, which is also involved in peripheral ulcerative keratitis, necrotizing scleritis and Mooren's ulcer. The characteristic ring-shaped lesions of some forms of infective keratitis (especially viral and fungal) are deposits of immune complex. Lens-induced endophthalmitis and some orbital inflammatory disorders are Type III reactions. The histological features of Type III hypersensitivity depend on several factors, particularly persistence of the circulating antigen and the size of the immune complex. If antibody is present in excess, the immune complexes are large and result in granulomatous inflammation. Equal amounts of antigen and antibody produce moderate-sized immune complexes and the inflammatory reaction is chronic but non-granulomatous. Excess antigen results in small immune complexes which produce an acute vasculitis. All three types of inflammatory response occur in lens-induced endophthalmitis.

Type IV hypersensitivity (cell-mediated, delayed type hypersensitivity – DTH) is delayed in that it takes more than 12 hours to develop. It is an antigen elicited, cellular immune reaction resulting in tissue damage. Unlike the other types of hypersensitivity it does not require the participation of antibodies, although there may be superimposed antibody reactions. After appropriate processing, MHC class II restricted antigen is presented to antigen-specific T lymphocytes that become activated and release lymphokines. This triggers a complex cellular response in which other lymphocytes, macrophages, fibroblasts and, to a lesser extent, neutrophils are recruited and activated. Tissue injury is caused by T lymphocytes and/or macrophages and results from cell-mediated cytotoxicity, phagocytosis, NK cell activity, enzyme release and, when antigen persists, aggregates of epithelioid cells (granulomatous inflammation).

Type IV hypersensitivity is the basis of the granulomatous inflammation of tuberculosis, leprosy and fungal infection, sympathetic ophthalmitis and the Vogt–Koyanagi–Harada syndrome. It may also be induced by viral infections, and occurs in corneal graft rejection, phlyctenulosis, optic neuritis, ocular myopathies, Sjögren's syndrome and contact allergy of the skin and conjunctiva. It plays a role in vernal keratoconjunctivitis and contact lens-related giant papillary conjunctivitis. The histological features of Type IV hypersensitivity depend on the inciting injury, but the earliest features are microvascular congestion and the perivascular accumulation of lymphocytes with associated tissue oedema and the deposition of fibrin. If antigen persists, the inflammation becomes granulomatous.

Ophthalmic hypersensitivity – allergic ophthalmic disease

Allergy means altered reaction, and is a term used synonymously with hypersensitivity. Allergic ophthalmic diseases are a group of external ocular conditions resulting from one or more types of hypersensitivity reactions to a known or presumed allergen. Approximately 20 per cent of the general population have some form of allergic disorder, and about a third of these have ophthalmic symptoms. Most individuals are only mildly affected, although some forms of ophthalmic allergy may be severe. Allergic ophthalmic disease most commonly affects the conjunctiva but other mucous membranes may also be affected, as may the cornea alone or in association with lid involvement. Widespread systemic allergic disease may also involve the lids, conjunctiva and cornea.

Allergic disease of the conjunctiva and other mucous membranes

Acute allergic conjunctivitis

Acute allergic conjunctivitis is the commonest allergic condition of the eye. It affects up to 10 per cent of the population, and is often associated with acute allergic rhinitis (acute allergic rhinoconjunctivitis). There is often a personal or family history of atopy including asthma and eczema. Itching is an important symptom, and is accompanied by lacrimation and redness of the lids and conjunctiva. Examination reveals hyperaemia and oedema, and possibly small conjunctival papillae beneath the upper lid. Symptoms may be seasonal (seasonal allergic conjunctivitis, hay fever conjunctivitis), perennial or sporadic. Severe sporadic cases may exhibit manifestations of anaphylaxis (angioneurotic oedema, bronchospasm, hypotension).

Acute allergic conjunctivitis is an IgE-mediated Type I hypersensitivity reaction to a known or presumed allergen in a sensitized individual. Various pollens are usually responsible for attacks with a seasonal peak, while house dust and animal danders are often the offending agents in perennial reactions. The identity of the allergen in sporadic cases is often not known, but possible candidates include drugs, cosmetics, insect bites, airborne allergens and certain foods.

Allergic granulomatous nodule

Allergic granulomatous nodules are nondescript lesions on the bulbar conjunctiva; the buccal mucous membrane can also be involved, and those affected may exhibit an allergic diathesis. Necrotizing granulomatous inflammation incorporates eosinophils, Charcot–Leyden crystals (eosinophilic crystalline material of uncertain nature) and other inflammatory cell debris (Fig. 2.28). The condition is otherwise known as the Splendore–Hoeppli phenomenon and, while the cause is unknown, helminth infection is a possibility. The mechanism is a Type III hypersensitivity.

Allergic disease of the lids, conjunctiva and cornea

Vernal keratoconjunctivitis (spring catarrh)

Vernal keratoconjunctivitis (VKC) is a chronic recurrent bilateral self-limiting inflammation that often shows a seasonal variation, being more common in the spring and summer. As with acute allergic conjunctivitis, there is often a personal or family history of atopy. The disease is widespread, but particularly prevalent in hot dry climates such as the Mediterranean area, the Middle East, West Africa, India and the southern United States. Most of those affected under the age of 10 are males, whereas after the onset of puberty males and females are equally affected. Symptoms include itching, foreign body sensation, photophobia, burning, lacrimation and a mucoid discharge. The conjunctiva and cornea are both involved. There are two forms of conjunctival involvement, the palpebral form and the limbal form, which may coexist.

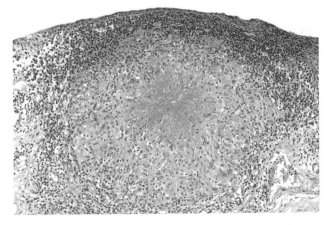

Figure 2.28 Allergic granulomatous nodule of conjunctiva. A central area of necrosis is surrounded by a granulomatous inflammatory reaction.

In the palpebral form, the upper tarsal conjunctiva is initially thickened, and papillae develop later and coalesce to form multiple giant flat-topped (cobblestone) structures (Fig. 2.29a) that may cause mechanical ptosis. Small papillae are sometimes present in the lower tarsal conjunctiva. Elsewhere the conjunctiva has a milky appearance and there are copious amounts of tenacious mucoid discharge. The limbal form is more common in black people, and is characterized by the presence of papillae, frequently superiorly; these papillae have a gelatinous appearance, coalesce to form a ridge and are topped by white dots (Horner–Trantas' dots – Fig. 2.29b).

Either form of conjunctival involvement may be associated with corneal changes involving particularly the upper half. Mild involvement includes punctate epithelial keratopathy characterized by small grey-white intraepithelial opacities (farinaceous epithelial keratopathy of Tobgy). These punctate erosions are usually transient and may enlarge into macroerosions, which can in turn, on rare occasions, develop into a shield ulcer. Shield ulcers are indolent superficial ulcerated areas with thickened edges and a plaque-like deposition (vernal plaque) that prevent re-epithelialization and resolve to form a ring-shaped scar within the superficial stroma. Other findings in the cornea include pannus formation and a peripheral arcus (pseudogerontoxon) resembling arcus senilis.

Histological examination of the conjunctival papillae in VKC reveals proliferation of the surface epithelial cells and an increased number of goblet cells. Downward extension of epithelium results in the formation of tubules and cysts (Fig. 2.29c). The stroma is hyperaemic and exhibits an inflammatory cell infiltrate consisting of mast cells, eosinophils, lymphocytes and plasma cells. Granulation and fibrous tissue subsequently form and the epithelium becomes atrophic and possibly keratinized. Limbal papillae contain less fibrous tissue than palpebral papillae and this accounts for their gelatinous appearance. Vernal plaque consists of stratified deposits of fibrin, cellular debris, IgA, IgG, fibronectin and complement adherent to Bowman's layer.

VKC involves Types I and IV hypersensitivity reactions. The cause is unknown, but pollens and animal danders may be involved. Eosinophils and free eosinophilic granules are characteristic findings in conjunctival scrapings and tears show elevated levels of IgE and/or IgG, histamine, eosinophilic major basic protein (EMBP), Charcot–Leyden crystal protein (found when eosinophils have undergone fragmentation), prostaglandins and leukotrienes. EMBP is cytotoxic and prevents epithelial healing, and this probably accounts for the corneal changes. All these findings are characteristic of

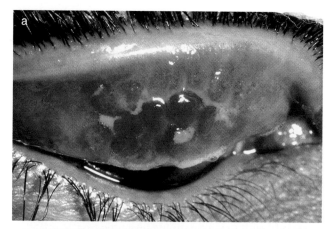

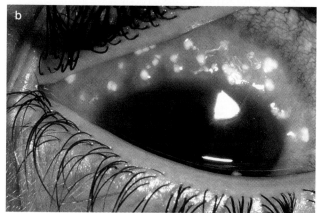

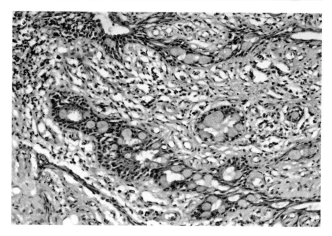

Figure 2.29 Vernal keratoconjunctivitis. (a) Cobblestone papillae of upper tarsal conjunctiva. (b) Horner–Trantas' dots. (c) Downward extension of epithelium with the formation of tubules and cysts.

a Type I mechanism, but a coexisting Type IV mechanism is suggested by the histological features.

Giant papillary conjunctivitis

Giant papillary conjunctivitis (GPC) is a chronic allergic conjunctivitis. It is usually due to contact lens wear (soft > hard), but is also seen in association with protruding corneal sutures, extruded scleral buckles, ocular prostheses, cyanoacrylate glue and other foreign bodies. The clinicopathological features are similar to those of VKC, but the symptoms are milder and precede the signs. If contact lenses are the cause, blurred vision and lens intolerance are characteristic.

Several factors may play a role in the pathogenesis. A possible antigenic stimulus is the proteinaceous, lipid and/or mineral deposit that accumulates on the surface of the foreign material, particularly when meibomian gland dysfunction coexists. Mechanical trauma to the conjunctiva may contribute by releasing neutrophil chemotactic factors and by disrupting the tight junctions between epithelial cells, thereby allowing penetration of antigen. The composition, size and shape of the foreign body may also be important. The hydrogels of soft contact lenses predispose more to GPC than the polymethylmethacrylate (PMMA) of hard lenses. Large, poorly fitting contact lenses, especially if worn for long periods, are associated with a higher incidence of GPC, possibly due to the greater surface area for deposition of antigenic material, increased ocular surface trauma or prolonged exposure to noxious stimuli. The immune mechanism responsible for GPC, like that of VKC, is a cell-mediated Type IV reaction with an IgE-mediated Type I component.

Phlyctenular keratoconjunctivitis (phlyctenulosis)

Phlyctenules (phlyctens) are nodular inflammatory lesions of the conjunctiva, limbus (Fig. 2.30) or cornea. They are commonly bilateral, and primarily affect children and young adults. When the conjunctiva alone is involved symptoms are relatively mild, with itching, lacrimation and irritation. Corneal phlyctenules produce more severe symptoms – foreign body sensation, photophobia, blepharospasm and lacrimation. Conjunctival

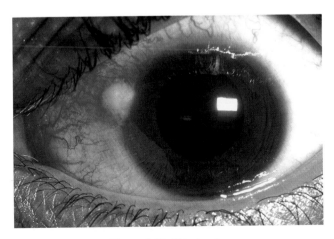

Figure 2.30 Phlyctenule.

and limbal phlyctenules are localized areas of hyperaemia with a white nodular thickening in the centre; this later becomes necrotic and ulcerated. Resolution without sequelae takes place in 2–3 weeks. Corneal lesions initially resemble marginal keratitis but are more severe, spread centrally and are associated with vascularization. Healing leaves characteristic triangular scars with the base at the limbus.

Phlyctenules are seen on microscopy to be accumulations of lymphocytes. The lesions represent a cell-mediated immune response in a previously sensitized host. Phlyctenulosis is commonly associated with staphylococcal antigen, but other causative antigens include those derived from *Candida* spp., *Coccidioides immitis*, nematodes, lymphogranuloma venereum, adenoviruses and herpes simplex virus. In the past the main cause of phlyctenular keratoconjunctivitis was tuberculosis.

Contact dermatoconjunctivitis/keratitis

Contact dermatoconjunctivitis/keratitis is an allergy that develops over a 48-hour period following exposure to a substance to which there has been previous sensitization. Contact sensitizing substances include locally applied drugs, particularly atropine and neomycin, EDTA and the preservatives in ophthalmic preparations (benzalkonium chloride, thiomersal). Other sensitizing substances include parabens (antimicrobial agents used in lotions, creams and cosmetics), lanolin (medication, cosmetics), nickel (jewellery), chromates (jewellery, leather products, fabrics) and p-phenylenediamine (hair sprays, fabrics, shoes).

Contact ophthalmic allergy involves acute and chronic lesions of the lids, conjunctiva and cornea. Itching is a prominent symptom. Acute dermatitis/blepharitis resembles acute eczema with erythema, vesicle formation, oedema, oozing and crusting. The acute response comprises injection and chemosis of the lower conjunctiva with a serous or mucoid discharge. Papillae develop over the entire conjunctiva, and as the condition becomes chronic the lids thicken and exhibit dryness, fissuring and crusting. Associated keratopathy includes superficial punctate epitheliopathy with erosion, subepithelial opacities, marginal infiltration and ulceration and, in severe disease, stromal oedema.

The contact sensitizing substances are generally haptens of low molecular weight that bind to tissue proteins to form antigens. Initial exposure sensitizes the immune system, and a Type IV hypersensitivity reaction ensues 48–72 hours after re-exposure to the antigen. The time taken for sensitization to develop depends on the strength and concentration of the sensitizing agent, the duration of exposure, the presence of any coexisting lid or ocular surface disease and individual susceptibility.

Allergic microbial blepharoconjunctivitis

Chronic low-grade inflammation of the lids and conjunctiva commonly results from hypersensitivity to staphylococcal infection of the anterior lid margin including the lash follicles, and/or the posterior lid margin including the meibomian glands. Symptoms are often disproportionate to the signs and overlap with the features due directly to infection. Anterior blepharitis is characterized by erythema and crusting, and collection of exudates around the base of the lashes. Lid scarring ensues and chronic problems arise due to the misdirection of the lashes. Signs of posterior blepharitis include hyperaemia, telangiectasis at the lid margin, and abnormalities of the meibomian glands and their secretions. Conjunctival signs include thickening, hyperaemia and a mixed papillary and follicular response involving mainly the lower fornix. Corneal abnormalities occur particularly with posterior blepharitis and include superficial punctate keratopathy, marginal keratitis, pannus formation and peripheral corneal degenerations.

The main histological features of allergic microbial blepharoconjunctivitis, apart from the lid abnormalities, are conjunctival papillary hyperplasia and scattered lymphoid follicles in the subepithelial stroma. Staphylococci are the organisms most frequently implicated, but others that may be involved include chlamydiae, fungi and protozoa. Staphylococcal antigens provoke immediate Type I hypersensitivity, but cell-mediated mechanisms are thought to account for the clinically less pronounced reactions to other organisms.

Marginal keratitis
(catarrhal infiltrates/keratitis)

Marginal keratitis is a corneal response to the microbial antigens present in association with a blepharoconjunctivitis. Clinical features include foreign body sensation, ocular discomfort, photophobia and redness. Initial lesions are isolated small round grey-white peripheral corneal infiltrates separated from the limbus by a 1–2-mm clear zone. The infiltrates extend circumferentially and later ulcerate. Adults are affected more often than children. The lesions usually resolve spontaneously within 4 weeks with little if any residual scarring or vascularization. The lesions themselves are sterile, but pathogens may be cultured from the lids or conjunctiva.

The corneal infiltrates are collections of neutrophils in a superficial area of stromal necrosis. Lymphocytes and plasma cells are present in the adjacent tissue. Staphylococcal cell wall antigens are the most likely causative agents. They bind to antibody to form an immune complex, which is deposited in the peripheral cornea and produces a Type III hypersensitivity reaction. Bacteria other than staphylococci implicated in marginal keratitis include *Streptococcus pneumoniae*, *Haemophilus aegyptius*, *Bacillus* spp., *Moraxella lacunata*, *Neisseria gonorrhoeae*, *Escherichia coli* and *Actinomyces* spp.

Allergic disease with cutaneous and/or systemic involvement

Atopic keratoconjunctivitis

Atopic keratoconjunctivitis (AKC) is a chronic manifestation of several ocular surface disorders in the presence of atopic dermatitis, an inflammatory reaction of the skin that usually begins in childhood and is associated with a personal or family history of one or more other atopic diseases. The skin lesions include erythematovesiculobullous elements, lichenification and nodular lesions. Ophthalmic disease occurs in up to 40 per cent of those with atopic dermatitis, who are predominantly male and between the ages of 30 and 50 years. It is bilateral and usually symmetric. Symptoms are perennial, although there may be seasonal exacerbations, and those affected may identify flare-ups with animal danders, house dust and certain foods. Itching, burning, tearing, photophobia, pain, eczematous changes such as thickening, scaling and lichenification of the lids, blepharitis, lash loss and meibomian gland dysfunction all occur. Pallor and thickening of the inferior conjunctiva is typical with acute exacerbations resulting in hyperaemia and chemosis. A mucus discharge is present and papillae are seen in both upper and lower fornices, and on the tarsal conjunctiva. These papillae are not as striking as those of VKC or GPC. Limbal papillae and Horner–Trantas' dots may also be present. Conjunctival scarring with subepithelial fibrosis, symblepharon, shallowing of the fornices and lid changes, particularly punctal ectropion with resultant epiphora, all develop. Corneal changes occur in 75 per cent of cases, and include punctate keratitis (especially involving the inferior third of the cornea), vascularization and shield-like ulceration with subsequent anterior stromal scarring. Associated conditions include keratoconus and cataract, either anterior subcapsular or posterior polar. Those with AKC are predisposed to herpes simplex viral and staphylococcal infections.

Mast cells and eosinophils invade the conjunctival epithelium, and degranulating mast cells, eosinophils and mononuclear cells infiltrate the subepithelial stroma. Epithelial and goblet cell proliferation result in the formation of epithelial-lined cysts and tubules, and there may be perivasculitis and granuloma formation. The pathogenesis is not clear, but those with atopic dermatitis have abnormal reactivity of the skin to various non-specific stimuli including harsh soaps and detergents, wool and nylon, and too frequent bathing. Specific provoking allergens cannot be identified in most instances, but when known include animal danders, house dust and certain foods. In the conjunctiva CD4+ cells far outnumber CD8+ cells, and the epithelium shows increased MHC class II expression as do the fibroblasts and vascular endothelium of the stroma. As in other ophthalmic allergic diseases, these findings are indicative of complicated immune activity in which both Types I and IV mechanisms are involved. Deficient immunoregulation with depressed T cell function may explain the predisposition to herpes simplex viral and staphylococcal infections.

Stevens–Johnson syndrome (erythema multiforme)

The Stevens–Johnson syndrome is characterized by vesiculobullous eruptions affecting the skin and mucous membranes including the conjunctiva. It forms part of a range of blistering disorders that includes erythema multiforme, in which mucous membranes are not involved, and toxic epidermal necrolysis, a rare severe life-threatening syndrome in which lesions develop in both skin and mucous membranes. The Stevens–Johnson syndrome can occur at any age, but children and young adults are those most frequently affected. The condition is self-limiting and any late ophthalmic damage is due to residual scarring rather than the initial disease process. Following a prodromal phase in which symptoms of upper respiratory tract infection are accompanied by fever and malaise, symmetrically distributed cutaneous lesions appear particularly on the extremities. Primary skin lesions are usually round erythematous macules that rapidly become papular. Vesicles and bullae form and give rise to a characteristic target lesion. Any mucous membrane may be involved, although the mouth and eyes are the most frequently and severely affected. Conjunctival involvement ranges from mild catarrhal inflammation to pseudomembrane formation. Ocular surface abnormalities result from the destruction of conjunctival goblet cells and the fibrotic obstruction of lacrimal and accessory lacrimal gland ducts. The cicatricial changes of the conjunctiva remain static once the acute stage has subsided.

The Stevens–Johnson syndrome results from a Type III and possibly a Type IV hypersensitivity reaction to some unknown but probably externally acquired antigen. Triggering factors include drugs, particularly sulphonamides and anticonvulsants, and infections such as those due to herpes simplex virus and *Mycoplasma pneumoniae*. There appears to be an underlying immune-complex mediated vasculitis or perivasculitis. Circulating immune complexes, C3, IgM, fibrin and occasionally IgG are deposited in the vascular walls of the dermis of the skin and the subepithelial stroma of the

conjunctiva. Immunoglobulin and complement are also deposited in the epidermal/basement membrane junction of the skin and the epithelial/basement membrane junction of mucous membranes. The predominance of T cells in the early stages suggests cell-mediated tissue injury. An immunogenetic susceptibility is inferred by the association of HLA-Bw44, the dominant sub-group of HLA-B12.

Kawasaki disease

Kawasaki disease is a multisystem inflammatory disorder affecting mucocutaneous surfaces, the cardiovascular, respiratory and gastrointestinal systems, and joints. It occurs predominantly in Japan. The major ocular feature is non-infective conjunctivitis. The cause is probably an underlying hypersensitivity to bacterial toxins acting as superantigens (proteins that can activate T cells in the absence of pre-existing immunity).

AUTOIMMUNITY

Autoimmunity results from failure of the development or maintenance of tolerance to self antigens. The causes of particular autoimmune disorders are often not clear. The association of some with genetic markers (ankylosing spondylitis with HLA-B27, Behçet's disease with HLA-B5, Graves' disease with HLA-B8 and DRw3 in white people) is indicative of a genetic component, while in others there may be a response to foreign antigens such as micro-organisms or drugs.

Mechanisms that lead to the breakdown of tolerance include molecular mimicry between foreign and self antigens, the activation of autoreactive T cells, the alteration of self antigens by viruses or drugs in such a way that they are not tolerated by the immune system, idiotype dysregulation and polyclonal B cell activation. The association of HLA antigens with certain autoimmune disorders is not adequately explicable. Postulated mechanisms can be categorized into two main groups: either the HLA antigens are directly involved in disease pathogenesis, or the true culprits are genes closely related to the HLA loci. In autoimmune disorders, any of the hypersensitivity mechanisms can cause tissue injury. The processes are usually initiated by CD4+ cells, although some autoantibodies cause cell damage and interfere with the physiology of cell surface receptors.

Autoimmune ophthalmic disorders are either localized and affect primarily the conjunctiva or the uvea, or are systemic conditions with ophthalmic manifestations. The division is not absolute, and ophthalmic disorders resulting from autoimmunity are best considered topographically.

Autoimmunity and the conjunctiva

Autoimmune disorders of the conjunctiva include ocular cicatricial pemphigoid and the now rarely seen practolol-induced ocular toxicity syndrome.

Ocular cicatricial pemphigoid (ocular pemphigoid, benign mucous membrane pemphigoid)

Ocular cicatricial pemphigoid (OCP) is a chronic bullous cicatrizing disorder that primarily affects mucous membranes, particularly the conjunctiva. It is related to and may be a variant of bullous pemphigoid, a skin disorder where cutaneous rather than mucous membrane lesions predominate. It is uncommon, and most of those affected are females over the age of 50 years. OCP is severe, debilitating and blinding. It may begin in one eye, but eventually both are involved. Initial symptoms include irritation, burning and a mucoid discharge. Early signs are a persistent conjunctivitis with subepithelial vesicles that may burst and give rise to ulcers and pseudo-membranes. This is followed by progressive conjunctival subepithelial fibrosis with resulting symblepharon, shallowing of the fornices, and restricted lid and ocular movements. Distortion of the lids, fibrosis of the lacrimal and accessory lacrimal ducts, and reduced conjunctival mucin secretion lead to dry eye syndrome with corneal ulceration and infection.

The histological features of OCP are similar to those of bullous pemphigoid and are characterized by subepithelial bullae. Neutrophils, lymphocytes, plasma cells and occasional eosinophils infiltrate beneath the conjunctival epithelium. Granulation tissue forms at an early stage and later fibrosis with scarring leads to conjunctival shrinkage. Associated changes include keratinization with parakeratosis (extension of nuclei into the keratin layer) of the surface epithelium and a marked reduction in the goblet cell population.

OCP is an autoimmune reaction to epithelial basement membrane. Tissue destruction results from a Type II hypersensitivity response. Direct immunofluorescence shows binding of IgG or IgA to the basement membrane proteoglycans (Fig. 2.31). Associations with HLA-B12, HLA-DR4 and other histocompatibility antigens suggest an immunogenetic susceptibility.

Autoimmunity and the corneoscleral coat

Autoimmune disorders of the corneoscleral coat include sterile peripheral ulcerative keratitis and scleritis, which are frequently associated with systemic disease; Mooren's ulcer, which is thought to be a purely corneal autoimmune response; Thygeson's superficial punctate keratopathy; Cogan's syndrome; and scleritis.

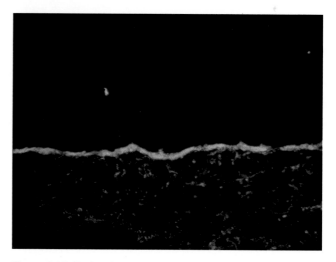

Figure 2.31 Ocular cicatricial pemphigoid. IgG at epithelial basement membrane. Immunofluorescence.

Sterile peripheral ulcerative keratitis (peripheral corneal melt)

Sterile peripheral ulcerative keratitis with or without adjacent scleritis is associated with autoimmune diseases such as rheumatoid arthritis, polyarteritis nodosa, Wegener's granulomatosis and systemic lupus erythematosus. Clinical features depend on the underlying disease. Symptoms can be relatively mild with little pain and minimal, if any, associated inflammation. Signs include peripheral and circumferential corneal furrowing, which may progress to focal loss of stroma, descemetocele formation and possible perforation. On other occasions thickening and opacification of the peripheral cornea (sclerosing keratitis) may precede peripheral and circumferential furrowing. Severe acute necrotizing sclerokeratitis, in which peripheral corneal ulceration accompanies necrotizing scleritis, may occur in exacerbations of any associated systemic disease. Vascularization, scarring and lipid keratopathy (see Fig. 5.41) may ensue. In all types of sterile peripheral ulcerative keratitis, deposition of immune complexes within the limbal vasculature leads to a Type III hypersensitivity response.

Mooren's ulcer

Mooren's ulcer is a progressive painful condition that affects otherwise healthy individuals. Ulceration starts at the corneal periphery and is associated with pain, photophobia and lacrimation. The ulcer spreads circumferentially and centrally, exhibits an undermined leading edge and may also slowly progress towards the sclera. Surrounding tissues are inflamed but perforation is unusual. Other features include anterior uveitis, secondary glaucoma and cataract. There are two clinical types of Mooren's ulcer: a unilateral type that occurs in older individuals and responds well to treatment, and a bilateral type seen in younger individuals, particularly black Africans, which is more aggressive and responds poorly to treatment. Injury, surgery or other ocular surface disorders may precede the onset of ulceration.

Neutrophils, lymphocytes and plasma cells infiltrate the corneal stroma and there is neovascularization with disruption of the mid-stromal collagen at the base of the ulcer. The cause of Mooren's ulcer is unknown, although evidence of an autoimmune aetiology with hypersensitivity against a corneal antigen is postulated. Adjacent basement membrane contains bound immunoglobulin and complement, and antibodies to conjunctival and corneal epithelium circulate together with immune complexes. The mechanisms of tissue destruction may involve a combination of Types II, III and IV reactions.

Thygeson's superficial punctate keratopathy

Thygeson's superficial punctate keratopathy is a rare insidious chronic epithelial keratitis exhibiting spontaneous exacerbations and remissions. All age groups and both sexes are affected. The condition is probably autoimmune, and there is no known association with any systemic disease. Symptoms include photophobia, foreign body sensation, burning and lacrimation. Clinical examination reveals groups of punctate intraepithelial corneal deposits. Corneal scrapings reveal atypical and vacuolated degenerate epithelial cells, occasional neutrophils, mononuclear cells and mucus.

Cogan's syndrome

Cogan's syndrome is an autoimmune inflammatory disorder in which an interstitial keratitis is accompanied by a Ménière-like vestibuloauditory dysfunction and possibly vascular inflammatory disease usually affecting large and medium-sized vessels. The average age of onset is 30 years. The commonest presenting symptoms are ocular discomfort and photophobia, with signs including conjunctival injection and a patchy granular infiltrate predominantly in the posterior cornea. Microscopy of the cornea reveals a thickened epithelium and lymphocytic infiltration, hyalinization and vascularization of the stroma.

Scleritis

Scleritis is a severe painful inflammation of the sclera. Like sterile peripheral ulcerative keratitis it is associated with systemic immune disorders, and in about 40 per cent of cases rheumatoid arthritis, polyarteritis nodosa, Wegener's granulomatosis, systemic lupus erythematosus or relapsing polychondritis coexist. Scleritis is an immune-mediated vasculitis with thrombotic occlusion

of the lumen and fibrinoid necrosis of the vessel wall. Types III and IV mechanisms are thought to be involved. Necrotizing granulomatous inflammation causes nodular thickening of the sclera (Fig. 2.32).

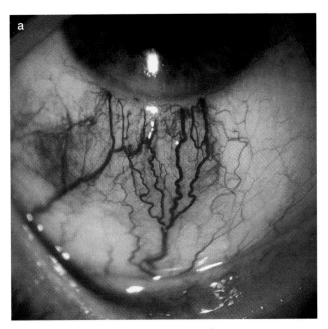

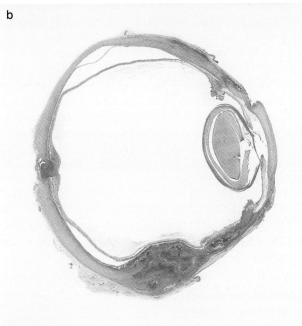

Figure 2.32 Scleritis. (a) Anterior vasocongestion and nodular thickening. (b) Equatorial nodular thickening due to granulomatous inflammation.

Autoimmunity and the uvea

Autoimmune disorders of the uvea are manifest as uveitis, which is classified as anterior or posterior according to the predominant site of involvement. Anterior uveitis is common, typically acute and self-limiting, and associated with MHC class I antigens, particularly HLA-B27. Most cases of acute anterior uveitis are isolated and of unknown cause, although some are associated with known or suspected autoimmune systemic diseases.

Posterior uveitis, unlike anterior uveitis, is relatively rare. It is often chronic and tends to be associated with MHC class II antigens. Posterior uveitis affects primarily the choroid, but may extend anteriorly to involve the ciliary body and iris with the development of a pan-uveitis. Examples of posterior/panuveitis include sympathetic ophthalmitis, the Vogt–Koyanagi–Harada syndrome and a wide variety of other acquired disorders of the posterior uvea, RPE and/or retina such as the white dot syndromes. Sympathetic ophthalmitis and the Vogt–Koyanagi–Harada syndrome share many clinical, histological and immunological features. They are both bilateral granulomatous inflammatory reactions resulting from autoimmunity to uveal/retinal antigens and have similar association with HLA haplotypes.

Acute anterior uveitis

Acute anterior uveitis (AAU) is relatively common. No underlying systemic disorder is present in most instances, but some cases are associated with systemic disorders such as the seronegative spondyloarthropathies. In the United Kingdom over 50 per cent of cases of AAU express HLA-B27 which is present in 8 per cent of the unaffected population. This association is even stronger in those in whom the AAU is recurrent, unilateral and of sudden onset. AAU is less common in countries such as Japan, and on the African continent where HLA-B27 is rare. The clinical features are those of acute unilateral anterior segment inflammation. There are well-recognized clinical types:

Isolated AAU

AAU in the absence of systemic disease accounts for at least 90 per cent of cases.

AAU and the seronegative spondyloarthropathies

About 10 per cent of cases of AAU are associated with the seronegative spondyloarthropathies, which include ankylosing spondylitis, reactive arthropathies, arthritis with inflammatory bowel disease, and psoriatic arthritis. Shared characteristics are the absence of rheumatoid factor (hence seronegative) and a strong association with certain HLA antigens, in particular HLA-B27. Common clinical features include predilection for axial skeletal involvement, asymmetric migratory oligoarthritis and enthesitis (inflammation of tendon insertions).

Ankylosing spondylitis (AS) affects the axial skeleton, where it causes ankylosis (bony fusion) of the apophyseal and sacroiliac joints. Young adult males are most frequently affected and symptoms include morning stiffness and low back pain. More advanced disease shows radiological evidence of sacroiliitis and spinal fusion. Ninety-five per cent of those with AS are HLA-B27 positive and approximately 25 per cent have an attack of AAU at some time during the course of their disease. The cause of AS is unknown, but *Klebsiella* spp. organisms may play a role.

Reactive arthritis is similar to AS, but more likely to involve the limbs than the spine. Joint involvement and AAU may follow certain infections, and pathogens include *Klebsiella* spp., *Salmonella* spp., *Shigella* spp., *Yersinia* spp., *Brucella* spp. and *Campylobacter* spp. in the gastrointestinal tract, and chlamydiae in the urethra. Reiter's syndrome is a triad of urethritis, arthritis and ophthalmic inflammation (conjunctivitis and/or AAU). It tends to be episodic and relapsing with fever and weight loss, and mucocutaneous lesions include conjunctivitis, painless oral ulcers, keratoderma blennorrhagica, dystrophic nail lesions, urethritis and circinate balanitis in men and cervicitis in women. The arthritis of Reiter's syndrome is a migratory asymmetric oligoarthritis affecting primarily the large joints (knees or ankles) at the lower extremities; other articular features include heel pain due to enthesitis, interphalangeal arthritis of the toes and/or fingers and sacroiliitis. The precise aetiology of Reiter's syndrome is unknown but infective agents such as chlamydiae play a role and, as with AS, there is a strong association with HLA-B27.

Arthritis and inflammatory bowel disease is a lower extremity large joint oligoarthritis or an HLA-B27 associated spondylitis that occurs in cases of Crohn's disease or ulcerative colitis. Ocular inflammation includes AAU and scleritis.

Psoriatic arthritis is manifest as either a monoarthritis or an asymmetric oligoarthritis of the interphalangeal joints of the hands and feet. It develops in 10–20 per cent of those with psoriasis. Ophthalmic features are less common than in the other seronegative spondyloarthropathies, but include conjunctivitis, HLA-B27 associated AAU and scleritis.

AAU associations

Many cases of AAU have a strong association with MHC class I antigens, and some are associated with systemic infections. Both groups illustrate possible pathogenetic mechanisms. The association of AAU and the seronegative spondyloarthropathies with HLA-B27 indicates a genetic predisposition and possibly helps to clarify immune mechanisms. The strongest association of AAU is with ankylosing spondylitis, in which over 90 per cent of affected Caucasians are HLA-B27 positive. At the molecular level, antigenic homology with a high degree of cross-reactivity exists between a peptide residue (B27PD) of MHC class I antigens and a uveitogenic peptide (PDS-Ag) derived from retinal S antigen (S-Ag). Tolerance to B27PD and other homologous peptides occurs after processing and presentation of MHC class II HLA antigens to HLA-peptide-specific T cells, which are either eliminated or down-regulated in the thymus. Failure of tolerance may result from infection, trauma or stress factors that stimulate normally suppressed T cell clones to recognize MHC molecules and cross-react with S-Ag peptide or other uveitogenic peptides presented by ocular APCs. Reactive arthritis and the accompanying AAU is known to be associated with gastrointestinal infections due to *Salmonella* spp., *Shigella* spp. and *Yersinia* spp.; Reiter's syndrome is associated with chlamydial urethritis. Reactive arthritis is sterile and usually occurs after the infection has resolved; hence it is presumed to be an immune phenomenon precipitated by infection in those with a genetic predisposition as indicated by the presence of HLA-B27. Occult or symptomatic gastrointestinal infection with Gram-negative bacteria, particularly *Klebsiella* spp. and *Salmonella* spp., is also associated with AAU, with or without AS. Some *Klebsiella* spp., protein residues share antigenic similarities with HLA-B27 and there is thus the potential for interaction between microbial antigens and MHC class I antigens, possibly resulting in the production of cross-reactive autoantibodies (molecular mimicry).

Chronic anterior uveitis

Chronic anterior uveitis may occur in association with systemic disorders such as juvenile chronic arthritis or sarcoidosis, or may be isolated as in Fuchs' uveitis syndrome.

Juvenile chronic arthritis

Juvenile chronic arthritis (JCA) is an inflammatory joint disease of at least 3 months' duration developing in children before the age of 16 years. The condition is pathogenetically and clinically distinct from rheumatoid arthritis. The three main clinical types are pauciarticular, polyarticular and systemic.

Pauciarticular (oligoarticular): four or fewer joints are involved, most commonly the knees. This type accounts for over half of the cases of JCA, and those most often affected are young girls.

Polyarticular: five or more joints are involved. This type accounts for 30–40 per cent of cases and, as with the pauciarticular type, is more common in young girls.

Systemic (Still's disease): this is the rarest type of JCA and can present at any age. Acute systemic symptoms and signs include fever, a transient maculopapular rash, generalized lymphadenopathy and hepatosplenomegaly, and occur before joint involvement. The number of arthritic joints varies and, while systemic features predominate in the early stages, a chronic polyarthritis predominates later.

Ocular manifestations of JCA-associated inflammation

The principal ocular manifestation of JCA-associated inflammation is bilateral chronic anterior uveitis which is usually asymptomatic, insidious in onset and only detectable on slit lamp examination. Risk factors include early age of onset (< 7 years), pauciarticular disease and positivity for antinuclear antibodies (ANA). Visual symptoms result from complications such as cataract, glaucoma and/or band keratopathy. In the systemic variant of JCA, chronic anterior uveitis is rare.

Cause of JCA

The cause of JCA is unknown. Autoimmunity is presumed, but the mechanism is unclear. Apart from JCA of polyarticular onset that develops late and probably represents a juvenile form of rheumatoid arthritis, all cases are seronegative for rheumatoid factor. ANAs are present in half of those with JCA of pauciarticular onset, and this correlates with the associated anterior uveitis. Those with JCA of pauciarticular onset and uveitis are usually also HLA-DR5 and DPw2 positive.

Classification of childhood arthritis

The International League of Associations for Rheumatology (ILAR) reviewed the classification of childhood arthritis in 1997. It was decided that the terms 'juvenile chronic arthritis' and 'juvenile rheumatoid arthritis' should be discarded, and that 'juvenile idiopathic arthritis' be adopted as an umbrella term to indicate disease of childhood onset characterized primarily by arthritis persisting for at least 6 weeks and of no known cause. The main subdivisions of juvenile idiopathic arthritis are systemic arthritis, oligoarthritis, polyarthritis (rheumatoid factor negative), polyarthritis (rheumatoid factor positive), psoriatic arthritis and enthesitis-related arthritis. This revised classification of arthritis is likely to have implications in the future classification of uveitis.

Fuchs' uveitis syndrome (Fuchs' heterochromic iridocyclitis)

Fuchs' uveitis syndrome accounts for approximately 2 per cent of uveitis cases. It occurs predominantly in the 20–35 age group, and males and females are equally affected. It is insidious in onset, usually unilateral, and visual symptoms are mild. Small stellate KPs are characteristic, but few cells are otherwise seen in the anterior chamber. Iris nodules are present and there is diffuse iris stromal atrophy. Iridolenticular adhesions are not seen, but cells are present in the vitreous. Gonioscopy reveals fine blood vessels in the filtration angle that are permeable to fluorescein and bleed readily if the intraocular pressure is lowered by paracentesis (Amsler's sign).

Light microscopy of the iris in Fuchs' uveitis syndrome reveals stromal atrophy with loss of pigment. Additional features include hyalinization of blood vessel walls, vascular endothelial cell proliferation, fibrosis and atrophy of the sphincter muscle, and patchy loss and vacuolation of the pigment epithelium. Eosinophils, mast cells, lymphocytes, plasma cells and Russell bodies are also present. Electron microscopy of the iris reveals small immature melanosomes in the melanocytes and degenerative changes in the nerve fibres. The cause of Fuchs' uveitis syndrome is unknown, but immunological and histological studies are consistent with an inflammatory process involving immune complexes in the aqueous. Complications of the disorder include cataract and glaucoma.

Posterior/panuveitis

Inflammation throughout the uvea may occur in systemic vasculitis (e.g. Behçet's disease). Other causes with known or presumed autoimmune aetiology include sympathetic ophthalmitis, the Vogt–Koyanagi–Harada syndrome and the white dot syndromes.

Sympathetic ophthalmitis

Sympathetic ophthalmitis is a rare, potentially blinding, bilateral intraocular inflammatory condition that can follow injury to one eye. Most cases are subsequent to perforating injuries in which the ciliary body is involved, but it can follow a wide variety of trauma, including elective surgical evisceration of the eye, subconjunctival rupture, contusion without perforation, and laser and cryosurgical procedures. Incarceration of uveal tissue or lens capsule in the wound is a predisposing factor, but its low incidence after filtering surgical procedures is probably explained by the known inhibitory property of aqueous on the function of immune cells. Although it can follow a perforating corneal ulcer, the association of

sympathetic ophthalmitis with intraocular infection is excessively rare.

After a latent period, usually of 2–12 weeks following the initial insult, the injured (exciting) eye becomes inflamed and exhibits the typical features of uveitis. Synchronously or very soon after, but occasionally years later, inflammation develops in the other (sympathizing) eye. The initial symptom is photophobia, and the signs are identical to those in the exciting eye. If untreated, severe bilateral panuveitis ensues and there may be exudative retinal detachment. Both eyes may become blind and painful. In some cases, small yellowish-white lesions (Dalén–Fuchs' nodules) are present in the mid-peripheral fundus at the level of the RPE. Systemic features occasionally noted include vitiligo, alopecia, poliosis, meningism, tinnitus, vertigo and deafness, all of which are conspicuous in the Vogt–Koyanagi–Harada syndrome.

Apart from any evidence of predisposing damage in the exciting eye, the histological picture of sympathetic ophthalmitis is identical in both eyes. The characteristic feature is a non-necrotizing granulomatous panuveitis (only rarely is the inflammation confined to the anterior or posterior uvea) with diffuse and massive lymphocytic infiltration, and scattered aggregates of epithelioid cells (Fig. 2.33a), many of which contain fine granules of phagocytosed melanin (Fig. 2.33b). Eosinophils are often present, and giant cells are occasionally seen. The lymphocytes are predominantly CD4+ cells in the early stages, but CD8+ cells dominate in the later stages. Dalén–Fuchs nodules (Fig. 2.33c) are granulomas located between Bruch's membrane and the RPE; they are not pathognomonic of sympathetic ophthalmitis and may occur in other forms of granulomatous uveitis. In advanced disease the nodules are associated with breaks in Bruch's membrane and degeneration of the RPE. Apart from Dalén–Fuchs' nodules, the retina is typically free from inflammation possibly due to the RPE secreting immunosuppressive factors such as TGF-β. Other features include destruction of the iris and ciliary epithelium, granulomatous foci within scleral neurovascular channels, and serous retinal detachment. In untreated cases the inflammation subsides to leave widespread scarring and marked loss of melanocytes. Phthisis bulbi may be the end result.

Sympathetic ophthalmitis is a T cell-mediated (Type IV) autoimmune response to one or more of several possible antigens including retinal S-antigen (located in the photoreceptor outer segment cell membrane), interphotoreceptor retinoid binding protein (IRBP), rhodopsin or recoverin (a retinal calcium-binding protein important in phototransduction). The rarity of the condition implies that factors other than exposure of antigen to the immune system are of aetiological importance. A genetic

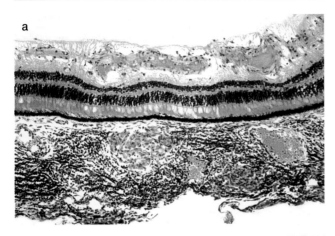

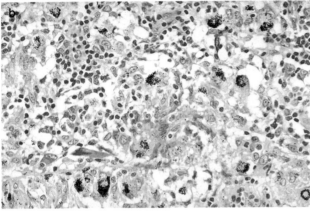

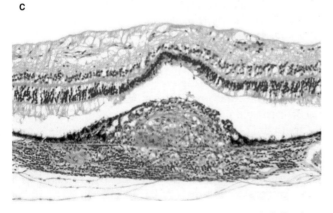

Figure 2.33 Sympathetic ophthalmitis. (a) Lymphocytic infiltration and granuloma formation in choroid. (b) Granulomatous inflammation with pigment phagocytosis. (c) A Dalén–Fuchs nodule.

predisposition is implied by the association with HLA-A11 and -DR4, and by certain racial variations. The association with non-surgical trauma suggests that other immune stimuli could act as adjuvants.

Vogt–Koyanagi–Harada syndrome

The Vogt–Koyanagi–Harada (VKH) syndrome comprises chronic uveitis and meningoencephalitis, and also involves the inner ear and skin. The auditory involvement is manifest as tinnitus, vertigo and deafness, and the cutaneous involvement as vitiligo, alopecia and poliosis. VKH occurs more frequently among Asians, Hispanics and native Americans, and affects predominantly the 20–40 age group. In the prodromal stage headaches, deep orbital pain, nausea, slight fever, occasional photophobia and lacrimation are characteristic, and in the uveitic (ophthalmic) stage bilateral granulomatous panuveitis may be associated with exudative retinal detachment. The uveitis is identical histologically to sympathetic ophthalmitis apart from a conspicuous plasma cell infiltrate. Weeks to months after the onset of symptoms the uveitis and neurological features resolve, although dysacusia, especially to high-frequency sounds, may persist. The fundus becomes depigmented but with mottling. Any exudative retinal detachment resolves spontaneously, but cataract and glaucoma are well-established complications. Recurrence at any time results in progression of pre-existing ocular damage.

The features of the prodromal stage suggest a viral infection, although no causative agent has yet been identified. The underlying mechanism of tissue damage is probably a Type IV autoimmune response to uveal antigens, possibly associated with melanocytes. As in sympathetic ophthalmitis, the strong association with HLA antigens, more evident in certain racial groups such as HLA-DR4 and DRw53 in the Japanese, is indicative of an immunogenetic predisposition.

White dot syndromes

A variety of presumed inflammatory conditions affect the choroid, RPE and/or the neurosensory retina, where they produce discrete white lesions. Such disorders, grouped together as white dot syndromes, include acute posterior multifocal placoid pigment epitheliopathy (APMPPE), acute retinal pigment epitheliitis, multiple evanescent white dot syndrome (MEWDS), punctate inner choroidopathy (PIC) and birdshot retinochoroidopathy. Similar lesions may be seen in conditions with an established inflammatory aetiology such as sympathetic ophthalmitis and the VKH syndrome due to autoimmunity, and cytomegalovirus and herpes simplex virus retinitis due to infection. Birdshot retinochoroidopathy is noteworthy in the context of autoimmunity, as it appears to be exclusively linked to HLA-A29.2 and shares some clinicopathological similarities with sympathetic ophthalmitis and the VKH syndrome. The pathogenesis of birdshot retinochoroidopathy is unknown, but it is thought to be an autoimmune response possibly to a retinal antigen.

Autoimmunity and the lens

Lens-induced endophthalmitis (phacoantigenic endophthalmitis)

Lens substance remaining in the eye following rupture of the capsule due to trauma or incomplete cataract extraction, or lens substance escaping through the degenerate capsule of a hypermature cataract, can, in certain individuals, provoke an inflammatory reaction of varying intensity. Symptoms usually commence within 2 weeks of the precipitating event, and range from a smouldering low-grade anterior segment reaction to intense ocular inflammation with pain, loss of vision, ciliary hyperaemia and hypopyon. Severe cases may lead to secondary glaucoma and ultimately phthisis bulbi. The condition may on rare occasions develop later in the fellow eye, thus clinically simulating sympathetic ophthalmitis.

The inflammatory reaction is centred on the iris–lens diaphragm. Neutrophils may invade the lens substance, and granulomatous inflammation exhibiting an infiltrate of neutrophils, eosinophils, lymphocytes, plasma cells, epithelioid cells and/or giant cells is seen in relation to extracapsular lens material (Fig. 2.34). This is surrounded by an area of granulation and/or fibrous tissue. Posterior segment findings include nodular or diffuse aggregates of inflammatory cells on the inner retinal surface and lymphocytic cuffing of the retinal vessels.

Lens-induced endophthalmitis results from a loss of immune tolerance to lens antigens. The factors that lead to a breakdown in the cellular mechanisms of immune tolerance are not clear, but there may be a genetic component or a relation to concurrent non-specific inflammation such as that produced by trauma or infection. The inflammation results from a Type III hypersensitivity in which immune complexes are produced by the reaction of immunoglobulin, particularly IgG, with lens protein. Any variation may relate to the production of different types of immune complexes.

Autoimmunity and the orbit

Autoimmune disorders affecting the different tissues and structures contained within the orbit include Wegener's granulomatosis (a vasculitis), myasthenia gravis (a disorder of the post-synaptic motor end plate), Sjögren's syndrome and dysthyroid orbitopathy.

Sjögren's syndrome

Primary Sjögren's syndrome (sicca syndrome) is an autoimmune disorder causing chronic inflammation of the lacrimal and salivary glands. It results in tear deficiency and dry eye (keratoconjunctivitis sicca), and saliva deficiency and dry mouth (xerostomia). Association with a

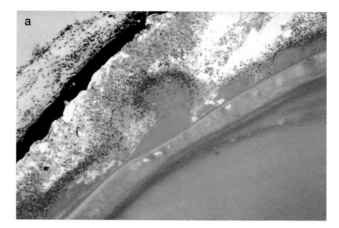

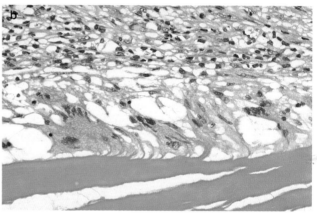

Figure 2.34 Lens-induced endophthalmitis. (a) Escaping lens material producing an inflammatory reaction. (b) Giant cells in relation to extracapsular lens material.

systemic immune disorder, particularly rheumatoid arthritis, designates Sjögren's syndrome as secondary. Sjögren's syndrome predominantly affects postmenopausal women, and has ophthalmic and oral manifestations.

Ophthalmic manifestations include foreign body sensation, burning, redness, itching and photophobia. The inferior tear meniscus is absent, and long strands of tenacious mucus are found in the conjunctival fornices. The tear film break-up time (TFBUT) is reduced and the precorneal tear film appears viscous with mucus strands and particulate debris. Punctate epithelial keratopathy is common, as are corneal filaments. Rose Bengal staining of the interpalpebral conjunctiva is characteristic, and decreased tear production is identified by the Schirmer test. In severe cases there may be corneal stromal infiltrates, peripheral thinning and ulceration with perforation. The principal oral features are dryness, dysphagia, dental caries and a susceptibility to infections.

Apart from the increased risk of conditions due directly to the ophthalmic and oral manifestations, Sjögren's syndrome has well defined associations with systemic autoimmune disorders such as rheumatoid arthritis, systemic lupus erythematosus, polyarteritis nodosa, scleroderma and polymyositis. Individuals with Sjögren's syndrome also have an increased risk of B cell lymphoma.

In Sjögren's syndrome histological changes are found in the lacrimal and salivary glands, and the conjunctiva. The normal tubuloacinar architecture of the lacrimal and salivary glands is disrupted by a dense lymphocytic infiltrate surrounding dilated epithelial ducts, which may be filled with inspissated secretion. In the lacrimal glands B cells form aggregates surrounded by CD4+ cells. A mixed response is also found in the salivary glands, although CD4+ cells predominate. Eventually the tubules, acini and interstitial tissue become atrophic. Accessory salivary glands are relatively easy to biopsy and may help in definitive diagnosis. Conjunctival impression cytology reveals loss of goblet cells, a reduced nuclear–cytoplasmic ratio in the epithelial cells, squamous metaplasia with mild keratinization and adherent mucus aggregates. Unlike the changes seen in OCP and the Stevens–Johnson syndrome, the tarsal conjunctiva is relatively spared. Lymphocytes (mostly T cells) infiltrate the conjunctival subepithelial stroma.

The events that precipitate the autoimmune response to lacrimal and salivary glands are unknown, but infection with Epstein–Barr virus and cytomegalovirus may be involved in genetically susceptible individuals, particularly those with HLA-B8, -DR3, and -DRw52 haplotypes (primary Sjögren's) and -DR4 (secondary Sjögren's). The tissue reaction is predominantly a Type IV hypersensitivity. Sjögren's syndrome is associated with the synthesis of multiple autoantibodies, including antinuclear antibodies (ANAs), rheumatoid factor (even in the absence of rheumatoid arthritis) and antibodies to the two Sjögren-specific antigens, Ro (SS-A) and La (SS-B).

Dysthyroid orbitopathy (Graves' orbitopathy, thyroid eye disease, endocrine exophthalmos)

Dysthyroid orbitopathy is an autoimmune disorder associated in the majority (75 per cent) of cases with thyroid disease, although some affected individuals may be euthyroid. It is most frequently associated with Graves' disease, but it may also occur in Hashimoto's thyroiditis, thyroid carcinoma, primary hyperthyroidism and following neck irradiation. It is more common in women, but tends to be more severe in men. There is a genetic predisposition, with up to 50 per cent concordance in identical twins and an increased prevalence of HLA-B8 and HLA-DR3 in those with Graves' disease and of HLA-DR5 in those with Hashimoto's thyroiditis.

In Graves' disease ophthalmic signs usually develop within 18 months of the onset of thyroid dysfunction, although they may occur simultaneously or precede it by many months. Dysthyroid orbitopathy is unpredictable but, following a varied course, it stabilizes and becomes inactive from 6 months to several years following onset. The clinical manifestations result from inflammation, oedema and secondary fibrosis of the orbital soft tissues. Swelling of the extraocular muscles leads to axial proptosis, which is typically symmetric and bilateral but may be asymmetric and unilateral. Ocular motility abnormalities cause diplopia, particularly on upward gaze. Other features include oedema and retraction of the lids, injection and oedema of the conjunctiva, and exposure keratitis. Enlarged extraocular muscles at the orbital apex may cause compressive optic neuropathy resulting in irreversible visual loss. There may be associated systemic features of thyroid dysfunction and an increased susceptibility to other autoimmune disorders.

The underlying pathology of dysthyroid orbitopathy is inflammation of the orbital soft tissues (Fig. 2.35) including the extraocular musculature. The inflammatory process is most pronounced in the endomysial connective tissue where fibroblasts are stimulated to produce collagen and glycosaminoglycans. The inflammatory cells are mostly lymphocytes and plasma cells, but there are occasional mast cells. The proptosis results from an increase in the volume of the orbital tissues consequent upon the oedema due to the inflammatory process and to the osmotic effect of the hydrophilic glycosaminoglycans. Enlargement of the superior rectus muscle may cause compression of the superior ophthalmic vein thereby reducing venous drainage and this, together with the absence of lymphatic drainage of the orbit, may contribute to the proptosis. As the condition advances, the secreted collagen organizes and contracts, and results in fibrosis and tethering.

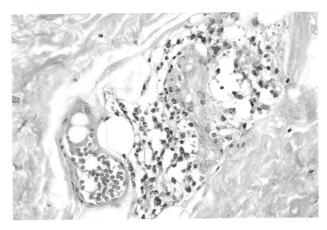

Figure 2.35 Dysthyroid orbitopathy. Inflammatory cells in vascularized fibrofatty orbital tissue.

In dysthyroid orbitopathy the target cells are the extraocular muscle cells and/or orbital fibroblasts. Cell-mediated immunity is an early event and a candidate antigen is a 64-kD protein found in the extraocular muscle cells and thyroid cell membranes. The events precipitating autoimmunity are unknown, but the association with certain HLA types indicates a genetic predisposition. Antigen-related activation of T and B cells leads to cytokine-mediated fibroblast proliferation with synthesis of collagen and glycosaminoglycans. In Graves' disease, antibodies may be directed against thyroid-stimulating hormone (TSH) receptors in the thyroid follicular cell. These antibodies include thyrotropin receptor antibodies (TRAbs), some of which are stimulatory (thyroid stimulating immunoglobulin or antibody – TSI or TSAb) and others inhibitory (thyroid binding inhibiting immunoglobulin or antibody – TBII or TBIA). Other antibodies are directed against thyroglobulin and thyroid mucosal cell surface antigen (thyroid pyroxidase).

Sclerosing orbital inflammation

Sclerosing orbital inflammation is a term much preferred to 'pseudotumour' for idiopathic non-specific inflammatory orbital disorders clinically simulating neoplasms. Those affected are usually between 20 and 50 years of age. Chronic progressive pain, proptosis, inflammation, restriction of ocular movement and visual loss are the presenting features. Most cases are unilateral, and the lacrimal gland region or the orbital apex (Tolosa–Hunt syndrome) are the sites most frequently affected. Microscopy of a biopsy shows significant fibrosis, a paucicellular infiltrate of lymphocytes, possibly with follicle formation, and plasma cells (Fig. 2.36).

IMMUNOLOGY OF TISSUE TRANSPLANTATION

Transplantation is the grafting into the body of a tissue or organ taken from another part of the body or from a different individual (donor). The aim is for the graft to become anatomically and physiologically integrated into the recipient. There are four types of graft:

Autograft: the graft is taken from and transplanted into the same individual; thus the donor is also the host. Examples of autografts include many types of skin graft, autokeratoplasty and autologous donor blood transfusion.

Isograft: the donor and recipient are separate individuals but genetically identical (i.e. identical twins).

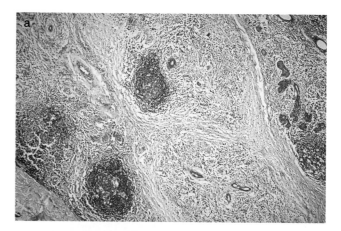

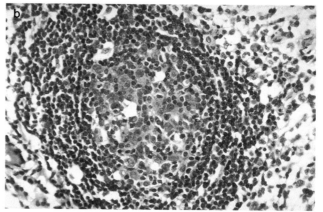

Figure 2.36 Sclerosing orbital inflammation. (a) Fibrosis and inflammatory cells with reactive follicles of lymphocytes. (b) Reactive lymphocytic germinal follicle with immature cells centrally and mature cells peripherally.

Allograft: the donor and recipient are of the same species but genetically different. Examples of allografts include blood transfusions, corneal grafts, amniotic membrane grafts, and kidney, heart and other organ transplantations.

Xenograft: the donor and recipient are of different species. Examples of xenografts include replacement of human heart valves with pig tissue.

Autografts and isografts cause no immune response from the recipient as they are antigenically identical to recipient tissue. Allografts and xenografts are antigenically different from recipient tissue and may elicit an immune response leading to the functional and structural destruction of donor tissue (rejection). Major histocompatibility antigens (HLAs), and to a lesser extent other cell surface glycoproteins such as ABO blood groups, are the principal mediators of tissue compatibility between donor and recipient. The closer the match between HLA antigens of donor and recipient, the greater the chance of survival of the grafted tissue.

Keratoplasty with corneal allografts is one of the most successful transplantation procedures, and more than 90 per cent of primary uncomplicated grafts survive 2 or more years without the need for systemic immunosuppressive therapy.

Tolerance of corneal allografts

The high rate of survival results from the unique relationship (immune privilege) of the eye to the systemic immune system. Important factors in corneal immune privilege and the survival of corneal allografts include:

1. The lack of blood vessels, lymphatics and inflammatory cells in the normal cornea.
2. The immunological difference between the central and peripheral cornea. Corneal stromal tissue acts as a barrier to the diffusion of soluble substances and the migration of cells originating from adjacent conjunctival lymphatics and blood vessels. Small and medium-sized molecules, such as IgG and IgA, and complement components C3, C4 and C5 can diffuse throughout the corneal stroma, but larger molecules, such as C1 and IgM, and Langerhans cells are less able to do so and are present in greatest concentrations at the periphery.
3. The presence of lymphocytotoxic antibodies to donor antigens.
4. Anterior chamber-associated immune deviation (ACAID).

Rejection of corneal allografts

Corneal graft rejection is due to tissue incompatibility which leads to a T cell mediated (Type IV) reaction. CD4 + (T_H) cells are activated by the immune stimulus of foreign MHC class II molecules or foreign MHC class I in conjunction with self MHC class II molecules after processing by host Langerhans cells. These activated cells release lymphokines (e.g. IL-2) that stimulate the proliferation and activation of more CD4 + (T_H) cells, CD8 + ($T_{C/S}$) cells, and B lymphocytes. Lysis of donor cells results from the activity of host NK cells and cytotoxic CD8 + cells that recognize foreign class I cell surface antigens. B cells synthesize antibodies that result in opsonization, complement binding and the facilitation of antibody-dependent cell-mediated cytotoxicity (NK cell activity). The immune response is modulated by suppressor T cells and further enhanced by the release of IFN-γ, which increases class II antigen expression on donor cells.

Class I and class II HLA and blood group antigens are found throughout the cornea but, because of corneal immune privilege, mismatch between host and donor antigens is less likely to result in rejection. Following corneal allografts, the development of antibodies to donor antigens may account for the increased risk of rejection in repeat grafts; HLA and ABO blood group matching is likely to reduce this risk. If the cornea is vascularized or oedematous, or if there is ongoing ocular inflammation, immune privilege may break down and immune/inflammatory cells and C1 and IgM pass into the central cornea. The risk of rejection is also greater with repeat or large eccentrically placed grafts.

Clinico-pathological features of corneal graft rejection

Immune graft rejection occurs after 2 weeks following transplantation. It is most common during the first 3–6 months, but may not develop until many years later. Without immunosuppressive therapy (corticosteroid eye drops), 80 per cent of grafts would be rejected. In corneal graft rejection all layers can be involved individually, simultaneously or sequentially.

Epithelial rejection is usually asymptomatic and begins as an elevated epithelial line that progresses across the graft. It occurs about 3 months after surgery, starts at the graft–host junction and affects up to 10 per cent of grafts. The line consists of neutrophils, lymphocytes and damaged epithelial cells. The host epithelium repairs any defects behind the advancing line, and the stroma is unaffected unless an epithelial defect persists. Subepithelial infiltrates in the donor tissue located below Bowman's layer resemble the keratopathy of epidemic keratoconjunctivitis and are thought to be a mild form of rejection. They are usually asymptomatic, occur about 10 months after surgery and affect up to 15 per cent of grafts.

Stromal rejection usually occurs in association with endothelial rejection and presents with loss of vision due to stromal oedema. The normal lamellar structure of the stroma is lost, the epithelial basement membrane is destroyed, monocytes, lymphocytes and plasma cells infiltrate the affected tissue, and fibroblasts proliferate.

Endothelial rejection is the commonest and most important form of graft rejection. It presents with sudden visual loss, pain and/or ocular inflammation usually about 8 months after surgery, although it may be delayed for many years. Early signs include anterior segment inflammation with circumcorneal injection. Lymphocytes may adhere to the endothelium to form a well-demarcated line (Khodadoust line) and advance in association with endothelial cell death. Alternatively, diffuse involvement is characterized by keratic precipitates scattered over the entire endothelial surface of the graft. Endothelial cell dysfunction and death lead to stromal oedema that may be permanent if treatment is delayed or inadequate.

Graft-versus-host reactions

Most immune reactions to transplanted tissue are a response of the host against the graft. The converse may occur when immunodeficient or bone-marrow-depleted recipients are transfused with allogenic blood products containing HLA-incompatible lymphocytes. Graft-versus-host disease (GVHD) is a cell-mediated/cytotoxic immune reaction that may have acute or chronic presentations. Acute GVHD presents early following transplantation, with involvement of the skin (erythema, bullae), liver dysfunction and diarrhoea. Chronic GVHD occurs later, with dermal sclerosis, sicca syndrome, gastrointestinal involvement, chronic hepatitis, pulmonary insufficiency, wasting and immunodeficiency.

Apart from keratoconjunctivitis sicca (due to chronic inflammation of the lacrimal glands), ophthalmic features of acute and chronic disease include conjunctivitis that varies from mild involvement to severe pseudomembranous/membranous inflammation with cicatrization. Uveitis may occur together with sequelae of cicatricial conjunctivitis. Conjunctivitis, particularly in acute disease, is an indicator of poor prognosis. Histological features indicate an immune response to epithelial cells and in the conjunctiva comprise lymphocyte migration into the basal epithelium. In more severe conjunctival disease, T lymphocytes infiltrate the substantia propria, subepithelial microvesicles form, and conjunctival epithelium is lost.

INFECTION

Infectious diseases are caused by organisms belonging to a variety of different groups including viruses, bacteria, fungi, protozoa, helminths and arthropods. In addition, several infectious diseases may be caused by prions, infective proteinaceous particles that lack the usual features of living organisms. Viruses are non-cellular, self-replicating infectious agents that contain genetic material but lack cell membranes and cytoplasm, and do not have the biochemical machinery necessary for synthesizing macromolecules; their survival and replication depends on symbiosis. Cellular organisms can be classified as prokaryotes and eukaryotes. Bacteria are prokaryotes and characteristically lack intracellular membrane-bound organelles including nuclei, but possess a protective cell wall covering their cell membranes. Fungi, protozoa, hel-

minths and arthropods are eukaryotes and are made up of cells that contain membrane-bound organelles.

The association and interaction of organisms of different species is termed symbiosis and is important in the consideration of infection. Symbiosis may be subdivided, according to the relative benefit obtained by each partner, into three broad categories: commensalism, mutualism and parasitism. Commensalism is where one species uses a larger species as its physical environment to acquire nutrients. The skin, lids, conjunctival sac, mouth and gastrointestinal tract are colonized by an extensive range of commensal organisms (particularly bacteria – the normal flora) that are usually harmless. A saprophyte is a commensal that digests dead or decaying organic matter. Mutualistic relationships convey reciprocal benefits to the two organisms and include those of the many species of bacteria that colonize the gut and prevent invasion by pathogens. The relationship is termed parasitic when one organism alone (the parasite) benefits from a relationship with another (the host). Parasites may or may not be harmful to the host, and the most successful association is when parasites achieve a balance with their host that ensures the survival of both. A parasite causing disease in the host is termed a pathogen. Organisms may change their behaviour; for example, changes in environmental conditions may cause commensals to become parasitic and give rise to opportunistic infections.

PRIONS

Prions (incorrectly referred to as slow viruses) are minute infectious agents that appear to be modified host glycoprotein (prion protein – PrP) and do not contain nucleic acid. They do not induce a detectable immune reaction, but can produce disease in humans after an incubation period of up to 30 years. Prions cause at least three human neurodegenerative disorders: Creutzfeldt–Jakob disease (CJD), the Gerstmann–Straussler–Streinker syndrome and kuru. Animal prion diseases include scrapie, bovine spongiform encephalopathy (BSE), transmissible mink encephalopathy and chronic wasting muscle diseases of deer and elk. Variant CJD (vCJD) is the human equivalent of BSE. CJD is not contagious but can probably be transmitted by the ingestion of infected foods and, on rare occasions, by transplantation of cornea and dura mater, by human-derived pituitary growth hormone and by contaminated surgical instruments and cortical electrodes. Molecular genetic data suggests that those with iatrogenic CJD probably harbour a genetic susceptibility to the disease. Prion diseases have few ophthalmic features apart from the neuro-ophthalmic manifestations of encephalopathy. Prions are highly resistant to conventional methods of sterilization.

VIRUSES

Viruses range in size from 10–300 nm and consist of single- or double-stranded, linear or circular nucleic acid (DNA or RNA) contained within a protein coat (capsid) composed of structured units (capsomeres). The complete unit of nucleic acid and capsid is known as the nucleocapsid (virion), which often has distinct symmetry depending on the way the capsomeres are assembled. Three types of symmetry are known: cubic, helical and complex. Nucleocapsids with cubic symmetry are typically icosahedral (20-sided) and consist of pentameric capsomeres at the corners and hexameric capsomeres elsewhere. Helical nucleocapsids are elongated and the capsomeres are arranged around a spiral of nucleic acid. Nucleocapsids with complex symmetry do not conform to either cubic or helical symmetry. Some viruses have an envelope which is usually a bilipid layer of host cell origin. Viruses are so small that they can be seen only by electron microscopy, although compact intracellular inclusions representing sites of viral synthesis and replication (inclusion bodies) can often be seen by conventional light microscopy. DNA viral-infected cells have intranuclear inclusion bodies while RNA inclusion bodies are usually intracytoplasmic.

Viruses gain access to the body by attaching themselves to receptor sites on the membranes of epidermal/epithelial cells of skin and mucous membranes via ligand molecules on their capsomeres. The envelope of enveloped viruses fuses with the cell membranes. Ligand-binding triggers receptor-mediated endocytosis and, once inside the cell, capsomeres dissociate as a result of lysosomal enzymatic activity. Replication of viruses within the host cell may result in cell death (cytopathic effect). Alternatively, the infected cell may remain apparently normal but the viral genome integrates with the host cell DNA (latent infection). Viral replication may be reactivated by external stimuli and recurrent infection results. Oncogenic viruses transform cells that they infect into cancerous cells with the production of a malignant neoplasm. Viral diseases may be localized to the site of entry where they result from the cytopathic effect. On occasions, local disease may be subclinical. A common mechanism for the release of virions is extrusion through the cell membrane with or without the acquisition of an envelope. Some viruses have genes for proteins (virokines) which combat host defences and help dissemination; systemic involvement may follow haematogenous (viraemia), lymphatic or neural spread. Viruses cannot be grown on artificial media and cell culture is required. Viruses are broadly classified into DNA or RNA viruses.

DNA viruses

Papovaviruses

Papovaviruses are a group of small (45–55 nm), non-enveloped icosahedral viruses. Their name derives from the three members: papilloma virus, polyoma virus and simian vacuolating virus. The papilloma and polyoma viruses are oncogenic; polyoma viruses are also associated with progressive multifocal leukoencephalopathy. At least 65 serotypes of human papilloma virus (HPV) infect epidermal/epithelial cells and are associated with a variety of epidermal/epithelial neoplasms of the lids and conjunctiva; non-ocular associations include intraepithelial neoplasms and infiltrating squamous cell carcinomas of the uterine cervix. Transmission of infection is through abrasion of the skin or mucous membranes, or by sexual contact.

Adenoviruses

Adenoviruses are medium-sized (70–90 nm), non-enveloped and icosahedral (Fig. 2.37). Because of their stability in the environment, they are easily transmitted. Their nucleocapsids consist of 252 capsomeres with fibre-like projections at each of the 12 vertices. The projections terminate in knob-like structures, which are important determinants of the biological properties of the virus. Six subgenera (A–F) and at least 47 serotypes of adenovirus have been identified. Adenoviruses are a common cause of follicular conjunctivitis and upper respiratory tract

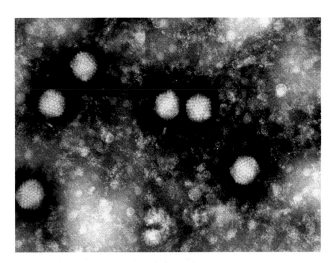

Figure 2.37 Adenovirus. 75 nm virus particles negatively stained with 1.5% phosphotungstic acid. TEM.

infections, particularly pharyngitis, and can also infect the gastrointestinal and urinary tracts. Well-defined syndromes of adenoviral infections associated with particular serotypes include epidemic keratoconjunctivitis, pharyngoconjunctival fever and chronic adenoviral conjunctivitis.

Epidemic keratoconjunctivitis

Epidemic keratoconjunctivitis (EKC) is a highly contagious disease occurring world-wide and affecting individuals of all ages. It is caused primarily by serotypes 8 and 19, and less commonly by types 2, 3, 4, 5, 7, 9, 10, 11, 14, 16, 21, 29 and 37. Epidemics are common but sporadic. Spread is usually by hand-to-eye contact, but contaminated instruments (e.g. tonometer heads) and topical medications (e.g. eye drops) are also sources of infection. EKC is characterized by acute follicular conjunctivitis with preauricular lymphadenopathy, and an upper respiratory illness and sometimes diarrhoea, particularly in children. Punctate epithelial keratitis developing 7–14 days following onset is caused by infection of corneal epithelial cells. Subepithelial infiltrates consisting of lymphocytes, occasional neutrophils and degenerate tissue develop later as a result of delayed hypersensitivity to viral antigen. Although EKC is self-limiting and resolves in approximately 2 weeks, the subepithelial infiltrates may persist for weeks to months and result in impaired vision.

Pharyngoconjunctival fever

Pharyngoconjunctival fever may be sporadic, but most commonly occurs in epidemics and mainly affects children of school age. It is usually caused by serotypes 3, 4 and 7, rarely by types 1, 5 and 14. Pharyngoconjunctival fever differs from EKC in that spread is by droplet transmission, although outbreaks can occur in the summer months due to the contamination of inadequately chlorinated swimming pools. Clinical manifestations include acute follicular conjunctivitis, preauricular lymphadenopathy, pharyngitis and short-lived systemic features including low-grade fever, malaise, myalgia and gastrointestinal disturbance. The conjunctivitis is self-limiting and resolves after 7–10 days. Keratitis, if present, is usually mild, resolves quickly and rarely affects vision.

Chronic adenoviral conjunctivitis

On rare occasions, chronic conjunctivitis and keratoconjunctivitis is caused by adenovirus serotypes 3, 4, 5 and 19. Clinical features include photophobia, lacrimation and conjunctival hyperaemia.

Investigations for adenoviral infections

Conjunctival scrapings in acute adenoviral conjunctivitis reveal a lymphocytic response. Definitive diagnosis of adenoviral infection can be made by the isolation of virus from conjunctival specimens during the first week of infection. Demonstration of a fourfold or greater increase in serum antibody titres to adenovirus is of diagnostic value. Viral nucleic acid can be detected by molecular methods and viral antigen by immunological techniques.

Herpesviruses

Herpesviruses are a group of large (180–200 nm) enveloped viruses (Fig. 2.38). Their icosahedral nucleocapsid consists of 162 capsomeres and contains a spool-like proteinaceous core on which the double-stranded DNA is wrapped. An amorphous asymmetric mass (the tegument) containing viral structural and regulatory proteins separates the nucleocapsid from the envelope. The envelope is composed of lipids derived from the host nuclear membrane, and glycoproteins, which are either synthesized by the virus or are modified host cell protein. The glycoproteins form distinct protrusions (spikes) dispersed over the surface of the

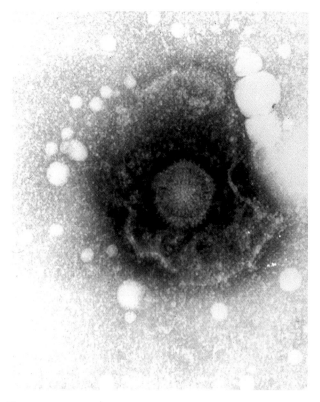

Figure 2.38 Herpesvirus. Virus particles negatively stained with 1.5% phosphotungstic acid. TEM.

envelope and account for the biological properties of the particular virus. There are eight serotypes of human herpesvirus (HHV-1–8). Those of importance to ophthalmologists are HHV-1 and -2 (herpes simplex virus HSV-1 and -2), HHV-3 (varicella zoster virus – VZV), HHV-4 (Epstein–Barr virus – EBV), HHV-5 (cytomegalovirus – CMV) and HHV-8 (Kaposi sarcoma virus – KSV). Almost all herpesviruses express common antigenic determinants and many produce eosinophilic intranuclear inclusions surrounded by a halo (Cowdry type A inclusions).

Herpes simplex virus

Herpes simplex virus (HSV) includes two antigenically distinct types (HSV-1 – HHV-1 and HSV-2 – HHV-2). HSV-1 is transmitted in oral secretions and causes ulcerative disease of the face, lips and eyes. Infection is widespread, mostly subclinical and occurs in childhood such that up to 80 per cent of adults have immunological evidence of infection. HSV-1 infection is more common than HSV-2, which is transmitted sexually and is responsible mainly for genital infections. HSV disease exhibits primary and latent phases followed by reactivation.

The primary phase occurs at the site of initial inoculation, where infection destroys epidermal/epithelial cells and leads to vesicle formation and ulceration. Cell necrosis (lytic infection) results in inflammation dominated initially by neutrophils; lymphocytes infiltrate later. Lesions may be subclinical but, if manifest, are mild and self-limiting. In lytic infection, the virus fuses with the cell surface membrane, loses its envelope and passes into the cytoplasm where the capsid is lost to expose viral DNA, which passes to the cell nucleus. Viral DNA encodes a series of intermediate early (alpha), early (beta) and late (gamma) genes that lead to the production of viral structural proteins within the cytoplasm and replication of viral DNA within the nucleus where nucleocapsids are assembled. An envelope is acquired as the nucleocapsid buds outwards through the nuclear membrane. The newly formed viruses then either pass out of the cell via the endoplasmic reticulum and Golgi apparatus or, if the intracellular viral mass is large, cause cell lysis. Free viruses infect adjacent cells or migrate to sensory nerve terminals and, by retrograde axonal transport mechanisms, pass to neuronal cell bodies in sensory and autonomic root ganglia where further viral replication may occur. Specific immunity develops during the primary phase.

The latent phase of herpetic disease is when viral DNA persists within infected neurons of the peripheral and autonomic nervous system. Virions cannot be detected and normal cellular function is maintained. Viral gene expression is almost completely repressed, but limited transcription generates a family of RNA molecules termed latency-associated transcripts (LATs); the function of LATs and the mechanism of latency are not clear. During the latent phase viruses do not actively replicate and are concealed from the immune system; therefore there can be no immune response, nor can antiviral agents be effective. The possibility of latent infection in non-neural tissue (extraneural latency) has yet to be confirmed.

Reactivation converts latent infection to active viral replication. The mechanisms governing reactivation are not clear, but triggering factors include sunlight, cold, pyrexia, menstruation, immunodeficiency and immunosuppression. The rate of recurrence may depend on the viral strain. Viruses are synthesized in nerve ganglia, distributed to peripheral tissues by anterograde axonal transport and shed from nerve terminals to invade adjacent cells, where further replication occurs with resultant recurrent disease. The features of recurrent disease depend on the particular nerve/tissue involved and the viral strain. Reactivation is manifest usually in adolescents or adults as mucocutaneous vesicular lesions (cold sores).

Ophthalmic herpes simplex

The primary phase of infection usually occurs in children and is generally due to HSV-1. Clinical features include vesicles on the lid margin, follicular conjunctivitis and punctate epithelial keratitis that may progress to a dendritic ulcer. Primary infection in neonates is usually due to HSV-2 transmitted from the maternal genital tract at the time of delivery. The lack of a mature immune system leads to a potentially fatal disseminated infection involving the lungs, liver, adrenal glands, CNS and eyes. The latent phase follows primary ocular and periocular infection, and the trigeminal, ciliary and superior cervical ganglia are affected. Transneuronal spread during the latent phase may result in recurrent infection at a site away from the primary infection; corneal infection (ophthalmic division of the trigeminal nerve) can thus be a consequence of initial infection of the facial area (maxillary division of the trigeminal nerve). Recurrent ophthalmic HSV infection is due to viral reactivation and is most commonly manifest as epithelial keratitis or stromal disease (stromal keratitis and disciform keratopathy), although blepharitis, conjunctivitis, uveitis and retinitis may also occur.

Epithelial keratitis follows reactivation of viral replication in the trigeminal ganglion. Viruses reach the cornea via the ophthalmic division of the trigeminal nerve and the ciliary nerves. Recurrent epithelial keratitis is manifest as focal loss of epithelium and dendritic ulcers, and is due to active viral replication within corneal epithelial cells, a process controlled by the host immune response. In the early stages, infected cells swell, their nuclear chromatin changes, nucleoli are lost, nuclear membranes swell and nuclear division in the absence of cell division leads to the formation of multinucleate epithelial cells. As infection advances, eosinophilic intranuclear inclusion bodies form, metabolism ceases and the cells become necrotic. HSV epithelial keratitis usually resolves spontaneously due to viral replication being controlled by immune mechanisms involving the activity of cytokines, principally interferon.

Stromal keratitis is usually indicative of prolonged and recurrent infection. Symptoms include pain, photophobia, redness and reduced vision. Ulceration, stromal necrosis, thinning, descemetocele formation and keratic precipitates may all occur, and the cornea may perforate. There is evidence that HSV stromal keratitis results from an immune response to viral antigen rather than from cellular destruction by replicating virus. In those with immunity to HSV, antibodies from the tears and limbal circulation diffuse into the cornea and combine with HSV antigen expressed by keratocytes. Complement is activated and cytokines induce migration of neutrophils and lymphocytes, and promote an inflammatory response. Plasma cells migrate to the limbal region and provide a local source of antibodies. Immune complexes form and there may be granuloma formation. Deep stromal involvement and rupture of Descemet's membrane may result in the appearance of giant cells (Fig. 2.39). As the antigenic load diminishes, stromal keratitis resolves with resultant scarring and vascularization. Lipid keratopathy (see Fig. 5.41) may develop later.

Disciform keratopathy presents with acute onset of blurred vision, mild conjunctival injection and minimal discomfort. Clinical examination reveals a centrally situated well-circumscribed round or oval area of epithelial

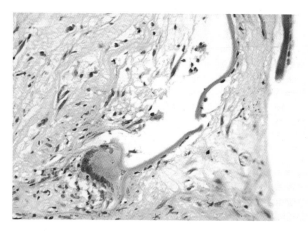

Figure 2.39 HSV keratitis. A giant cell in relation to disrupted Descemet's membrane.

and stromal oedema with associated anterior uveal inflammation. The oedema results from endothelial dysfunction thought to be secondary to an immune response to viral antigen within the stroma or, more probably, the endothelium. Disciform keratopathy usually resolves spontaneously or following topical corticosteroid medication, although some cases are more aggressive and lead to scarring and thinning, or to epithelial or stromal keratitis. Lesions tend to recur and may eventually produce endothelial damage.

Post-herpetic (metaherpetic) keratopathy is the persistence of epithelial and/or stromal lesions after active viral replication and inflammation have subsided. The epithelium fails to heal completely. Factors contributing to this include corneal anaesthesia, poor cellular adhesion due to herpetic damage of the underlying basement membrane, tear film instability due to damaged epithelial microvilli, and secondary bacterial infection. The epithelium in affected areas is degenerate and disorganized with loss of polarity. The basement membrane and Bowman's layer are disrupted or absent, and the underlying stromal collagen is disorganized. Stromal necrosis results in part from lytic enzymes, particularly collagenases, released from abnormal epithelial cells, keratocytes and chronic inflammatory cells.

Investigations for ophthalmic herpes simplex

The clinical features of most HSV infections are sufficient for diagnosis, but in equivocal cases conjunctival swabs, corneal epithelial and stromal biopsies, keratoplasty specimens and aqueous may be submitted for investigation. Cytology of corneal epithelium shows multinucleate cells and eosinophilic intranuclear inclusions surrounded by a clear zone (Cowdry type A inclusions). Electron microscopy may reveal virus particles. HSV can be grown in cell culture, viral antigen can be detected by immunological methods and nucleic acid by molecular methods. Serological investigation is of limited value because of the near universality of primary infection after the age of 5 years.

Varicella zoster virus

Varicella zoster virus (VZV – HHV-3) is identical in morphology and similar in pathobiology to HSV. It is thought to enter through the nasopharyngeal mucosa where it replicates before passing into the blood stream and lymphatics. VZV causes varicella and herpes zoster, both of which have ophthalmic manifestations. On first exposure, usually in childhood, VZV causes varicella (chicken pox), an acute systemic febrile illness characterized by a generalized vesicular skin eruption. Ophthalmic involvement includes lid vesicles, conjunctivitis, punctate epithelial keratitis and dendritic ulceration. Following primary infection with VZV, the virus becomes latent in sensory root ganglia. Reactivation results in herpes zoster (shingles), a localized vesicular skin eruption in the affected dermatome that may be associated with viraemia and systemic manifestations.

Herpes zoster ophthalmicus

Herpes zoster ophthalmicus (HZO) accounts for 10–25 per cent of all cases of herpes zoster and is a significant cause of morbidity. Those affected are usually elderly and present with prodromal fever, malaise, headache and dysthesia of the affected dermatome. One to four days later, grouped vesicular cutaneous lesions develop, become pustular and crust in 7–10 days. HZO is due to reactivation of virus latent in the sensory root ganglion of the trigeminal nerve; the ophthalmic division is more frequently and severely affected than the others and, if the nasociliary division is involved, up to 50 per cent of those with HZO develop ophthalmic complications. The clinical features are diverse and depend on the predominant nerve involved, the various pathogenetic mechanisms and the individual's immune response. The lids become erythematous and swollen, and a vesicular rash develops in the distribution of the ophthalmic division of the trigeminal nerve. Mucopurulent conjunctivitis is common, conjunctival vesicles develop and these may rupture when abraded by lid movement. Over half of those affected have corneal involvement that presents as punctate epithelial keratitis, which may develop into dendritic ulceration. Stromal inflammatory disease is manifest as nummular keratitis (fine granular deposits surrounded by a circular haze) or disciform keratitis. Other ocular manifestations of HZO include episcleritis, scleritis, anterior uveitis and secondary glaucoma (due to associated trabeculitis or post-inflammatory cicatricial closure of the filtration angle). Skin eruptions tend to leave pits, scars and areas of altered pigmentation, and corneal stromal lesions become scarred and vascularized. Long-term sequelae of HZO include keratoconjunctivitis sicca, exposure keratopathy, lipid keratopathy (see Fig. 5.41) and post-herpetic neuralgia.

The skin lesions of varicella and herpes zoster (including HZO) are indistinguishable on histological examination. Vesicles filled with neutrophils and inflammatory debris become pustules and erode to form shallow ulcers. Multinucleate giant epithelial cells with characteristic eosinophilic intranuclear inclusions surrounded by a clear zone (Cowdry type A inclusions) are present. Corneal inflammatory changes lead to scarring, vascularization and lipid keratopathy. The uvea exhibits a lymphocytic cellular infiltrate that extends into the trabecular meshwork. The pathogenesis of the ophthalmic manifestations of HZO is complex and incompletely understood. During the early stages of the disease when the virus is actively replicating, vasculitis, neuritis and other inflammatory responses lead to tissue damage. The virus can be isolated from the eye in acute disease but cannot be identified in the chronic stage, thus suggesting that the delayed manifestations are immune phenomena.

Epstein–Barr virus

Epstein–Barr virus (EBV – HHV-4) is ubiquitous and more than 95 per cent of the adult population is seropositive. It causes infectious mononucleosis (glandular fever) and is associated with Burkitt's lymphoma and nasopharyngeal carcinoma. Ophthalmic involvement with EBV infection is rarely diagnosed, but manifestations include follicular conjunctivitis, Parinaud's oculoglandular syndrome, punctate epithelial keratitis, uveitis and choroidoretinitis. Lymphocytosis is present in 70 per cent of cases of active infection. Serological diagnosis is based on the distribution of antibodies to various viral components including viral capsid antigen (VCA), Epstein–Barr nuclear antigen (EBNA) and early antigen (EA). Those with recently acquired EBV infection have elevated levels of IgM and IgG to VCA and EA. Serum positive for EBNA is indicative of previous infection.

Cytomegalovirus

Cytomegalovirus (CMV – HHV-5) is ubiquitous. Diseases associated with CMV infection, although rare, are often devastating. In most instances initial infection is subclinical, and occurs usually in utero or shortly after birth but invariably before puberty. As with HSV and VZV infections, recurrence of active disease is due to reactivation of the latent virus. Sources of the virus include saliva, urine, tears, breast milk, cervical and vaginal secretions, faeces and blood. Transmission is by direct or indirect contact. Evidence of CMV infection can be found in almost every organ of the body, and the disorders caused depend largely on the immune state of the host. The fetus and the immunocompromised are particularly vulnerable. A feature common to all CMV infections is the characteristic cytopathic effect, which is manifest as marked cellular enlargement (cytomegalic cells) and eosinophilic intranuclear inclusions surrounded by a clear zone giving rise to an owl's eye appearance.

CMV is transmitted across the placenta and involves 0.5–2 per cent of all fetuses; of these 10–20 per cent have signs of infection. In primary maternal infections the fetus is at risk because of its relative lack of immune defences and the inability of maternally derived CMV antibodies to cross the placenta. The commonest sites of fetal involvement are the brain, eyes, inner ears, liver and bone marrow. Those affected present at or soon after birth with hepatosplenomegaly, jaundice, pete-chiae, respiratory distress and neurological defects ranging from mild learning difficulties to profound disability. Otherwise asymptomatic children may develop late sensorineural hearing loss or mental retardation.

Primary infection after birth is asymptomatic, or in older children and adults presents as an atypical mononucleosis. Symptoms include fever, lymphadenopathy, pharyngitis and rubelliform rashes. Lymphocytosis with atypical lymphocytes is common. Primary infection is followed by the development of specific immunity, and it is assumed that further involvement is due to reactivation of latent infection.

Disseminated CMV infections cause serious disease in the immunocompromised and usually result from reactivation of latent infection, although on rare occasions the virus may originate from exogenous sources. Organ transplant recipients and those with AIDS are at risk of multiple organ involvement manifest as retinochoroiditis, pneumonitis, encephalitis, enterocolitis, hepatitis and adrenalitis; individuals with AIDS are at particular risk of developing CMV retinitis.

Kaposi sarcoma virus

Kaposi sarcoma virus (KSV – HHV-8) is present in Kaposi sarcoma and appears to be confined to those who acquired HIV by sexual contact.

Herpesvirus retinitis

HSV, VZV and CMV may all cause necrotizing retinitis. In HSV and VZV infections the necrosis is acute, whereas CMV retinitis is only slowly progressive.

Acute retinal necrosis (ARN – BARN if it is bilateral) is due to HSV and VZV infection. Discretely demarcated areas of retinal necrosis (Fig. 2.40a) at the periphery are followed by rapid circumferential spread and subsequent retinal detachment. The vitreous and anterior segment are inflamed and optic neuropathy may also occur. The pathological features described relate to VZV retinitis (the histological changes of HSV retinitis are not fully established). In the active phase, diffuse necrotizing retinitis occurs together with occlusive vasculitis, optic neuritis and papillitis associated with chronic panuveitis in which lymphocytes and plasma cells predominate. Eosinophilic inclusions are found in mononuclear cells, mainly in the peripheral choroid. Electron microscopy reveals large quantities of virus particles in all layers of the neurosensory retina. Late stages of the disease are characterized by extensive glial scarring, epiretinal membrane formation and ischaemic optic atrophy.

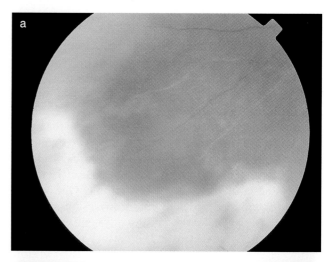

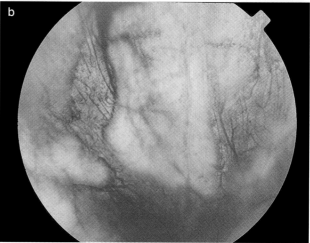

Figure 2.40 HSV retinitis. (a) Acute retinal necrosis. (b) Progressive outer retinal necrosis.

Vitrectomy specimens can be used for culture, nucleic acid detection and the demonstration of viral antibody.

Progressive outer retinal necrosis (PORN) is due to VZV infection and occurs in the immunocompromised, particularly those with AIDS. A bilateral rapidly progressive deep retinitis presents with minimal evidence of vitritis or retinal vasculopathy (Fig. 2.40b). There is multifocal full thickness or outer retinal necrosis and occasional retinal vasculopathy, and retinal detachment occurs in 70 per cent of affected eyes. Optic nerve abnormalities are rare. Investigations are similar to those for acute retinal necrosis.

CMV retinitis develops only in those who are severely immunocompromised and is particularly associated with AIDS, where it affects up to 50 per cent of cases and is indicative of a poor life expectancy. Affected individuals may be asymptomatic, but in more advanced cases symptoms include floaters, scotomata and reduced visual acuity. Fundus examination reveals white areas of retinal necrosis, haemorrhages and vascular sheathing ('pizza-pie' or 'cottage-cheese' and 'tomato ketchup' fundus – Fig. 2.41a). The retinopathy starts as one or two foci that progressively enlarge, particularly towards the ora serrata, and the fovea is often spared until late in the disease. Rhegmatogenous retinal detachment occurs in up to 30 per cent of cases. In AIDS, untreated CMV retinitis is relentlessly progressive and leads to total retinal necrosis within 6 months of onset. Moderate uveitis and vitreous inflammatory activity may be present. Resolution of retinal lesions reveals local atrophy and pigment dispersion. Histological examination of CMV retinitis demonstrates the characteristic cytomegalic cells (Fig. 2.41b) and eosinophilic intranuclear owl's eye inclusions. The retina is necrotic with destruction of all layers, and is eventually replaced by a thin glial membrane. CMV viral particles and antigen can be identified in a patchy distribution throughout the retina by electron microscopy (Fig. 2.41c) and immunohistochemistry respectively. The presence of neutrophils is characteristic of CMV retinitis in AIDS but not in other immunodeficiency states; this is attributed to preserved granulocyte function in AIDS. CMV reaches the eye by haematogenous spread and the predisposition of those with AIDS to CMV retinitis is thought to be related to the coexistence of HIV microvasculopathy, which allows access of CMV to retinal tissue through the damaged vascular wall. The only systemic risk factor clearly associated with the development of CMV retinitis in those with HIV infection is a CD4 + lymphocyte count < 50 per mm^3.

Poxviruses

Poxviruses are the largest (200–300 nm) and most complicated of all viruses. They are elliptical or brick-shaped, contain double-stranded DNA, and a double membrane envelops the nucleocapsid. Poxviruses replicate within the cytoplasm of the host cell and appear as inclusion bodies. Human poxvirus diseases include smallpox, vaccinia, molluscum contagiosum and orf (contagious pustular dermatitis), an infection of sheep and goats that is occasionally transmitted to animal workers, where self-limiting pustular lesions can involve the lids.

Molluscum contagiosum is a cutaneous lesion that can occur on most parts of the body, including the lids. It is caused by the molluscum contagiosum virus, which infects epidermal cells. It is the commonest poxvirus associated with ophthalmic infection, and is spread by direct contact or fomites. After an incubation period of about 2 weeks, infected cells proliferate and enlarge, becoming filled with eosinophilic inclusions containing

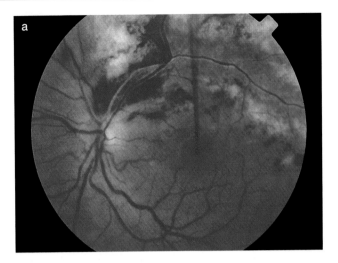

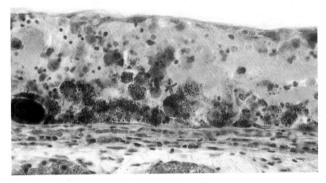

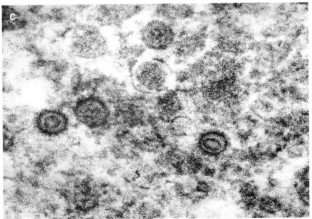

Figure 2.41 CMV retinitis. (a) Fundus appearance. (b) Large cytomegalic cells. (c) Inclusion bodies; owl's-eye appearance. TEM.

viral DNA. The result is the formation of a nodular lobulated mass 2–5 mm in diameter with an umbilicated centre from which white cheesy material (infected degenerate cells) can be expressed. The lesions are self-limiting and usually disappear in 2–3 months, although they may persist for up to 4 years.

Follicular conjunctivitis and punctate epithelial keratitis may accompany lid involvement and are probably related to virus particles shed into the tear film. Histological examination of lesions excised *in toto* shows thickening of the epidermis and a central pit (Fig. 2.42a). The epidermal cells are enlarged and contain eccentrically placed eosinophilic intracytoplasmic inclusions (molluscum bodies) that displace the nucleus. Smears of material expressed from the central core show similar inclusion-bearing cells (Fig. 2.42b).

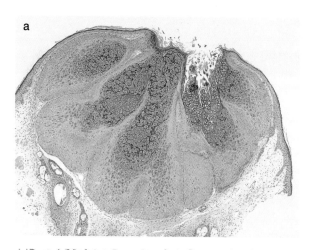

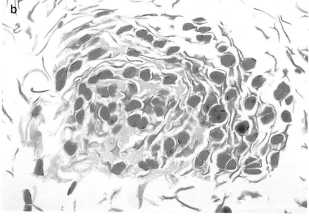

Figure 2.42 Molluscum contagiosum. (a) Epidermal thickening and a central pit. (b) Numerous eosinophilic inclusions (molluscum bodies).

RNA viruses

Picornaviruses

Picornaviruses are small (25–30 nm), non-enveloped and icosahedral. They are important causes of systemic diseases involving the CNS, gastrointestinal tract, respiratory tract and heart. They include polioviruses, coxsackieviruses, enteroviruses and rhinoviruses. The commonest ophthalmic manifestation of infection is con-

junctivitis. Coxsackievirus type A-24 and enterovirus type 70 cause acute haemorrhagic conjunctivitis, which occurs predominantly in Africa, Asia, South America, the Caribbean and the southern United States.

Paramyxoviruses

Paramyxoviruses are medium-sized (45–55 nm), enveloped and helical, and cause measles, mumps and Newcastle disease.

Measles (rubeola) is a highly contagious infection characterized by upper respiratory tract symptoms, fever and a rash. In the very young and malnourished it is particularly severe, and can have a mortality rate of up to 25 per cent. Ophthalmic involvement is common and includes mucopurulent conjunctivitis and keratitis. The keratitis is potentially blinding, particularly if there is concurrent vitamin A deficiency as is common in underdeveloped countries, and takes the form of punctate epithelial lesions that progress to ulceration and possibly perforation. Subsequent corneal scarring may be severe and lead to post-measles blindness. The measles virus is also responsible for subacute sclerosing panencephalitis, a rare progressive neurodegenerative disease characterized in the eye by a macular choroidoretinopathy with superficial retinal haemorrhages, oedema and retinal folds; measles antigen can be detected in infected retinal cells.

Mumps (infectious parotitis) is an acute systemic infection characterized by swelling of the parotid glands and meningoencephalitis. It affects children and young adults. Initial infection of the respiratory tract epithelium leads to dissemination of virus through the blood and lymphatic systems to infect other sites, notably the salivary and lacrimal glands, CNS, pancreas and testes. The commonest ophthalmic manifestations are acute dacryoadenitis (Fig. 2.43) and acute catarrhal conjunctivitis. Other manifestations are less common, but include diffuse episcleritis, scleritis, interstitial keratitis and anterior uveitis.

Newcastle disease (fowl pest) may occur in those who come into contact with infected birds, particularly chickens. It is characterized by a mild follicular conjunctivitis and preauricular lymphadenopathy.

Togaviruses

Togaviruses are medium-sized (60–70 nm), enveloped and icosahedral, and cause various diseases including rubella (German measles), which is a relatively mild self-limiting disorder. In rubella, after an incubation period of 2–3 weeks, initial malaise and lymphadenopathy is followed by a maculopapular rash spreading from the

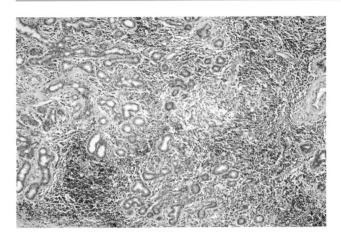

Figure 2.43 Dacryoadenitis. Lacrimal gland stroma infiltrated by inflammatory cells.

face to the trunk. A mild follicular conjunctivitis may precede the rash and last for several days. If rubella virus is contracted by a mother during the first trimester of pregnancy, the unborn child may develop congenital defects (congenital rubella syndrome). Infection after 20 weeks of gestation is unlikely to cause any serious malformation but, once infected, the virus remains within the fetus and may be detected in the nasopharynx and urine of up to 80 per cent of affected neonates.

Congenital rubella syndrome (Rubella embryopathy): maternal viraemia may lead to placental infection and subsequent fetal viraemia. The virus may disseminate to many fetal tissues and, depending on the time of infection with respect to fetal development, causes a variable constellation of congenital defects. The congenital rubella syndrome is characterized by retardation of intrauterine growth, retinopathy, cataracts, deafness, congenital heart disease, microcephaly and mental retardation. Other features include corneal oedema, anterior chamber anomalies, glaucoma and microphthalmos. Retinopathy is the commonest ocular manifestation and usually presents as a salt and pepper appearance of the fundus with depigmentation of the RPE. The cataract in the congenital rubella syndrome is dense centrally but less opaque at the periphery and is due to viral infection, which reduces the replication rate of lens cells and causes retention of cell nuclei. Virus persists in lens fibres for at least a year after birth and may cause severe intraocular inflammation following cataract surgery.

Orthomyxoviruses

Orthomyxoviruses are medium-sized (80–120 nm), enveloped and helical, and cause influenza, the ophthalmic manifestations of which are conjunctivitis and, on rare occasions, mild uveitis.

Retroviruses

Retroviruses are medium-sized (80–120 nm), enveloped and icosahedral. They contain two identical copies of single-stranded RNA and a reverse transcriptase, which promotes synthesis of double-stranded DNA from the viral RNA template. The synthesized viral DNA is then incorporated permanently into the DNA of the host cell. Retroviruses include HIV and human T cell lymphotropic viruses 1 and 2 (HTLV-1 and -2), which are oncogenic.

BACTERIA

Bacteria are prokaryotic organisms, contain DNA and RNA, and include rickettsiae, chlamydiae, mycoplasmas, cocci and bacilli, mycobacteria and spiral bacteria.

Rickettsiae

Rickettsiae are small (300–2000 nm) aerobic coccobacillary (short bacilli) organisms that are incapable of replication outside the host cell because they do not generate their own ATP. The organisms replicate in the salivary glands and alimentary canals of blood-sucking arthropod vectors such as ticks, mites and lice. Human rickettsial diseases follow a bite by the vector and are traditionally divided into spotted fever and typhus groups (Table 2.3). The rickettsiae replicate in vascular endothelial cells, which initially proliferate and subsequently degenerate. Clinical features of rickettsial diseases include headache, myalgia and fever followed by a rash. Conjunctivitis and/or keratitis, and anterior and posterior uveitis are the main ophthalmic manifestations but retinal arteriolar and venous occlusions, cotton-wool spots, retinal haemorrhages, oedema and exudates, perivasculitis and optic disc oedema all reflect the vascular involvement. Rickettsiae can only be grown in cell culture or experimental animals, and the diagnosis of infection is based on serology.

Table 2.3 Rickettsial diseases

Group	Agent	Vector	Disease
Spotted fever	*Rickettsia rickettsii*	Tick	Rocky Mountain spotted fever
	Rickettsia conorii	Tick	Boutonneuse fever
Typhus	*Rickettsia prowazekii*	Louse	Epidemic typhus
	Rickettsia typhi	Louse	Murine typhus
	Rickettsia tsutsugamushi	Mite	Scrub typhus

Chlamydiae

Chlamydiae, like rickettsiae, can only replicate inside eukaryotic host cells. They lack the enzymes necessary to synthesize ATP; hence the necessity to parasitize the metabolic machinery of a host cell in order to reproduce. There are four species of chlamydiae: *Chlamydia trachomatis, Chlamydia pneumoniae, Chlamydia psittaci* and *Chlamydia pectorum*. *C. trachomatis* and *C. pneumoniae* are human pathogens; *C. psittaci* only occasionally infects humans but affects a wide variety of wild and domesticated birds and animals; *C. pectorum* causes infection in ruminants. There are 15 types of *C. trachomatis* – types A, B, Ba and C, and types D–K belong to the trachoma biovar; types L1, L2 and L3 belong to the more invasive LGV biovar. Types A, B, Ba and C cause trachoma and types D–K cause chlamydial oculogenital disease and neonatal conjunctivitis. Diseases caused by the LGV biovar include lymphogranuloma venereum (an uncommon sexually transmitted disease) and, occasionally, Parinaud's oculoglandular syndrome. The life cycle of chlamydiae is unique and complex. Two basic developmental and morphological forms, the elementary body and the reticulate body, differ in their structure and metabolism. The elementary body (300–400 nm) is the extracellular metabolically inert infectious particle. The DNA of an elementary body has a dense central core and 60 per cent of the mass of the cell wall is made up of a cysteine-rich protein, known as the major outer membrane protein (MOMP); multiple disulphide cross-linkages within the MOMP confer rigidity to the elementary body. The cell walls contain lipopolysaccharide and an abundant cysteine-rich protein, known as OMP2. The reticulate body (800–1000 nm) is intracellular and metabolically active, and replicates by binary fission within an intracytoplasmic inclusion in the host cell. Chlamydiae are actively taken up by the epithelial cells of the conjunctiva and genital tract, but the mechanisms by which they attach themselves to and enter host cells has not been clearly established. Soon after internalization the elementary body starts to differentiate into the larger metabolically active reticulate body, which grows and divides by binary fission until, after 25–30 hours, some reverse into elementary bodies. By 48 hours post-infection, the chlamydial inclusions may contain more than 1000 chlamydiae, mostly as elementary bodies. The infected cell usually lyses by 72 hours post-infection with release of the chlamydiae. The necrotic cellular debris produced and the immune responses against chlamydial antigen result in inflammation and further tissue damage. *C. trachomatis* inclusions are round or oval and sufficiently rigid to deform or displace the nucleus of the infected cell; the inclusions also contain glycogen and stain positively with Giemsa and iodine. Chlamydiae, like rickettsiae, require cell culture and do not grow on artificial media. Chlamydial infection of the eye takes the form of oculogenital disease or trachoma, the disease produced depending on the type of infecting organism and host factors such as age, nutrition and immune status. Initial infection produces an acute self-limiting response (chlamydial oculogenital disease), but repeated infection results in a delayed type of hypersensitivity (trachoma).

Chlamydial oculogenital disease

Genital epithelial infection with *C. trachomatis* serovars D–K is the commonest sexually transmitted disease in developed countries. Many infected individuals are asymptomatic but, when symptomatic, infection in men is characterized by urethritis and sometimes prostatitis, epididymitis and proctitis; symptomatic women usually have a cervicitis that may progress to endometritis, salpingitis and generalized pelvic inflammatory disease. The cervix of infected women is the main reservoir of the organism. Spread to the conjunctiva may occur in the adult and the neonate.

Adult chlamydial conjunctivitis results from direct inoculation by genital secretions, fomites or infected water, which may be found in swimming pools. Affected individuals are usually aged 15–40 years and present with acute and often asymmetrical follicular conjunctivitis with preauricular lymphadenopathy. Corneal involvement includes epithelial keratitis, marginal and central infiltrates, and subepithelial opacities similar to those of epidemic keratoconjunctivitis. Most cases resolve without sequelae, but occasionally a picture resembling trachoma can develop. Coexisting genital infection is usually present.

Neonatal chlamydial conjunctivitis results from contact with the organism in the secretions of an infected birth canal. Of those neonates at risk, 60–70 per cent develop conjunctivitis. Acute bilateral infection occurs 5–19 days after birth and is characterized by a mucopurulent discharge, swollen lids and conjunctival hyperaemia. As in adult infection, keratitis may develop. There may be associated upper respiratory tract infection, pneumonitis or genital infection.

Trachoma

Trachoma is a chronic cicatrizing conjunctivitis that leads to progressive scarring of the lids and cornea. It is a major cause of blindness in many underdeveloped countries, such as parts of the Middle East, Africa and Asia, where hygiene is poor and medical care of a low standard. Trachoma is caused by *C. trachomatis* serovars A, B, Ba and C, and infection is spread by direct eye to eye transmission, and by flies, fomites and contaminated water. *C. trachomatis* infects the conjunctival epithelium and produces a conjunctivitis characterized by the presence of tarsal follicles and papillae that may obscure underlying blood vessels. The onset is frequently during the first year of life, and may go unnoticed. The cornea may be involved during the acute inflammatory stage with superficial punctate keratitis and superficial neovascularization. Lymphoid follicles may develop at the limbus and, on resolution, leave characteristic depressions (Herbert's pits – Fig. 2.44). Slow progression over many years results in conjunctival scarring, symblepharon, entropion, trichiasis and dry eye. Severe disease results in corneal scarring, ulceration, a predisposition to secondary bacterial infection and blindness. The degree of scarring is related to the cellular immune response and is more severe in those with impaired cellular immunity.

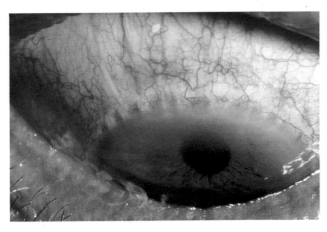

Figure 2.44 Herbert's pits.

Investigations for chlamydial disease

Microscopy of conjunctival scrapings reveals inflammatory cells and epithelial cells that, in neonatal conjunctivitis, may contain intracytoplasmic inclusions (Fig. 2.45a, 2.45b). Inclusions are not usually seen in adult chlamydial conjunctivitis or trachoma. The isolation of chlamydiae in cell culture remains the most specific method for accurate diagnosis. Chlamydial antigen is detectable by immunological methods (Fig. 2.45c) and nucleic acid by molecular methods. Serological tests are of limited value as many individuals have pre-existing antibodies. Although sophisticated laboratory tests have replaced the older cytological investigations, the latter still have a role in developing countries where resources are limited.

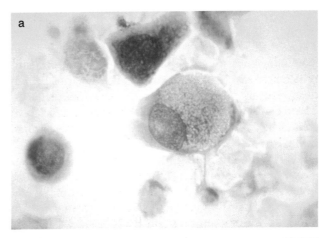

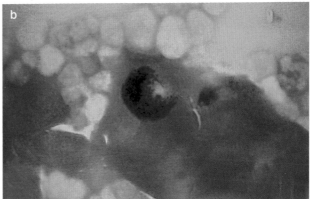

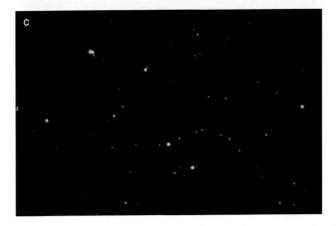

Figure 2.45 Chlamydia. (a) Inclusion body; ovoid structure adjacent to the nucleus of an epithelial cell. Giemsa stain. (b) Inclusion body. Iodine stain. (c) Elementary bodies. Direct immunofluorescence.

Mycoplasmas

Mycoplasmas are amongst the smallest free-living organisms known, and measure up to $0.3\ \mu$m in diameter. They are pleomorphic, and lack a true cell wall and consequent rigidity. *Mycoplasma pneumoniae* is implicated in the Stevens–Johnson syndrome and *Ureaplasma urealyticum* in Reiter's syndrome. Mycoplasmas need complex cultures and soft agar.

Cocci and bacilli

The cytoplasm of these bacteria is enclosed by a cell membrane consisting of a bilayer of phospholipids and proteins which carry out many of the metabolic functions that, in eukaryotes, are performed by organelles. The membrane is the major barrier to the passage of solutes between the cell and the environment. The cell wall is external to the cell membrane and comprises a sac of peptidoglycan that is thick (20–80 nm) in Gram-positive organisms but relatively thin (≤ 10 nm) in Gram-negative organisms. Teichoic acids found among the peptidoglycan of most Gram-positive organisms are important surface antigens and are believed to facilitate the passage of ions. Gram-negative organisms have a second membrane external to the peptidoglycan sac and anchored to it by lipoprotein bridges consisting of lipopolysaccharide, phospholipid and a number of proteins. The polysaccharide chains of lipopolysaccharide are important antigenic determinants. The region between the cell membrane and the peptidoglycan sac is the periplasmic space, which contains digestive enzymes and other proteins that capture specific nutrients such as amino acids, sugars and ions, and directs them to active transport systems.

A glycocalyx, fimbriae and flagellae may be present on the surface of some cocci and bacilli. The glycocalyx (the terms 'capsule' and 'slime layer' are sometimes used) is a coating of polysaccharide and is important in adherence, in resisting desiccation and as a camouflage against phagocytes. Fimbriae are hair-like structures that facilitate adherence to host cells. Flagellae are long helical filaments anchored beneath the cell wall and are distributed in either a polar or peritrichous fashion; they are the commonest mechanism of propulsion and are important antigens.

Genetic information is carried in a long double-stranded DNA molecule (chromosome). There is no nuclear membrane and there are no introns, and the DNA, which is tightly coiled into a region known as the nucleoid, comprises a continuous sequence of genes. Extrachromosomal DNA is found in the cytoplasm as circular strands known as plasmids which replicate independently of the main chromosome. Many plasmids direct the formation of sex pili, which can be regarded as long fimbriae. Functionally, the tip of a sex pilus binds to a recipient bacterial cell, the pilus retracts and the cells are pulled together. This leads to the formation of a cytoplasmic tunnel and DNA transfer between cells, a process that can spread genes and control new phenotypic characteristics. Resistance to antibiotics is acquired in this way. DNA may also be carried between cells by viruses (bacteriophages).

Metabolism

Carbon, nitrogen, sulphur and oxygen are necessary for bacterial metabolism. Carbon is obtained from organic nutrients, and nitrogen and sulphur from inorganic nitrates and sulphates. Oxygen is obtained from organic nutrients or water, or is taken up as free oxygen. The major organic constituents of bacteria are nucleic acids, proteins, polysaccharides and complex lipids, and the energy required for their biosynthesis is supplied principally as ATP, which is produced by oxidative phosphorylation (respiration) or substrate level phosphorylation (fermentation). In respiration, free oxygen is commonly used (aerobic respiration), but a few organisms do not use oxygen (anaerobic respiration). Organisms that use aerobic respiration only are known as aerobes, while those that use fermentation only and for which free oxygen is toxic are known as anaerobes. Microaerophilic organisms require limited amounts of oxygen, while facultative anaerobes are able to grow in the presence or absence of free oxygen. All organisms require carbon dioxide for metabolism, but those that need a considerable amount are termed capnophilic.

Growth and culture

Most cocci and bacilli multiply rapidly when nutrients are available, some having a doubling time as short as 20 minutes. Environmental factors that influence growth include temperature, acidity, osmotic pressure, ionic strength and the availability of nutrients. Most pathogens can be cultured on artificial media and grow in the dark at a temperature of 37°C and at a pH range 6–8 on solid and liquid phase media. Solid phase media include blood agar (nutrient agar containing 5–20 per cent horse blood) and chocolate agar (heated blood agar). Liquid phase media include Robertson's cooked meat, thioglycollate broth and brain–heart infusion.

Spore formation

Under adverse conditions certain Gram-positive organisms form spores. In spore formation a daughter chromosome is isolated, an envelope containing peptidoglycan is synthesized and the spore is liberated on autolysis of the parent cell. Cytoplasmic components are degraded, a gel of calcium dipicolonate forms and a reduced water content contributes to heat resistance. Germination of spores necessitates cracking of the envelope by sublethal exposure to heat, enzymes or chemicals.

Gram reaction

The chemical rationale of the Gram reaction is obscure, but is probably due to a mixture of factors including the thickness, chemical composition and functional integrity of the cell wall of Gram-positive organisms. Staining involves the use of crystal violet or methyl violet, Lugol's iodine followed by decolourizing with acetone or alcohol, and counterstaining with carbol fuchsin or neutral red. Gram-positive organisms resist decolourization and appear blue-black, while Gram-negative organisms are readily decolourized and appear red. When Gram-positive organisms die they become Gram-negative.

Pathogenicity

The pathogenicity of cocci and bacilli is dependent on the balance between the virulence of the invading organism and the immune state of the host. All are potentially pathogenic and some, following adhesion to host cell membranes, enter the cells where they divide and multiply within endocytic vacuoles. Intracellular organisms either remain within the vacuoles or lyse their membranes and escape to the cytoplasm. Some remain extracellular but, when established, multiply and cause disease locally by direct invasion or systemically by vascular or lymphatic spread. Most cause disease by the production of adhesins, aggressins or toxins, and by the undesirable consequences of host immune responses.

Adhesins are recognition molecules of lectins coated on the surface of fimbriae. They interact with host cell surface receptors, which are usually the sugar moiety of a glycoprotein or glycolipid. Polymorphisms of these receptors render some individuals more susceptible to certain types of infection.

Aggressins are synthesized by organisms and act predominantly in the local tissue environment in a way that favours their proliferation and spread. Aggressins include components of the glycocalyx, and enzymes such as coagulase, streptokinase, collagenase and hyaluronidase.

Toxins are of two types: exotoxins and endotoxins. Exotoxins are liberated from organisms and are antigenic, extremely potent and have wide-ranging effects at the site of bacterial growth or distally. Endotoxins are derived from lysed or dead bacteria. The endotoxin of Gram-negative organisms is the lipid moiety of the lipopolysaccharide in the cell wall, whereas the endotoxins of Gram-positive organisms include the peptidoglycan component of the cell wall. Endotoxins activate the alternative complement pathway, leading to inflammatory damage, and the coagulation system, which causes intravascular coagulation. Endotoxins also induce leukocytes to secrete large amounts of cytokines, which cause fever and possibly endotoxic shock.

Harmful host immune responses include hypersensitivity reactions to bacterial toxins, cell-mediated immune responses, insoluble immune complex formation resulting from antigens combining with host antibodies, and immune cross-reactions if host tissues have antigenic similarities to invading bacteria, so enabling defensive antibodies to cross-react with normal tissue antigens.

Classification

Classification of cocci and bacilli is difficult, and in the present context it is best to use phenotypic rather than genotypic data. Morphology and Gram reactions are the main criteria, but developments in molecular genetics may change or at least modify the currently established system. In broad general terms, cocci and bacilli are regarded as Gram-positive or Gram-negative.

Cocci

Cocci are spherical and Gram-positive or Gram-negative.

Gram-positive cocci

Staphylococcus **spp.** contain at least 15 different species. They measure approximately 1 μm in diameter and are capable of both aerobic and anaerobic respiration. Their appearance in smears as clusters (Fig. 2.46a) reflects their ability to divide in more than one plane. Two important members of the group are *S. aureus* and *S. epidermidis*, which share many morphological and cultural characteristics but are differentiated biochemically. *S. aureus* produces coagulase (coagulase positive), which induces the coagulation of fibrin that localizes the infection and protects the organism from phagocytosis. *S. epidermidis* does not produce coagulase (coagulase negative). Staphylococci colonize the nares and skin, and frequently infect the lids (anterior blepharitis, external and internal hordeolum) and conjunctiva (chronic conjunctivitis). Corneal infection is less common, but results in severe purulent keratitis. Immune responses to staphylococcal toxins may be manifest as allergic microbial blepharoconjunctivitis, marginal keratitis and phlyctenular keratoconjunctivitis. Micrococci are similar to *S. epidermidis* but smaller.

Streptococcus **spp.** are widely distributed in nature, 0.5–1 μm in diameter and capable of both aerobic and anaerobic respiration. Their appearance in smears as pairs or chains (Fig. 2.46b) reflects their ability to divide in one plane only. The medically significant streptococci are categorized on the basis of haemolysis on blood agar (complete haemolysis – β; partial haemolysis – α; no haemolysis – γ) or by the presence or absence of group-

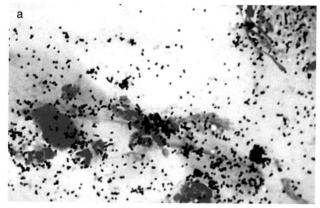

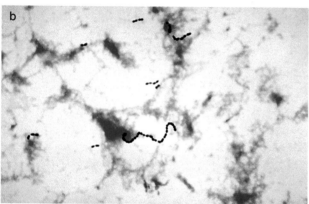

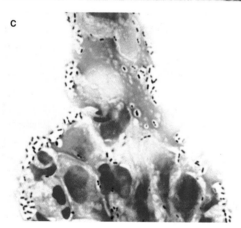

Figure 2.46 Gram-positive cocci. (a) *Staphylococcus aureus*. Corneal smear. (b) *Streptococcus pyogenes*. Vitreous smear. (c) *Streptococcus pneumoniae* (pneumococci). Corneal smear.

specific carbohydrate antigens (Lancefield Groups A–S). Important members of the group are *S. pyogenes*, *S. pneumoniae* (pneumococci) and oral streptococci. *S. pyogenes* appears as chains and produces β-haemolysis, and the majority belong to Lancefield Group A. Ophthalmic infections produced by *S. pyogenes* include conjunctivitis, keratitis and endophthalmitis. *S. pneumoniae* (Fig. 2.46c) are diplococci (pairs) and produce α-haemolysis. The organism is relatively resistant to phagocytosis by virtue of its capsule. It is a common cause of bacterial

conjunctivitis, and can also cause keratitis and intraocular infection. Oral streptococci include species of α-haemolytic streptococci other than *S. pneumoniae* and non-haemolytic streptococci previously known as viridans streptococci. Most are mouth commensals and associated with dental caries and bacterial endocarditis. On rare occasions they infect the outer eye, and they may be responsible for post-surgical endophthalmitis or appear as opportunistic pathogens in pre-existing disease.

Gram-negative cocci

***Neisseria* spp.** include two important human pathogens, *N. meningitidis* (meningococcus) and *N. gonorrhoeae* (gonococcus). *N. meningitidis* is capsulate but *N. gonorrhoeae* is not. Both appear in smears as diplococci. When seen in smears, *N. meningitidis* is both extracellular and intracellular (within neutrophils) whereas *N. gonorrhoeae* is intracellular (Fig. 2.47). *Neisseria* spp. are capnophilic, grow best on chocolate agar and are differentiated by their sugar utilization pattern. *N. gonorrhoeae* may be carried in the nasopharynx, genital tract and anal canal, and is spread by sexual or other intimate contact. It is a major cause of acute purulent bacterial conjunctivitis, including neonatal conjunctivitis, and it can invade intact corneal epithelium with ulceration, proceeding rapidly and possibly leading to perforation and endophthalmitis. *N. meningitidis* is also carried in the nasopharynx, is spread by droplets and may cause bacterial conjunctivitis in addition to meningitis.

Branhamella catarrhalis is now sometimes classified with *Moraxella*. It is morphologically similar to *Neisseria*, but with less fastidious growth requirements. It occurs as a commensal in the respiratory tract, and is not infrequently cultured from infections of the outer eye.

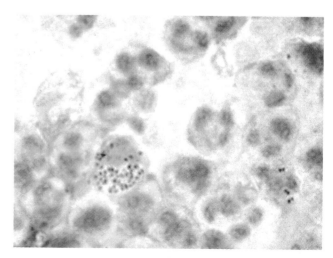

Figure 2.47 Gram-negative coccus. *Neisseria gonorrhoeae* (gonococci). Intracellular organisms in the purulent exudate of neonatal conjunctivitis.

Bacilli

Bacilli are rod-shaped and, like cocci, are Gram-positive or Gram-negative.

Gram-positive bacilli

***Bacillus* spp.** are aerobic and frequently spore-forming. They are widely distributed in nature, being commonly found in soil. *B. anthracis* causes anthrax, while *B. subtilis* and *B. cereus* are common pathogens in intraocular infections following perforating injury.

***Corynebacterium* spp.** are capable of aerobic and anaerobic respiration. They are widely distributed in nature, and those of ophthalmic importance are *C. xerosis* and *C. diphtheriae*. *C. xerosis* is frequently part of the normal conjunctival flora and usually non-pathogenic. Other similar but unclassified bacilli, together with *C. xerosis*, are collectively referred to as diphtheroids. *C. diphtheriae* is the cause of diphtheria, the ophthalmic manifestation of which is membranous conjunctivitis. It can occasionally infect the cornea and penetrate an intact epithelium to cause ulceration and possibly perforation. The mediator for its pathogenicity is an exotoxin that inhibits protein synthesis and causes death of mucosal and other cells.

***Listeria* spp.** are short rod-shaped organisms, often coccobacillary, and of uncertain affiliation. Although microaerophilic, they are similar in other respects to the *Corynebacterium* spp. *L. monocytogenes*, an infrequent cause of ocular inflammation, can breach an intact corneal epithelium. It is implicated in Parinaud's oculoglandular syndrome, and is a rare cause of endogenous endophthalmitis.

***Proprionibacterium* spp.** are small bacilli sometimes classified as anaerobic diphtheroids. They are found in hair follicles, and sweat and sebaceous glands as commensals. *P. acnes* is a cause of late post-surgical endophthalmitis.

***Clostridium* spp.** are ubiquitous, anaerobic and spore-forming. They are widely distributed in soil, and form part of the normal flora of the lower intestinal tract of humans and animals. They elaborate potent exotoxins that cause severe disease, including gas gangrene and food poisoning (*C. perfringens*), tetanus (*C. tetani*) and botulism (*C. botulinum*). *C. perfringens* may cause gas gangrene endophthalmitis.

***Nocardia* spp.** are aerobic, thin branching filamentous organisms. They are widespread in the environment and are opportunistic pathogens. *N. asteroides* can cause keratitis and endophthalmitis. Like mycobacteria, *Nocardia* spp. are often acid-fast.

***Actinomyces* spp.** are anaerobic and filamentous. They include *A. israelii* and *Tropheryoma whippeli*. *A. israelii*

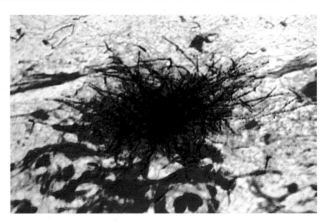

Figure 2.48 Gram-positive bacillus. *Actinomyces israelii*. Smear from lacrimal canaliculus.

(formerly known as streptothrix) causes actinomycosis and lacrimal caniculitis (Fig. 2.48). *T. whippeli* causes Whipple's disease, a disorder that affects the small bowel (steatorrhoea), the CNS (dementia, ophthalmoplegia, myoclonus), the joints (arthralgia, arthritis) and the skin (hyperpigmentation).

Gram-negative bacilli

***Pseudomonas* spp.** are aerobic and comprise a complex group of opportunistic pathogens of plants and animals including humans. The pathogen of major importance is *Ps. aeruginosa* (Fig. 2.49a) a ubiquitous motile organism that flourishes in many conditions including soil and vegetation, and moist situations in the hospital environment. It also colonizes the gastrointestinal tract. The widespread distribution of *Ps. aeruginosa* is made possible by its simple growth requirements, the possession of structural factors, and toxins that enhance virulence and render it resistant to many antibiotics. Most strains produce a blue-green pigment (pyocyanin) and a characteristic offensive odour in routine culture. Fimbriae-mediated adherence is a feature of its pathogenicity. Pseudomonas infections are primarily opportunistic, *Ps. aeruginosa* being a common cause of keratitis and endophthalmitis in eyes compromised by trauma or pre-existing disease. The source of the organism is often tap water or contaminated eye drops.

***Moraxella* spp.** are aerobic and frequently observed as diplobacilli (paired bacilli attached to each other – Fig. 2.49b). They share morphological features with *Neisseria* and *Branhamella*, and some confusion exists over their clas-sification. *M. lacunata* (Morax–Axenfeld diplobacillus) is a frequent cause of conjunctivitis and keratitis.

Enterobacteriaceae are facultative anaerobic or microaerophilic, and form the largest collection of important Gram-negative bacilli. A total of 30 genera and over

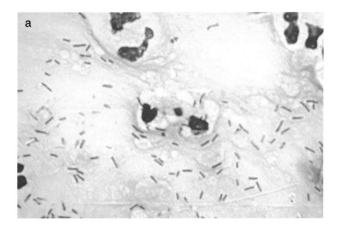

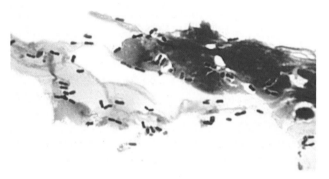

Figure 2.49 Gram-negative bacilli. (a) *Pseudomonas aeruginosa.* Vitreous smear. (b) *Moraxella spp.* Corneal smear.

120 species have been described, but more than 95 per cent of the important isolates belong to only 10 of the genera and constitute fewer than 25 species. Enterobacteriaceae occur in soil, water and vegetation, and are an important component of the intestinal flora where they are outnumbered only by Gram-negative aerobes such as *Bacterioides*. With the exception of *Salmonella* spp. and *Shigella* spp., most enterobacteriaceae, although non-pathogenic in the bowel, are important opportunistic ocular pathogens. *Escherichia coli*, *Klebsiella pneumoniae*, *Enterobacter aerogenes*, *Enterobacter cloacae* and *Proteus* spp. (*P. mirabilis*, *P. morgagni*) may all produce keratitis, while *Serratia marcescens* is a frequent contaminant of contact lens solutions.

Haemophilus spp. are aerobic and comprise many members, but only *H. influenzae* and *H. ducreyi* are of significance. *H. influenzae* is frequently coccobacillary, with six antigenic serotypes (a–f) and nine biotypes (I–VIII and *aegyptius*). *H. influenzae* can be isolated from the normal conjunctiva but, particularly in children in warmer climates, may cause acute conjunctivitis characterized by a mucopurulent discharge and petechial haemorrhages;

infection due to type b is particularly severe with the possible development of meningitis, septic arthritis or endophthalmitis. *H. influenza aegyptius* (Koch–Weeks bacillus) is a common pathogen in acute purulent conjunctivitis, and may occasionally cause severe keratitis by direct infiltration through intact corneal epithelium. In areas of endemic trachoma, *Haemophilus* spp. are associated with seasonal waves of epidemic conjunctivitis and may contribute to the intensity of trachomatous conjunctival inflammation. *H. ducreyi*, the causative organism of chancroid, can also cause Parinaud's oculoglandular syndrome.

Acinetobacter spp. are aerobic bacilli or diplobacilli. They are distributed in soil and water, and form part of the normal flora of the skin, nose, pharynx and gastro-intestinal tract. Ophthalmic infections due to these organisms include conjunctivitis, keratitis and endophthalmitis.

Francisella spp. are aerobic and include *F. tularensis*, which is widely distributed in nature among wild rodents, sheep and game birds. In humans, it is one of the causes of Parinaud's oculoglandular syndrome, less frequent causes of which are the related organisms *Yersinia* and *Pasteurella*.

Bartonella spp. are aerobes found in a variety of animal reservoirs. Insect vectors are known or have been implicated in human infections. *B. henselae* (the cat-scratch bacillus) causes cat-scratch disease, a subacute infection of the skin, soft tissues and regional lymph nodes that may follow contact with a cat or kitten. The ophthalmic manifestations of cat-scratch disease are those of Parinaud's oculoglandular syndrome.

Cocci, bacilli and ophthalmic infection

Conjunctivitis

Conjunctivitis, due to a multitude of Gram-positive and Gram-negative cocci and bacilli, is the commonest infective condition of the eye. It may be acute or chronic. It is usually acquired by hand to eye contact, but transmission may also be by fomites including contact lenses and vectors such as flies. Predisposing causes include coexistent acute or chronic upper respiratory infection, blepharitis, nasolacrimal duct obstruction, previous viral or chlamydial ophthalmic infection and contact lens wear. Acute conjunctivitis is characterized by foreign body sensation, lacrimation and redness accompanied by chemosis and lid swelling, stickiness of the lids and a mucopurulent or purulent discharge and, depending on the severity of the infection, membrane or pseudomembrane formation.

Infection is usually due to *S. aureus*, *S. epidermidis*, *S. pneumoniae*, *H. influenzae*, *M. lacunata* or *N. gonorrhoeae*. *S. aureus* conjunctivitis may be associated with staphylococcal blepharitis and *H. influenzae* infection occurs particularly in children. Contact lens wearers may develop infection due to *Ps. aeruginosa*, *Klebsiella* spp., *E. coli* and other coliforms. Membrane formation is associated with *C. diphtheriae* and *S. pyogenes*, while pseudomembrane formation is most commonly due to *S. pyogenes* and *N. gonorrhoeae*.

Infection lasting longer than 4 weeks is defined as chronic and is often associated with blepharitis or chronic dacryocystitis. The commonest causative organisms of chronic infection are *S. aureus* and *M. lacunata*.

Neonatal conjunctivitis (ophthalmia neonatorum) is a purulent discharge from the eye during the first 28 days of life. Geographic variations are evident in the causative agent but, in addition to *C. trachomatis*, *N. gonorrhoeae* is an important cause as it may lead to ocular perforation. Other causative agents include *Haemophilus* spp., *Staphylococcus* spp., *Streptococcus* spp., HSV and irritants such as silver nitrate and antiseptics used prophylactically at birth.

Investigations of bacterial conjunctivitis: conjunctival cultures should be taken prior to the start of therapy. Cultures from other sites may also be required, and these include the lid margins and meibomian secretion if there is associated blepharitis and/or meibomitis, the cervix and/or urethra if *N. gonorrhoeae* or *C. trachomatis* have been isolated, and the nasopharynx if *N. meningitidis* or *H. influenzae* are the cause. Culture of fomites may be necessary, and these include contact lenses, their solutions and cases, local medications and their containers, and ocular prostheses if their use parallels the duration of the conjunctivitis. In neonatal conjunctivitis, the examination of a Gram-stained smear of the discharge, conjunctival culture and culture of the maternal cervix are indicated.

Canaliculitis/dacryocystitis

Partial or complete blockage of the lacrimal drainage system predisposes to infection of the canaliculi (canaliculitis) and the lacrimal sac (dacryocystitis). Inflammation may be acute with abscess formation or chronic, and is typically associated with epiphora. Histological examination of excised sacs reveals acute and/or chronic inflammatory cells, granulation tissue and fibrous thickening of the sac wall. The epithelial lining may exhibit squamous metaplasia with an increased goblet cell population, and the causative organism may be demonstrable. *A. israelii* is the characteristic aetiological agent, particularly of canaliculitis, while infection of the sac is frequently due to *S. aureus* or streptococci. If the contents of the sac become inspissated, a small foreign body can act as a nidus for the formation of a dacryolith or concretions. Concretions are similar to a dacryolith, but are smaller and can sometimes be expressed from the canaliculus. Microscopy of dacryoliths and concretions may reveal the causative organism (often *A. israelii*) in association with large eosinophilic crystals, the nature of which is uncertain.

Keratitis

Gram-positive cocci (*S. aureus*, *S. epidermidis*, *S. pneumoniae*, *S. pyogenes*, *S. viridans*), Gram-negative cocci (*N. gonorrhoeae*, *N. meningitidis*), Gram-positive bacilli (*C. diphtheriae*, diphtheroids), Gram-negative bacilli (*Moraxella* spp., *Acinetobacter* spp., *E. coli*, *K. pneumoniae*, *Proteus* spp., *Ps. aeruginosa*, *S. marcescens* and other enteric bacteria) and Gram-positive filamentous bacilli (*N. asteroides*) all cause keratitis. *S. aureus*, *S. pneumoniae* and *Ps. aeruginosa* are among the commonest pathogens. Local predisposing causes of keratitis include trauma, contact lens wear and ocular surface disorders. Trauma may be mechanical or non-mechanical, all types of contact lenses have been implicated, and the ocular surface lesions that predispose to corneal infection include dry eye syndromes and other disorders that result in conjunctival scarring such as trachoma, ocular cicatricial pemphigoid and the Stevens–Johnson syndrome. Chronic alcoholics, sufferers from Parkinson's disease and those with debilitating or age changes who may have altered host defences such as reduced blinking, decreased tear flow, lowered tear lysozyme, chronic blepharitis, lid malposition with corneal exposure, and reduced corneal sensation are also all predisposed to keratitis. The immune state of the host probably determines the severity but not the susceptibility to corneal infection, which in the immunocompromised has a fulminant and prolonged course. Malnutrition, particularly if associated with xerophthalmia due to vitamin A deficiency, impairs defence mechanisms to post-traumatic infection. Symptoms of corneal infection include foreign body sensation, pain, photophobia and blepharospasm. Red swollen lids are accompanied by a purulent discharge. Clinical examination of the cornea reveals suppuration, usually centrally, with an overlying epithelial defect and adherent mucopurulent or purulent exudate. Intraocular involvement results in hypopyon, possibly secondary glaucoma and a mild vitritis. Keratitis with perforation can proceed to endophthalmitis.

Investigations of bacterial keratitis: the causative organisms may be demonstrable in corneal scrapes or cultured on appropriate media. Nucleic acid detection may be of value if the organism is not otherwise identifiable.

Endophthalmitis/panophthalmitis

Bacterial infection is the commonest cause, and may be exogenous or endogenous. Clinical features include pain, loss of vision, redness, and swelling of the lids and conjunctiva. Cells are present in the aqueous and may be sufficiently abundant to form a hypopyon, while the vitreous is invariably cloudy or opaque due to abscess formation (Fig. 2.50). Organization may result in phthisis bulbi.

Exogenous endophthalmitis develops when organisms enter the eye following perforation consequent upon infection of the cornea, injury or surgery. In the aphakic or pseudophakic eye with a posterior capsulotomy, access to the vitreous is facilitated and infection in the posterior segment readily follows that in the anterior segment. The incidence of endophthalmitis following perforating ocular trauma is variable, being reported as between 10 per cent and 65 per cent in different series. *Bacillus* spp. are frequent causative organisms; *S. aureus*, streptococci and coliforms are less common. Post-surgical endophthalmitis is rare and, while it can develop after any intraocular operation, the commonest surgical procedure that results in intraocular infection is cataract extraction with implantation of an intraocular lens. Sources of organisms include the patient (lid and conjunctival flora), the surgeon (hands, gloves, nares), contaminated instruments, implants, drugs, irrigations and infusions, and environmental airborne flora; pathogens include *S. aureus*, *S. pyogenes*, *S. pneumoniae* and enter-

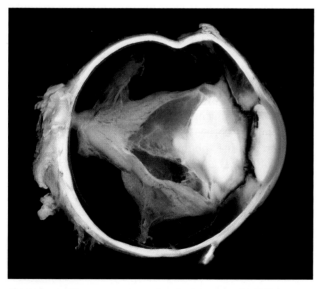

Figure 2.50 Exogenous endophthalmitis. Total hypopyon and vitreous abscess.

obacteriaceae. Some individuals do not develop post-surgical endophthalmitis for many months, and in these cases the most common organisms found are *P. acnes* and *S. epidermidis*. Fistula-producing procedures carried out for glaucoma are a constant concern because in the long term, bacteria (usually conjunctival flora) may infect the filtering bleb and enter the eye to produce endophthalmitis.

Endogenous endophthalmitis results from the haematogenous spread of organisms to the eye from a site of infection elsewhere in the body, or from contaminated intravenous catheters or needles. Meningitis, pneumonitis, urinary tract infections, endocarditis, septic arthritis, gastrointestinal infections and infected skin wounds may all lead to endogenous endophthalmitis, and the immunocompromised, the aged, diabetics and chronic alcoholics are the most susceptible. Organisms enter the eye through the retinal or uveal circulation, but in order to invade the ocular tissues and produce infection they must cross one of the blood–ocular barriers and establish a septic focus before breaking through into the aqueous or vitreous to produce a true endophthalmitis.

Investigations of bacterial endophthalmitis/panophthalmitis: microscopy of aqueous or vitreous taps may reveal the causative organism, which can be cultured on appropriate media. In chronic cases, culture may not be fruitful and nucleic acid detection may be required to identify the underlying pathogen.

Orbital cellulitis

Orbital cellulitis is usually secondary to infection in the ethmoid or maxillary sinus, but other causes include trauma (lacerations, insect bites, puncture wounds) and preseptal cellulitis resulting from an inflamed lid or lacrimal sac. Post-operative infection is rare, but may follow retinal detachment, strabismus or orbital surgery. Causative organisms include *S. aureus*, *S. pneumoniae*, *S. pyogenes* and *H. influenzae*; infection by *Clostridia* spp. can result in gas gangrene.

Gram-negative bacilli, autoimmune uveitis and arthritis

Infection with *Klebsiella* spp., *Salmonella* spp., *Shigella* spp., *Yersinia* spp., *Brucella* spp. (organisms found in cattle, sheep and goats that cause brucellosis) and *Campylobacter* spp. (curved organisms that cause gastrointestinal disease) has been implicated in the aetiology of autoimmune uveitis and reactive arthritis. An association with HLA-B27 may be due to the antibodies produced in response to infection cross-reacting with cell surface antigens.

Mycobacteria

Mycobacteria are non-motile, non-spore-forming aerobic bacilli, 1–10 μm in length. Over 74 species have been identified, but most human infections are due to *M. tuberculosis* (tuberculosis) or *M. leprae* (leprosy). Atypical mycobacteria including *M. avium*, *M. intracellulare*, *M. fortuitum* and *M. chelonae* are of importance in the immunocompromised. The cell walls of mycobacteria contain long-chain fatty acids (mycolic acids), which makes Gram staining difficult. *M. tuberculosis* and atypical mycobacteria resist decolourizing with acid and alcohol, and are thus acid- and alcohol-fast (AAFB) and are stained with Ziehl–Neelsen (Fig. 2.51a). *M. leprae* is only acid-fast (AFB) and is stained with Wade–Fite (Fig. 2.51b). *M. tuberculosis* and atypical mycobacteria are generally slow growing, and culture requires Löwenstein Jensen medium (glycerol, malachite green and whole egg). *M. leprae* cannot be cultured on artificial media.

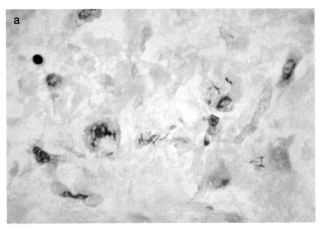

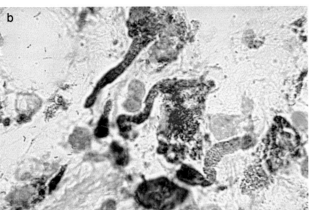

Figure 2.51 Mycobacteria. (a) *M. tuberculosis*. Bacilli in a granuloma. Ziehl–Neelsen stain. (b) *M. leprae*. Bacilli in uveal stroma. Wade–Fite stain.

Tuberculosis

M. tuberculosis is the principal causative organism of tuberculosis, a chronic necrotizing granulomatous disease. It is estimated that one-third of the world's population is infected, with 8 million new cases and 3 million deaths being reported each year. During the twentieth century the incidence of tuberculosis in developed countries declined until the mid-1980s. An apparent increase since then has been attributed to immigration from countries where the disease is endemic, to the increase in the number of those who are immunocompromised and to the possible increase in the prevalence of antibiotic-resistant strains.

Primary infection by *M. tuberculosis* in previously unexposed individuals is usually via the lungs, but other sites of entry include the gastrointestinal tract and skin. The organisms penetrate into macrophages and replicate. The macrophages migrate to the draining lymph nodes where secondary lesions develop. The characteristic histological lesion is a caseating granuloma (tubercle) which develops soon after the initial infection. In the lung, infection takes the form of a primary complex which comprises a small local granulomatous lesion (Ghon focus) and marked enlargement of the hilar lymph nodes. Those affected are usually children or young adults who are either asymptomatic or have a relatively mild fever. Subsequent events depend on the immune state of the individual. If the cell-mediated response is sufficiently aggressive, bacterial multiplication ceases, the organisms remain localized and the primary lesion heals by fibrosis, often with calcification and viable organisms sequestered within. If the primary immune response is insufficient to halt bacterial replication, areas of caseation undergo liquefaction due to the release of hydrolytic enzymes from macrophages. Multiplying mycobacteria then spread locally within the lungs or via the blood stream to be disseminated throughout the body. Local pulmonary involvement is manifest as pneumonitis, and haematogenous dissemination results in multi-organ involvement.

Infection in an individual with a past history of primary infection produces post-primary disease, which is exogenous or endogenous. Exogenous post-primary disease originates from inhaled mycobacteria, while endogenous post-primary disease arises from multiplication of mycobacteria lying dormant within primary lesions. In post-primary disease, necrosis is more extensive and lesions enlarge to form tumour-like masses (tuberculomas). The extensive necrosis is due to the release of TNFs, proteases and other digestive enzymes from activated macrophages. Pulmonary involvement is manifest as chronic progressive pneumonitis with abscess formation and cavitation. Extrapulmonary disease includes scrofula (painless lymphadenitis, usually cervical), peritonitis, pericarditis, genitourinary involvement, spondylitis (Pott's disease), articular and osseous tuberculosis, chronic skin disease (lupus vulgaris), CNS involvement (meningitis, intracranial tuberculomas) and infection of the eye and ocular adnexae.

Ophthalmic tuberculosis

The incidence of ophthalmic tuberculosis mirrors that of systemic disease and arises from active infection or an immune response to local or systemic infection. Active infection may follow direct inoculation, contiguous spread from adjacent structures, or haematogenous dissemination from other infected pulmonary or extrapulmonary sites. The lids, conjunctiva and orbit, the cornea, episclera and sclera, and the uvea, retina and optic nerve may all be involved.

Primary infection of the lids is rare, and lid involvement is usually secondary to contiguous spread of lupus vulgaris. Tuberculosis of the conjunctiva results from primary inoculation, secondary spread from the face or adjacent sinuses, or haematogenous dissemination. Features vary from acute purulent or pseudomembranous conjunctivitis to chronic granulomatous inflammation. Primary conjunctivitis may be accompanied by lymphadenopathy (Parinaud's oculoglandular syndrome) but, in secondary tuberculous infection, lymph node involvement is unusual. Orbital infection is the result of local infiltration or haematogenous spread, and can present as chronic cellulitis, periostitis, osteomyelitis, abscess formation and chronic dacryoadenitis.

Corneal involvement is relatively common in tuberculous infection. It is usually due to an immune-mediated reaction (phlyctenular keratoconjunctivitis, interstitial keratitis), but may be secondary to spread from adjacent structures (sclerokeratitis). Episcleritis results from hypersensitivity to mycobacterial antigens, while tuberculous scleritis may follow contiguous spread from adjacent tissue or haematogenous dissemination.

Any part of the uvea may be affected, but the choroid is particularly vulnerable because of its rich blood supply. Solitary or multiple choroidal granulomas, yellowish-white nodules with indistinct borders ranging in size from 0.5 mm–2 cm in diameter, are the commonest ocular manifestation of tuberculosis. They are usually unilateral, fewer than five in number and affect the posterior pole. Spontaneous resolution leaves choroidoretinal scars. Isolated retinal tuberculosis is rare and retinal involvement is usually the result of extension from choroidal disease, which may be associated with exudative retinal detachment and possibly severe endophthalmitis. Retinal vasculitis is probably an immune-mediated reaction. Inflammatory tuberculous optic neuropathy is due to infiltration of the nerve secondary to tuberculous meningitis. Papilloedema may be a consequence of increased intracranial pressure.

Investigations for tuberculosis

Chest X-ray and sputum examination are standard investigative procedures in suspected tuberculous disease. In the Mantoux skin test, tuberculin antigen (purified protein derivative – PPD) is injected intradermally and a firm swelling, maximal at 48–72 hours after injection, is indicative of prior exposure to *M. tuberculosis*. Accessible localized suspected tuberculous lesions can be investigated histologically and material can be taken for culture and nucleic acid detection.

Leprosy

M. leprae is the causative organism of leprosy (Hansen's disease), a chronic, slowly progressive destructive disease of the skin, mucous membranes and peripheral nerves. The organism replicates only very slowly and is grown in experimental animals (e.g. armadillos, mice) at peripheral sites (e.g. the footpad) that are cooler than core body temperature. Leprosy is not easily transmitted, and years of contact with infected individuals are often necessary for the disease to become established. The mycobacteria are shed in nasal secretions or from cutaneous lesions and probably enter the body via breaks in the skin or mucous membranes. Leprosy is rare in developed countries but endemic in parts of Africa, Asia, and Central and South America, where there are an estimated 15 million cases. Most individuals have a natural protective immunity and only a small proportion of those exposed to infection are at risk of developing the disease. During an incubation period of many years, *M. leprae* grows within epidermal/epithelial cells, macrophages and the Schwann cells of peripheral nerves. The onset of disease is gradual, with a range of inflammatory activity depending on the degree of cell-mediated immunity. Clinical features and biopsy results allow for classification into three overlapping forms: lepromatous, borderline and tuberculoid (Madrid classification), with further subdivision into intermediate forms, borderline tuberculoid and borderline lepromatous (modified Ridley and Jopling classification – Table 2.4). A further indeterminate early form of the disease cannot be classified.

Lepromatous leprosy (LL) develops when an adequate immune response to *M. leprae* fails to develop and proliferation of the organism continues relentlessly over many years. The lesions are multiple and diffuse, and initially affect the skin and peripheral nerves of the cooler portions of the body. Skin lesions are seen as multiple erythematous macules, papules or nodules,

Table 2.4 Modified Ridley and Jopling classification of leprosy

		Cell-mediated immunity	Presence of *M. leprae*
Lepromatous	LL	+	+ + + + (multibacillary)
Borderline lepromatous	BL	+ +	+ + + +
Borderline	BB	+ + +	+ + +
Borderline tuberculoid	BT	+ + + +	+ +
Tuberculoid	TT	+ + + + +	+ (paucibacillary)

and the facial skin thickens to produce the characteristic lion-like facial appearance (leonine facies). Extensive destruction of cartilage and bone leads to a saddle-nose, pendulous ear lobes, claw-shaped hands, hammer toes and other deformities. Neural involvement results in patchy sensory loss. Multiple, highly infectious, tumour-like lesions are present in the skin, eyes, testes, nerves, lymph nodes and spleen. Foamy (lipid-laden) macrophages form nodular or diffuse infiltrates and contain large numbers of mycobacteria (multibacillary), but an inflammatory response is lacking.

Tuberculoid leprosy (TT) occurs in infected individuals who exhibit a brisk cell-mediated immune response. The resulting granulomatous inflammation limits bacterial proliferation and thereby confines the disease to the skin and cutaneous nerves. Skin lesions are few in number, and consist of well-defined erythematous or hypopigmented plaques with flat centres. Involvement of peripheral nerves leads to their visible enlargement and complete sensory loss. Ophthalmic involvement is less common than in the lepromatous form. The lesions cause little disfigurement and are not infectious. The granulomatous response resembles that of tuberculosis, and only a few mycobacteria are seen (paucibacillary).

Borderline leprosy (BB) has characteristics of both the tuberculoid and lepromatous forms of the disease with intermediate clinical, histological and immunological features. There are variable presentations of skin and peripheral nerve involvement with internal organ and ophthalmic manifestations. Affected individuals may remain stable or progress towards one of the polar forms when their condition may be classified as borderline tuberculoid (BT) or borderline lepromatous (BL). The histological appearance of the lesions has the characteristics of the polar forms of the disease, with a mixture of macrophages and lymphocytes and a variable number of *M. leprae*.

Reactions or reactional states are episodes of acute or chronic inflammation resulting in sudden worsening of symptoms and can occur in any type of leprosy (except indeterminate). They usually follow treatment but may be spontaneous and are probably manifestations of the immune response to components of disrupted and dying mycobacteria. The two main groups are non-lepromatous and lepromatous lepra reactions.

Non-lepromatous lepra reactions (reversal, upgrading, Jopling Type I reactions) occur in BT, BB and BL weeks to months after starting treatment. Lesions become swollen and erythematous and may ulcerate and lead to unsightly scarring. A painful neuritis may develop and can present as a facial nerve palsy. The reaction usually lasts for several months, after which the disease often changes in character towards tuberculoid.

Lepromatous lepra reactions (erythema nodosum leprosum, Jopling Type 2 reactions) occur only at the LL end of the spectrum where up to 50 per cent of those treated suffer from one or more episodes. It presents on the extensor surfaces of the limbs with rapid onset of painful erythematous papules, which gradually subside to leave dark staining of the skin. Associated features include malaise, afternoon fever, bone pain, painful neuritis, acute lymphadenitis, epididymo-orchitis, large-joint arthritis, nephritis and uveitis. The severity ranges from a mild acute illness to severe life-threatening disease. The histological appearance of the lesions resembles the Arthus phenomenon, with a polymorphonuclear cellular infiltrate, vasculitis and degenerating foam cells in addition to resolving lepromatous granulomas with identifiable *M. leprae*.

Ophthalmic leprosy

Ophthalmic leprosy is a potentially blinding condition and, in endemic areas, a significant cause of preventable visual disability. The predilection for the eye probably relates to the preference for *M. leprae* to grow optimally at cooler temperatures. The different types of systemic disease exhibit considerable overlap in their ophthalmic features. Ophthalmic involvement is more common in LL, in which intraocular complications, particularly the various forms of uveitis, are frequent. Those with TT tend to have external eye disease such as lagophthalmos, exposure keratitis and corneal opacities.

Madarosis is a common manifestation, particularly of tuberculoid leprosy. Lagophthalmos and lower lid entropion result from VIIth cranial nerve involvement, which tends to occur early in tuberculoid disease but late in the lepromatous form. Lid nodules may develop in lepromatous disease in which *M. leprae* infiltrate the marginal and pretarsal fibres of the orbicularis oculi muscle, leading to loss of skin elasticity and muscle tone, dermatochalasis and heavy drooping upper lids, ectropion, entropion and trichiasis. Lacrimal gland and meibomian gland involvement result in dry eye. Exposure keratopathy is common and can lead to secondary bacterial infection, perforation and blindness. Involvement of the Vth cranial nerve, particularly in lepromatous disease, causes conjunctival and corneal anaesthesia with subsequent neuropathic damage, and this is further compounded by pre-existing lid disease, trichiasis and dry eye syndrome. Intraneural spread of *M. leprae* into the cornea results in enlarged oedematous beaded corneal nerves (string of pearls) due to granulomatous inflammation; this appearance is pathognomonic of leprosy and may be the first clinical sign of the disease. Avascular keratitis, interstitial keratitis and corneal lepromas (large granulomas) may also develop. Episcleritis and scleritis are common, and may be due to direct bacillary invasion or immune mechanisms such as the deposition of immune complexes. Focal lepromas develop in the cooler interpalpebral region and present as nodular episcleritis. Chronic or recurrent scleritis in leprosy results in scleromalacia, staphyloma or phthisis bulbi.

There may be an acute fulminant anterior and intermediate uveitis or a chronic low-grade insidious anterior uveitis. Acute fulminant anterior and intermediate uveitis is severe and occurs in the erythema nodosum leprosum reaction, probably as the result of a hypersensitivity reaction. It usually occurs at the start of therapy or follows termination of treatment, and is characterized by an abrupt onset with rapid progression to hypopyon, iridolenticular adhesion, elevated intraocular pressure and occasionally spontaneous hyphaema. Chronic low-grade insidious anterior uveitis in LL is a frequent cause of blindness. An insidious anterior uveitis and local sympathetic autonomic neuropathy result in iris atrophy and constricted non-reactive pupils. Signs of acute inflammation are minimal, with few anterior chamber cells, mild to moderate aqueous flare and no or few iridolenticular adhesions. A few scattered fine keratic precipitates may be present. Iris pearls are microlepromas, appearing as superficial chalky white particles on the iris surface, at the pupillary margin or in the inferior angle, and are pathognomonic for ocular leprosy. Cataract or secondary glaucoma may ensue. The ocular changes result from direct invasion of *M. leprae* or immune reactions to bacterial antigens. Macrophages, lymphocytes and plasma cells are seen and *M. leprae* are demonstrable.

Spiral bacteria (spirochaetes)

Spiral bacteria are thin helical bacilli, 5–20 μm in length, with flagellate-like structures that permit spiral motility. They share many features with Gram-negative bacilli and are a significant cause of disease world-wide. They include *Treponema pallidum*, *Borrelia burgdoferi* and *Leptospira interrogans*. *T. pallidum* cannot be grown on artificial media. It is too thin to be seen by light micro-

scopy in Gram- or Giemsa-stained sections, and silver impregnation (Warthin–Starry stain) or electron microscopy is necessary (Fig. 2.52). Motile organisms in infected secretions can be identified by darkground illumination or immunofluorescence. The organism is fragile and susceptible to heat or drying, and transmission necessitates close contact such as occurs in sexual intercourse. *B. burgdoferi* is transmitted by ticks of the *Ixodes* genus and is the cause of Lyme disease. *L. interrogans* is the cause of leptospirosis in wild and domestic animals. The principal reservoirs are rats, dogs, cats, pigs, cattle and horses. Human infection (Weil's disease) is the result of inoculation of mucous membranes, such as the conjunctiva, by infected urine. The predominant ophthalmic manifestation of Weil's disease is haemorrhagic conjunctivitis.

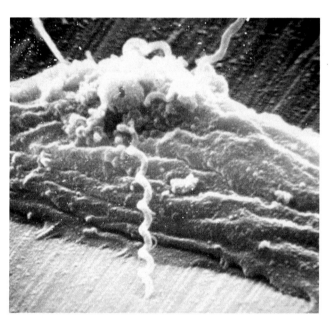

Figure 2.52 Spiral bacteria. *Treponema pallidum*. SEM.

Syphilis

T. pallidum is the causative organism of syphilis, a sexually transmitted disease that is now uncommon in developed countries, but remains an important cause of disease elsewhere, with an estimated 12 million new cases occurring each year. Syphilis may be acquired or congenital, and ophthalmic manifestations occur in both.

Acquired syphilis

Acquired syphilis is almost always sexually transmitted. There are three stages: primary, secondary and tertiary.

In primary syphilis, *T. pallidum* enters the body through small breaks in the skin or mucous membranes and slowly replicates. After an incubation period of 2–10 weeks, a painless ulcerated papule (chancre) develops at the site of inoculation. Regional lymph nodes are enlarged, but the lesions resolve spontaneously. Histological examination in the early stages reveals neutrophils, a fibrinous exudate and numerous organisms. Later, the picture is one of an endarteritis; lymphocytes, plasma cells and macrophages are seen, the endothelium of the small vessels is swollen and the obliterated vascular lumen results in tissue necrosis. At the time of primary infection spirochaetes invade regional lymph nodes where they proliferate. Two to three months later some of those affected develop secondary syphilis, a febrile illness comprising generalized lymphadenopathy, headache, myalgia and a maculopapular skin rash. Other lesions include condylomata lata (exudative lesions containing a large number of spirochaetes affecting the perineum, vulva or scrotum), follicular syphilids (papular lesions around hair follicles causing hair loss) and nummular syphilids (circular lesions of the face and perineum). Whitish patches develop on the mucous membranes of the mouth, conjunctiva and pharynx, and may progress into snail track ulcers.

If secondary syphilis is untreated, spirochaetes either lie dormant or continue to multiply and slowly give rise to the lesions of tertiary syphilis. There is often a latent period of years or decades before clinical features become manifest, and any organ of the body may be affected. Most of the lesions result from focal ischaemic necrosis secondary to obliterative endarteritis. The three principal manifestations of tertiary syphilis are cardiovascular syphilis, neurosyphilis and progressive destructive disease. Cardiovascular syphilis is due to obliterative endarteritis of the vasa vasora of the aorta, and results in aortitis, aortic aneurysm and aortic valve incompetence. Neurosyphilis comprises a range of disorders resulting from slowly progressive involvement of the CNS, and includes meningitis, meningovascular neurosyphilis with cerebrovascular occlusions, and parenchymatous neurosyphilis that results in tabes dorsalis (spinal cord involvement) and general paralysis of the insane (cerebral cortex involvement). Progressive destructive disease results from gumma formation (granulomatous inflammation) in any tissue, but particularly in the skin, bone and joints.

Congenital syphilis

Transplacental transmission of *T. pallidum* may occur throughout pregnancy, but the fetus is affected only after the third month when its immune system is developed. The fetus may abort, the child may be stillborn or die shortly after birth, or the lesions of congenital syphilis may appear. The skin and mucous membranes and the bones, liver, lungs and teeth may all be affected, as may the eyes. Early congenital syphilis appears within 3 weeks of birth with mucocutaneous lesions and osteochondritis. Disseminated disease causes hepatosplenomegaly, anaemia, thrombocytopenia, pneumonitis. Rhinitis (snuffles) and osteitis of the nasal bones result in the characteristic saddle-nose deformity and hypertelorism. Other stigmata include deformities of bone (sabre shins) and teeth (Hutchinson's teeth), bilateral knee effusions (Clutton's joints) and deafness.

Ophthalmic syphilis

Acquired disease

All three stages of acquired syphilis can involve ophthalmic structures. Chancres of the lid and conjunctiva are very rare but not unknown. In secondary syphilis, the lid skin may exhibit a maculopapular rash and there may be associated papillary conjunctivitis. In tertiary syphilis, gummas may affect the lids. Corneal involvement in primary and secondary syphilis is rare, but unilateral stromal (interstitial) keratitis occurs in tertiary syphilis. Episcleritis can occur in secondary syphilis while in tertiary syphilis scleritis, although rare, may be the only clinical manifestation.

Anterior and/or posterior uveitis occurs in the secondary and tertiary stages of syphilis. In secondary syphilis, anterior uveitis begins as an acute unilateral iritis or iridocyclitis of varying severity. Posterior uveitis during secondary syphilis is either diffuse or localized, and may develop into lesions that clinically resemble retinitis pigmentosa. In tertiary syphilis the severity of the inflammation, particularly in the anterior segment, is variable, with Koeppe and Busacca nodules and solitary or miliary granulomas being seen. Posterior uveitis in tertiary syphilis can lead to breaks in Bruch's membrane that predispose to subretinal neovascularization. Neuroretinitis occurs in association with neurosyphilis. Papillitis with venous engorgement is seen together with flame-shaped haemorrhages, arteriolar sheathing, retinal thickening and exudates. Residual changes include optic atrophy and pigment mottling. Cranial nerve palsies are a complication of basilar meningitis. Visual field defects can result from occlusive vasculitis affecting visual pathways. The Argyll–Robertson pupil, a miotic pupil that reacts to accommodation but not to light, is probably due to degenerative changes in the rostral mid-brain.

Congenital disease

Ophthalmic complications of early congenital syphilis are analogous to those of acquired secondary syphilis and the commonest manifestation is uveitis, usually posterior, which begins as subclinical multifocal inflammation of the choriocapillaris. Post-inflammatory changes are seen as diffusely scattered foci of choroidoretinal atrophy, patchy proliferation of the RPE and attenuated retinal blood vessels, giving rise to the characteristic salt and pepper fundal appearance. Histological features include choroidoretinal adhesion, outer retinal atrophy and RPE disturbance. Anterior uveitis may be acute and results in complications such as glaucoma and cataract. In late congenital syphilis the commonest inflammatory feature is bilateral (cf. acquired syphilis) non-ulcerative stromal (interstitial) keratitis, which affects 40 per cent of surviving untreated cases. It usually presents between the ages of 5 and 25 years with pain and blurred vision. The corneal mid-stroma is oedematous and infiltrated by lymphocytes and plasma cells. Later, the central area becomes vascularized (salmon-patch appearance). If untreated the keratitis may last for several months, but it usually regresses to leave a scarred cornea with vascular remnants (ghost vessels).

Investigations for syphilis

T. pallidum is poorly staining and not visualized by conventional light microscopy. The organisms can be demonstrated in material obtained from the infectious sites of primary and secondary syphilis, and can be seen using darkground illumination, phase contrast microscopy, silver staining, fluorescent microscopy and electron microscopy. Serological tests of importance in establishing a diagnosis fall into two groups: non-treponemal and treponemal tests. Non-treponemal tests detect IgG and IgM antilipoidal antibodies produced in response to the membrane lipids of *T. pallidum*. The Venereal Disease Research Laboratory (VDRL) is one such test, but lacks specificity and may give false positive reactions, particularly in infectious mononucleosis, viral hepatitis, leprosy and autoimmune disease. Treponemal tests detect specific IgG and IgM antitreponemal antibodies. The *T. pallidum* immobilization (TPI) and fluorescent treponemal antibody absorption (FTA-Abs) tests are those most often used. The FTA-Abs is the first to become positive in syphilis, and usually remains positive after treatment.

Lyme disease

Lyme disease, a chronic staged progressive infection caused by *B. burgdoferi*, is characterized by remissions and exacerbations. It occurs world-wide, with endemic foci distributed throughout North America, Europe and Northern Asia. The organism reproduces locally at the site of inoculation, spreads to regional lymph nodes and is disseminated in the blood. Localized infection (stage 1) is characterized by a rash (erythema migrans) at the site of inoculation and regional lymphadenopathy. Systemic features include fever, malaise, headache and arthralgia. There are no ophthalmic manifestations. Systemic infection (stage 2) begins several weeks to months after the initial rash, with migratory musculoskeletal pains, CNS involvement (meningitis, cranial nerve palsies) and cardiac abnormalities (atrioventricular block, left ventricular dysfunction, acute myopericarditis and pancarditis). Apart from neuro-ophthalmic abnormalities (optic neuropathy, pupillary anomalies, blepharospasm) associated with CNS infection, ophthalmic involvement includes follicular conjunctivitis and uveitis (anterior, posterior and panuveitis). Persistent infection (stage 3) begins months to years after inoculation, and is characterized by arthritis (large joint arthritis), dermatitis (acrodermatitis chronica atrophicans) and variable CNS manifestations (paraesthesiae, encephalitis, transverse myelitis). Ophthalmic involvement includes episcleritis, stromal keratitis, orbital myositis and cortical blindness. IgM and IgG antibodies to *B. burgdoferi* can be detected by direct immunofluorescence or enzyme immunoassay.

FUNGI

Fungi are eukaryotes varying in size from 2 μm upwards. They occur widely in nature, but relatively few cause disease in humans although increasing numbers are being recognized as opportunistic pathogens. They have multiple chromosomes containing both DNA and RNA, and their rigid cell walls consist of chitin or cellulose in a mixture of proteins and lipids. Fungi exist as mycelia or yeasts, but these terms are not formal taxons. A mycelium is a multinucleate mass of cytoplasm enclosed within a filamentous system of tubes that arises when spores germinate and put out long threads (hyphae) that branch as they elongate. Yeasts do not have the mycelial pattern but are ovoid structures and reproduce by budding. Some fungi can switch between a mycelial and yeast form depending on environmental conditions such as temperature. Reproduction of fungi is asexual or sexual, and their morphology exhibits marked variations during their life cycle. The form appearing after asexual division (anamorph) is often distinct from the form appearing after sexual reproduction (teleomorph). The same fungus may exist in both forms. Asexual spores form at the tips of hyphae and are of two general types, conidia and sporangiospores: conidia are naked, whereas sporangiospores are produced within a sac-like structure known as a sporangium. Most fungi require contact between two compatible mycelia for sexual reproduction, although some produce two kinds of sex cells on a single mycelium.

Growth and culture

The growth and cultural requirements of fungi are similar to those of cocci and bacilli. They grow best on Sabouraud's medium (glucose–peptone agar, pH 5.6, enriched with yeast extract and chloramphenicol) and in brain–heart infusion.

Staining

Fungi are best demonstrated in smears and tissues with Grocott's hexamine (methenamine) silver, which stains their cell walls black, and periodic acid-Schiff (PAS), which stains them magenta. Most yeasts are also Gram-positive.

Fungal infection in ophthalmology

Fungi form part of the normal flora of the lids and conjunctiva in about 20–25 per cent of the population, and are commoner in warmer climates and in those who work outdoors. Most fungal infections of the eye result from spores produced by anamorphs of opportunistic fungi. It is rare for more than one strain to be involved, and only the anamorph is seen in smears and cultures. Factors that predispose to fungal infection of the eye (oculomycosis) include pre-existing lesions such as corneal epithelial defects, reduced local defences as may occur with the local use of antibiotics or corticosteroids, and a compromised immune system as may result from immunosuppressive therapy or a disease such as AIDS. Fungi gain access to the eye and orbital tissues by direct inoculation, spread from adjacent structures, or haematogenous spread from a distant site. In the immunocompromised virtually any species of fungus is capable of causing infection of the eye and orbit, and the commonest that do so are commensals of the conjunctiva and the respiratory, gastrointestinal and female genital tracts. Pathogenic fungi may cause direct physical damage relating to adherence, penetration and replication of the organism. Tissue injury also results from the production of toxins (mycotoxins) and enzymes by the fungi and from the host response.

Classification

Fungal classification is complex and largely based on the mechanism of spore formation. Various systems of classification exist, but essentially there is a primary division into lower and higher fungi.

Lower fungi (zygomycetes)

These form sporangiospores and have non-septate hyphae. When hyphae of two compatible strains of zygomycetes meet, each produces a short branch, which divides to form cells known as gametangia. The gametangia fuse to produce a thick-walled zygospore. Meiosis occurs when the zygospore germinates, the growing hypha produces a sporangium and its haploid spores develop into mycelia. Lower fungi include *Rhizopus*, *Absidia* and *Mucor*, *Pneumocystis carinii* and *Rhinosporidium seeberi*.

Rhizopus, Absidia and Mucor are ubiquitous in soil and vegetable material. They are among the normal flora of the nose and pharynx, and can be cultured from almost any body orifice. The metabolically inert sporangiospores are routinely inhaled but, in healthy individuals, fail to germinate. Should they germinate, they cause mucormycosis, the patterns of which include rhino-orbito-cerebral, gastrointestinal, pulmonary and cutaneous forms. The rhino-orbito-cerebral type is the commonest and the one with ophthalmic manifestations.

Pneumocystis carinii grows slowly in the alveoli of the lungs of immunocompetent individuals. The organism is widespread throughout the world, and a large proportion of the population has antibodies to it. It causes a pneumonitis-like condition which is usually asymptomatic but is manifest in up to 85 per cent of those with AIDS. Extrapulmonary involvement is rare and results from haematogenous dissemination. Choroidal pneumocystosis in AIDS is usually asymptomatic, bilateral and characterized by one or more discrete yellow-white subretinal plaques at the posterior pole. The lesions enlarge as the organisms invade the adjacent choroid but resolve to leave large areas of choroidal atrophy. CMV retinitis may coexist. Microscopy of lesions reveals collections of *P. carinii* surrounded by a frothy material; inflammatory activity is absent.

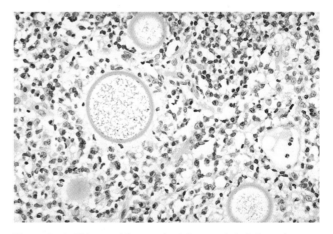

Figure 2.53 *Rhinosporidium seeberi*. Sporangia in inflamed conjunctival stroma.

Rhinosporidium seeberi infects the nasal mucosa and conjunctiva, where polyps form and appear as solid, irregularly lobulated pinkish-red masses. *R. seeberi* are seen within the polyps as white spherical structures containing sporangiospores (Fig. 2.53).

Higher fungi (ascomycetes, basidiomycetes and conidial fungi)

These form conidia on the tips of septate hyphae, but are not considered as multicellular because each septum has a pore that allows free movement of cytoplasm and nuclei. Based on the mechanism of reproduction, higher fungi are classified as ascomycetes, basidiomycetes or conidial fungi.

Ascomycetes have distinct male or female structures – i.e. they are heterothallic. When strains of opposite sex come into contact, the structures fuse to form a multi-nucleated zygote (ascogonium). A short hypha containing a nucleus sprouts from each parent in the ascogonium, the nuclei fuse, and genetic recombination is followed by meiosis and mitosis. Spores are produced endogenously in the elongating hypha, which is termed an ascus. The ascus ruptures, spores are released and a new round of haploid growth commences.

Basidiomycetes also reproduce sexually. Mycelia of suitably mating types fuse to form a club-shaped structure (basidium). Fusion of nuclei is followed by meiosis and mitosis leading to the production of four spores attached to the end of the basidium. A droplet of liquid appears at each point of attachment, hydrostatic pressure builds up and the spores break away.

Conidial fungi are otherwise known as imperfect fungi. A sexual cycle has not been observed in their reproduction, but most are considered to be heterothallic ascomycetes that either have strict mating requirements or have lost the ability to produce sexual spores. Conidial fungi are regarded as a provisional group only, and the discovery of a sexual stage in their reproduction will lead to them being moved into the ascomycetes or basidiomycetes group.

Higher fungi include *Fusarium* spp., *Aspergillus* spp., *Histoplasma capsulatum*, *Candida* spp., *Cryptococcus neoformans* and *Coccidioides immitis*.

***Fusarium* spp.** commonly grow on vegetable material and many are plant pathogens. *F. solani* is an anamorph; its teleomorph is an ascomycete. It is one of the commonest ocular fungal pathogens and causes keratitis and endophthalmitis.

***Aspergillus* spp.** are anamorphs; their teleomorphs are ascomycetes. *A. fumigatus* and *A. flavus* are important ophthalmic pathogens and cause keratitis (Fig. 2.54), endophthalmitis and orbital cellulitis.

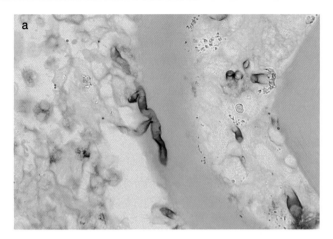
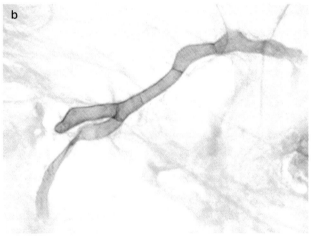

Figure 2.54 *Aspergillus spp.* (a) *A. fumigatus*. Corneal smear. Grocott hexamine (methenamine) silver stain. (b) *A. flavus*. Corneal smear. PAS stain.

Histoplasma capsulatum is an anamorph and grows as a yeast at 37°C and as a mycelium in soil; its teleomorph is an ascomycete. *H. capsulatum* is endemic to the central and south-eastern United States (particularly the Mississippi and Ohio River Valleys), Puerto Rico, and parts of Central America, Asia, Italy, Turkey, Israel and Australia. Human infection may result from the inhalation of the organism. Most cases are asymptomatic, but an acute pneumonitis (infectious histoplasmosis) occurs in about 5 per cent of infections. The manifestations of ocular involvement are infectious endophthalmitis, solitary choroidoretinal granulomas and the presumed ocular histoplasmosis syndrome. Histoplasma endophthalmitis and solitary choroidoretinal granulomas (histoplasmomas) are rare but occur in the immunocompromised. Choroidal granulomas may clinically mimic ocular toxocariasis.

Presumed ocular histoplasmosis syndrome (POHS) is a multifocal choroidopathy (Fig. 2.55) associated with *H. capsulatum*. Koch's postulates have not as yet been

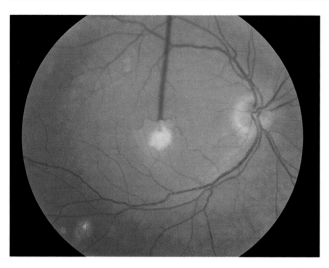

Figure 2.55 *Histoplasma capsulatum*. Presumed ocular histoplasmosis syndrome; maculopathy and histo spot.

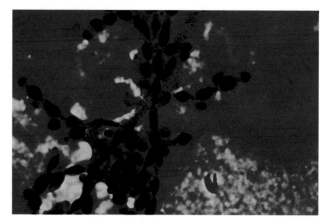

Figure 2.56 *Candida albicans*. Culture from a corneal ulcer. Gram stain.

fulfilled, and identical clinical features are found in non-endemic areas in those with no immunological evidence of previous exposure to *H. capsulatum*. POHS is more common than infectious histoplasmosis and, in those cases where previous histoplasma infection can be demonstrated, it is thought to be immune-mediated. The initial infection is accompanied by transient fungaemia and the organisms are taken up by the choroidal vascular endothelium, resulting in a bilateral asymptomatic multifocal choroiditis that heals to leave atrophic scars (histo spots). Five to fifteen years later, principally in the 20–45 years age group, macular scars become symptomatic due to the development of choroidal neovascularization that leads to a subretinal membrane or plaque interposed between Bruch's membrane and the RPE. Lesions in the region of the optic disc result in peripapillary atrophy. The pathogenic mechanism is unknown, but there is a significant association with HLA-B7 and HLA-DRw2 haplotypes, particularly in disease with choroidal neovascularization.

Candida spp. are yeast-like conidial fungi. *C. albicans* is part of the normal flora of the mouth, gastrointestinal tract and vagina. It is an important ocular pathogen causing keratitis (Fig. 2.56) and intraocular infection.

Cryptococcus neoformans is a yeast-like anamorph in the same family as *Candida albicans*; the teleomorph is a basidiomycete. *C. neoformans*, the causative agent of cryptococcosis, is found in many natural environments and grows particularly well in bird droppings. It is an important CNS pathogen in the immunocompromised and causes meningitis, which frequently results in papilloedema, optic neuropathy and chiasmal involvement;

other neuro-ophthalmic manifestations include cranial nerve palsies, nystagmus and internuclear ophthalmoplegia. The commonest intraocular lesion in cryptococcosis is choroidoretinitis. The organism can be grown from the CSF in cryptococcal meningitis.

Coccidioides immitis is a fungus that grows as a mycelium with arthrospores in soil and as a spherule with endospores in tissue. It occurs in arid climates such as those of Central and South America, and Mexico. It is the causative agent of coccidioidomycosis, the ophthalmic manifestations of which include lid infection, conjunctivitis and choroidoretinitis.

Fungal keratitis

Fungal infection of the cornea is unusual, but may follow trauma (often trivial) associated with plant material. The causative organisms include *Candida* spp., *Fusarium* spp. and *Aspergillus* spp. The onset is insidious, with clinical features becoming manifest days or weeks following inoculation. The corneal surface is dry and rough, appearing dirty white or grey, and the margins of the infected area are irregular with grey lines radiating outwards. Satellite microabscesses develop and eventually central sloughing leaves a deep ulcer. A descemetocele may form and the cornea may perforate. Scarring is ultimately severe, but vascularization is not a conspicuous feature. The histological features are non-specific; neutrophils infiltrate from the limbal vascular arcades and the precorneal tear film, and the enzymes produced, together with mycotoxins, bring about the destruction of tissue. Fungal elements may be seen (Fig. 2.57). The causative organisms may be demonstrable on microscopy of corneal scrapes, and can be cultured on appropriate media.

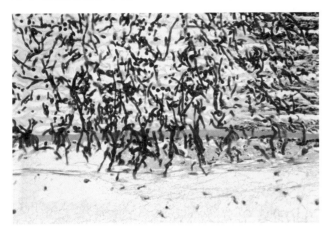

Figure 2.57 Fungal keratitis. Fungal elements in deep corneal stroma. PAS stain.

Fungal endophthalmitis

Fungal endophthalmitis is exogenous or endogenous. Hypopyon and vitreous abscess develop, and phthisis bulbi may be the end result. Clinical diagnosis is often delayed because the cause is not suspected, but organisms may be visible on microscopy of anterior chamber and vitreous taps and may be grown on appropriate media. The reaction seen histologically is often granulomatous.

Exogenous endophthalmitis occurs when fungi, usually *Candida* spp., *Fusarium* spp. or *Aspergillus* spp., enter the eye following fungal keratitis with perforation. Implantation of plant fibre (particularly wood) due to a perforating injury may also lead to fungal endophthalmitis, but post-surgical fungal endophthalmitis is exceptionally rare.

Endogenous endophthalmitis occurs when fungal elements reach the eye via the blood stream. It is invariably produced by one of the *Candida* spp., nearly always *C. albicans*. Predisposing factors include the use of broad spectrum antibiotics; indwelling intravenous catheters; recent major surgery, particularly of the gastrointestinal tract; a compromised immune system associated with malnutrition, debilitating disease, corticosteroid use and AIDS; and contaminated self-administered injections by intravenous drug abusers.

Fungal orbital cellulitis

Fungal orbital cellulitis is classified as aspergillosis (due to *Aspergillus* spp.) or mucormycosis (due to *Rhizopus*, *Absidia*, *Mucor* and other zygomycetes). Both are more common in the immunocompromised.

Aspergillosis is usually secondary to direct extension of infection from the paranasal sinuses, in particular the maxillary sinus. In immune competent individuals it occurs most often in tropical environments and is only slowly progressive, possibly being asymptomatic for many years. An allergic diathesis, a deviated nasal septum and nasal polyps predispose to sinus infection. The clinical manifestations include visual loss, proptosis and pain. The histological reaction is granulomatous. Aspergillosis as an opportunistic infection in the immunocompromised produces a different histological picture, as those affected may be incapable of mounting a delayed hypersensitivity response; the reaction is nongranulomatous and tissue necrosis is more evident. The diagnosis of aspergillosis necessitates biopsy and culture.

Mucormycosis is a highly aggressive infection. Diabetes mellitus is the commonest predisposing condition, but others include renal failure, lymphoproliferative disorders, extensive malignancies, hepatic and gastrointestinal diseases, severe burns and malnutrition. Visual complications result from obstruction of the ophthalmic arteries and involvement of the vasa vasora of the IIIrd, IVth and VIth cranial nerves. Black necrotic eschars and black pus formation in the nares and on the palate are characteristic of associated nasal involvement, and extensive bone destruction may be evident on radiological examination. Mucormycosis agents are extremely difficult to culture, and the diagnosis depends on histological evaluation of biopsy material. Unlike other fungi, the organisms are easily seen in routinely stained haematoxylin and eosin preparations.

PROTOZOA

Protozoa are unicellular eukaryotes, 1–50 μm in size, and humans are often an intermediate host in their life cycle. They include *Plasmodium* spp. (malaria), *Leishmania* spp. (visceral and cutaneous leishmaniasis), *Trypanosoma* spp. (trypanosomiasis), *Toxoplasma gondii* (toxoplasmosis), *Acanthamoeba* spp. (acanthamoebic keratitis), *Nosema* spp. (keratitis), *Isospora belli* (gastrointestinal disease) and *Cryptosporidium* spp. (gastrointestinal disease). Malarial infection has an adverse effect on erythrocyte behaviour; the ophthalmic effects of this include subconjunctival and retinal haemorrhages resulting from haemolytic anaemia, and cranial nerve palsies as a consequence of cerebral hypoxia due to intravascular coagulopathy. Cutaneous leishmaniasis may involve the lids and trypanosomiasis can result in urticarial lid swelling, preauricular lymphadenopathy and uveitis. The most important protozoal pathogens of concern to ophthalmologists are *Toxoplasma gondii*, *Acanthamoeba* spp. and *Nosema* spp. *Nosema* spp. are microsporidial protozoa. Infection (nosematosis) is consequent upon direct inoculation from domestic animals, and the majority of cases involve the cornea of the immunocompromised.

Toxoplasma gondii

This is an obligate intracellular protozoon. The definitive host is the cat. Intermediate hosts include humans, sheep, pigs, cattle and many rodents. The organism exists as sporozoites, bradyzoites and tachyzoites. Sporozoites are contained within an oocyst (sporocyst) and result from sexual reproduction of the organisms within the intestinal mucosa of the cat. Up to 10 million oocysts a day are excreted in cat faeces and may remain viable in moist soil for up to 2 years. Bradyzoites are relatively inactive and contained within tissue cysts that develop within any organ but commonly the brain, eye, heart, skeletal muscles and lymph nodes. The cysts contain up to 3000 bradyzoites and may lie dormant for years without provoking an inflammatory reaction. Bradyzoites increase in number within the cysts and, when the cyst wall breaks down, escape and become tachyzoites, which invade contiguous cells and cause inflammation. Tachyzoites (trophozoites) are the free motile proliferating forms (Fig. 2.58a) responsible for active disease. They can be visualized in tissue sections with Giemsa stain, and may undergo asexual replication (endodyogeny) in all cells. Humans are most commonly infected by ingesting undercooked meat containing bradyzoites. Infection by oocysts from contaminated hands or food, such as vegetables or unpasteurized milk, is much less common. Rarer forms of transmission include inoculation by penetrating trauma, transplantation of infected tissues and blood transfusion. Following ingestion, oocysts and bradyzoites release tachyzoites that pass through the intestinal wall and enter circulating leukocytes to be disseminated throughout the body, and it is at this stage that antibodies are produced. Transplacental transmission can lead to congenital toxoplasmosis.

Toxoplasmosis

T. gondii causes toxoplasmosis, which may be primary or result from the reactivation of dormant encysted bradyzoites which themselves are acquired either in utero or after birth. Primary acquired infection in the adult is either asymptomatic or presents as a febrile illness similar to infectious mononucleosis. The commonest manifestation is asymptomatic cervical lymphadenopathy with affected nodes exhibiting a characteristic histological appearance comprising follicular hyperplasia, adjacent granulomas and sinus distension. Primary acquired infection in the immunocompetent is self-limiting, but in the immunocompromised may cause severe disease man-

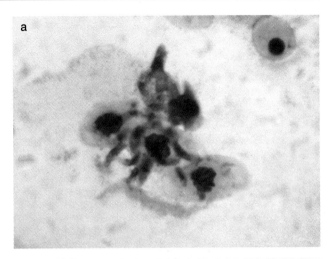

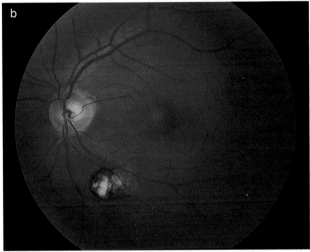

Figure 2.58 *Toxoplasma gondii.* (a) Tachyzoites. Giemsa stain. (b) Fundus appearance of an inactive retinochoroidal lesion.

ifest as fever, myocarditis, pneumonitis and encephalitis. Reactivation of latent infection with similar systemic manifestations occurs in the immunocompromised, AIDS being particularly associated with multifocal encephalitis. Congenital toxoplasmosis results from transplacental migration in infected pregnant women. The severity of disease depends on the developmental stage of the fetus. Infection during the first trimester results in spontaneous abortion, stillbirth or severe disease. If infection occurs after the first trimester, infants may appear unaffected at birth but manifestations of infection appear months or years later. The commonest presentation of congenital toxoplasmosis is with retinochoroiditis or neurological disorders including psychomotor or mental retardation, seizures, microcephaly and deafness; other manifestations include intracranial calcification, hydrocephalus, anaemia, jaundice, rash, pneumonitis, diarrhoea and hypothermia.

Ocular toxoplasmosis

Ocular toxoplasmosis (Fig. 2.58b) follows congenital or acquired systemic disease. The commonest manifestation is retinochoroiditis, which appears as a white fluffy retinal lesion surrounded by oedema. Histological examination of retinal lesions reveals a sharply demarcated granuloma with central coagulative necrosis and a cellular infiltrate of macrophages, lymphocytes and plasma cells. Healing of the acute lesion results in a glial scar, vaso-obliteration, RPE proliferation and possibly calcification. Burnt-out lesions appear as punched-out scars with exposure of the underlying sclera and pigment proliferation. Viable toxoplasma cysts may remain within the scar but elicit little reaction. The factors leading to reactivation of *T. gondii* tachyzoites from these cysts is not known, but their release stimulates a marked inflammatory response. Recurrent infection occurs at the border of existing scars or as new satellite lesions. The predisposition for infection at the macular and juxtapapillary regions may be a consequence of the entrapment of free organisms or infected macrophages in the terminal capillaries of these areas. The vitreous and anterior uvea may also be involved in ocular toxoplasmosis, inflammation at these sites being either secondary to that in adjacent tissues or a hypersensitivity reaction to *T. gondii* antigen.

Investigations for toxoplasmosis

The diagnosis of toxoplasmosis can be confirmed by laboratory investigations, including the detection of toxoplasma antigens and antibodies in body fluids and tissue specimens. In systemic disease, where biopsy material is available, the histological appearance of lymph node and other tissue biopsies may be helpful. Serum titres of antibodies may be low, but nevertheless serological tests help confirm past exposure and, as in other infections, the type of antibody produced relates to the chronicity of infection. IgG antibodies appear at 1–2 weeks after infection and peak at 1–2 months before falling, but remain detectable throughout life. IgM antibodies also appear at 1–2 weeks after infection and can persist in low titres for up to a year. IgA antibodies indicate recent infection and their presence is helpful in the diagnosis of congenital infection in the fetus and newborn; they usually disappear after about 7 months. IgE antibodies are also markers of recent infection, but are detectable for shorter periods.

The value of serological tests is limited by the high prevalence of toxoplasma antibodies in certain communities and the persistence of high titres in otherwise normal individuals. Recent infection is supported by demonstrating high titres of IgG and IgM antibodies, although this finding is not diagnostic. Serologic tests for toxoplasmosis include the Sabin–Feldman dye test, enzyme immunosorbent assay, indirect fluorescent antibody, indirect haemagglutination tests and immunosorbent agglutination assay.

The Sabin–Feldman dye test is the standard reference test against which all other serological tests are compared. It is a neutralization test in which live organisms are exposed to serum and complement. If specific IgG antibodies are present in the serum, the cell membranes of the organisms are lysed and fail to stain with methylene blue. Titres are determined by the dilution at which 50 per cent of organisms are stained. Antibodies appear from 1 week post-infection and reach high titres ($> 1:1024$) in 6–8 weeks. Thereafter titres gradually decline over a period of months to a year, but may remain positive at a low level ($1:4$–$1:64$) for life. There is no correlation with the strength of the response and the clinical severity of the disease or the activity of ocular lesions.

Enzyme immunosorbent assay (EIA) detects IgG and IgM and can be used for serum and aqueous. False positives may occur in those with rheumatoid factor.

Indirect fluorescent antibody (IFA) tests are carried out by incubating a slide preparation of killed tachyzoites with serum and antihuman globulin labelled with fluorescein. IgG and IgM can be detected, but false positives occur in those with antinuclear antibodies or rheumatoid factor and false negatives in those with high levels of IgG. The advantages of the test are that it is easier to perform, safer and more economical than the dye test.

The indirect haemagglutination test utilizes erythrocytes coated with *T. gondii* antigen. Agglutination occurs in the presence of IgG antibodies in test serum, but the test is not helpful in screening because of the large number of false positives.

The immunosorbent agglutination assay (ISAGA) is used to detect IgG, IgM, IgA and IgE. It is a sensitive and specific technique not affected by the presence of antinuclear antibodies or rheumatoid factor.

Negative tests

Tests reported as negative should be repeated on undiluted serum if there is a high clinical suspicion of infection. The Sabin–Feldman dye test is the only one used to test undiluted serum, there being an extremely high rate of false results with the others. A negative dye test on undiluted serum makes the diagnosis of toxoplasma retinochoroiditis highly unlikely. Toxoplasma antigen and nucleic acid detection tests are not currently used in routine practice, although they can be helpful in diagnosing uveitis and other inflammatory conditions where the aetiology is obscure.

Acanthamoeba spp.

Acanthamoeba spp. are a significant component of the protozoal fauna of soil and water including domestic water supplies, swimming pools, fresh water ponds, lakes and mineral water. Subclinical exposure is common, and the organisms may be isolated from the nose and throat of asymptomatic individuals. *Acanthamoeba* spp. cause severe keratitis, particularly in contact lens wearers, and potentially fatal infections of the CNS. Classification of the organisms is confusing, and many were previously known as *Hartmanella*. Differences in size and cyst morphology are the basis of current classification, but variation within species makes precise morphological identification impossible; the problem will be solved by molecular biological methods. Organisms range in size from 10–50 μm. They replicate by simple binary fission and exist as trophozoites and cysts. Trophozoites are active and infective, and feed by phagocytosing other micro-organisms including bacteria and fungi. A characteristic feature of trophozoites is the presence of a contracting vacuole and a large number of slender needle-like pseudopodial projections (acanthopodia) at the anterior end in the direction of movement. Mitotic division occurs when environmental conditions are suitable. Under adverse conditions the trophozoite transforms into a double-walled cyst 15–30 μm in size. Cysts are resistant to cold, dehydration and many antimicrobial agents. The outer wall (ectocyst) is wrinkled and follows the contour of the inner wall (endocyst). The endocyst varies in shape from circular to polygonal or stellate with intermittent junctions (ostioles) with the ectocyst. The ostioles are plugged by opercula that dissolve at excystation when the amoeba detaches itself from the endocyst and escapes through an ostiole.

Acanthamoebic keratitis

Keratitis is the main manifestation of ophthalmic infection, although there may be nodular anterior scleritis, posterior scleritis and optic neuritis. Of the 20 or more named species of *Acanthamoebae*, five (*A. castellanii*, *A. hatchetti*, *A. polyphaga*, *A. rhysodes* and *A. culbertsoni*) are known to cause ophthalmic disease. Corneal epithelial trauma predisposes to infection. The trauma may be overt and involve organic material, or minor in the form of microabrasions associated with contact lens wear, particularly daily-wear or extended-wear soft lenses and the use of non-sterile home-made saline. Cysts and trophozoites adhere to soft contact lenses and are frequent con-

taminants of lens care systems, particularly if bacterial and/or fungal contamination coexists. Trophozoites attach to the injured epithelium, multiply and cause cytolysis, their attachment depending on adhesion molecules, pseudopodia and an intact cytoskeletal system. They then migrate into the corneal stroma and induce an inflammatory response and tissue necrosis by the elaboration of lytic enzymes.

Most of those infected with *Acanthamoeba* spp. are young and healthy, and give a history of a known risk factor. The keratitis is usually unilateral and severe pain is out of proportion to the physical signs. The corneal epithelium shows dendritiform irregularity, oedema and necrosis, and, with progression, conjunctival injection becomes severe and associated with chemosis. Radial keratoneuritis (Fig. 2.59a) is common and appears as linear midstromal infiltrates following the course of the corneal nerves. Patchy crescentic anterior corneal stromal infiltrates become confluent and form the ring-shaped appearance (Fig. 2.59b) of advanced infection. Neovascularization is unusual, but inflammatory activity in the anterior chamber may be severe enough to produce hypopyon. Associated anterior nodular scleritis may

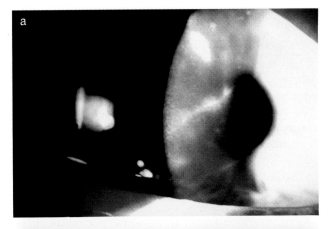

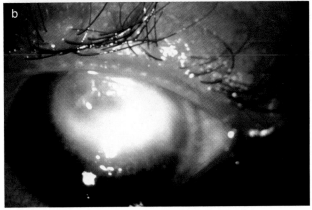

Figure 2.59 Acanthamoebic keratitis. (a) Radial keratoneuritis. (b) Ring ulcer.

account for the pain. Histological examination of involved corneas reveals stromal necrosis, neutrophils and acanthamoebae, usually cysts. If Descemet's membrane is involved, multinucleate giant cells may be seen.

Investigations for acanthamoebic keratitis

Acanthamoeba spp. may be grown from corneal scrapes and biopsies, keratoplasty specimens, and contact lenses and their cases and solutions. Non-nutrient agar is inoculated and seeded with *E. coli*, which serves as a food source for the amoebae, leaving identifiable tracks on the culture plate. Organisms, usually cysts, may be found in wet-mount preparations of contact lens soaking solutions (Fig. 2.60a), and in corneal scrapes and tissue stained with periodic acid-Schiff, Grocott hexamine (methenamine) silver (Fig. 2.60b), calcofluor white and fluorescein-labelled antibodies directed against *Acanthamoeba* spp. (Fig. 2.60c). Electron microscopy may also be helpful (Fig. 2.60d). Definitive diagnosis of

acanthamoebic keratitis is only made when organisms are identified by microscopy or culture of corneal scrapes or biopsies, or keratoplasty specimens.

HELMINTHS

Helminths are worms, a number of which are responsible for disease. They fall into three groups: nematodes (roundworms), trematodes (flukes) and cestodes (tapeworms). Adult worms may be centimetres or even metres in length although larvae may measure only 100–200 μm. Humans are essential in the life cycle of some helminths, but in others human infection is accidental. The outer surface of nematodes is a tough collagenous cuticle which, although antigenic, is largely resistant to immune attack, whereas the surface of trematodes and cestodes is a complex plasma membrane which prevents the host damaging the outer surface. Worms release large

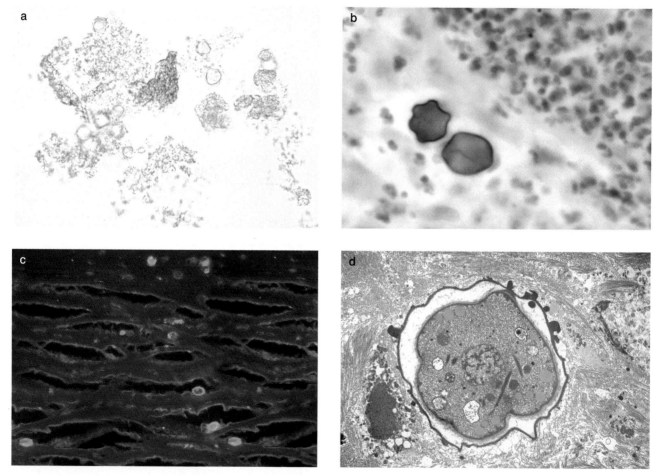

Figure 2.60 Acanthamoebic cysts. (a) Wet-mount preparation. (b) In corneal stroma. Grocott hexamine (methenamine) silver stain. (c) In corneal stroma. Immunofluorescence. (d) Transmission electron micrograph.

amounts of antigenic material in their secretions and excretions, and this plays an important role in immune reactions. Disease attributable to helminths arises in several ways, but the most important ocular manifestations are due to mechanical disturbances or immunological responses including IgE mediated allergic reactions, the production of specific IgG and IgM antibodies, and active cell-mediated immunity.

Nematodes

Nematodes have cylindrical bodies and a complete tubular digestive system. Those of ophthalmic importance include *Toxocara* spp. (toxocariasis), *Trichinella spiralis* (trichinosis), *Onchocerca volvulus* (onchocerciasis), *Loa loa* (loaiasis) and *Wuchereria bancrofti* (Bancroftian filariasis).

Toxocara spp.

Toxocara spp. include *T. canis* and *T. cati*. Human infection is associated with *T. canis*, a ubiquitous canine nematode affecting dogs (12–15 per cent), wolves and foxes. The complete life cycle occurs only in the host animal, and in humans maturation does not proceed beyond the larval stage, the larvae becoming dormant or encysted. In pregnant bitches, larvae are activated and, by transplacental migration, infect the puppies in utero. The presence of infection in puppies during their first 6 months of life is of particular importance, as infection in humans is virtually confined to young children and occurs by the ingestion of ova present in faecal-contaminated play areas and on the coats of infected pets. Many of those affected give a history of having played with puppies as children. Following human ingestion, second stage larvae emerge in the gut and penetrate the mucosa to enter the portal circulation and intestinal lymphatics. Many of these larvae then lodge in the liver and spleen, but others may reach the lungs, brain or eyes. Generalized infection with *T. canis* is usually asymptomatic, but disseminating larvae may cause visceral larva migrans (VLM), an illness characterized by fever, hepatosplenomegaly, pulmonary infiltrations and encephalopathy.

Ocular toxocariasis

Ocular toxocariasis is always unilateral and any associated VLM is subclinical. The larvae reach the eye via the ophthalmic artery and enter the retinal and possibly the uveal circulation. Presenting features depend on the site involved. Local inflammation in the peripheral retina results in the formation of a whitish mass. Vision remains normal, and the condition may go undetected for many years. If the retina at the posterior pole is involved a similar mass forms but vision is affected, and in children strabismus may develop. For reasons not understood, infection may present as severe endophthalmitis (Fig. 2.61a) and the retinal involvement is not recognized until the inflammation regresses spontaneously. Neovascular glaucoma and phthisis bulbi may result if the inflammation does not subside. Granulomatous inflammatory foci in relation to the larvae exhibit eosinophilic abscess formation surrounded by epithelioid cells, giant cells, lymphocytes, plasma cells and fibroblasts (Fig. 2.61b). Finding the larva in enucleated eyes often requires the cutting of a large number of sections.

Investigations for toxocariasis

VLM causes leukocytosis with eosinophilia and raised serum IgG, IgM and IgA. Serological diagnosis only confirms previous exposure and does not establish

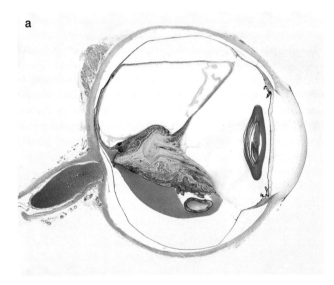

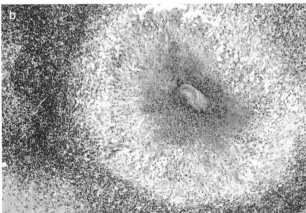

Figure 2.61 *Toxocara canis.* (a) Endophthalmitis. Inflammatory mass and total retinal detachment. (b) Granulomatous inflammation with larva centrally.

whether or not a particular intraocular lesion is due to toxocariasis. Intraocular fluid aspirates may contain eosinophils and antigen.

Trichinella spiralis

T. spiralis is the cause of trichinosis, which results from eating undercooked pork or game. The organism has a world-wide distribution, and outbreaks of trichinosis can occur in any population that consumes pork products. After consumption, larvae in the gastrointestinal tract mature into adult worms, which lay eggs. The eggs hatch and larvae migrate into the blood through the intestinal wall and cause a febrile illness with myalgia and marked eosinophilia. Severe infections may be fatal. Clinical features include lid oedema, conjunctivitis and painful proptosis, which is usually the result of larval infiltration of the extraocular muscles. Encysted larvae may be seen in muscle biopsy specimens.

Onchocerca volvulus

O. volvulus is the cause of onchocerciasis (river blindness). Humans are the natural host of the adult worm, the intermediate host being biting blackflies of the genus *Simulium*. Onchocerciasis is endemic across equatorial Africa and in circumscribed areas of Central and South America. Foci of disease are always located in the vicinity of rivers or streams that form the breeding sites of the blackflies. Adult *O. volvulus* reside in dense fibrous subcutaneous nodules (onchocercomata). Fertilized females within these nodules produce first stage larvae (microfilariae – Fig. 2.62) which migrate through the superficial dermis, from where they are ingested by feeding blackflies. Within the flies, second and third stage

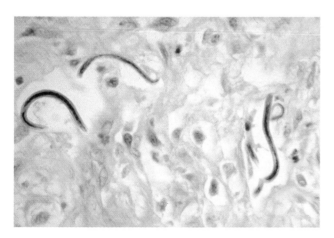

Figure 2.62 *Onchocerca volvulus.* Microfilariae. Giemsa stain.

larvae develop and infect other humans when the flies bite again. Onchocercomata develop and the life cycle is completed.

Onchocerciasis

The bite of the blackfly may produce a painful wheal that develops quickly and resolves in 2–3 days. The commonest initial manifestation is pruritus, but this may not occur until 6 months to 2 years after the initial infection. Pruritus is followed by a maculopapular rash and more severe skin changes (onchodermatitis) characterized by thickening of the skin with lichenification and scaling, crusted papules and deeper erosions with surrounding inflammation. Over several years skin pigmentation may alter with areas of hyper- and hypopigmentation and possibly a leopard-skin appearance of the shins. In the early stages, histological examination shows a perivasculitis. Microfilariae are later found at the epidermal/dermal junction and, if dying or dead, are associated with an intense eosinophilic cellular infiltrate. Onchodermatitis is manifest as thickening of the epidermis, inflammation and fibrosis, and in the later stages microfilariae are found. Pigment changes parallel the clinical picture. Onchocercomata are firm round masses in the subcutaneous tissue or fascial planes firmly attached to periosteum or joint capsules, mostly around the pelvis but also in the head and shoulder region. They are formed of dense fibrous scar tissue that encases the adult worms, which lie coiled up like a ball of string. Inflammatory cells infiltrate and occasional areas of necrosis and liquefaction may be present. Lymph nodes draining areas of onchodermatitis become firm and discrete. Microscopy shows capsular fibrosis, atrophic follicles and dilated subcapsular sinusoids, and granulomatous inflammation may be associated with the presence of microfilariae.

Ocular onchocerciasis

Circulating microfilariae can enter the eye and affect both the anterior and posterior segments. They can also reach the cornea and aqueous from the periorbital skin and conjunctiva. Live microfilariae can be seen in the aqueous and are associated with anterior uveitis. Dying or dead microfilariae in the cornea result in punctate keratitis due to focal collections of lymphocytes and eosinophils with local oedema. Posterior segment lesions are the result of invasion by microfilariae from the orbit along the sheaths of the ciliary vessels and nerves, or via the blood stream. Early changes involve the RPE and a characteristic pigmentary retinopathy develops. Lymphocytes, plasma cells and eosinophils infiltrate the choroid.

Investigations for onchocerciasis

The adult worm can be found in excised onchocercomata and microfilariae may be seen in skin snips or ocular samples. If they are not readily found, nucleic acid detection can be helpful. Serum antibodies may be detected by immunological methods.

Loa loa (the African eyeworm)

Loa loa (Fig. 2.63) is the cause of loaiasis, which is prevalent in West and Central Africa and is transmitted by the bloodsucking mangrove fly (*Chrysops* spp.). Adult worms reside in subcutaneous connective tissue and microfilariae are disseminated in the blood. The worms develop slowly and symptoms may not appear until at least a year after the initial bite by the vector. One of the first signs of infection is the presence of transient swellings (Calabar swellings) in the extremities as the worms migrate through subcutaneous tissues. Adult worms can migrate beneath the conjunctiva and cause acute inflammation, chemosis and itching. Intraocular invasion by adult worms or microfilariae is rare.

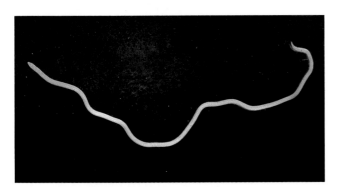

Figure 2.63 *Loa loa*. The adult worm × 2.

Wuchereria bancrofti

W. bancrofti is spread by the mosquito and is prevalent in the tropics, where it causes Bancroftian filariasis. The adult worm is responsible for most of the general manifestations, which include lymphoedema (elephantiasis). Intraocular lesions (anterior uveitis, subretinal inflammation) are due to direct invasion by microfilariae following haematogenous dissemination. Conjunctival oedema may accompany recurrent allergic episodes provoked by the death of adult worms.

Trematodes

Trematodes cause significant human disease. They have a number of characteristics, including two muscular suckers – a ventral sucker for attachment and an oral sucker, which is the opening of an incomplete digestive tract that ends in a blind loop. All trematodes have complex life cycles requiring one or more intermediate hosts, the first of which is invariably a mollusc (snail or clam). Schistosomes are the only trematodes that cause ophthalmic disease.

Schistosoma mansoni, S. haematobium and S. japonicum

These all cause schistosomiasis. The organisms differ from other trematodes in that they are not hermaphrodite but exist in separate male and female forms. The adult worms are obligate intravascular parasites with a unique mode of transmission. The larval stage (cercariae) emerge from snails, penetrate the epidermis of the skin and enter the lymphatics and capillaries. They reach the lungs and mature before being disseminated. An allergic reaction results in headache, fever, joint pains and widespread oedema. The lids share in the generalized oedema, and nodules in the subconjunctival stroma are seen histologically as eosinophilic granulomas with central necrosis (Splendore–Hoeppli phenomenon).

Cestodes

The bodies of cestodes are ribbon-like and composed of segments (proglottids). The head (scolex) has organs of attachment comprising four suckers and a crown of hooklets. The worms absorb food in the host intestine through their body wall. All species are hermaphrodite, and both sets of reproductive organs are found in each mature proglottid. *Taenia solium* (cysticercosis) and *Echinococcus granulosus* (hydatid disease) are two cestodes that produce disease with ophthalmic manifestations.

Taenia solium (pork tapeworm)

T. solium in its larval stage is found in raw or undercooked pork, and causes cysticercosis. Ocular involvement in cysticercosis results from direct invasion by blood-borne larvae. Fully developed cysticerci form within the eye and enter the subretinal space and vitreous. The clinical manifestations are initially due to mechanical disturbances, but later, exudative choroidoretinitis is caused by an immune response to *T. solium* antigen.

Echinococcus granulosus

E. granulosus causes hydatid disease. Dogs are the primary host for the worms, the ova of which are ingested by sheep, and less commonly humans. Hydatid cysts develop, most frequently in the liver but also elsewhere, including the orbit, where they can cause painless proptosis. Invasion into the eye is very unusual. In the Casoni test, sterile fluid from the cyst is injected intradermally and, in positive cases, an immediate wheal and flare reaction indicates an IgE response. The demonstration of IgG antibodies to echinococcal antigen in the serum is a more reliable and safer test.

ARTHROPODS

Arthropods have a chitinous exoskeleton, jointed appendages and a segmented body. They develop from egg to adult by a process of metamorphosis in which intermediate morphological stages include larvae, nymphs and pupae. Species belonging to two classes (Insecta and Arachnida) may cause ophthalmic disease.

Insecta

Diptera (flies)

These act as vectors in the transmission of some bacterial and helminth infections (e.g. trachoma, onchocerciaris, Bancroftian filariasis). Direct infection is rare but larvae (maggots), frequently those of *Oestrus ovis* (Fig. 2.64), can provoke external ophthalmomyasis. Penetration of the globe by larvae, especially *Hypoderma bovis*, results in internal ophthalmomyasis.

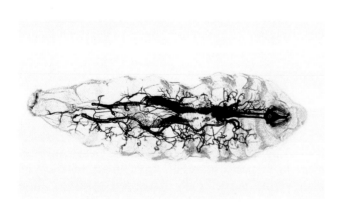

Figure 2.64 *Oestrus ovis*; larval form.

Phthirus pubis and Phthirus capitis (pubic and head lice)

These insects cling to coarse hairs including the eyebrows and lashes by using terminal claws on their legs. Following the deposition of ova (nits) and larval stages, mature insects emerge. *P. pubis* (Fig. 2.65) is seen more often on the eyebrows and lashes than *P. capitis*. Infestations with lice may result in secondary bacterial infection.

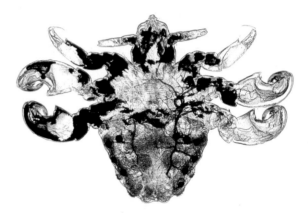

Figure 2.65 Phthirus pubis (pubic louse).

Arachnida

Demodex folliculorum

D. folliculorum is a mite commonly seen as a commensal in histological sections of skin (Fig. 2.66), especially of the face, where it infests hair follicles. It has a questionable role in the development of blepharitis.

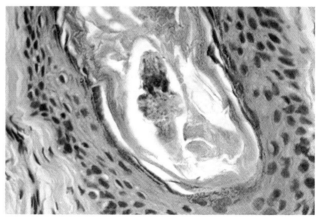

Figure 2.66 *Demodex folliculorum*; larva within a hair follicle.

Ixodidiae (ticks)

Ixodidiae spp. (Fig. 2.67) do not directly cause ophthalmic disease, but act as vectors for the organisms causing Lyme disease and some rickettsial infections.

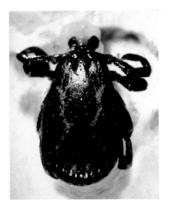

Figure 2.67 *Ixodes* spp. (tick).

Chapter 3

Genetics

Introduction

Basic principles

DNA
   Chromosomes
      Genes
   Non-chromosomal DNA
RNA
Interpreting the genetic code: protein synthesis
Mutations

Genetic abnormalities and inherited disorders

Chromosomal abnormalities
   Numerical abnormalities
   Structural abnormalities
   Mosaicism
The effects of chromosomal abnormalities
Syndromes associated with numerical chromosomal
   abnormalities

Syndromes associated with structural chromosomal
   abnormalities
Single gene defects
   Autosomal dominant disorders
      Autosomal dominant disorders of connective
         tissue
   Autosomal recessive disorders
      Autosomal recessive disorders of metabolism
      Disorders of amino acid metabolism
      Disorders of carbohydrate metabolism
      Disorders of lipid metabolism
      Disorders of mineral metabolism
      Lysosomal storage diseases: sphingolipidoses,
         mucopolysaccharidoses and mucolipidoses
      Disorders of DNA repair
   X-linked disorders
      X-linked dominant disorders
      X-linked recessive disorders
Disorders of mitochondrial inheritance
Multifactorial inheritance
Somatic mutations

INTRODUCTION

Many disorders of the eye, the visual system and ocular adnexae have a genetic component in their aetiology. Affected individuals have an abnormality in the structure or expression of their genetic code. The genetic code is a manifestation of deoxyribonucleic acid (DNA), a nucleic acid that encodes all the information necessary for the formation and functioning of a living cell and for transmitting characteristics to successive generations. Some genetic disorders show a clear pattern of inheritance and, although many such disorders exist, their frequency in the population is low. In developed countries, approximately $4:1000$ children suffer from disorders that result in severe visual handicap and at least half of these are inherited. It is important to appreciate, however, that some inherited genetic disorders do not present until later in life and that a number of common conditions such as glaucoma, cataract and refractive error also have a genetic component in their aetiology. A large number of genetic disorders can be diagnosed by combining clinical examination with laboratory investigations, which include an ever-increasing number of tests based on DNA analysis. Molecular genetics currently allows for carrier detection, prenatal or presymptomatic diagnosis and genetic counselling in some disorders while future developments may conceivably result in the treatment or even elimination of genetic disorders.

BASIC PRINCIPLES

Nucleic acids are present within all living cells. The two main types are deoxyribonucleic acid (DNA) and ribonucleic acid (RNA). Both consist of a sugar–phosphate backbone with projecting nitrogenous bases which are either purines (adenine and guanine in both DNA and RNA) or pyrimidines (cytosine in both DNA and RNA, thymine in DNA, uracil in RNA). A unit of base, sugar and phosphate is termed a nucleotide.

DNA

The DNA molecule is a double helix formed by two nucleotide chains coiled around each other and held together by hydrogen bonds between specific pairs of bases; adenine or guanine of one chain pair respectively with thymine and cytosine of the other. The sugar component is deoxyribose. The unit length of DNA is the base pair (bp). One thousand bp constitute a kilobase (kb); a megabase (Mb) is 10^6 bp. The total length of nuclear DNA in a somatic cell is 6000 Mb which, if continuous and fully extended, would be approximately 3 m. The functions of DNA are to encode genetic information and to transmit it to subsequent generations.

Chromosomes

DNA molecules are packaged into the chromosomes present in all nucleated cells. The structure of chromosomes is extremely complex, but essentially each consists of a strand of DNA coiled around a basic unit or elementary fibre consisting of repeated units (nucleosomes) each comprising eight molecules of the protein histone. These elementary fibres are further coiled on themselves to form the chromatin fibre, which can be resolved by electron microscopy. Human somatic cells contain 46 chromosomes. There are 22 pairs of autosomes and one pair of sex chromosomes; the latter are an X and a Y in males and two X in females. Members of a pair of autosomes are termed homologous, and each is derived from one parent. If in cell culture mitosis is arrested at metaphase by the use of a drug such as colchicine, chromosomes can be identified by Giemsa and other stains. This identification allows for the classification of chromosomes according to their length and the position of the centromere, which is a visible constriction at the point of attachment of two identical DNA molecules (sister chromatids) seen during the mitotic process. Autosomes are numbered from 1 to 22 as they decrease in size (i.e. the higher the number the smaller the chromosome), and each has a short and a long arm, designated respectively 'p' and 'q'. The X and Y chromosomes are strikingly different. The X chromosome is the larger and contains 6 per cent of the total nuclear DNA, encoding over 50 genes, whereas the Y chromosome is small and has only two genes mapped to it; one of these is the testis-determining gene. As with autosomes, each sex chromosome is derived from one parent. This difference in the size of the sex chromosomes accounts in part for the characteristics of X-linked inheritance. Compaction of chromosomes occurs during the metaphase of cell division during which genetic material is accurately allocated to daughter cells.

Genes

Genes are functional units of DNA that direct the formation of a protein; they have a structural, enzymatic or regulatory function. It is estimated that in humans there are 100 000 pairs of genes. Expression of a gene depends on the type of cell or tissue, although some (housekeeping genes) are expressed universally. A gene is composed of coding sequences of DNA (exons) interrupted at intervals by non-coding sequences (introns). In addition, regulatory sequences located in and around the gene control its expression. Of all DNA only about 10 per cent has a clearly identified function. The function of the remaining 90 per cent is not clear, and the nucleotide sequence is subject to immense variation between individuals. The entire complement of DNA for a somatic cell, and therefore the whole body excluding the gonads, is termed the genome (genotype). Interaction of the genotype with the environment results in the physical, physiological and biochemical characteristics (phenotype) of the individual.

Genes are present in pairs located in the same position (locus) on two homologous autosomes or X chromosomes. Each member of a pair is termed an allele; if two alleles are identical the individual is homozygous for that gene, while if they are different the individual is heterozygous. In normal mitosis (somatic cell division) an identical set of alleles passes to the daughter cells and is contained in paired (diploid) sets of chromosomes. In meiosis (germ cell formation) reciprocal exchange of alleles takes place between homologous chromosomes (recombination); cell division results in daughter cells containing a single set of alleles (segregation) in an unpaired (haploid) set of chromosomes. At fertilization the haploid number of chromosomes from paternal and maternal gametes combine in the formation of the zygote, which thus has a diploid complement. All subsequent somatic cells of the conceptus are derived from mitosis of this single cell.

Non-chromosomal DNA

While most DNA is packaged into the nuclear chromosomes, a small amount is contained within the mitochondria present in cell cytoplasm (mitochondrial DNA-mtDNA). No paternal mtDNA passes to the zygote at fertilization (the head of the sperm is too small to contain mitochondria), so all mtDNA is of maternal origin. The mtDNA molecule takes the form of a loop similar to a bacterial plasmid. The entire mitochondrial genome consists of 16 569 bp encoding the 13 genes essential for the respiratory chain. In addition, mitochondria also contain ribosomes and are self-sufficient for the expression of the genes encoded by their DNA. The other proteins and co-factors required for oxidative phosphorylation are encoded by nuclear DNA and are transported into the mitochondria. Disordered oxidative phosphorylation may therefore result from an abnormality of either mtDNA or nuclear DNA.

RNA

RNA differs from DNA in that it is single stranded, the sugar is ribose rather than deoxyribose, and uracil replaces thymine. Whereas the function of DNA is to encode genetic information and transmit it to subsequent generations, the function of RNA is to read and translate the genetic code. There are several types of RNA, including messenger RNA (mRNA), transfer RNA (tRNA), ribosomal RNA (rRNA) and heterogeneous RNA (hRNA).

INTERPRETING THE GENETIC CODE: PROTEIN SYNTHESIS

The fundamental coding unit of DNA is termed a codon and comprises three nucleotide bases. There are 64 possible codons; each either corresponds to one of the 20 amino acids in a polypeptide chain or acts as a signal to start or stop protein synthesis. The basic processes involved are transcription, post-transcriptional modification, translation and post-translational modification. Transcription is the first stage, where the sequence of base pairs of a gene is transcribed into a length of mRNA. The two strands of DNA separate in the region of a gene; one strand then acts as a template for the formation of a complementary strand of hRNA under the influence of the enzyme RNA polymerase II. Both coding and non-coding sequences of DNA are transcribed into hRNA, which is later modified into mRNA by the enzymatic removal of non-coding sequences. Translation of mRNA into protein occurs in the cytoplasm and involves both tRNA and rRNA. Each tRNA molecule has two parts; one binds a specific amino acid and the other, consisting of three bases, forms an anticodon, which binds to a complementary mRNA codon. One or more ribosomes (composed of rRNA) attaches to a strand of mRNA, tRNA molecules are aligned on each ribosome according to the mRNA codon sequence, and peptide bonds between adjacent amino acid molecules carried by the tRNA form a polypeptide chain. In the stage of post-translational modification, proteins are modified within the endoplasmic reticulum or Golgi apparatus before reaching their final form.

MUTATIONS

Mutations are stable heritable changes in DNA produced by the action of mutagens, which are external factors (e.g. radiation and chemicals) that damage DNA and result in genetic alterations. Mutagens that act during embryogenesis may lead to congenital malformations and are thus teratogenic. DNA damaged during embryogenesis is not repaired, either because it is not recognized as damaged or because the repair mechanism is faulty, and this results in disorders that can themselves become inherited. Mutagens can also be oncogenic and lead to the formation of neoplasms. The two broad categories of mutation are length mutations and point mutations.

Length mutations (in which there can be either gain or loss of genetic material) include deletions, duplications and insertions of DNA sequences. Depending upon the amount of DNA involved, length mutations form a continuum with structural chromosomal abnormalities.

Point mutations (in which there are alterations in the genetic code but genetic material is neither gained nor lost) occur as the result of a change of the nucleotide base, and the effects may occur at any stage in the processes of transcription or translation, resulting in unstable mRNA or in mRNA that cannot be translated into a functional polypeptide. Point mutations may cause a mis-sense translation in which the mutant codon codes for a different amino acid in a polypeptide. Similarly, a nonsense mutation may result in the generation of a termination codon, alterations of initiator codons, codons at splicing sites and disruption of promoter sequences.

Deletions and insertions, if not a multiple of three, result in misreading of the genetic code (frameshift mutation) and, if more extensive, may damage whole genes or extensive parts of a gene, thereby severely disrupting protein synthesis. Mutations may also be silent; an example of this is when the base sequence of a codon changes into another which codes for the same amino acid. The same clinical disorder may result from mutation of different genes (genetic heterogeneity). Conversely, different diseases may result from different mutations of the same gene (allelic heterogeneity).

GENETIC ABNORMALITIES AND INHERITED DISORDERS

Genetic disorders are due to chromosomal abnormalities, single gene defects, mitochondrial inheritance, multifactorial inheritance or somatic mutations. Inheritance may be Mendelian (according to the rules first described by Gregor Mendel) or non-Mendelian. Disorders of Mendelian inheritance are single gene defects whereas disorders of non-Mendelian inheritance are usually chromosomal abnormalities (some of these can exhibit Mendelian inheritance), defects of mtDNA or disorders of multifactorial inheritance.

CHROMOSOMAL ABNORMALITIES

Chromosomal abnormalities may occur in both somatic and germ cells. Apart from their role in oncogenesis, those arising in somatic cells are of little clinical significance. Those arising during gametogenesis, however, can have profound effects because they are transmitted to every somatic cell of the offspring and the consequence is heritable disease. Chromosomal aberrations are common and affect approximately 7.5 per cent of all conceptions. As many of them are lethal, only approximately 0.6 per cent of live births are affected. Chromosomal abnormalities are numerical or structural or, less commonly, result from mosaicism.

Numerical abnormalities

Any deviation from the normal diploid complement of 22 pairs of autosomes and one pair of sex chromosomes, which is not an exact multiple of the diploid number, is termed aneuploidy. Of the specific types of aneuploidy, trisomy and monosomy are relatively common. In trisomy a chromosome is added, while in monosomy a chromosome is absent – a situation that, apart from when the sex chromosomes are involved, is usually lethal. Polyploidy describes the presence of a multiple of the haploid number of chromosomes (23) within a cell, and such states are also usually lethal. Numerical chromosomal abnormalities arise from nondisjunction, i.e. the failure of paired chromosomes to separate during the anaphase of mitosis or meiosis. The cause is not clear, although increased maternal age is a consistent association, particularly with trisomy.

Structural abnormalities

Mutations can involve segments of DNA that are sufficiently large to be visible under the light microscope as chromosomal aberrations. With conventional techniques the smallest aberration visible corresponds to approximately 0.13 per cent of the genome (8 Mb). Structural abnormalities may result from chromosome breakage followed possibly by reconstruction in an abnormal combination. The distinct types of such abnormalities are translocations, inversions and deletions.

Translocation: pairing of homologous chromosomes with exchange and rearrangement of genetic material (crossing-over or recombination) occurs during meiosis.

Translocation is the abnormal transfer of part of one chromosome to a non-homologous chromosome. In the majority of cases the translocation is balanced, i.e. genetic material is not lost and the affected person is phenotypically normal. Carriers of balanced translocations are, however, at risk of producing offspring with unbalanced karyotypes and severe phenotypic abnormalities. Occasionally gain or loss of genetic material results in an unbalanced translocation. Duplication is an unbalanced translocation where a DNA sequence is repeated and can occur within the same chromosome (tandem duplication) giving rise to a partial trisomy.

Inversion: this results from a break in a chromosome at two places followed by reconstruction, but with the removed segment the opposite way round. Affected individuals are phenotypically normal but, because of disrupted meiosis, produce gametes with unbalanced abnormalities; their children are thus usually severely abnormal.

Deletion: disturbance during meiosis (or mitosis in somatic cells) may result in the formation of fragments that are not incorporated into any of the chromosomes and are lost in subsequent cell divisions. This loss or deletion of a portion of a chromosome can involve either a terminal or a middle (intercalary or interstitial) segment. Terminal deletions of both ends can lead to fusion of the ends to form a ring chromosome. The manifestations of deletions depend on the amount of genetic material lost.

Mosaicism

Mosaicism is the presence of at least two cell lines that, although derived from a single zygote, differ in genetic constitution. Mosaicism originates from errors of mitosis after fertilization, and may arise at any stage of development. It is not infrequent and can occur in any form of genetic abnormality ranging from trisomies to single gene defects. In numeric chromosomal abnormalities such as Turner's and Down's syndromes the phenotype is less severe than in the non-mosaic forms.

The effects of chromosomal abnormalities

Major chromosomal abnormalities are usually incompatible with life and lead to fetal death and early spontaneous abortion. Exceptions compatible with survival involve the smaller chromosomes such as the X chromosome and chromosome 21 that have proportionately smaller amounts of genetic material. Monosomy of the X chromosome causes Turner's syndrome, and trisomy of chromosome 21 causes Down's syndrome. Autosomal chromosomal abnormalities involve large numbers of genes and are therefore associated with multiple congenital anomalies which follow a consistent pattern that depends on the nature of the abnormality. Features of different chromosomal syndromes often overlap: microcephaly, mental retardation, short stature, congenital heart defects and ophthalmic abnormalities including microphthalmos and colobomas are common to many syndromes associated with autosomal defects.

Syndromes associated with numerical chromosomal abnormalities

In liveborn infants, syndromes associated with numerical chromosomal abnormalities are virtually all trisomies. Trisomy of chromosome 21 (Down's syndrome) is the most common, Trisomy 18 (Edward's syndrome) is much less common, and Trisomy 13 (Patau's syndrome) is very rare. Trisomy 21 has a relatively long survival, but Trisomy 18 and Trisomy 13 are usually fatal within the first year. All three exhibit ophthalmic manifestations.

Trisomy 21 (Down's syndrome)

Trisomy of chromosome 21 is a major cause of mental retardation. The overall incidence depends on maternal age and is approximately 1 : 800 live births increasing to approximately 1 : 40 live births in mothers aged 45 years or older. At least 90 per cent of those with Down's syndrome have trisomy of chromosome 21; approximately 5 per cent have only a partial trisomy as the result of a structural unbalanced translocation defect in the long arm of chromosome 21, while a small proportion of cases are mosaics resulting from nondisjunction during mitosis of a somatic cell in early embryogenesis. Chromosome 21, being one of the smaller human autosomes, contains less than 2 per cent of the human genome and this may account for the relatively less severe defects of Down's syndrome as compared to those that occur in abnormalities involving the larger chromosomes.

Affected individuals are of small stature and mentally retarded. They may exhibit hypertelorism and a characteristic facial appearance that includes epicanthic folds, up-slanting of the palpebral fissures (Mongoloid slant), a flat nasal root and round cheeks. The neck is short, and abnormalities in the upper limbs include short broad hands with a simian crease, abnormal dermatoglyphics and short fifth fingers with clinodactyly. Congenital heart disease affects approximately 35 per cent of cases and accounts for most of the deaths in childhood. After 10 years of age, the estimated life expectancy is 55 years. Clinical and histological features of Alzheimer's disease are universal by the age of 35 years.

The ophthalmic manifestations of Trisomy 21 are generally relatively minor and do not form any characteristic pattern. It has been suggested that the chromosomal abnormality affects the eye relatively late in development. The commonest features, in addition to the craniofacial anomalies, are iris hypoplasia (95 per cent) and Brushfield's spots (85–90 per cent); Brushfield's spots are coloured spots in the periphery of the iris seen histologically as areas of normal stroma surrounded by a ring of hypoplasia. Cataract formation is frequent (60–85 per cent), and there is an increased incidence of keratoconus. Other features include fundus hypopigmentation, an abnormal number of optic disc vessels, colobomas, myopia and retinal detachment.

Trisomy 18 (Edward's syndrome)
Trisomy of chromosome 18 has an incidence of 1 : 8000 live births and is usually lethal within the first year. Systemic features include a female predominance, mental deficiency and delay of psychomotor development, a prominent occiput, microstomia and micrognathia, epicanthic folds, narrow palpebral fissures, a short sternum and rocker-bottom feet. There is muscular hypertonia, the limbs being flexed and the hands clenched. Congenital heart disease is present in 90 per cent of cases and is the major cause of death. Ptosis and microphthalmos are characteristic ophthalmic manifestations, together with corneal opacities, cataracts and colobomas. It has been suggested that the effect of the chromosomal abnormality is to initiate widespread cellular hyperplasia and hypertrophy; histologically, the commonest findings are retinal folds and dysplasia, immaturity of the drainage angle and ciliary body, and thickening and hyperplasia of both the epithelium and endothelium of the cornea.

Trisomy 13 (Patau's syndrome)
The majority of cases of Patau's syndrome die within the first year of life and, although rare (1 : 20 000 live births), it is the chromosomal defect most consistently associated with severe ophthalmic abnormalities. Malformations include holoprosencephaly and other CSN anomalies, inguinal and umbilical hernias, cleft lip and palate, and congenital heart disease. Those affected fail to thrive and die in infancy. Bilateral ophthalmic manifestations occur in all cases. Microphthalmos is characteristic, and associated colobomas of the iris and ciliary body suggest that the developmental anomaly disrupts normal invagination of the optic vesicle. Mesodermal tissue at or near the site of the coloboma undergoes metaplasia, with the resultant formation of cartilage. There are cataracts, a persistent hyperplastic primary vitreous, retinal dysplasia and, occasionally, cyclopia.

Syndromes associated with structural chromosomal abnormalities

Structural chromosomal abnormalities occur with a frequency of approximately 1 : 500 live births and those of the greatest significance are deletions, which are usually sporadic, although in some syndromes it may be possible to demonstrate a reciprocal translocation in the parents. The majority of deletion syndromes are characterized by general features such as low birth weight, mental retardation, and craniofacial and skeletal abnormalities. Many syndromes with ophthalmic features have been described, but the most important are those associated with deletions of 11p13 and 13q14. Other ophthalmic lesions associated with structural abnormalities of chromosomes include Rieger's anomaly (del 4q, del 4p, dup 3p), congenital cystic eye (del 12p) and cyclopia (del 18p).

11p13 deletion syndrome
Deletion of the short arm of chromosome 11, specifically band 13, is associated with a sporadic form of aniridia. Other features include mental retardation, micro- or macrocephaly, and skeletal and genitourinary malformations. In addition there is a high risk of developing Wilms' tumour (nephroblastoma) before the age of 3 years; this forms part of the WAGR syndrome (Wilms' tumour, aniridia, genitourinary abnormalities and mental retardation).

13q14 deletion syndrome
Interstitial deletion of band 14 of the long arm of chromosome 13 results in a syndrome characterized by severe mental retardation, microcephaly, facial and orbital abnormalities, and short stature. Congenital heart defects, cryptorchidism, anal atresia and absent thumbs are also features, as is the frequent association of retinoblastoma. The degree of systemic abnormality depends on the size of the deletion, and it is possible that a very small deletion of band 14 may exist in those with retinoblastoma who have an otherwise normal phenotype. This deletion may be detectable in up to 5 per cent of retinoblastoma cases. As the enzyme esterase D is assigned to band 14 and is present in lower concentrations in 13q14 deletion, its assay is of some value in the diagnosis of retinoblastoma and in genetic screening.

SINGLE GENE DEFECTS

Most abnormalities in the genetic code are silent and do not result in inherited disorders. When a single gene defect has a biological effect it may act at any level of protein synthesis. The manifestations of the

Table 3.1 Autosomal dominant disorders of ophthalmic importance

Disorder	Gene locus	Gene
Cataract, posterior polar	1p	
Ehlers–Danlos syndrome	1p	PLOD
Cataract, nuclear	1p36	
Schnyder's central crystalline distrophy	1p36-p34	
Retinitis pigmentosa	1q13-q23	RP18
Cataract, zonular pulverulent	1q21-q25	GJA8
Juvenile glaucoma	1q23	GLC1A
Age-related macular degeneration	1q25-q31	ARMD1
Iris coloboma	2pter-p25.1	
Aniridia	2p25	
Cataract, anterior polar	2p25	
Dominant drusen	2p21-p16	EFEMP1
Primary open-angle glaucoma	2cen-q13	GLC1B
Ehlers–Danlos syndrome	2q31-q32.3	COL3A1
Cataract, Coppock-like	2q34-q35	CRYG4
Waardenburg syndrome	2q35	
von Hippel–Lindau disease	3p25-p24	
Congenital stationary night blindness	3p21	GNAT1
Macular dystrophy/spinocerebellar atrophy	3p13-p12	SCA7
Congenital stationary night blindness	3q21-q24	RHO
Retinitis pigmentosa	3q21-q24	RHO
Primary open-angle glaucoma	3q21-q24	GLC1C
Optic atrophy (Kjer type)	3q28-q29	OPA1
Stargardt-like macular dystrophy	4p	STGD4
Congenital stationary night blindness	4p16.3	PDE6B
Rieger's syndrome	4q25	RIEG1
GM2-gangliosidosis, AB variant	5	
Wagner's syndrome	5q13-q14	WGN1
Familial polyposis coli	5q21-q22	
Lattice/granular corneal dystrophy	5q31	TGFB1
Treacher Collins' syndrome	5q32-q33	TCOF1
Glaucoma with iris/angle anomalies	6p25	
Retinitis pigmentosa	6p21.2-cen	RDS
Macular dystrophy	6p21.2-cen	RDS
Cone-rod dystrophy	6p21.2-cen	RDS
Adult vitelliform macular dystrophy	6p21.2-cen	RDS
Cone dystrophy	6p21.1	GUCA1A
Cone-rod dystrophy	6p	CORD7
Macular dystrophy, Stargardt-like	6q11-q15	STGD3
North Carolina macular dystrophy	6q14-q16.2	MCDR1
Progressive bifocal choroidoretinal atrophy	6q14-q16	MCDR1
Cone dystrophy	6q25-q26	RCD1
Goldenhar's syndrome	7p	
Dominant cystoid macular oedema	7p21-p15	CYMD
Retinitis pigmentosa	7p15-p13	RP9
MPS VII	7q21.3-q22.1	
Retinitis pigmentosa	7q31.3	RP10
Tritanopia	7q31.3-q32	BCP
Pigment dispersion glaucoma	7q35-q36	
Retinitis pigmentosa	8q11-q13	RP1
Primary open-angle glaucoma	8q23	GLC1D
Tuberous sclerosis	9q33-q34	
Nail-patella glaucoma syndrome	9q34	LMX1B
Ehlers–Danlos syndromes	9q34.2-q34.3	COL5A1
Atypical Marfan's syndrome	9q34.2-q34.3	
Osteogenesis imperfecta	9q34.2-q34.3	
Renal-coloboma syndrome	10q25	PAX2
Helicoid peripapillary choroidoretinal dystrophy	11p15	AA
Aniridia + Wilms' etc.	11p13	PAX6
Best's disease	11q13	VMD2
Neovascular inflammatory vitreoretinopathy	11q13	VRN1
Retinitis pigmentosa	11q13	ROM1

Table 3.1 Continued

Disorder	Gene locus	Gene
Familial exudative vitreoretinopathy	11q13-q23	EVR1
Tuberous sclerosis	11q23	
Stickler's syndrome	12q1.23	COL2A1
Cataract, polymorphous	13q	
Reiger's syndrome	13q14	RIEG2
Retinoblastoma	13q14.2	RB1
Macular dystrophy, Stargardt-type	13q34	STGD2
Retinitis pigmentosa	14q11.2	NRL
Marfan's syndrome	15q21.1	FBN1
Tuberous sclerosis	16p13	
Cataract, nuclear	16q22	
Niemann–Pick disease	17	
Cataract, anterior polar	17p13	
Retinitis pigmentosa	17p13.3	RP13
Cone dystrophy	17p13-p12	CORD5
Central areolar choroidal dystrophy	17p13	CACD
Cone dystrophy	17q	CORD4
Neurofibromatosis (type 1)	17q11.2	NF1
Cataract, zonular sutural	17q11-q12	CRYBA1
Ehlers–Danlos syndromes	17q21.3-q22.05	
Atypical Marfan's syndrome	17q21.3-q22.05	
Osteogenesis imperfecta	17q21.3-q22.05	
Retinitis pigmentosa	17q22	RP17
Cataract, cerulean	17q24	
Cone-rod dystrophy	18q21.1-q22.3	CORD1
Myotonic dystrophy	19q13.1	
Cone-rod dystrophy	19q13.3	CRX
Leber's congenital amaurosis	19q13.3	CRX
Retinitis pigmentosa	19q13.3	CRX
Retinitis pigmentosa	19q13.4	RP11
Arteriohepatic dysplasia (Alagille's syndrome)	20p12	JAG1
Posterior polymorphous dystrophy	20q11	
Congenital hereditary endothelial dystrophy	20q11	
Cataract, nuclear	21q22.3	CRYAA
Cataract, cerulean	22q	CRYBB2
Neurofibromatosis (type 2)	22q11.21-q11.23	NF2
Sorsby's fundus dystrophy	22q12.1-q13.2	TIMP3

defect depend on the function of the particular protein involved and, because of the large number of different proteins and their functions, the spectrum of disease is wide-ranging. Defects on the autosomes and sex chromosomes are most frequently transmitted by Mendelian inheritance, whereas in mutations of non-chromosomal (mitochondrial) DNA the inheritance is non-Mendelian. Disorders of Mendelian inheritance are numerous and often severe, there being over 4000 listed types. The risk of transmission to offspring is high and genetic counselling is possible if a precise diagnosis can be made and a clear pattern of inheritance established. Single gene defects may be autosomal (dominant or recessive), X-linked (dominant or recessive) or mitochondrial. The type of Mendelian inheritance depends on the location of the defective gene on an autosome or the X chromosome (genes on the small Y chromosome are of little importance) and on the expression of the allelic genes, which may be dominant or recessive. As a general rule, autosomal dominant conditions cause either anatomical defects or involve structural proteins, while autosomal recessive conditions are usually enzyme deficiencies, metabolic disorders or disorders of DNA repair. The clinical features of a genetic defect depend on penetrance and expressivity. Penetrance is the probability that an abnormal genotype will result in an abnormal phenotype. An individual with the abnormal gene may not manifest a partially penetrant disorder, yet will transmit the gene to a child who may be affected. If a disorder has variable expressivity, although the disease will be manifest in all individuals possessing the gene, there may be considerable variation in the clinical features.

Autosomal dominant disorders

The characteristic feature of autosomal dominant inheritance is expression of the trait in a heterozygote – i.e. only one of a pair of alleles need be abnormal for the expression of the disorder. Key features are:

1. Equal transmission to males and females in affected families because the affected gene is located on one of the 22 autosomes and not on the sex chromosomes.
2. Affected individuals usually have an affected parent and, unless the disorder interferes with the ability to reproduce, there is transmission to successive generations.
3. On average 50 per cent of the offspring of a heterozygote and a normal mate are affected.
4. Most unaffected families do not carry the gene and, unless there has been a new mutation, it is unlikely that transmission to offspring will occur. All those affected have an affected parent. The clinical features will depend on penetrance and expressivity.
5. Homozygosity for dominant genes is uncommon but often lethal and requires that both parents are heterozygous for the condition and therefore have the disease.

A wide range of autosomal dominant disorders are known (Table 3.1) and many are described elsewhere in this book. Ophthalmic disorders include retinal dystrophies (e.g. the various forms of retinitis pigmentosa, the cone-rod dystrophies, Best's vitelliform macular dystrophy, dominant drusen), the phakomatoses, congenital cataracts and myotonic dystrophy.

Autosomal dominant disorders of connective tissue

The autosomal dominant disorders of connective tissue (Marfan's syndrome, Stickler's syndrome, pseudoxanthoma elasticum, the Ehlers–Danlos syndromes) form a group of systemic disorders with important ophthalmic manifestations.

Marfan's syndrome

Marfan's syndrome is characterized by skeletal, cardiovascular and ophthalmic defects. Its prevalence is approximately 1–5 : 50 000, it has variable expressivity and approximately a third of cases are new mutations. Those affected are of tall stature with long limbs (Fig. 3.1), the arm span being greater than the height.

Arachnodactyly, pectus excavatum, scoliosis and joint laxity are among other features, while cardiovascular defects include aortic, mitral or combined valve incompetence and dilatation of the ascending aorta that can lead to a dissecting aneurysm. Ophthalmic manifesta-

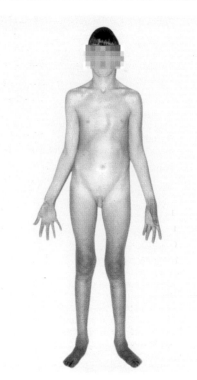

Figure 3.1 Marfan's syndrome.

tions affect the lens, the cornea and the size of the globe, and reflect the intrinsic lesion of connective tissue. Lens abnormalities include bilateral supero-temporal subluxation in 60–80 per cent of cases in childhood. The zonular fibres remain intact although they are abnormal, being composed almost entirely of microfibrillar fibres containing fibrillin. Microspherophakia is also described. Corneal abnormalities include megalocornea, cornea plana and keratoconus. Axial myopia is frequent. Retinal detachment occurs in 9 per cent of eyes with subluxated lenses. Glaucoma develops in 8 per cent of cases due to drainage angle anomalies, including abnormal iris insertions or subluxated lenses. Poor mydriasis results from hypoplasia of the iris dilator muscle.

The most frequent mutation in Marfan's syndrome is that of the fibrillin gene, which has been mapped to chromosome 15 (15q21.1). Fibrillin is a structural protein similar to collagen and forms microfibrils that act as a scaffold for the deposition of elastin during embryogenesis. The abnormality of these fibres results in an inability of elastic fibres to resist normal mechanical stress and this leads to the characteristic clinical features.

Stickler's syndrome

Stickler's syndrome, the commonest autosomal dominant disorder of connective tissue, is frequently underdiagnosed. Its prevalence is estimated at 1 : 10 000. Systemic features include loss of hearing; facial anomalies such as maxillary hypoplasia, micrognathia and a depressed nasal bridge; cleft palate; and skeletal abnormalities including joint laxity and arthritis. Characteristic ophthalmic manifestations include an optically empty vitreous, atrophy of the neurosensory retina, RPE hyperplasia, and lattice-like perivascular pigmentation. Retinal hole formation leads to retinal detachment in 30 per cent of cases. Other features resemble those of Marfan's syndrome, and include congenital high myopia, ectopia lentis and glaucoma consequent upon anomalies of the drainage angle. Characteristic wedge or fleck-shaped lens opacities occur in up to 50 per cent of cases.

Stickler's syndrome is genetically heterogeneous and arises from mutations in the structural gene for Type II procollagen located on chromosome 12 (12q1.23). Such mutations either prevent normal collagen synthesis or result in an abnormal gene product. The association of vitreous and joint abnormalities is explained by the presence of Type II collagen at both sites.

Pseudoxanthoma elasticum

Pseudoxanthoma elasticum is a genetically heterogeneous disorder of elastic tissue that may be inherited as autosomal dominant or autosomal recessive. At least four types have been described. The molecular basis is unknown at present. Cutaneous abnormalities include skin laxity and yellowish papules or a macular rash involving predominantly the side of the neck and skin flexures. Internal organs may also be involved, and lesions in the walls of the coronary arteries and the renal vasculature lead to secondary systemic complications. In the eye angioid streaks (see Fig. 5.16a) develop in 85 per cent of cases. Elastic fibres degenerate and swell, disintegrate and become calcified; these characteristic histological features occur in the dermis of the skin (Fig. 3.2) and in the medial coat of affected blood vessels. Angioid streaks represent calcification and breaks in Bruch's membrane (see Fig. 5.16b), thus allowing fibrovascular tissue to grow through from the choroid and to extend beneath the RPE; subsequent exudation and haemorrhage results in a submacular scar.

Ehlers–Danlos syndromes

Ehlers–Danlos syndromes comprise a rare group of at least 10 clinically and genetically heterogeneous disorders of connective tissue. The majority are autosomal dominant, but autosomal recessive and X-linked types are known. The common pathogenetic mechanism is the production of defective or deficient collagen, which results in skin hyperelasticity and fragility, joint hyperextensibility and often a bleeding diathesis. Ophthalmic features depend on the specific type of syndrome, but reflect the basic connective tissue defect. Accordingly there may be epicanthal folds, high myopia, keratoconus, blue sclera, lens subluxation, retinal detachment

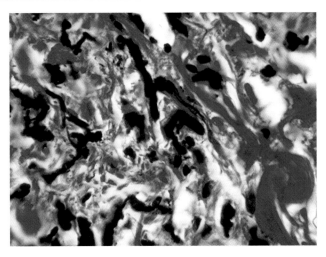

Figure 3.2 Pseudoxanthoma elasticum. Thickened fragmented fibres in dermis of skin. Verhoeff stain.

and angioid streaks (see Fig. 5.16). Specific biochemical abnormalities identified in some cases include deficiencies of lysyl oxidase and lysyl hydroxylase, abnormalities of the amino-terminal cleavage site of the procollagen chains of Type I collagen and abnormalities in the structure of Type II collagen.

Autosomal recessive disorders

Clinical features develop in an autosomal recessive disorder only if those affected are homozygous for the defective gene (Table 3.2). Key features are:

1. Affected families exhibit equal transmission to males and females.
2. Both parents are usually heterozygous for the trait and clinically normal. There is often no family history of the disorder.
3. The proportion of affected offspring is, on average, 25 per cent; one-half of all offspring will be heterozygous and therefore asymptomatic carriers of the trait. The disorder usually only occurs within one group of brothers and sisters.
4. Autosomal recessive disorders are more common in consanguineous marriages, for in such families there is a greater probability of related parents being heterozygous for the trait.
5. The clinical features of autosomal recessive disorders differ from those of autosomal dominant disorders in that they are usually less variable and are more evident in childhood, thus allowing for earlier diagnosis.
6. Most autosomal recessive genes are rare in the general population because homozygotes tend to die before reproductive age.
7. The majority of inherited metabolic diseases are autosomal recessive.

Table 3.2 Autosomal recessive disorders of ophthalmic importance

Disorder	Gene locus	Gene
Congenital glaucoma	1p36	GLC3B
Neuroblastoma	1p32	
Neuronal ceroid-lipofuscinosis CLN1 (Infantile Batten's disease)	1p32	
Leber's congenital amaurosis	1p31	RPE65
Retinitis pigmentosa	1p31	RPE65
Retinitis pigmentosa	1p22-p21	ABCA4
Stargardt's disease	1p22-p21	ABCA4
RP + para-arteriolar preservation of RPE (RP12)	1q31-q32.1	CRB1
Usher's syndrome	1q41	USH2A
Chediak–Higashi syndrome	1q43	
Alstrom's syndrome	2p14-p13	ALMS1
Congenital glaucoma	2p21	GLC3A
Retinitis pigmentosa	2p16-p11	RP28
Achromatopsia	2p11	CNGA3
Xeroderma pigmentosum	2q21	
Retinitis pigmentosa	2q31-q33	RP26
Oguchi's disease	2q37	SAG
Usher's syndrome, type 2	3p24.2-p23	USH2B
GM1-gangliosidosis	3p21-cent	
Morquio's syndrome B	3p21-cent	MPS IVB
Bardet–Biedl syndrome	3p13-p12	BBS3
Retinitis pigmentosa	3q21-q24	RHO
Usher's syndrome, type 3	3q21-q25	USH3A
Retinitis pigmentosa	4p16.3	PDE6B
Retinitis pigmentosa	4p12-cen	CNGA1
Mucolipidosis II & III	4q21-q23	
Bassen–Kornzweig syndrome	4q24	MTP
GM2-gangliosidosis, AB variant (Tay–Sachs disease AB variant)	5	
Maroteaux–Lamy syndrome (MPS VI)	5q11-q13	
Sandhoff's disease	5q11-q13	
Retinitis pigmentosa	5q31.2-q34	PDE6A
Retinitis pigmentosa	6p21.3	TULP1
Retinitis pigmentosa	6cen-q15	RP25
Zellweger's syndrome	7q11.12-q11.23	
Refsum's disease	7q21-q22	PEX1
Retinitis pigmentosa	8q13.1-q13.3	TTPA
Achromatopsia	8q21-q22	ACHM3
Galactosaemia	9p13	
Oculocutaneous albinism (OCA3)	9p3	TRP-1
Xeroderma pigmentosum	9q34.1	
Usher's syndrome, type 1f	10	USH1F
Refsum's disease	10p15.3-p12.2	PHYH
Usher's syndrome, type 1d	10q	USH1D
Metachromatic leukodystrophy	10q21-q24	
Retinitis pigmentosa	10q23	RGR
Hermansky–Pudlak syndrome	10q23.1-q23.3	
Retinitis pigmentosa	10q24	RBP4
Crouzon's craniofacial dysostosis	10q25-q26	FGFR2
Gyrate atrophy	10q26	OAT
Usher's syndrome, Acadian	11p15.1	USH1C
Bardet–Biedl syndrome	11q13	BBS1
Usher's syndrome, type1	11q13.5	MYO7A
Oculocutaneous albinism (OCA1)	11q14-q21	TYR
Ataxia telangiectasia	11q22-q23	
Fundus albipunctatus	12q13-q14	RDH5
Sanfilippo's syndrome	12q14	
Phenylketonuria	12q22-q24.1	
Wilson's disease	13q14-q21	
Oguchi's disease	13q34	RHOK
Hers' disease (glycogen storage disease IV)	14	
Rod monochromacy	14	ACHM1
Leber's congenital amaurosis	14q24	LCA3
Microphthalmos	14q32	
Usher's syndrome, French	14q32	USH1A

Table 3.2 Continued

Disorder	Gene locus	Gene
Oculocutaneous albinism (OCA2)	15q11.2-q12	
Bardet–Biedl syndrome	15q22.3-q23	BBS4
Tay–Sachs disease, GM$_2$-gangliosidoses, juvenile and adult forms	15q22-q25.1	
Retinal dystrophy, retardation, spasticity	15q24	MRST
Retinitis pigmentosa	15q26	RLBP1
Retinitis pigmentosa	16p12.3-p12.1	RP22
Neuronal ceroid-lipofuscinosis CLN3 (Batten's disease)	16p12.1	CLN3
Bardet–Biedl syndrome	16q21	BBS2
Macular corneal dystrophy	16q22	
Tyrosinaemia type II	16q22.1	
Krabbe's disease	17	
Cone-rod dystrophy (CORD6)	17p13	GUCY2D
Leber's congenital amaurosis	17p13	GUCY2D
Pompe's disease	17q23	
Galactokinase deficiency	17q23-q25	
Green/blue eye colour	19	
Mannosidosis	19p13.1-p12	
Xeroderma pigmentosum	19q13.2	
Optic atrophy with ataxia and 3-methylglutaconic aciduria	19q13.2-q13.3	OPA3
Usher's syndrome, type 1	21q21	USH1E
Homocystinuria	21q22.3	
Hurler; Scheie; Hurler–Scheie syndrome	22q11	
Metachromatic leukodystrophy	22q13.31-qter	

Autosomal recessive disorders of metabolism

Autosomal recessive disorders include inherited metabolic disorders of amino acids (e.g. albinism, homocystinuria, alkaptonuria), carbohydrates (e.g. galactosaemia), lipids (e.g. neuronal ceroid lipofuscinoses) and minerals (e.g. Wilson's disease), lysosomal storage disorders (sphingolipidoses, mucopolysaccharidoses, mucolipidoses) and disorders of DNA repair (ataxia telangiectasia, xeroderma pigmentosum). The majority of autosomal recessive metabolic and storage disorders result from an abnormality in enzyme function, and several general principles underlie their pathophysiology:

1. Enzyme deficiency is almost always autosomal recessive. Most enzymes are synthesized in quantities exceeding the minimum biochemical requirements and heterozygotes, who have approximately 50 per cent activity of the affected enzyme, are therefore clinically normal. In most metabolic pathways the enzyme deficiency is overcome by compensatory mechanisms such as an increase in the amount of substrate. In the homozygous state, where both alleles are abnormal, enzyme activity is completely absent. This cannot be compensated for and the result is that the normal product of the affected enzyme is absent, thus allowing substrates or intermediate compounds to accumulate.

2. Substrate accumulation and/or product deficiency are the underlying mechanisms of disorders resulting from enzyme deficiencies; enzymes convert a substrate into a product and abnormal enzyme function upsets the balance of the equation.

3. The physical properties of the substrate molecule determine the features of the disorder. Small soluble molecules, such as phenylalanine, diffuse out of cells where they are normally metabolized and cause damage throughout the body. Large non-diffusible macromolecules remain trapped within an organelle or cell and damage the tissues in which they accumulate. This is exemplified in the lysosomal storage disorders, which are a group of conditions that result from mutations in genes that encode for lysosomal acid hydrolases, the enzymes that degrade biological molecules. Enzyme deficiency leads to the accumulation of normal substrates in lysosomes and cellular dysfunction results.

4. Both the clinical and pathological features may be similar in different enzyme deficiencies; this is known as phenotypic homology and may occur if the substrates of the enzymes are metabolically similar.

5. More than one enzyme can be involved in a single gene defect if:
   a) A co-factor common to several enzymes is involved.

b) There is an abnormality in a subunit shared by different enzymes.

c) Multiple enzymes are processed by a single enzyme that is defective.

d) There is an abnormality in the organelle that usually contains a group of enzymes.

Disorders of amino acid metabolism

Many inherited disorders of amino acid metabolism are known. Those of ophthalmic importance include albinism, alkaptonuria, homocystinuria and cystinosis.

Albinism

Albinism is a heterogeneous group of at least 10 inherited disorders characterized by hypopigmentation resulting from a defect in the synthesis of melanin. The incidence is variable but is of the order of 1 : 20 000 of the general population. Ophthalmic manifestations are common, and albinism accounts for about 9 per cent of severe visual handicap in children. Most types are inherited as autosomal recessive. Albinism is classified into two broad clinical types: oculocutaneous albinism (OCA), in which there is hypopigmentation of the eyes, skin and hair (Fig. 3.3), and ocular albinism (OA), in which the eyes alone are affected. OA can also be inherited as an X-linked recessive (Nettleship–Falls albinism). Features common to both OCA and OA include decreased visual acuity, photophobia, iris transillumination, foveal hypoplasia, nystagmus and an abnormal decussation of nerve fibres at the optic chiasm. Albinos are susceptible to premature actinic skin damage and ultraviolet light-induced cutaneous malignancies due to the absence of melanin. The subgroups of OCA depend on the activity of tyrosinase, which is an enzyme in the pathway that converts 1-tyrosine to 3, 4 dihydroxyphenylalanine (DOPA) and subsequently to melanin. The tyrosinase gene is located on chromosome 11 (11q14-q21), and its activity can be determined by the hair bulb incubation test in which the roots of a plucked hair are incubated in a solution containing tyrosine; normal tyrosinase activity results in intense pigmentation but if tyrosinase activity is reduced, pigment production is also reduced. The ophthalmic features of albinism are similar among the subgroups but may vary in degree and are possibly due to developmental abnormalities that include underdevelopment of the central retina and reduced numbers of rod photoreceptors and ganglion cells. There are three types of OCA:

Type I OCA

In type I OCA (OCA1), tyrosinase activity is completely or partially inhibited as the result of a mutation in the tyrosinase gene. The various types of OCA1 include OCA1a (complete absence of pigment), OCA1b (yellow OCA), OCA1-MP (minimal pigment albinism) and OCA1-TP (temperature dependent albinism). OCA1 can alternatively be referred to as tyrosinase negative.

Type II OCA

In type II OCA (OCA2), tyrosinase activity is normal (tyrosinase positive OCA). It is caused by mutations at the P locus on chromosome 15 (15q11.2-q12); the role of the P protein is unknown. In those affected, pigmentation increases with age and ephelides and lentigines appear but the skin does not tan.

Type III OCA

In type III OCA (OCA3), although tyrosinase is found in normal amounts its activity is reduced due to the absence of tyrosinase-related protein (TRP-1), the gene of which maps to chromosome 9 (9p23). OCA3, also known as brown OCA, is described only in Africans and is characterized by light brown skin and hair, moderate tanning ability, blue-grey irises and iris transillumination. Rufous oculocutaneous albinism (ROCA) is also ascribed to TRP-1 mutations and is characterized by bright copper-red skin and hair, and reduced iris pigmentation. Those with ROCA have no visual pathway abnormalities.

Hermansky–Pudlak syndrome

The Hermansky–Pudlak syndrome maps to chromosome 10 (10q23.1-q23.3) and has a variable pigment phenotype; affected individuals do not tan. The disorder is characterized by albinism, abnormal platelet agglutination and abnormal tissue ceroid accumulation. Restrictive lung disease and ulcerative colitis can develop later.

Chediak–Higashi syndrome

The Chediak–Higashi syndrome maps to chromosome 1 (1q43) and is characterized by albinism and increased susceptibility to infection due to leukocyte dysfunction,

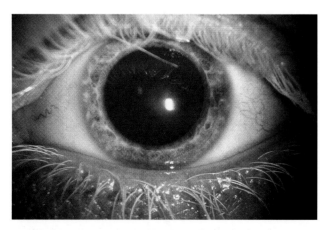

Figure 3.3 Oculocutaneous albinism. Iris transillumination and pale lashes.

and a predisposition to lymphoreticular malignancy and early death.

Alkaptonuria (ochronosis)

Alkaptonuria results from a deficiency of homogentisic acid oxidase with a consequent increase in the body of homogentisic acid, a degradation product of phenylalanine and tyrosine. Homogentisic acid is excreted in the urine where it is oxidized to ochronotic pigment, which is deposited in connective tissues (see Fig. 5.38).

Homocystinuria

Homocystinuria is a disorder of amino acid metabolism that exhibits clinical features in common with Marfan's syndrome. It affects 1 : 200 000 live births, but there are racial variations (e.g. it is commoner in the Irish). The skeletal, nervous and vascular systems are all involved. Affected individuals are often tall with skeletal malformations including arachnodactyly. Other features include a malar flush, fair hair and seizures, and approximately half of the cases exhibit progressive mental retardation. Increased platelet stickiness predisposes to arterial thrombosis and thromboembolism, which makes general anaesthesia hazardous. Ectopia lentis occurs in 90 per cent of cases; characteristically, but not exclusively, the lens dislocates inferonasally. Other features include myopia, retinal detachment, strabismus and retinal vascular occlusions.

In homocystinuria, the enzyme cystathione β-synthetase (which controls the synthesis of cystathionine, an intermediate in the conversion of homocystine to cysteine) is deficient and the result is a build-up of homocystine and homocystine precursors. The gene for the enzyme is located on chromosome 21 (21q22.3). The cause of the ectopia lentis is an abnormality of the zonular fibres, which have a matted appearance and are irregularly distributed; short broken filaments remain attached to the lens capsule but the bulk of fibres retract to the basement membrane of the non-pigmented ciliary epithelium (Fig. 3.4). Amino acid electrophoresis and chromatography of urine and plasma are useful in establishing the diagnosis.

Cystinosis

Cystinosis is characterized by the intracellular accumulation of cystine at levels up to 100 times the normal. This results from impaired transportation of cystine across lysosomal membranes. The high intracellular concentration of cystine leads to crystallization of the amino acid within lysosomes of many body tissues, including the abdominal viscera, the thyroid and the reticuloendothelial system. The ophthalmic tissues involved are the conjunctiva, cornea, iris, lens capsule and RPE.

Three clinical types of cystinosis are described: infantile, juvenile and adult. The infantile type is the most

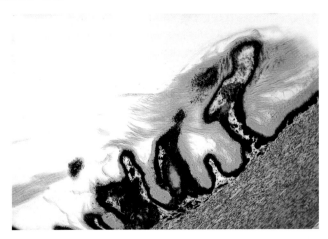

Figure 3.4 Homocystinuria. Thick matted zonular fibres lying over the ciliary epithelium.

severe, with onset during the first year of life. There is renal tubular dysfunction and later massive and widespread cystine deposition. Renal failure necessitating transplantation occurs by the end of the first decade. Extrarenal complications such as hypothyroidism and diabetes mellitus are common. Crystalline deposits within the conjunctiva and cornea are the cause of the distressing photophobia. If those affected survive into adulthood, retinal degeneration and glaucoma develop. Microscopy reveals rectangular or hexagonal crystals in the conjunctiva and needle-shaped crystals within the cornea. Crystals are also present within the RPE, which shows focal areas of degeneration. Elevated levels of cystine in cultured fibroblasts and neutrophils assist in confirmation of the diagnosis. Heterozygotes have half normal lysosomal cystine transport and mildly elevated cystine levels in fibroblasts and polymorphonuclear leukocytes, thus allowing for carrier detection.

Disorders of carbohydrate metabolism

The numerous disorders of carbohydrate metabolism include the glycogen storage diseases (e.g. von Gierke's, Pompe, Andersen and McArdle diseases), but few have significant ophthalmic features. Galactosaemia, a potentially treatable cause of childhood cataract, is an exception.

Galactosaemia

Lactose, the principal carbohydrate of mammalian milk, is a disaccharide composed of galactose and glucose. Galactose must first be converted to glucose before it can be metabolized via the Embden–Meyerhof pathway. There are three stages in the conversion, involving the enzymes galactokinase (GK), galactose-1-phosphate uridyl transferase (GPUT) and uridine diphosphate galactose-4-epimerase. Galactosaemia and galactosuria result if galactose is not converted into glucose because of a lack of GK or GPUT.

GK deficiency is inherited as an autosomal recessive, the locus for the GK gene being on chromosome 17 (17q23-q25). The disorder has a relatively benign course, with affected babies being well apart from cataract formation during the first year of life.

GPUT deficiency (classic galactosaemia) is inherited as an autosomal recessive with a genetic locus for the enzyme on chromosome 9 (9p13). The disorder presents in the neonate within a few days of milk ingestion. Clinical features include diarrhoea and vomiting, jaundice, hypoglycaemia, hepatosplenomegaly, mental retardation and cataracts. The elevated levels of galactose-1-phosphate account for the widespread tissue damage. The liver is particularly involved, with accumulation of fat, cholestasis, and later cirrhosis. If untreated, the disorder is rapidly fatal.

Mechanism of cataract formation in galactosaemia
Accumulation of galactose leads to the formation of the sugar alcohol, dulcitol (galactitol). This cannot cross cell membranes, and its accumulation within the lens fibres increases the intracellular osmotic pressure, resulting in fluid accumulation and cell swelling. This can be seen within the first few weeks of life as an oil-drop cataract, which is not a true cataract but an optical phenomenon due to the altered refractive index of the lens consequent upon swelling of the lens fibres. It is reversible if dietary control of the galactosaemia is prompt. Later, disruption of lens fibres with the formation of clefts containing precipitated lens protein leads to permanent opacification (Fig. 3.5). An increased suscept-

ibility to the development of bilateral presenile posterior subcapsular cataracts and of secondary cataracts consequent upon insults such as trauma, inflammation and diabetes mellitus is seen particularly in GK deficient heterozygotes.

Disorders of lipid metabolism

Abnormalities of lipids and lipoproteins are a heterogeneous group that includes the familial hyperlipidaemias, the hypolipoproteinaemias and the neuronal ceroid lipofuscinoses; the latter are of considerable ophthalmic importance.

Neuronal ceroid lipofuscinoses (Batten's disease)
The significant feature of the neuronal ceroid lipofuscinoses (NCL) is the accumulation of ceroid, an autofluorescent conjugated lipopigment in neural (including retinal) and other tissues. Varying degrees of progressive encephalopathy, seizures and loss of vision are characteristic. The pathogenesis is obscure.

The infantile and late infantile forms present with neurological features including developmental regression, behavioural problems, dementia, myoclonus and visual failure. A rapid downhill course leads to death between the ages of 4 and 10 years. Blindness is the result of widespread retinal degeneration, initially most marked posteriorly, where there is often a bull's eye maculopathy. Other retinal lesions include clumped pigment, narrow arterioles and optic atrophy.

The juvenile form is one of the commoner neurodegenerative diseases of childhood and presents between 5 and 8 years of age with central visual loss and night blindness. The ophthalmic manifestations progress more slowly than in the earlier onset types but maculopathy, retinopathy and optic atrophy are characteristic. Neurological features include behavioural changes followed by the development of seizures and progressive dementia. Death occurs before the third decade.

In NCL, abnormal lipopigment is stored in membrane-bound cytosomic inclusions that vary in their morphology according to the disease type. Dense granular osmiophilic deposits occur predominantly in the infantile forms; those with curvilinear profiles are characteristic of the late infantile type (Fig. 3.6), while lamellar structures occur predominantly in the juvenile type. Lymphocytes containing vacuoles filled with lipopigment found in the peripheral blood are characteristic of the juvenile type. Diagnosis can be confirmed by finding the characteristic intracellular inclusions on electron microscopical examination of biopsies of the rectum, skeletal muscle, skin or conjunctiva.

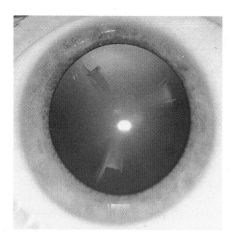

Figure 3.5 Galactosaemic cataract.

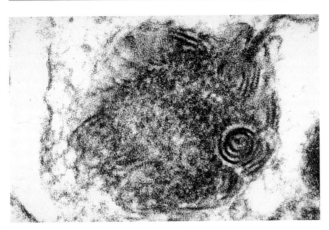

Figure 3.6 Neuronal ceroid lipofuscinosis, late infantile type. Intracellular curvilinear inclusions. TEM.

Disorders of mineral metabolism

Deficiencies and excess of both major and minor (trace) minerals cause systemic disease. Of particular ophthalmic importance is the disorder of copper metabolism that results in Wilson's disease.

Wilson's disease (hepatolenticular degeneration)

Wilson's disease is a rare autosomal recessive disorder of copper metabolism. The synonym hepatolenticular degeneration indicates specifically the involvement of the liver and the lentiform nucleus of the basal ganglia (not the lens of the eye). The ophthalmic and neurological manifestations are closely associated but are not specific for Wilson's disease and may develop in cholestatic liver disease in which copper accumulates. The ophthalmic changes can also occur in chalcosis due to the intraocular retention of a copper-containing foreign body.

The daily requirement of copper (1–2 mg) is necessary for the synthesis of copper-containing enzymes such as cytochrome oxidase and superoxide dismutase. The dietary intake of copper is much greater than the requirement and the excess is bound into caeruloplasmin, an alpha-2-globulin present in the blood. In Wilson's disease the circulating caeruloplasmin is reduced, the consequence being increased concentration of free copper which becomes loosely bound to albumin, in which form it is deposited in the tissues. A genetic locus for the disorder has been assigned to chromosome 13 (13q14-q21). Paradoxically, the gene for caeruloplasmin is located on chromosome 3 and it is clear that the primary lesion is not simply a reduced level of caeruloplasmin but a more complex abnormality of the biliary excretion of copper. The mechanism by which an excess of copper damages cells is not clear.

Wilson's disease becomes symptomatic during adolescence or early adulthood. The majority present with features related to chronic liver disease, but a small number present with neurological and/or psychological manifestations. Inco-ordination and tremor progress to disabling dystonia and spasticity with dysarthria and dysphagia. Dementia and psychiatric disorders, such as behavioural abnormalities, may also develop. Post-mortem examination of the brain of those affected reveals a reddish-brown discoloration of the basal ganglia in which loss of neurons is associated with astrocytic proliferation. Cortical atrophy is common, and there is spongy softening and cavitation of the white matter. Copper-induced damage can also affect the kidneys, with resultant glomerular and tubular dysfunction. Acute haemolytic episodes and skeletal lesions such as osteoporosis and arthropathies may also be present.

The characteristic ophthalmic lesion of Wilson's disease is the Kayser–Fleischer ring (see Fig. 5.35), a golden brown deposit of metallic copper in the periphery of Descemet's membrane. The deposits are arranged in a linear fashion and are thought to result from an active metabolic process within the endothelium. Most of those affected with Wilson's disease develop a Kayser–Fleischer ring, and a relatively small number also develop a green anterior subcapsular sunflower cataract due to the deposition of copper between the capsule and the epithelium of the lens. The corneal and lens involvement are of diagnostic value.

Lysosomal storage diseases: sphingolipidoses, mucopolysaccharidoses and mucolipidoses

Lysosomal storage diseases are a group of predominantly autosomal recessive conditions that result from mutations in genes that encode for lysosomal acid hydrolases, the enzymes that degrade essentially all biological macromolecules. Enzyme deficiency leads to the accumulation (hence the term 'storage') of normal substrates in lysosomes, and cellular dysfunction results. The brain and heart are particularly involved, and the disorders are ultimately fatal. Although rare, more than 30 distinct types of lysosomal storage diseases have been described and are classified according to the material retained within the lysosomes. Those that affect the eye fall into three broad categories: sphingolipidoses, mucopolysaccharidoses and mucolipidoses.

Sphingolipidoses

The sphingolipidoses result from defects in the catabolic pathway of substances derived from cell membranes, such as gangliosides, cerebrosides, sphingomyelin and sulphatides. Intermediate lipids accumulate and progressive degeneration within the CNS is characterized by epilepsy, ataxia, paralysis, hyper-reflexia and dementia.

Blindness is common, and ophthalmoscopic findings include a cherry-red spot at the macula and optic atrophy. The sphingolipidoses include the gangliosidoses (Tay–Sachs disease, Sandhoff's disease, the GM_1 galactosidoses) and the Niemann–Pick lipidoses.

Gangliosidoses

The gangliosidoses are a group of rare autosomal recessive disorders resulting from deficiency of lysosomal hydrolase. At least seven different disorders are known, of which the most important are Tay–Sachs disease, Sandhoff's disease and the GM_1 galactosidoses. The ganglioside GM_1 is converted into GM_2 by the enzyme β-galactosidase. The subsequent catabolism of GM_2 is dependent on the enzymes hexosaminidase A and hexosaminidase B. The underlying defect in Tay–Sachs disease is faulty synthesis of hexosaminidase A caused by a genetic abnormality on chromosome 15 (15q22-q25.1). A separate mutation that renders both hexosaminidase A and hexosaminidase B defective gives rise to Sandhoff's disease.

Tay–Sachs disease (GM₂ Type I) is the infantile form of the gangliosidoses. Prior to the onset of screening programmes and appropriate counselling, it was more common among Ashkenazi Jews; in non-Jewish Western populations its incidence is less than $1 : 10\,000$. GM_2 accumulates in lysosomes throughout the body but more especially in the neurons of the CNS and retina, which are distended by the deposits (Fig. 3.7a). Electron microscopy reveals these deposits to be composed of concentric whorls of lamellae (membranous cytoplasmic bodies – Fig. 3.7b). Later, when the cells degenerate, strongly birefringent extracellular deposits of the material are characteristic. In the eye, degeneration of the swollen ganglion cells results in atrophy of the retinal nerve fibre layer and optic nerve.

During the first year of life there is an exaggerated startle reflex, hypotonia, progressive weakness, loss of acquired skills and decreased attentiveness. Motor and mental deterioration are rapidly progressive. Seizures develop, the head enlarges and the child usually dies before 10 years of age. In association with the psychomotor deterioration, vision becomes seriously impaired. Ophthalmoscopy (Fig. 3.7c) in the early stages reveals a pale fundus due to ganglioside accumulation in the retinal ganglion cells, which consequently become distended. A characteristic cherry-red spot at the macula is due to the absence of ganglion cells at this site and the normal choroidal circulation showing through. As the disease progresses, the ganglion cells die, the cherry-red spot becomes less apparent and optic atrophy becomes the principal feature.

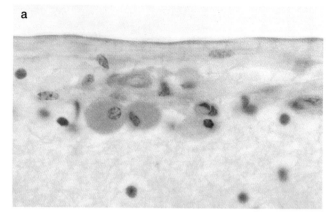

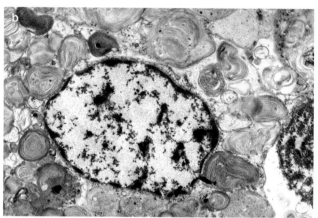

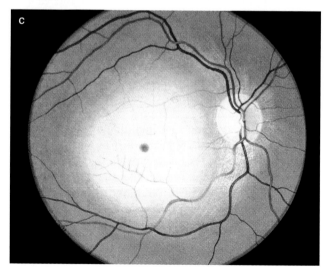

Figure 3.7 Tay–Sachs disease. (a) GM_2 in retinal ganglion cells. PAS stain. (b) Membranous cytoplasmic bodies. TEM. (c) Fundus appearance.

Sandhoff's disease (GM₂ Type II) is probably more common in the non-Jewish population. Clinically similar to Tay–Sachs disease, both hexosaminidase A and hexosaminidase B are deficient.

GM₁ galactosidoses are rare and result from abnormal synthesis of β-galactosidase. There are three types: infantile, juvenile and adult (GM₁ – Types I, II, III). GM₁ – Type I (infantile) is the least rare of the galactosidoses and is the only form to have significant ophthalmic involvement. It is caused by a mutation in the β-galactosidase gene located on chromosome 3 (3p21-cent). The defect leads to storage of several types of macromolecules of complex carbohydrates including GM₁ galactoside, which accumulates in cells throughout the body but particularly in the CNS and the autonomic nervous system, and in the retinal ganglion cells. Those affected present at birth with hypotonia, limb oedema and failure to thrive. They are dysmorphic with hepatosplenomegaly and a cherry-red spot at the macula resembling that seen in the other gangliosidoses. Corneal clouding has been described. Blindness occurs early and psychomotor development ceases at 3–6 months. Spasticity ensues, the infant may develop seizures and later becomes decerebrate. Death usually occurs by 2 years of age. Characteristic haematological findings are vacuolated lymphocytes in the peripheral blood and large foamy histiocytes in the bone marrow.

Niemann–Pick lipidoses

The Niemann–Pick lipidoses are a group of lysosomal storage disorders in which sphingomyelin, cholesterol and other lipids accumulate within brain cells and hepatocytes, and within macrophages in many organs throughout the body. There are two groups:

Group I in which sphingomyelinase is deficient due to mutations in the sphingomyelinase gene. The two types in the group are Type A (neurovisceral) and Type B (visceral only).

Group II in which sphingomyelinase activity is normal but in which the metabolic defect is thought to involve the intracellular esterification of cholesterol. As in Group I, there are two types: Type C (neurovisceral ophthalmoplegic lipidosis) and Type D (a juvenile variant).

The majority of individuals with Niemann–Pick lipidosis fall into group I, Type A. Ashkenazi Jews are those most frequently affected and presentation is in early infancy with failure to thrive, conspicuous hepatosplenomegaly and progressive psychomotor retardation. A cherry-red spot at the macula is present in up to 50 per cent of cases. Other types may have a retinopathy, and in Type C disease there is a vertical ophthalmoplegia. Death in the Niemann–Pick lipidoses occurs before the age of 5 years.

The characteristic histological feature is the foam cell – a macrophage distended by cytoplasmic vacuoles containing sphingomyelin and cholesterol. The whorled lamellar structures within the vacuoles, also seen in other storage diseases, are revealed by electron microscopy. Foam cells are particularly abundant in the liver, spleen, bone marrow and lymph nodes. Neurons in the CNS and the ganglion cells of the retina are initially distended with the stored material but later become atrophic.

Mucopolysaccharidoses

The mucopolysaccharidoses (MPS) are a group of lysosomal storage disorders caused by a deficiency in one of the enzymes involved in the catabolism of the mucopolysaccharides (glycosaminoglycans – GAGs) dermatan sulphate, heparan sulphate, chondroitin sulphate and keratan sulphate. Incompletely degraded GAGs are secreted in the urine and are stored within cells of most organs of the body; neurons, connective tissue cells, cardiac muscle, endothelial cells, hepatocytes and macrophages are particularly involved. The MPS include the syndromes of Hurler, Scheie, Hunter, Sanfilippo and Morquio. With the exception of the Hunter syndrome, which is an X-linked recessive disorder, all are inherited as autosomal recessives. The MPS have systemic and ophthalmic manifestations.

Systemic manifestations involve the CNS, skeleton and viscera. Initially intracellular accumulation of GAGs predominates within the CNS, but as the disorder advances neurons are progressively lost and gliosis, cortical atrophy and communicating hydrocephalus ensue. GAGs within chondrocytes interfere with eventual ossification, resulting in the characteristic deformities (e.g. the gargoyle facies). GAGs within cardiac muscle lead to distortion of the heart valves and, within the endocardium, to thickening and consequent narrowing of the coronary arteries. GAGs within the hepatocytes and Kupffer cells of the liver and within the macrophages of the spleen lead to hepatosplenomegaly.

The ophthalmic manifestations are corneal clouding, pigmentary retinal degeneration, glaucoma and optic atrophy. Corneal clouding, manifest as a ground glass appearance, is seen in all forms of MPS except Hunter's and Sanfilippo's syndromes. Although the epithelium and endothelium appear clinically normal, GAGs infiltrate all layers of the cornea except Descemet's membrane. Characteristic intracellular inclusions may be demonstrable by microscopy of corneal epithelial biopsies. Pigmentary retinal degeneration may occur in all forms of MPS except Morquio's syndrome. The characteristic bone spicule pigmentation is associated with narrowing of the retinal vessels and optic atrophy. The visual fields are constricted and there is night blindness. Open angle glaucoma probably occurs in MPS because

GAG-laden cells obstruct the trabecular meshwork. Optic atrophy can develop as a result of glaucoma, degeneration of the ganglion cell and nerve fibre layers of the retina, optic disc swelling (which may result from communicating hydrocephalus) or, if there is scleral involvement, from constriction of the intrascleral portion of the optic nerve.

Mucolipidoses

The mucolipidoses are a rare group of lysosomal storage disorders with features intermediate between the sphingolipidoses and the mucopolysaccharidoses. Classification of the disorders is difficult, with frequent overlap in the clinical and biochemical findings. The ophthalmic manifestations include a cherry-red spot at the macula, retinal degeneration, granular corneal deposits and corneal clouding.

Disorders of DNA repair

Ataxia telangiectasia (Louis–Bar syndrome)
Ataxia telangiectasia is characterized by progressive cerebellar ataxia, dry skin, recurrent respiratory infections and the frequent occurrence of lymphomas. The principal ophthalmic features are telangiectasia of the conjunctival capillaries (Fig. 3.8) and abnormalities of ophthalmic motility such as nystagmus and ophthalmoplegia. The defect in DNA repair results in chromosomal breakage.

Xeroderma pigmentosum
Xeroderma pigmentosum affects children between 2 and 5 years of age. Presentation is with neoplastic and non-neoplastic manifestations of UV light damage, including freckling, poikiloderma and atrophy of light-exposed skin, which has the appearance of a 60–70 year old. Actinic keratosis, basal cell carcinoma, squamous cell carcinoma and melanoma develop later in childhood or in early adult life. The cause is an inability to excise UV-damaged segments of DNA resulting from defective UV endonuclease the genetic loci for which are on chromosomes 9(9q34.1), 2(2q21) and 19(19q13.2).

X-linked disorders

A disorder is termed X-linked when the causative gene is located on the X chromosome. Males and females are affected differently. All normal females have two X chromosomes and they may be homozygous or heterozygous for a particular trait. Clinical expression is variable and depends upon the trait being dominant or recessive. In general, X-linked disorders are intermediate in severity between autosomal recessive (severe) and autosomal dominant (less severe) traits.

X-linked dominant disorders

X-linked dominant disorders are manifest in both females and males, and pedigrees superficially resemble those of autosomal dominant disorders. Key features are:

1. Absence of male-to-male transmission. An affected male transmits the disorder only to his daughters.
2. A heterozygous female transmits the condition to half her children, whether male or female.
3. Homozygous states are often lethal. Affected females are therefore aborted or stillborn.
4. As a consequence of the foregoing, in an affected family there are on average twice as many affected females as males.

X-linked dominant disorders are few in number, but rare and severe. Those of ophthalmic importance include incontinentia pigmenti and Aicardi's syndrome.

Incontinentia pigmenti
Incontinentia pigmenti is usually lethal to affected males. In female neonates, intraepidermal vesicles on the extremities progress to warty outgrowths that later become pigmented. Mesodermal defects involving the eyes, teeth, skeleton and heart may become manifest later in childhood. CNS involvement occurs in approximately one-third of cases and results in seizures, spasticity, paresis and mental retardation. Ophthalmic manifestations occur in one-third of cases and can lead to blindness. Cataract, nystagmus and strabismus are common. Corneal opacities, uveitis, microphthalmos, retinal pigmentary changes and vascular anomalies can also be seen as can retinal detachment, which may lead to the formation of a retrolental mass, leukocoria and phthisis bulbi. In incontinentia pigmenti, melanin pigment in the basal

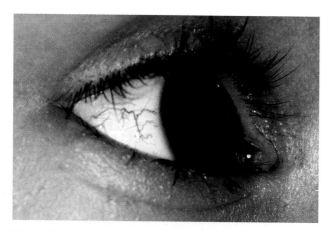

Figure 3.8 Ataxia telangiectasia. Dilated conjunctival capillaries.

layers of the epidermis is diminished or even absent but the amount in the upper dermis is increased; it was at one time thought that the basal cells were 'incontinent' of pigment, which dropped into the dermis – hence the name of the condition. In the eye, the RPE proliferates and, as the RPE exerts an organizing influence on the developing retina, there is often associated retinal dysplasia.

Aicardi's syndrome

Aicardi's syndrome is a rare and serious neuro-ophthalmic disorder which is lethal to males in utero. Affected females suffer serious malformations of the CNS, including agenesis of the corpus callosum, and die within the first few years of life. Ophthalmic manifestations are common, and include optic disc colobomas, choroidoretinal atrophy, persistent pupillary membranes and microphthalmos.

X-linked recessive disorders

X-linked recessive disorders form the majority of X-linked conditions with ophthalmic manifestations. Key features are:

1. Males always express the trait as they have a single X chromosome.
2. Unaffected males cannot transmit the trait.
3. Male-to-male transmission is impossible because the father contributes only his normal Y chromosome to male offspring.
4. Affected males in a family are either brothers or related through carrier females (e.g. maternal uncles).
5. Carrier females do not usually manifest clinical disease or, if manifestations are present, they are usually mild.
6. All daughters of an affected male will be obligate carriers of the trait because the father's abnormal X chromosome is passed on to female offspring.
7. On average, half the sons of a carrier female will be affected and half her daughters will be carriers (assuming that the father is unaffected).

Females may be symptomatic for a number of reasons:

1. They may be homozygous for the condition as the result of having an affected father and a carrier mother.
2. Unbalanced inactivation of the normal X chromosome (lyonization) can result in mild clinical manifestations of the trait, such as the fundal appearances in carriers of X-linked ocular albinism, choroideraemia and retinitis pigmentosa.
3. The second X chromosome may be absent, as in Turner's syndrome.

4. Translocation of the X chromosome can result in a copy of the gene being located on an autosome.

X-linked recessive disorders are relatively common, and many are of ophthalmic importance (Table 3.3).

Norrie's disease

Norrie's disease is a rare X-linked recessive condition that presents with blindness in male children at or soon after birth. Systemic features include mental retardation (25 per cent) and the later development of cochlear deafness (30 per cent). The ophthalmic manifestations are due to bilateral retinal folds and detachments, and vitreous haemorrhage with the formation of a retrolental mass (Fig. 3.9). The histological features are those of retinal dysplasia with absence of the retinal vasculature. A candidate gene (NDP) has been identified on the X chromosome near to the centromere (Xp11.3) and within a region containing the loci for X-linked retinitis pigmentosa, congenital stationary night blindness, X-linked cone dystrophy and familial exudative retinopathy. The Norrie's disease gene product (norrin) is similar to certain nerve growth factors and may be involved in retinal development.

Fabry's disease (angiokeratoma diffusum, galactosidase deficiency)

Fabry's disease is a glycolipidosis resulting from deficiency of α-galactosidase A, an enzyme that splits the sugar molecule from the lipid moiety in the natural breakdown process of hexosylceramides, which are

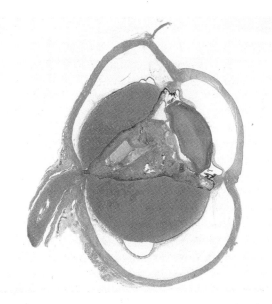

Figure 3.9 Norrie's disease. Detached dysplastic retina forming a retrolental mass.

Table 3.3 X-linked recessive disorders of ophthalmic importance

Disorder	Gene locus	Gene
Ocular albinism	Xp22.3-p22.2	OA1
X-linked juvenile retinoschisis	Xp22.2	RS1
Corneal dermoids	Xp22.2-p22.1	
Retinitis pigmentosa	Xp22.13-p22.11	RP15
Retinitis pigmentosa	Xp22	RP23
Retinitis pigmentosa	Xp21.3-p21.2	RP6
Oregon eye disease	Xp21.2	DMD
Retinitis pigmentosa	Xp21.1	RP3
Congenital stationary night blindness	Xp21	CSNB2
Cone dystrophy	Xp11.4	COD1
Åland Island eye disease	Xp11.4-q21	ÅIED
Congenital stationary night blindness	Xp11.4-p11.3	CSNB4
Congenital stationary night blindness	Xp11.4-p11.3	CSNB1
Optic atrophy	Xp11.4-p11.2	OPA2
Retinitis pigmentosa (RP2)	Xp11.3	RP2
Retinal dysplasia, primary	Xp11.3-p11.23	PRD
Coats' disease	Xp11.3	NDP
Familial exudative vitreoretinopathy	Xp11.3	NDP
Norrie's disease	Xp11.3	NDP
Retinitis pigmentosa	Xp11.3	RP2
Congenital stationary night blindness	Xp11.23	CACNA1F
X-linked megalocornea	Xq13.3-q25	
Choroideraemia	Xq21.1-q21.3	CHM
Fabry's disease	Xq21.22-q21.33	
Alport's syndrome	Xq22.3	
Lowe's oculocerebral syndrome	Xq25-q26.1	
Retinitis pigmentosa	Xq26-q27	RP24
Cone dystrophy	Xq27	COD2
Hunter's disease	Xq27	
X-linked anophthalmos	Xq27-q28	
Protanopia	Xq28	RCP
Blue cone monochromatism	Xq28	GCP
GPD6 deficiency	Xq28	

normal components of cell membranes. The gene for the enzyme is located on the X chromosome (Xq21.22-q21.33) and mutations result in deficiency of the enzyme with consequent accumulation of hexosylceramides throughout the tissues of the body. The disorder is X-linked recessive, with the full-blown syndrome being seen in males, in whom episodic burning pain in the limbs is often accompanied by fever. Cutaneous lesions in the form of clusters of punctate dark red telangiectases occur in the bathing trunk area, and aneurysmal lesions may develop on mucous membranes. Renal, cardiovascular and cerebrovascular complications are common and reduce life expectancy to 40–50 years. Females may be affected by similar but less severe manifestations. In the eye, finely divided white to yellow-brown deposits form in both the epithelial and subepithelial layers of the conjunctiva and cornea. The corneal lesions exhibit a whorl-like pattern similar to those of drug-induced cornea verticillata and are a helpful diagnostic sign, particularly in carrier females. Other manifestations include lens opacities, retinal vascular abnormalities and abnormalities secondary to neurological disease.

DISORDERS OF MITOCHONDRIAL INHERITANCE

As all mtDNA is inherited from the mother, it is only daughters who can pass mitochondrial genetic defects to their descendants. The DNA of each mitochondrion within the oocyte may be different, and this results in genetic heterogeneity between daughters. There may also be heterogeneity of mtDNA between cells of the same individual. The consequence of this heteroplasmy (multiple alleles of the mitochondrial genome) is variable expressivity within a family according to the amount of the abnormal alleles present in the critical cell or tissue. It may therefore be difficult to distinguish mitochondrial inheritance from any of the types of Mendelian inheritance. Mitochondrial disorders are most likely to affect metabolically active tissues that rely on aerobic oxidation and ATP production, such as the brain, skeletal muscle, cardiac muscle and the eye. With the exception of Leber's hereditary optic neuropathy, all disorders due to mutations of mtDNA are associated with myopathy. The two mtDNA abnormalities of particular importance to the ophthalmologist are Leber's hereditary optic neuropathy and chronic progressive ophthalmoplegia/ Kearns–Sayre syndrome. Gyrate atrophy may also be considered a mitochondrial disease as the defective enzyme (ornithine aminotransferase – OAT) is present in the mitochondrial matrix; the OAT gene, however, is encoded in nuclear DNA and its mode of inheritance is therefore Mendelian.

MULTIFACTORIAL INHERITANCE

Disorders with multifactorial (polygenic) inheritance are caused by the interaction of more than one gene together with an effect from the environment. Because of the many variables within a disease and the lack of any clear pattern of inheritance it is often difficult to identify such disorders, although they are thought to be common. The risk of transmitting these diseases is less than those attributable to single gene defects, and most affected individuals tend to be first degree relatives. Some forms of glaucoma and myopia are thought to be inherited in this way, as are systemic hypertension and diabetes mellitus.

SOMATIC MUTATIONS

Acquired genetic abnormalities of somatic cells are associated with the development of neoplasms.

Chapter 4

Growth, differentiation and development

General principles and definitions

The cell cycle
Growth
  Hypertrophy
  Hyperplasia
Determination and differentiation
Morphogenesis
Congenital malformations
  Teratogens
  Types of malformation
    Agenesis
    Atresia
    Hypoplasia
    Dysgenesis
    Heterotopia, ectopia and choristomas
    Hamartomas
Tumours
Abnormal differentiation and growth in mature tissue
  Metaplasia
  Dysplasia
  Neoplasia
    Classification and nomenclature of neoplasms
    Biological characteristics of neoplastic cells
    Behaviour of neoplasms
  The effects of neoplasms on the host
    Local effects
    Systemic effects
  Oncogenesis and carcinogenesis
    Carcinogens
    Host factors
    Genetic basis of oncogenesis
    The oncogenic process

Developmental anomalies

Chronology of gestational development
  The pre-embryonic period
  The embryonic period
  The fetal period
Embryogenesis and organogenesis
  Normal organogenesis
  Anomalies of organogenesis
    Failure of development of the optic vesicle and anterior neural tube: regression of the optic vesicle
    Anomalies arising during mid-line differentiation
    Anomalies of invagination of the optic vesicle
    Failure of closure of the embryonic fissure
The corneoscleral coat and the anterior segment
  Normal development
    Anterior chamber and drainage angle
    Sclera
    Iris
  Anomalies of development
    Corneal developmental anomalies
    Anterior chamber dysgenesis
    Iris developmental anomalies
The lens
  Normal development
  Anomalies of development
    Anomaly of formation: congenital aphakia
    Anomalies of size and shape
    Anomaly of position: congenital ectopia lentis
    Anomaly of transparency: congenital cataract
The vitreous and the vasculature
  Normal development
  Anomalies of development
The retina
  Normal development
  Anomalies of development

Anomalies of development of the outer layer of
the optic vesicle
Anomalies of development of the inner layer of
the optic vesicle
The optic disc and optic nerve
Normal development
Anomalies of development
Abnormalities in the size of the eye
The ocular adnexae
Normal development
Anomalies of development

Disorders of postnatal cell and tissue growth

The lids
Cysts and choristomas
Epidermoid cyst
Dermoid cyst
Leaking cysts
'Meibomian cyst'
Sweat gland cyst
Benign proliferations of keratinocytes
Basal cell papilloma
Inverted follicular keratosis
Squamous cell papilloma
Keratoacanthoma
Molluscum contagiosum
Intraepidermal proliferations of keratinocytes
Actinic keratosis
Carcinoma *in situ*
Malignant infiltrating proliferations of keratinocytes
Basal cell carcinoma
Squamous cell carcinoma
Benign proliferations of epidermal melanocytes
Melanocytic naevi
Intraepidermal proliferations of epidermal
melanocytes
Lentigo
Melanoma *in situ*
Malignant infiltrating proliferation of epidermal
melanocytes
Melanoma
Proliferation of Merkel cells
Merkel cell carcinoma
Sebaceous gland proliferations
Sebaceous hyperplasia
Sebaceous adenoma
Sebaceous carcinoma
Sweat gland proliferations
Apocrine cystadenoma
Cylindroma
Papillary syringocystadenoma
Syringoma
Eccrine poroma
Clear cell hidradenoma
Pleomorphic adenoma
Sweat gland carcinoma

Hair follicle proliferations
Trichofolliculoma
Trichoepithelioma
Trichilemmoma
Pilomatricoma
Vascular proliferations
Capillary haemangioma
Naevus flammeus
Cavernous haemangioma
Neural proliferations
Neurofibromas and schwannomas
Proliferation of dermal melanocytes
Blue naevi
The conjunctiva
Cysts and choristomas
Epithelial cyst
Dermoid
Dermolipoma
Complex choristoma
Epibulbar osseous choristoma
Intrascleral nerve loop
Benign proliferation of epithelial cells
Squamous cell papilloma
Intraepithelial proliferations of epithelial cells
Malignant infiltrating proliferations of epithelial cells
Squamous cell carcinoma
Mucoepidermoid carcinoma
Benign proliferations of epithelial melanocytes
Melanocytic naevi
Intraepithelial proliferations of epithelial melanocytes
Malignant infiltrating proliferation of epithelial
melanocytes
Melanoma
Vascular proliferations
Telangiectasia
Pyogenic granuloma
Kaposi sarcoma
Lymphatic proliferations
Lymphangioma and lymphangiectasia
Accessory lacrimal gland proliferations
Oncocytoma
Non-epithelial melanocytic proliferations
Ocular melanocytosis
Oculodermal melanocytosis
The lacrimal sac
The orbit
Cysts and choristomas
Dermoid cyst
Epidermoid cyst
Lymphangioma
Teratoma
Other cystic lesions
Lacrimal gland proliferations
Pleomorphic adenoma
Other benign lesions
Adenoid cystic carcinoma
Pleomorphic carcinoma
Other carcinomas

Vascular proliferations
  Cavernous haemangioma
  Capillary haemangioma
  Arteriovenous fistulae
  Racemose haemangioma
  Varices
  Haemangiopericytoma
Neural proliferations
  Meningioma
  Juvenile optic nerve glioma
  Adult optic nerve glioma
  Neurofibroma
  Schwannoma
Other soft tissue proliferations
  Embryonal sarcoma
Osseous and cartilaginous proliferations
The eye
  Cysts, hyperplasias and choristomas
    Iris cysts
    Fuchs' 'adenoma'
    Pseudoadenomatous hyperplasia of the ciliary
      epithelium
    Ringschwiele
    Congenital hypertrophy of the RPE
    Osseous choristoma of the choroid
  Melanocytic proliferations
    Naevi and melanocytomas
    Melanomas
  Neuroepithelial proliferations
    Retinoblastoma
    Trilateral retinoblastoma
    Retinocytoma
    Medulloepithelioma
    Other neuroepithelial neoplasms
  Vascular proliferations
    Choroidal haemangioma
    Retinal haemangioblastoma
    Retinal cavernous haemangioma
    Retinal racemose haemangioma
  Neural proliferations
    Uveal neurofibroma

Uveal schwannoma
Retinal astrocytoma
Smooth muscle proliferations
Lymphoproliferative lesions, fibroblastic and histiocytic
proliferations, plasma cell accumulations and
leukaemic deposits
  Lymphoproliferative lesions
    Lymphoma
    Reactive lymphoid hyperplasia
    Ophthalmic manifestations of lymphoproliferative
      lesions
  Fibroblastic and histiocytic proliferations
    Fibrous histiocytoma
    Nodular fasciitis
    Xanthelasma
    Juvenile xanthogranuloma
    Sinus histiocytosis with massive
      lymphadenopathy
    Langerhans cell histiocytosis
  Plasma cell accumulations
    Plasmacytoma
  Leukaemic deposits
Syndromes associated with disorders of cell and tissue
growth
  The phakomatoses
    von Hippel–Lindau disease
    Sturge–Weber syndrome
    Wyburn–Mason syndrome
    Neurofibromatosis type 1
    Neurofibromatosis type 2
    Tuberous sclerosis
  Other syndromes
    Gorlin–Goltz syndrome
    Muir–Torre syndrome
    Cowden's disease
    Goldenhar's syndrome
    Gardner's and Turcot's syndromes
Secondary neoplasms
  Local infiltration
  Metastases

GENERAL PRINCIPLES AND DEFINITIONS

The fertilized ovum undergoes complex processes of growth, differentiation and morphogenesis to develop into the co-ordinated groups of cells, tissues and organs that comprise all complex living creatures. Once formed, the cells of many adult tissues continue to grow and differentiate as part of a constant cycle of cellular death and replacement in response to normal and pathological events. Abnormalities of growth, differentiation and development can occur at any stage from the time of fertilization into adult life. Changes during intrauterine development can lead to congenital abnormalities that may be so severe as to cause death of the fetus. During postnatal and adult life some variations in growth and differentiation may be a response to physiological stimuli (e.g. changes in cardiac and skeletal muscle in response to exercise), whereas abnormalities of growth and differentiation may give rise to cancer and related conditions.

THE CELL CYCLE

Cells replicate by mitosis. The cell cycle is the time between two successive divisions, and is divided into four unequal phases. The M (mitotic) phase, comprising division of the nucleus (mitosis) and the cytoplasm (cytokinesis), is followed by the first gap (G_1) phase during which the cell devotes itself to its own specialized activities, if any. After a variable time G_1 is followed by a period of DNA synthesis (S phase, in which all chromosomes are replicated) and then a second gap (G_2) phase. The next M phase follows. During normal development, the replicative characteristics of cells depend on differentiation and cell type. In mature normal tissues, cells are classified as labile, stable and permanent. In labile cells, one daughter cell differentiates while the other will continue cycling. Stable cells enter a resting (G_0) phase after an M phase and do not re-enter the cell cycle unless stimulated. Permanent cells become terminally differentiated after mitosis and cannot re-enter the cell cycle. The duration of S, G_2 and M phases is relatively constant, but that of G_1 varies from hours (e.g. corneal epithelial cells) to many months.

GROWTH

Growth is the process in which increased size and/or weight of a biological unit results from the synthesis of tissue components. The biological units may range from cells and cell components to tissues, organs, organisms and populations of organisms. The growth of a cellular aggregate may be multiplicative (due to an increase in cell number resulting from mitotic division), auxetic (due to an increase in cell size) or accretionary (resulting from the accumulation of extracellular tissue such as bone). All three mechanisms may coexist. Atrophy is the opposite of growth. Both growth and atrophy occur during development and in mature tissues in response to injury or changing environmental conditions.

Hypertrophy is the enlargement of individual cells.

Hyperplasia is an increase in the number of cells, and frequently occurs concurrently with hypertrophy. Examples of hyperplasias include cutaneous epidermal and conjunctival epithelial hyperplasias, and pseudoadenomatous hyperplasia of the ciliary epithelium, all of which may be a response to chronic inflammation; Ringschwiele (hyperplasia of the ciliary epithelium and peripheral RPE) occurs in association with retinal detachment, and meningeal hyperplasia with juvenile optic nerve glioma. Hyperplasias may resemble neoplasms, and on occasions discriminating between the two may be difficult, even on histological grounds; this difficulty is exemplified in many lymphoproliferative lesions and with the meningeal hyperplasia associated with juvenile optic nerve glioma. An important functional component of hyperplasia is a decrease of cell loss by apoptosis, but the mechanisms of this are unclear.

DETERMINATION AND DIFFERENTIATION

Differentiation is the process by which cells in a developing multicellular organism become specialized from an undifferentiated parent into cells with specific morphology and/or function. Cells may be determined or differentiated. Determined cells have entered the process of differentiation but are not yet distinguishable from parent cells; they persist into adult life and include stem cells such as the basal cells of the epidermis and mucous membranes, and haemopoietic stem cells. Differentiated cells are distinguishable from parent cells. The process of differentiation involves a progressive restriction in genomic expression at the transcription stage but without a change in the number of genes present in the differentiating cell. Control of normal differentiation is genetic and environmental: a small number of control genes (e.g. homeobox-containing genes) produce regulatory proteins which influence expression of other genes; the pattern of differentiation of one cell type may be controlled by another (induction) or be influenced by endocrine and other humoral factors.

MORPHOGENESIS

Morphogenesis is the development of structure and form of an embryo from primitive cell masses. A fertilized ovum initially divides into totipotent cells that differentiate into ectoderm, mesoderm and endoderm, cells of each lineage being pluripotent and capable of forming several cell types. A period of organogenesis follows in which organs or their primordia form as a consequence of the interaction of cells from ectoderm, mesoderm and endoderm, each of which is committed to a specific fate. Each cell then undergoes a process of determination, differentiation and maturation to reach its final state. Morphogenesis requires co-ordinated growth, differentiation, migration and apoptosis of cells.

CONGENITAL MALFORMATIONS

Spontaneous abortion is the usual outcome of human conception with up to an 80 per cent loss, mainly as a consequence of chromosomal abnormalities. Those that survive are usually normal, although a significant proportion have congenital malformations (anatomical developmental anomalies present at birth) which may be isolated or multiple and form part of a syndrome. Their incidence in full-term neonates is approximately 5 per cent, but for stillborn and premature infants this may be as high as 25 per cent. Many congenital malformations (40–65 per cent) are multifactorial or of unknown cause. Known causes are chromosomal abnormalities (15–28 per cent), single gene defects (15–25 per cent) and teratogens (8–10 per cent).

Teratogens

Teratogens are physical, chemical or biological agents that act directly on the tissues of the developing embryo or fetus to produce a congenital malformation. The extent and severity of the abnormality produced depends on the nature of the teratogen and the developmental stage when exposure occurs. Physical teratogens include mechanical trauma and radiation. Chemical teratogens include drugs such as alcohol, tobacco, thalidomide, lysergic acid diethylamide (LSD), folic acid antagonists, anticonvulsants, warfarin, testosterone, protamine zinc insulin, diuretics

and corticosteroids. Non-pharmacological teratogens include environmental pollutants. Biological teratogens include infective agents (e.g. herpes simplex virus, rubella virus, *Treponema pallidum*, *Toxoplasma gondii*) and maternal nutritional and metabolic disorders (e.g. hyper- and hypovitaminosis A, low iodine levels, folic acid deficiency, diabetes mellitus, phenylketonuria). Some teratogens are also mutagenic and cause chromosomal abnormalities and single gene defects.

Types of malformation

Disruption of morphogenesis may occur throughout fetal development, and the outcome depends on the stage of development and the characteristics of the cause. The following types of defect are of particular importance.

Agenesis (aplasia) is the failure of development of a structure. Examples include anencephaly and anophthalmos.

Atresia is the failure of the development of a lumen in tubular epithelial structures. Examples include some forms of congenital nasolacrimal stenosis, and oesophageal and biliary atresia.

Hypoplasia is the failure of an organ or structure to develop to its normal size. It differs from atrophy in that it is developmental, whereas atrophy is an acquired reduction in the size of a previously normal structure. Examples of hypoplasia include microphthalmos, and hypoplasias of the optic nerve and retina.

Dysgenesis (maldifferentiation) is the failure of normal differentiation of an organ or structure, which may retain some primitive embryonal elements. Examples include the anterior chamber dysgeneses.

Heterotopia, ectopia and choristomas: heterotopia is the presence of a tissue in an abnormal location as a result of a developmental anomaly. Ectopia is congenital displacement or malposition of a structure (e.g. ectopia lentis, ectopic pregnancy). Choristomas are heterotopias in which anomalous differentiation at the stem cell stage of development results in a congenital mass containing tissue not normally present at the site affected. Although not always clinically apparent at birth, the underlying lesion from which they develop is congenital. Examples include dermoid cysts, osseous choristomas of the choroid and complex choristomas of the conjunctiva.

Hamartomas are abnormal tissue masses, the growth of which is co-ordinated with that of the individual. The constituents of a hamartoma are fully differentiated and normally found in the tissue or organ in which it develops. As with choristomas, hamartomas are congenital but may not be clinically apparent at birth. Common examples are the vascular hamartomas and melanocytic naevi.

TUMOURS

A tumour is an abnormal tissue swelling (space-occupying lesion). The term does not imply aetiology, and the assumption that all tumours are neoplasms is erroneous. All disorders of cell growth, other than metaplasia, lead to proliferations, and those involving solid tissues produce tumours. Causes of tumours other than disorders of growth include immune-mediated and infective inflammatory lesions, vascular leakage (haematomas) and cysts (a circumscribed collection of material produced by the cells lining its wall). The specific names of tumours of whatever aetiology often ends with the suffix '-oma'. This includes choristomas, hamartomas, neoplasms and swellings of an inflammatory nature such as granulomas and tuberculomas.

ABNORMAL DIFFERENTIATION AND GROWTH IN MATURE TISSUE

Labile and stable cells maintain their population by steady replication according to the cell cycle. Their growth and differentiation is appropriate to the tissue of which they are part. Under adverse conditions and in response to noxious stimuli, cells may break free of the normal regulatory mechanisms controlling their replication and differentiate abnormally.

Metaplasia

Metaplasia is the reversible transformation of one type of fully differentiated cell into another fully differentiated type. It is often an adaptive response to adverse conditions that the metaplastic cells are better able to withstand. Metaplasia results from the activation and/or suppression of groups of genes involved in the maintenance of cellular differentiation. Metaplasia may occur in neoplasms, but is best regarded as a change that takes place in non-neoplastic tissue.

Ophthalmic examples include metaplasia of the conjunctival and corneal epithelium from non-keratinized to keratinized in the dry eye syndromes; metaplasia of lens epithelium into fibroblasts leading to subepithelial fibrosis (a cause of posterior capsular opacification following cataract surgery); and metaplasia of lacrimal gland duct epithelium and acinar myoepithelium into cells that produce the mesenchymal component of pleomorphic adenomas. Chronic inflammation of mesenchymal tissue can result in bone formation (osseous metaplasia).

Dysplasia

Dysplasia is the alteration of the size, morphology and organization of the cellular components of a tissue. It is characterized by increased cell growth and histological features including loss of cell polarity (disturbance of the normally structured and recognized layers of a tissue – Fig. 4.1a), cellular atypia with pleomorphism (variation in the shape of the cells and their nuclei), a high nuclear/cytoplasmic ratio and increased nuclear DNA (recognized by hyperchromatism, i.e. more darkly staining nuclei). Dysplastic epidermal and epithelial surfaces may also exhibit dyskeratosis (the production of keratin other than on the surface – Fig. 4.1b) and parakeratosis (the retention of nuclei into the layer of surface keratin – Fig. 4.1c; in parakeratosis the granular cell layer is usually absent). Dysplasia is a pre-malignant condition, and while early forms may be reversible, severe dysplasia can lead to the development of a malignant neoplasm unless it is adequately treated. Examples of dysplastic processes include actinic keratosis and carcinoma *in situ* of the skin and intraepithelial neoplasia of the conjunctiva.

Neoplasia

Neoplasia means new growth. A neoplasm is defined as an abnormal tissue mass, the growth of which exceeds and is unco-ordinated with that of normal tissues, and which persists and grows in the same excessive manner after cessation of the provoking stimulus. Cell growth is autonomous and has escaped from the normal regulatory mechanisms.

Classification and nomenclature of neoplasms

Neoplasms are classified according to their cell or tissue of origin and their behaviour (Table 4.1). All solid neoplasms have the suffix '-oma', but not all lesions with this suffix are neoplasms. In broad terms, neoplasms of mature tissue are of either epithelial or mesenchymal

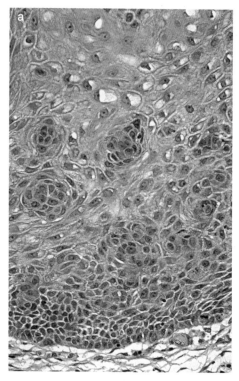

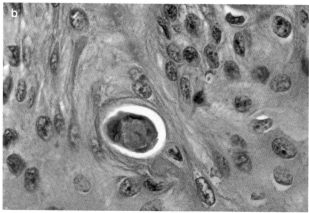

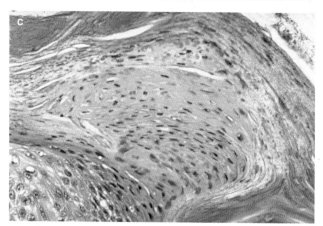

Figure 4.1 Dysplasia. (a) Loss of cell polarity. (b) Dyskeratosis; an epithelial cell not on the surface but producing keratin. (c) Parakeratosis; the retention of nuclei into the surface keratin.

origin; most can be benign or malignant. Bone marrow malignancies (e.g. leukaemias, lymphomas) and embryonal neoplasms, other than teratomas, have no benign counterparts. Malignant embryonal neoplasms have the suffix '-blastoma' after the structure from which they originate. All malignancy is collectively referred to as cancer.

Benign epithelial neoplasms are termed papillomas if their growth is papillary, or adenomas if their cells are glandular (endocrine or exocrine). Malignant epithelial neoplasms are carcinomas. Carcinoma *in situ* is a term applied to an epithelial neoplasm that exhibits cellular features associated with malignancy but has not invaded through the basement membrane separating it from underlying tissue in which there are potential routes of metastasis, such as lymphatic and blood vessels.

Benign melanocytic proliferations (melanocytic naevi) in humans are hamartomas and not true neoplasms. Melanomas are malignant neoplasms of melanocytes and have no benign counterpart in humans.

Benign mesenchymal neoplasms are named according to cell type followed by the suffix '-oma' (e.g. angioma, lipoma). Malignant mesenchymal neoplasms are sarcomas and are named as their benign counterparts but with the suffix '-sarcoma' (e.g. angiosarcoma, liposarcoma).

Some malignant neoplasms are so poorly differentiated that their origin is not readily recognized in routine histological preparations, and in such instances immunohistochemistry may be helpful.

Table 4.1 Classification of cell and tissue proliferations of mature tissue, excluding those of lymphoid and haemopoietic tissue

Cell/tissue of origin	Benign	Malignant
Epithelium		
Skin and mucous membranes	Papilloma	Carcinoma
Glandular structures	Adenoma	Adenocarcinoma
Mesenchyme		
Melanocyte	Naevus	Melanoma
Schwann cell	Schwannoma	Malignant schwannoma
Smooth muscle	Leiomyoma	Leiomyosarcoma
Striated muscle	Rhabdomyoma	Rhabdomyosarcoma
Fibrocyte	Fibroma	Fibrosarcoma
Lipocyte	Lipoma	Liposarcoma
Chondrocyte	Chondroma	Chondrosarcoma
Osteocyte	Osteoma	Osteosarcoma
Vascular tissue	Angioma	Angiosarcoma

Biological characteristics of neoplastic cells

Neoplastic cells result from the monoclonal proliferation of a single cell, and their unique feature is autonomy. Their degree of differentiation varies, and most reproduce to a variable extent the growth pattern and the synthetic activity of their cell of origin. Undifferentiated neoplasms are referred to as anaplastic. Products such as keratin, mucin or collagen may accumulate within a neoplasm, while humoral factors may be secreted into the blood stream to produce systemic effects.

Autonomy of growth is relative for most neoplastic cells, which still require some stimulation from growth factors (e.g. PDGF, IGFs) and hormones (e.g. oestrogens for breast and endometrial carcinoma, androgens for prostatic carcinoma). Lymphocytes in the stroma reflect the host's immune response to the neoplasm.

Genetic abnormalities

The molecular lesion of neoplasia lies within the genome, and its inheritance by subsequent generations of cells explains the persistent proliferation following withdrawal of the initiating stimulus. Neoplastic cells are genetically unstable in that genetic abnormalities continue to be acquired and expressed in addition to those of the initial carcinogenic process. The many clones of cells within a lesion are reflected in the histological appearance, which may show a heterogeneous pattern exhibiting varying degrees of differentiation; it is this instability and heterogeneity that enable some neoplasms to resist chemotherapy. The accumulation of genetic abnormalities may be manifest in neoplastic cells as chromosomal abnormalities (polyploidy, aneuploidy) and other abnormalities of DNA (nuclear pleomorphism, hyperchromatism, abnormal chromatin distribution, multiple or enlarged nucleoli).

Proliferation

Increased mitotic activity accounts for neoplasms behaving as expanding masses of tissue. Uncontrolled proliferation of neoplastic cells results from the loss of normal contact inhibition, while abnormal intercellular and cell-matrix adhesion allows some types of neoplastic cells to metastasize. Most neoplastic cells rapidly undergo apoptosis and expansion is less than expected. Apoptosis is a mechanism that is controlled by many of the genes that also control proliferation. Some neoplastic cells have defective apoptotic mechanisms (e.g. melanomas, some low-grade B cell lymphomas).

Metabolic abnormalities

Neoplastic cells tend to be resistant to hypoxia because of their tendency to utilize anaerobic glycolysis. Protein synthesis may be abnormal in that proteins normal for the tissue may be overproduced, and some not normally synthesized in that tissue may be produced (e.g. ACTH in bronchogenic carcinoma).

Tissue interactions

Neoplastic cells require metabolic and structural support from surrounding tissues and are able to stimulate the proliferation of fibrovascular tissue (stroma) in which they become embedded. The formation of stroma is termed a desmoplastic reaction, and is induced by growth factors produced by the neoplastic cells. If metabolic support is insufficient, growth either ceases or the neoplasm becomes necrotic.

Behaviour of neoplasms

Neoplasms have a parasitic relationship with the body. They affect the host to varying degrees, and are classified as benign or malignant (Table 4.2). The principal distinguishing feature is invasiveness.

Benign neoplasms

Benign neoplasms have an expansile growth pattern often associated with the formation of a capsule derived from surrounding connective tissue. Benign neoplastic cells show no tendency to invade the surrounding tissue, and never spread (metastasize) to distant sites. Mitosis is infrequent and growth is usually slow. Benign neoplasms are well differentiated, often closely resembling their tissue of origin.

Table 4.2 Behaviour of neoplasms

Feature	Benign	Malignant
Growth rate	Slow	Rapid
Growth pattern	Locally expansile	Invasive and metastatic
Differentiation	Well differentiated	Often poorly differentiated
Necrosis	Rare	Common
Border	Often encapsulated	Often poorly defined
Cell morphology	Normal	Large and pleomorphic – increased nuclear/cytoplasmic ratio
Nuclear morphology	Normal	Irregular and hyperchromatic with multiple nucleoli
Mitotic activity	Low	High – some abnormal

Malignant neoplasms

Malignant cells and the structures they form show evidence of increased cell turnover and incomplete differentiation. Increased cell turnover is manifest as a large number of mitoses, many cells having abnormal appearances with tripolar, quadripolar and ring mitotic figures being present (Fig. 4.2a). Malignant cells tend to be larger than their normal counterparts and show pleomorphism; multinucleate cells are sometimes present. The nuclear/cytoplasmic ratio is increased, i.e. the nuclei occupy a greater proportion of the cell volume than is normal, the DNA content of the nuclei is greater than normal (evident as hyperchromatism – Fig. 4.2b), and chromosomal analysis often shows loss of normal ploidy. Malignant cells grow in such a way that the normal orderly relationship is lost, i.e. differentiation is incomplete and may in some instances be so poor that recognizable structures are not formed. Malignant neoplasms are invasive and may infiltrate adjacent tissues and/or metastasize to distant sites where subpopulations of malignant cells proliferate.

Local invasion occurs by direct extension and is determined by a number of factors, which include:

1. Less cohesion due to a greater negative surface electrostatic charge than normal. In the case of epithelial neoplasms, the number of intercellular bridges (desmosomes) is reduced and defective basement membrane substances, which fail to arrest growth, are produced.
2. The increased motility resulting from the production by neoplastic cells of an autocrine motility factor that stimulates cell locomotion.
3. The secretion of integrins, a family of glycoprotein adhesion molecules, that bind to the extracellular matrix components of the tissue being invaded.
4. The secretion of proteinases that degrade the matrix proteins posing a barrier to the spread of neoplastic cells.

Local invasion is characteristic of basal cell carcinoma. Pagetoid spread (named after Paget's disease of the nipple) is a particular form of local invasion in which malignant cells spread into the adjacent epithelium, and is commonly seen in sebaceous carcinoma. Other examples of direct extension include the perineural infiltration by adenoid cystic carcinomas of the lacrimal gland and the extension of retinoblastomas through the parenchyma of the optic nerve.

Metastasis is the process whereby neoplasms spread from their site of origin (the primary neoplasm) to distant sites (secondary neoplasms). In most cases it depends on the ability of neoplastic cells to invade vascular channels. Carcinomatosis is extensive metastatic disease. Important routes of metastasis are the lymphatics, blood vessels and the body cavities. Metastasis may be surgically induced.

Lymphatics: afferent lymphatic channels carry malignant cells to the regional lymph nodes, where they may form secondary neoplasms. Lid and conjunctival malignant neoplasms can disseminate in this way, but orbital and intraocular malignancies cannot do so as there are no lymphatic channels in the orbit or eye.

Blood vessels: the blood stream carries malignant cells to form secondary neoplasms in the organs perfused by blood that has drained the primary neoplasm.

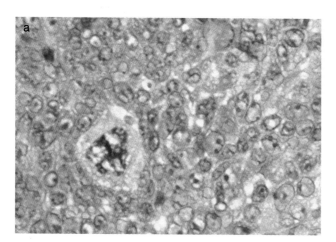
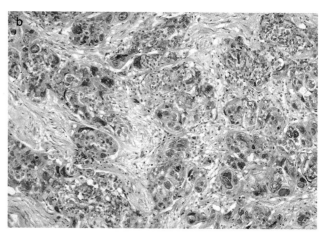

Figure 4.2 Malignant neoplasia. (a) Abnormal mitosis in an epidermal cell. (b) Pleomorphic hyperchromatic nuclei with an increased nuclear/cytoplasmic ratio.

Haematogenous metastases most commonly occur in bone, lung, liver and brain.

Body cavities: neoplastic cells can spread within the serous cavities of the body and within the subarachnoid space and ventricular system of the CNS, where malignant neoplasms such as retinoblastomas may disseminate within the CSF.

Surgically-induced metastasis: neoplastic cells may spread via lymphatics and blood vessels and by dissemination within body cavities as a consequence of manipulative procedures carried out during surgery.

Metastatic deposits

Neoplastic cells that penetrate lymphatic and vascular channels eventually reach the systemic circulation, but < 0.1 per cent of them survive to establish a new colony. These are mechanically arrested in arterioles, capillaries and venules, the vascular endothelium retracts and the neoplastic cells infiltrate adjacent tissues before growing locally as a metastatic deposit. A new vascular supply is necessary, and growth factors secreted by the neoplastic cells stimulate angiogenesis in the host tissues. Malignant neoplasms may recur both locally and at metastatic sites many years after surgical removal; this dormancy may be due to immunologic suppression, to a lack of growth factors or to inadequate vascularity.

The effects of neoplasms on the host

The effects of neoplasms on the host are local and/or systemic.

Local effects

Local effects result from the mechanical consequences of an expanding mass or from tissue destruction and infiltration. The causative lesion may be a primary or secondary neoplasm. The effect of an expanding mass depends on its anatomical site and on its size and rate of growth. A small lesion in an anatomically confined space (such as a meningioma within the optic canal) may have serious consequences, whereas a large lesion at a site that will tolerate expansion (such as a neurofibroma of the lid) has little consequence. Neoplasms may destroy tissue as a result of pressure atrophy or, in the case of malignancy, by infiltration; thus benign adenomas of the pituitary gland may destroy the pituitary fossa by pressure while basal cell carcinomas or other malignant neoplasms may destroy a lid by infiltration.

Systemic effects

Systemic effects include fever, anorexia, weight loss and cachexia, immune responses and paraneoplastic syndromes.

Fever may result from the release of pyrogens by the neoplastic cells or from the production of cytokines by inflammatory cells.

Anorexia, weight loss and cachexia are common in those with malignant neoplasms. The mechanisms accounting for these features are poorly understood, but it is thought that they result from secretion of tumour necrosis factors (TNFs) or other factors by neoplastic cells.

Immune responses occur because the cells of a malignant neoplasm express antigens recognized as foreign by the immune system of the host. A cell-mediated immune response characterized by the presence of CD4 + (T_H) and CD8 + ($T_{C/S}$) lymphocytes, macrophages and NK cells results, and in some instances this correlates with a more favourable prognosis. Oncodevelopmental antigens such as alpha-fetoprotein and carcinoembryonic antigen are sometimes expressed by malignant neoplasms, particularly when they become dedifferentiated and more primitive (fetal dedifferentiation) and, although they probably do not play any role in immune responses, their identification in blood is of diagnostic value.

Paraneoplastic syndromes result from neoplastic cells producing hormones or cytokines, or provoking an immune response; they are not attributable to invasion or metastasis by neoplastic cells. The range of paraneoplastic syndromes is very wide and includes endocrine, neurological, muscular, haematological, immune, gastrointestinal, dermatological and ocular syndromes. Neuromuscular syndromes and cancer- and melanoma-associated retinopathies are the most relevant to ophthalmologists.

Neuromuscular syndromes include central and peripheral neuropathies, myasthenia gravis and the Lambert–Eaton syndrome, the latter being most frequently associated with small cell carcinoma of the lung.

Cancer-associated retinopathy (CAR) occurs most frequently in association with small cell carcinoma of the lung but has also been described in other malignancies, including carcinomas of the breast, uterine cervix, endometrium and prostate. It presents with an acute onset of rapid, progressive and relentless bilateral visual loss. Initial signs include a mild vitritis, attenuation of the retinal vessels and pigmentary retinopathy. The pathogenesis is thought to involve the ectopic synthesis by neoplastic cells of the photoreceptor molecule recoverin;

antibodies are produced and cross-react with photoreceptor recoverin, thereby damaging the retina.

Melanoma-associated retinopathy (MAR) may occur with cutaneous melanoma. Acute onset of photopsia and night blindness develop without visible retinopathy. It is thought that antibodies to cutaneous melanoma cross the blood–retinal barriers and impair bipolar cell function but do not cause cell death. MAR is more rod-specific than CAR.

Oncogenesis and carcinogenesis

Oncogenesis is the term used for the pathogenesis of all neoplasms, both benign and malignant. Carcinogenesis applies to the pathogenesis of malignant neoplasms. Neoplasia is a genetic disease caused by changes in critical genes such as those related to cell development, differentiation, proliferation, survival, senescence and genetic repair. At least five genetic changes are necessary for a cell to alter in such a way as to escape the normal growth control mechanisms and undergo sustainable clonal proliferation. The causes of the initiating genetic defects are predominantly environmental, although there is interplay with inherited or other constitutional risks. Most neoplasms occur in cells that are actively replicating (e.g. skin epidermis, gut epithelium). Postmitotic cells (e.g. nerve, skeletal muscle) rarely undergo neoplastic transformation.

Carcinogens

Carcinogens are chemical, physical and biological mutagenic agents known or alleged to alter DNA in such a way as to cause neoplasms.

Chemical agents

Chemical carcinogens are many and varied. The major classes are polycyclic aromatic hydrocarbons, aromatic amines, nitrosamines, azo dyes and alkylating agents. The carcinogenic risk cannot be predicted from the structural formula of the chemicals, and even apparently closely related compounds have different effects. Some chemical carcinogens act directly and require no metabolic conversion, while others, known as procarcinogens, require enzymatic conversion into ultimate carcinogens. If the substance required for this conversion is ubiquitous within tissues, neoplasms develop at the site of contact or entry. Other procarcinogens require conversion by enzymes confined to certain organs and so often only induce the formation of neoplasms remote from the site of entry.

Physical agents

Radiation is here defined as energy emitted from a source that is transmitted through an intervening medium and absorbed by a body. It includes the entire electromagnetic spectrum and charged particles emitted from radioactive sources. Radiation is the most important physical carcinogen, although only that of higher energy is carcinogenic. DNA damage results either by direct absorption of radiation or indirectly by the generation of free radicals that react with DNA. UV light is a major cause of skin malignancies (basal and squamous cell carcinoma, melanoma), especially in fair-skinned people who lack the protective effect of the higher melanin content of pigmented skin. The risk is greatly exaggerated in those with xeroderma pigmentosum due to the inability to repair UV light-induced DNA damage. Ionizing radiation is carcinogenic, especially in high dosage but probably also in low dosage. Haemopoietic tissues, the thyroid, breast and bone are particularly sensitive. The high incidence of orbital and facial malignancy in those with retinoblastoma may in part be induced by the radiotherapy used to treat the original neoplasm, combined with genetic predisposition. A number of physical agents such as asbestos and other foreign substances are carcinogenic.

Biological agents

Oncogenic viruses cause neoplasia. They are found among all families of DNA viruses, but retroviruses are the only oncogenic RNA viruses. Oncogenic viral DNA is incorporated directly into host cell DNA, while oncogenic viral RNA is transcribed by reverse transcriptase prior to incorporation. Integration of the viral genome can then alter the expression of host genes and so induce neoplasia. Viruses may also enhance the formation of neoplasms by indirect mechanisms. This occurs in HIV infection, where immunosuppression with the development of AIDS results in the appearance of viral-associated neoplasms such as non-Hodgkin lymphoma. Important oncogenic viruses include the human papilloma virus, the Epstein–Barr virus and a number of retroviruses.

Human papilloma virus (HPV) (of which there are over 50 strains) induces benign and malignant epithelial neoplasms, including those of the lids and conjunctiva. They produce proteins that inhibit the function of p53 and Rb1 gene products.

Epstein–Barr virus (EBV) in addition to causing infectious mononucleosis (glandular fever) is the agent that induces nasopharyngeal carcinoma and Burkitt's lymphoma when associated with a cofactor, probably malaria in certain regions of Africa.

Retroviruses that give rise to oncogenes include human T cell lymphotropic viruses (HTLVs) associated with T cell lymphomas. HTLV1 is endemic in the West Indies, parts of Africa and Japan, and is possibly involved in the aetiology of uveitis in certain ethnic groups.

Host factors

Age, race, diet, genetic factors and endocrine and immune status are host factors that influence oncogenesis. Neoplastic disease is primarily a disorder of the elderly and probably reflects the cumulative effect of carcinogens. A familial predisposition is associated with onset at an earlier age then sporadic neoplasia. Racial differences in the distribution of neoplastic disease relate to differences in genetic makeup and environmental factors such as different dietary customs and differing exposure to carcinogens. A brisk immune response may modify neoplastic behaviour. Immunodeficiency is known to be associated with a high risk of neoplasia (probably due to an inadequate immune response to oncogenic viruses).

Genetic basis of oncogenesis

Genetic abnormalities may predispose to neoplasia and may be also be observed in neoplastic cells. Malignant neoplastic cells in particular have unstable DNA, and random chromosomal abnormalities are common. Gross DNA defects, manifest as chromosomal abnormalities, are associated with some neoplasms of ophthalmic importance; these include uveal melanoma (chromosomes 3, 8, 9, 13, 17), retinoblastoma (chromosome 13), von Hippel–Lindau disease (chromosome 3) and chronic myeloid leukaemia (Philadelphia chromosome, a unique small chromosome resulting from a reciprocal translocation between chromosomes 9 and 22). Despite the apparent rarity of familial transmission, neoplasia is fundamentally a genetic disorder caused by the effects of at least three types of genes: oncogenes, anti-oncogenes and genes involved in DNA repair.

Oncogenes

Oncogenes are genes that cause malignant transformation of normal cells. Most oncogenes are mutated (activated) forms of one of at least 60 normal genes (proto-oncogenes) involved in the control of cell proliferation and differentiation. Activation of proto-oncogenes results from structural or regulatory mutation, translocation, gene amplification or other genetic damage, and results in altered, enhanced or inappropriate expression of a gene product (oncoprotein) that initiates a chain of events leading to neoplasia. Oncogenes act dominantly within somatic cells, thereby causing sporadic neoplasia. Germ-line mutations are less common, but cause inherited neoplasia. Oncogenes are found in both the human/animal genome (cellular oncogenes – c-onc) and in oncogenic RNA retroviruses (viral oncogenes – v-onc). The enzyme reverse transcriptase contained in retroviruses enables viral RNA to be transcribed into complementary DNA, which is then incorporated into the genome of an infected cell. Many proto-oncogenes are related to specific RNA oncogenic viruses.

Anti-oncogenes

Anti-oncogenes (tumour-suppressor genes) have the opposite effect to oncogenes; i.e. they control cell proliferation and block malignant transformation. They act recessively, and the loss or inactivation of both copies of the autosomal gene may result in neoplasia. Important anti-oncogenes include the retinoblastoma (Rb1) gene located on chromosome 13 (13q14.2) and p53, a gene located on the short arm of chromosome 17 the product of which causes cells with damaged DNA to undergo apoptosis. Mutation of p53 results in the accumulation of damaged DNA and increases the risk of neoplastic transformation. Anti-oncogenes may not be specific for one type of neoplasm; the Rb1 gene, which is undoubtedly associated with retinoblastoma, is also expressed in the cells of lung cancers; p53 mutations occur in many epithelial and other malignancies.

Genes involved in DNA repair

Mutations of these genes result in accumulation of damaged DNA, and include those located on chromosomes 9 (9q34.1), 2 (2q21) and 19 (19q13.2) in xeroderma pigmentosum and on chromosome 11 (11q22-q23) in ataxia telangiectasia.

The oncogenic process

Neoplasms result from a complex multistage process involving exposure to environmental mutagens, somatic mutation and genetic predisposition. Oncogenesis is initiated by two or more events that can involve oncogenes and anti-oncogenes. Expression of oncogenes and/or inhibition of anti-oncogenes leads to cells lacking the normal mechanisms that control proliferation and differentiation. Neoplastic cells undergo unrestrained clonal proliferation to cause a spectrum of disease with behaviour ranging from benign to malignant.

Six sequential stages are described:

1. Initiation. Mutations from carcinogens change the growth characteristics of a cell, which may show an altered response to its microenvironment and a selective growth advantage over normal cells. DNA repair mechanisms may repair the defect or the cell may undergo apoptosis or be eliminated by the immune system.

2. Growth. Initiated cells undergo clonal proliferation, which may be facilitated by environmental physical, biological and chemical factors. Growth merges with the promotion stage.

3. Promotion. Clonal proliferation continues and altered gene expression occurs in response to continued exposure to carcinogenic agents. This stage is reversible, but is a stage at which more genetic mutations are accumulated by the cell.

4. Conversion. Irreversible neoplastic changes occur within a cluster (10 to 1000) of cells. These changes relate to the microenvironment with little influence of external factors.

5. Propagation. Neoplastic cells proliferate autonomously to form a mass of perhaps 10^6 cells. The condition remains subclinical.

6. Progression (invasion and metastasis) The neoplastic cell mass continues to expand and becomes clinically apparent. For malignant neoplasms, cells separate from the primary mass to infiltrate surrounding tissues and invade blood and lymphatic vessels and metastasize to distant sites. Changes in the karyotype of malignant cells is characteristic of this stage, as are increase in cell mass and increasing cellular autonomy.

DEVELOPMENTAL ANOMALIES

CHRONOLOGY OF GESTATIONAL DEVELOPMENT

The three important developmental periods are the pre-embryonic period, the embryonic period and the fetal period.

The pre-embryonic period

This is the first 4 weeks following conception. During this period the tissue primordia are induced, and any insult usually results in death of the conceptus. Occasionally gross anomalies such as primary anophthalmos and cyclopia develop.

The embryonic period

This period extends from 4 to 8 weeks of gestation, and is characterized by the development of specific tissues and organs from the three primitive germ layers. It is also known as the period of organogenesis, and is when the basic structures of the eye develop. Insults result in major malformations such as primary anophthalmos, congenital cystic eyes and congenital non-attachment of the retina. Organogenesis is also occurring throughout the body at this time, so multisystem malformations may coexist. The important transition between the embryonic period and the subsequent fetal period is marked at 6 gestational weeks by the commencement of closure of the fetal fissure; failure of closure results in colobomatous defects.

The fetal period

This extends from the second gestational month to full term. During this period the intraocular tissues grow and develop, and any insult results in specific and localized ophthalmic lesions. Four main mechanisms are involved and result in specific malformations:

1. Retardation of growth and/or suppression of differentiation. This can result in malformations such as aniridia.
2. Abnormal growth and/or development resulting, for example, in anterior chamber dysgenesis.
3. Failure of atrophy of a transient structure, of which persistent hyperplastic primary vitreous is an example.
4. Failure of canalization of a duct, resulting in abnormalities such as congenital nasolacrimal stenosis.

EMBRYOGENESIS AND ORGANOGENESIS

Normal organogenesis

Ocular development commences during the initial 2 weeks of gestation. The eyes are derived from paired grooves (optic sulci) that form the cranial end of that part of the developing neural tube destined to become the diencephalon. With the closure of this tube the sulci develop into the optic vesicles which, by elongation of the stalks connecting them to the diencephalon, move towards the surface ectoderm where they initiate lens development. At the same time neural crest cells destined to become the connective tissue and skeletal components of the face, lids, conjunctiva and orbit migrate ventrally from their origin along the dorsolateral part of the neural tube to surround the developing eye and brain. At 4–6 weeks, the optic vesicle invaginates to form the double-walled optic cup. A transient defect, the embryonic fissure, develops along the ventral part of this cup and its stalk, allowing ingrowth of the hyaloid vasculature and development of the optic nerve. The fissure closes at approximately 6 weeks, commencing in its central part and extending simultaneously anteriorly and posteriorly, to envelop mesenchyme of neural crest origin; this includes the mesenchyme that will give rise to the hyaloid vasculature. The posterior, intermediate and anterior portions of the inner layer of the cup differentiate into the neurosensory retina, the non-pigmented epithelium of the ciliary body and the posterior pigment epithelial layer of the iris. The outer layer of the optic cup forms the RPE, the pigment epithelium of the ciliary body and the anterior pigment epithelial layer of the iris. Neural crest cells surrounding the differentiating optic cup form the remainder of the iris and ciliary body, and the choroid and sclera. Closure of the embryonic fissure occurs at an important time in development of both the eye and other organs when the primordia of most tissues have been formed, and marks the watershed between organogenesis and histogenesis (i.e. tissue differentiation and maturation). If insults occur before the fissure closes the consequence is major structural anomalies, whereas insults after the fissure closes result in less severe anomalies.

Anomalies of organogenesis

During the period of embryogenesis and organogenesis the optic vesicle may fail to develop or, if formed, it may either regress or fail to invaginate. There may be more widespread developmental failure of the anterior neural tube, anomalies may arise during mid-line differentiation or the embryonic fissure may fail to close.

Failure of development of the optic vesicle and anterior neural tube: regression of the optic vesicle

Anophthalmos

Anophthalmos is the absence of an eye. It is rare, but may occur either because the optic vesicle fails to form (primary anophthalmos) or because of widespread developmental failure of the anterior neural tube (secondary anophthalmos); regression of the optic vesicle also results in anophthalmos (degenerative anophthalmos). Primary and degenerative anophthalmos is bilateral in 75 per cent of cases and is usually sporadic, although autosomal dominant, autosomal recessive and X-linked patterns of inheritance have been described. Secondary anophthalmos is lethal. Anophthalmos differs from cryptophthalmos, an abnormality in which the palpebral fissure, lids and lashes are absent and the eye, although sometimes normal in size, is usually microphthalmic and abnormal.

Anomalies arising during mid-line differentiation

Cyclopia and synophthalmos

Cyclopia (a single median eye) and synophthalmos (partial fusion of ocular structures – Fig. 4.3) result from anomalies occurring during mid-line differentiation within the first gestational month. There may be an associated single orbit, a proboscis (anomalous nasal structure) and gross CNS malformations, including absence of the optic chiasm and a brain that has failed to develop into two hemispheres (holoprosencephaly, syn. arhinencephaly). Affected fetuses are either stillborn or die shortly after birth. Cyclopia and synophthalmos may be isolated or associated with a deletion of chromosome 18. The lack of major abnormalities below the diencephalon and in the rest of the body is characteristic. The tissues of the eye, although grossly abnormal in form, develop normally, thus suggesting that the anomalies occur at an early stage among pluripotential cells which when they start to differentiate form mature tissue.

Anomalies of invagination of the optic vesicle

Congenital cystic eye

Congenital cystic eye is rare and results from failed invagination of the optic vesicle, which persists and develops into a small congenital cyst composed of a fibrous coat that may or may not be connected to extraocular muscles and which is devoid of neuroectodermal elements.

Congenital non-attachment of the retina

Congenital non-attachment of the retina results from failed attachment of the primitive neurosensory retina to the developing RPE, the subretinal space being the remnant of the cavity of the optic vesicle. Congenital non-attachment of the retina may coexist with other ocular developmental anomalies such as persistent hyperplastic primary vitreous.

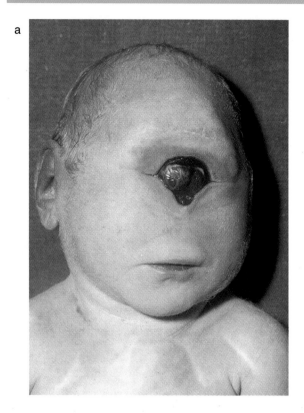

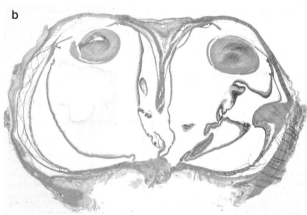

Figure 4.3 Synophthalmos.(a) Gross post-mortem appearance. (b) Histology.

Failure of closure of the embryonic fissure

Colobomas

A coloboma is the absence of part of an ocular or related structure. Colobomas are described as typical when occurring along the line of the embryonic fissure, and as atypical when they occur elsewhere. In the fully developed eye the site of the embryonic fissure is inferior and slightly nasal, and it extends from the optic nerve to the margin of the pupil (anterior part of the optic cup). A colobomatous defect may extend throughout the entire length of the fissure (complete coloboma); alternatively it may occur in the iris, ciliary body, choroid/retina or optic nerve, or at several sites. Colobomas are relatively common but, because of the sequence of the closure of the embryonic fissure, those at anterior and posterior sites are more common than those at mid-peripheral sites. They are usually bilateral but often asymmetrical and sporadic, although incompletely penetrant autosomal dominant forms are described. As a rule no other ocular malformations coexist, but colobomas may occur as features of Trisomy 13, and of thalidomide and LSD embryopathies. Many other colobomatous defects described at various sites are probably not colobomas but the result of unusual maldevelopment.

Typical iris colobomas are keyhole-shaped defects extending inferonasally from the pupil margin to the iris root (Fig. 4.4). The adjacent tissue is thinned, and delicate remnants of embryonic mesoderm may bridge the defect; the remainder of the iris tissue is normal.

Typical ciliary body colobomas are rare but invariably found in Trisomy 13. The defect is filled with connective tissue that may extend to an associated persistent hyperplastic primary vitreous. The colobomatous defect results in abnormal development of the zonule, leading to a lens coloboma.

Typical fundus colobomas are evident as white sharply demarcated defects in the inferonasal quadrant, and vary in size from an almost undetectable lesion (coloboma spurium) to one extending the full length of the embryonic fissure. They may be bisected by a bridge of apparently normal tissue. The retina is thinned and in extreme cases reduced to a delicate glial membrane; the RPE is absent or degenerate, there may be retinal dysplasia, and in later life a retinal hole may develop and rhegmatogen-

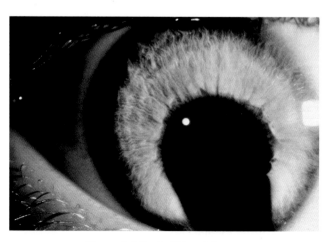

Figure 4.4 Typical iris coloboma.

ous detachment may ensue. The adjacent sclera usually retains its normal appearance but may be sufficiently thinned to form a staphyloma which can be so pronounced as to form an orbital cyst into which ocular contents herniate to such an extent that the cyst replaces the eye (ectatic colobomatous cyst).

Typical optic disc and nerve colobomas are inferior, grey-white and surrounded by clumps of pigment. They vary from an almost imperceptible lesion to a large defect involving the entire nerve head (Fig. 4.5) to produce the features seen in the Morning glory syndrome. Some forms of congenital tilted discs are thought to be colobomas.

Atypical colobomas are developmental defects occurring at a site other than along the line of the embryonic fissure. They resemble typical colobomas, and may form by anomalous closure of an abnormally placed optic fissure.

Macular 'colobomas' are unlikely to be true colobomas, and result possibly from photoreceptor dystrophies or inflammatory lesions due to maternal infections.

THE CORNEOSCLERAL COAT AND THE ANTERIOR SEGMENT

Normal development

At approximately the fourth to fifth week of gestation, following the separation of the lens vesicle from the surface ectoderm, mesenchymal tissue (derived at least in part from neural crest cells) accumulates between the ectoderm that ultimately forms both the epithelium of the cornea and the anterior part of the lens vesicle.

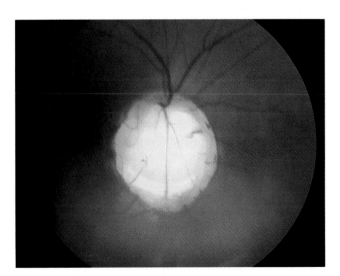

Figure 4.5 Typical optic disc coloboma.

From the sixth week onwards, this mesenchyme shows three waves of increased activity.

The first wave begins at the sixth week. Multiplication and migration of cells deep to the surface ectoderm lead to the formation of a solid disc of tissue that will become the endothelium of the cornea and trabecular meshwork. The endothelial cells have a high metabolic rate, and from the eighth week onwards secrete the lamellar component of Descemet's membrane.

The second wave commences at the seventh week, when mesenchymal cells move in several directions. Anteriorly they move between the epithelium and endothelium of the cornea to form the stromal keratocytes, stromal collagen and Bowman's layer. They also move between the corneal endothelium and the developing lens to form the pupillary membrane. Posteriorly they migrate to form the sclera.

The third wave is when the mesenchymal cells migrate to lie anterior to the lens and distal to the margin of the optic cup, and develop into the iris stroma. Differential growth of the eye results in the formation of a narrow slit-like space, the developing anterior chamber, between the corneal endothelium and the iris stroma. Until the 28th week the chamber is lined by mesothelium.

Anterior chamber and drainage angle

The anterior chamber and drainage angle form by a process of differential growth and/or reorganization, and not by cleavage. Formation of the anterior chamber begins at approximately the seventh week, and is associated with development of the fetal blood supply and differentiation of the corneal stroma. The rudimentary drainage angle and trabecular meshwork are not developed before the 12th week, and arise from the second wave of mesenchymal cell migration. The angle is formed initially by loosely organized undifferentiated neural crest cells and is covered by a layer of polyhedral cells continuous with the corneal endothelium and extending on to the anterior iris surface. During the fourth month, at the same time as the iris develops from the anterior rim of the optic cup, the meshwork differentiates into corneoscleral and uveal components; Schlemm's canal appears in the deepest part of the drainage angle anterior to the scleral spur. During the fifth month, the future angle lies at the junction of the iris root and corneal endothelium, and the ciliary body overlies the site of the trabecular meshwork. The angle develops further when the iris root and ciliary body slide posteriorly to the level of the scleral spur and expose the developing trabecular meshwork. At this time the endothelium lining Schlemm's canal becomes vacuolated, and this coincides with the differentiation of the ciliary body and the onset of aqueous secretion. The outflow facility of the trabecular meshwork probably reaches postnatal values by the 32nd week. By the seventh month the apex of the angle has reached the level of Schlemm's canal, and at birth it is at the level of the scleral spur. Deepening of the anterior chamber continues into postnatal life, and the angle reaches its adult appearance 6–12 months after birth.

Sclera

The sclera is formed from the cells that move posteriorly during the second wave of mesenchymal migration. Initially presenting as a condensation at the primitive limbus near the future insertion of the rectus muscles, the cells reach the posterior pole by 12 weeks and penetrate the optic nerve by the fourth month. Unlike the corneal collagen, the scleral collagen develops with random orientation.

Iris

The iris develops both from the anterior margin of the embryonic optic cup (neuroectoderm) and from the mesenchyme of neural crest origin. At 6 weeks the anterior chamber is bounded anteriorly by the corneal endothelium and posteriorly by a thin layer of vascularized mesenchyme, the anterior part of the tunica vasculosa lentis, which becomes the pupillary membrane. At about 3 months, the anterior walls of the optic cup grow rapidly forwards over the surface of the lens and within the pupillary membrane; capillaries proliferate and changes in the associated mesenchyme lead to the formation of the iris stroma, which then grows in association with the posterior neuroectodermal component that becomes the epithelium. Myofibrils that form the sphincter muscle can be recognized by 5 months, and those that form the dilator muscle by 6 months. Pigmentation of the epithelium starts at 4–5 months, and is complete by 7 months. The pupillary membrane begins to resorb during the sixth month and is complete by 8 months.

Anomalies of development

The co-ordinated integrated manner in which the cornea, trabecular meshwork and iris develop is subject to common influences, so that developmental anomalies of one are frequently accompanied by anomalies of the others, and there is considerable overlap with all three structures often being to some extent involved. Malformations may arise from an abnormality in any of the three waves of mesenchymal migration and, while aetiological factors are known in some instances, different factors may lead to identical features and the disorders are best classified in a descriptive manner rather than being grouped according to putative mechanisms. They affect the cornea, anterior chamber and iris.

Corneal developmental anomalies

Microcornea

Microcornea is a corneal diameter < 10.5 mm. It is seen in microphthalmos, and is commonly associated with malformation of the anterior segment. Microcornea is due to failure of growth of the optic cup.

Megalocornea

Megalocornea is a large cornea, i.e. adult size at birth or > 13 mm by 2 years. In the absence of buphthalmos it is usually bilateral and non-progressive and, apart from astigmatism, iris atrophy and occasionally lens subluxation, the rest of the eye is usually normal. Megalocornea can develop either in isolation or is inherited as an autosomal or X-linked recessive; there may be association with Marfan's syndrome, mental retardation or craniosynostosis.

Abnormalities of corneal curvature

These include an abnormally flat cornea (cornea plana), a condition that occurs in association with other disorders such as microphthalmos. Differences in the curvature of the corneal meridians give rise to astigmatism, but while this may be considered as a variant of the normal, some severe forms of astigmatism are inherited, usually as autosomal dominant. Other abnormalities of corneal curvature such as keratoconus and keratoglobus are regarded as degenerations.

Sclerocornea

Sclerocornea describes encroachment of scleral tissue into the cornea with obliteration of the limbus. Usually bilateral, the condition is associated with other ocular developmental anomalies such as microphthalmos, anterior chamber dysgenesis and cornea plana. It is more commonly sporadic, but inherited forms may also occur. Sclerocornea probably results from an abnormality of differentiation during the second wave of mesenchymal migration, with differentiation being into tissue similar to sclera rather than cornea.

Anterior chamber dysgenesis

Anterior chamber dysgenesis comprises a spectrum of abnormalities arising during the development of the anterior segment. They include Peter's anomaly, posterior keratoconus, posterior embryotoxon, and Axenfeld's and Rieger's anomalies and syndromes. Structures of both mesodermal and ectodermal origin (i.e. the lens and corneal epithelium) are involved and, as the anterior chamber does not result from cleavage of tissue, terms such as anterior chamber cleavage syndrome, mesodermal dysgenesis and neural crestopathies are not accurate. The descriptive term anterior chamber dysgenesis is probably more appropriate. A common underlying genetic mechanism is known for Peter's anomaly, autosomal dominant 'keratitis' and aniridia in which there are mutations of the PAX6 gene located on chromosome 11 (11p13). Rieger's syndrome, although genetically heterogeneous, is associated with mutations of the gene RIEG1 (4q25) which, like PAX6, is a regulatory gene important in ocular embryogenesis.

Peter's anomaly

Peter's anomaly is a rare sporadic and frequently bilateral disorder with a poor visual prognosis. Glaucoma complicates 50–70 per cent of cases. Peter's anomaly results from delay or failure of separation of the lens vesicle from the surface ectoderm, and leads to a persistent adhesion or stalk between the cornea and lens. Migration of mesenchyme is impeded by this adhesion and results in the characteristic features of the anomaly, including opacity of the central cornea, absence of Descemet's membrane and corneal endothelium (first wave of migration), thinning of the central cornea (second wave of migration) with oedema, and disorganization of normal lamellar structure. Fibrovascular pannus may replace Bowman's layer in the area of thinning. Throughout fetal life, the anterior chamber remains shallow and central or peripheral iridocorneal adhesions may result from aberrant and persistent tissue or faulty migration and induction of mesenchyme. In some cases the posterior corneal surface is in contact with a morphologically normal lens, suggesting that keratolenticular adhesion occurred later in development. Two types of Peter's anomaly are recognized.

Type I: a corneal opacity is present on the pupillary axis, the border of the opacity being connected to the colarette by strands of iris. The lens is uninvolved and, although there may be other ocular and systemic anomalies, the disorder is usually isolated and is probably the same as the 'internal ulcer' described by von Hippel.

Type II: the features of Type I are present together with lens abnormalities such as keratolenticular adhesion. This type is more frequently bilateral and is commonly associated with systemic and other ocular abnormalities including microphthalmos, aniridia and colobomas.

Posterior keratoconus

Posterior keratoconus may represent a mild form of Peter's anomaly. Sporadic and usually compatible with relatively normal vision, it comprises a circumscribed concavity of the posterior cornea, the stroma of which may be hazy, and thinning of Descemet's membrane associated with endothelial abnormality.

Posterior embryotoxon

Posterior embryotoxon is an anteriorly displaced and thickened Schwalbe's line (the peripheral end of Descemet's membrane). It is visible clinically without gonioscopy, and is present in up to 30 per cent of normal eyes. Posterior embryotoxon may be transmitted as an autosomal dominant.

Axenfeld's anomaly

Axenfeld's anomaly results when strands of abnormal iris tissue extend across the anterior chamber to insert into a posterior embryotoxon. If associated with glaucoma, it is termed Axenfeld's syndrome.

Rieger's anomaly

Rieger's anomaly results when Axenfeld's anomaly is associated with hypoplasia of the anterior iris stroma. This often leads to full thickness iris holes (pseudopolycoria) and displacement of the pupil (corectopia). Glaucoma occurs in approximately 60 per cent of cases. Rieger's syndrome comprises Rieger's anomaly and systemic malformations involving structures of neural crest origin such as the face and teeth; a broad nasal bridge, telecanthus, microdontia and maxillary hypoplasia are characteristic.

Rieger's syndrome is a genetically heterogeneous autosomal dominant disorder associated with deletions of chromosomes 4 and 13, and single gene mutations with loci at 4q25, 13q14 and 6p25. The gene mapped to 4q25 (RIEG1) encodes a regulatory factor (solurshin) that, like the gene product of PAX6, is important in normal ocular embryogenesis.

Iris developmental anomalies

Aniridia

The term aniridia is a misnomer as iris tissue is usually present, albeit in vestigial form; nevertheless it covers a group of disorders characterized by iris hypoplasia. Its incidence is between 1 : 64–100 000 live births. It may be inherited as an autosomal dominant form or, less commonly, is sporadic. The sporadic forms may represent new mutations or chromosomal deletions. Aniridia is not an isolated finding but is the most obvious feature of a panocular condition which, in addition to iris hypoplasia, includes any of the following:

1. Poor vision associated with pendular nystagmus and macular hypoplasia.
2. Glaucoma developing in up to 75 per cent of cases either as a result of a primary angle anomaly or because of progressive angle closure by peripheral iridocorneal adhesions.
3. Cataract (Fig. 4.6).
4. Ciliary body hypoplasia.
5. Corneal changes, including thick progressive fibrovascular pannus, abnormalities of Bowman's layer, Peter's anomaly and other anterior segment malformations.
6. Optic nerve hypoplasia.

The pathogenesis of aniridia is not known, but interference at 8 weeks' gestation may hinder the development of the iris epithelium, and at 12–14 weeks the neuroectodermal component. Deletions involving the short arm of chromosome 11 exhibit a high incidence of aniridia as part of the WAGR syndrome while other loci, particularly on chromosomes 1 and 2, are thought also to be associated with iris development. Mutations in the PAX6 gene (11p13) are associated with aniridia together with Peter's anomaly and autosomal dominant 'keratitis'.

In most cases the iris is reduced to a small stump and smooth muscle is absent. The angle may be anomalous and the retina may extend anteriorly as far as the pars plicata of the ciliary body. Later changes include the development of peripheral iridocorneal adhesions with growth of corneal endothelium into the angle and the subsequent development of glaucoma.

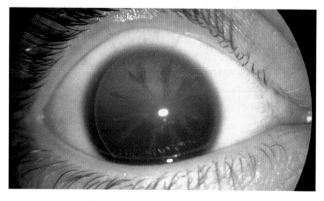

Figure 4.6 Aniridia with cataract.

Brushfield's spots

Brushfield's spots lie close to the pupillary margin. Most occur in Trisomy 21 and are seen as normal or hypercellular areas of iris tissue surrounding relative stromal hypoplasia.

Persistent pupillary membrane

Persistent pupillary membranes may be associated with anomalies of the vitreous and vasculature.

THE LENS

Normal development

The lens originates from ectodermal tissue. With the formation of the optic vesicle at about 28 days' gestation the overlying surface ectoderm thickens to form the lens placode, which rapidly invaginates to form the lens pit. The edges of the pit fuse to form the lens vesicle, which detaches itself from the surface ectoderm and remains suspended in the mesenchyme within the developing optic cup. The hyaloid vascular system develops through the mesenchyme and supplies the inner layer of the cup, the mesenchyme itself and the developing lens. The anterior wall of the lens vesicle becomes the anterior epithelium of the lens while the cells of the posterior wall elongate to form the primary lens fibres, which grow into and obliterate the cavity. All subsequent lens growth, beginning at 7 weeks of gestation and continuing throughout life, occurs from secondary lens fibre formation by elongation of epithelial cells in the equatorial zone. Secondary fibres pass from the anterior to the posterior pole of the lens and insert into the Y-sutures. After the third month the lens becomes isolated antigenically from the rest of the eye by the development of a basement membrane, which becomes the lens capsule. Throughout most of its intrauterine development the lens is invested by the tunica vasculosa lentis, a vascular mesenchymal layer supplied by the hyaloid vascular system, the portion anterior to the lens being the pupillary membrane. Development of the zonule of Zinn from the non-pigmented epithelium of the ciliary body occurs during the fifth month.

Anomalies of development

Anomalies of development are categorized as those of formation, size and shape, position and transparency.

Anomaly of formation: congenital aphakia

Congenital aphakia is rare and usually associated with other ocular anomalies. It may be primary, when the lens vesicle fails to form, or secondary, when the presumably abnormally developing lens is spontaneously absorbed.

Anomalies of size and shape

Microspherophakia (spherophakia)

Microspherophakia is usually bilateral, the lens being reduced in diameter and spherical in form. It may be an isolated phenomenon, but more commonly it occurs as part of the syndromes of Weill–Marchesani, Marfan and Alport (anterior lenticonus, hereditary nephritis and deafness). It results from arrested development of secondary lens fibres at approximately 5–6 months.

Lenticonus and lentiglobus

Lenticonus and lentiglobus are conical and hemispherical anomalies respectively. Both occur axially and affect the posterior or, less commonly, the anterior surface of the lens. Anterior lenticonus is part of Alport's syndrome, and may result from a central abnormality of the anterior capsule. A localized lens opacity may coexist.

Lens coloboma

Lens colobomas are either notch-like defects in the equatorial region or merely localized flattened areas of the equatorial curve. They are associated with failure of zonular development.

Anomaly of position: congenital ectopia lentis

Congenital ectopia lentis results from a developmental or inherited anomaly of the suspensory apparatus, and may be associated with anomalies of the iris such as corectopia. Zonular fibres are usually present but are few in number and are spaced far apart.

Anomaly of transparency: congenital cataract

Congenital lens opacities affect up to 0.4 per cent of neonates and can be a significant cause of visual disability in children because of their intrinsic effects on vision and the associated development of amblyopia. They may result from abnormal development or degeneration of normally formed lens tissue. Many causes have been identified, and congenital cataracts may occur as part of a syndrome or in isolation (non-syndromic). Their morphology may vary widely and is determined by the timing rather than the nature of the insult. There are a number of types.

Nuclear cataracts result from transient abnormal growth during the early stages of lens formation when the embryonic nucleus is developing.

Sutural and axial cataracts result from abnormal fusion of secondary lens fibres.

Lamellar cataracts result from a transient insult occurring later in the development of an otherwise normal lens, and are due to an abnormality of the fibres encircling the embryonic nucleus. The time of the insult during intrauterine growth determines the position of the cataractous layer in the lens cortex, and the duration of the insult its thickness. Areas of lens outside the lamellae may also be involved, and are seen clinically as radial opacities (riders).

Polar cataracts may be anterior or posterior. Congenital anterior polar cataracts are usually remnants of the embryonic pupillary membrane, although they may also occur if, during early development, there is an anomaly of closure or separation of the lens vesicle. A plaque of connective tissue forms in an area of fibrous metaplasia associated with a break in the anterior epithelium. Such cataracts may be dominantly inherited, but an acquired unilateral form can result from intrauterine ocular perforation such as may occur in amniocentesis. Congenital posterior polar cataracts may result from a disturbance in the regression of the tunica vasculosa lentis in which the posterior subcapsular lens cortex degenerates. Subsequently the lens epithelial cells, which migrate posteriorly, enlarge and become vacuolated (bladder cells or Wedl cells).

Total cataracts reflect an abnormality involving most of the lens fibres, which have developed anomalously or have been damaged by a cause present throughout development or occurring towards the end of gestation. The lens may have a milky appearance with liquefaction of the lens substance; vacuoles form in the equatorial region and epithelial cells migrate on to the posterior capsule. Abnormal lens protein may resorb, leaving the capsule and some cellular remnants (membranous cataract). The tunica vasculosa lentis may persist in association with a cataractous lens (cataracta vasculosa). Absence of lens substance centrally, resulting for example from primary aplasia of the lens nucleus or selective resorption of the nucleus, leads to the formation of an annular cataract resembling a Soemmering's ring.

Transient neonatal lens vacuoles are fluid-filled vacuoles in the region of the sutures of the posterior cortex. A common finding in premature infants and seen clinically as lens opacities at approximately 1–2 weeks postnatally, they resolve completely after about 2 weeks.

Inherited congenital cataracts

Approximately one-third of congenital cataracts occur in the absence of other abnormalities and are inherited. Several forms of autosomal dominant congenital cataracts are associated with genetic defects that cause abnormalities in human lens crystallin proteins (Table 4.3). Cerulean cataracts have bluish-white lamellar opacifications, and at least one form is associated with a mutation in the β-crystallin gene CRYBB2 (22q), which results in reduced synthesis of the protein. The Coppock cataract, an autosomal dominant congenital cataract involving the embryonic lens, is linked to the region of chromosome 2 that contains the multigene family of γ-crystallin genes (2q34-q35).

Table 4.3 Autosomal dominant congenital cataracts

Cataract morphology	Locus	Gene
Posterior polar	1p	
Nuclear	1p36	
Zonular pulverulent	1q21-q25	GJA8
Anterior polar	2p25	
Coppock-like (embryonic nucleus)	2q34-q35	CRYG4
Polymorphous	13q	
Nuclear	16q22	
Anterior polar	17p13	
Zonular sutural	17q11-q12	CRYBA1
Cerulean	17q24	
Nuclear	21q22.3	CRYAA
Cerulean	22q	CRYBB2

THE VITREOUS AND THE VASCULATURE

Normal development

During the third week of embryonic life, the terminal branch of the primitive ophthalmic artery invades the embryonic fissure to form the hyaloid artery. Following the closure of the fissure at 5–7 weeks the hyaloid artery remains within the optic cup and sends branches into the primary vitreous, which is mesenchyme of neural crest cell origin that has collected between the primitive retina and the lens vesicle. The richly vascularized primary vitreous is fully developed by the eighth week. The developing capillary system initially invests the posterior lens capsule, but later completely encloses the developing lens as the tunica vasculosa lentis, the anterior part of which is termed the pupillary membrane. Coincidental with this, at about 6 weeks, the acellular secondary vitreous begins to appear between the primary vitreous and the developing retina. The secondary vitreous is avascular apart from the hyaloid artery that traverses it as it passes from the optic disc to the primary vitreous. The hyaloid vascular system, including the tunica vasculosa lentis, begins to degenerate during the fourth month and is lost by 28–33 weeks, leaving a remnant seen clinically as Cloquet's canal. During the fourth

month, the primary vitreous along with the hyaloid vascular system degenerates other than where the latter emerges from the optic disc and from where the retinal vessels develop. The developing vessels push into the retinal nerve fibre layer to form a polygonal network that reaches the ora serrata, initially nasally and later temporally. Retinal vascularization may not be complete, particularly on the temporal side, until 1 month post-term.

Anomalies of development

Anomalies of development of the vitreous and components of the ocular vascular system are intimately related.

Persistent hyperplastic primary vitreous

Persistent hyperplastic primary vitreous (PHPV) is a congenital anomaly that results from failure of regression of the primary vitreous. Usually unilateral (except when associated with Trisomy 13), it presents at birth with leukocoria. Two forms, anterior and posterior, are described.

Anterior PHPV is the most frequent. The affected eye is microphthalmic, with a shallow anterior chamber and a vascularized retrolental mass to which abnormally elongated ciliary processes may be attached. Posterior subcortical cataract usually develops at an early stage. Ultrasonography reveals a persistent trunk of the hyaloid artery. With differential growth of the eye, contraction of the retrolental mass and progression of the cataract, the anterior chamber becomes shallow and pupil block glaucoma may ensue. Fibrovascular tissue extends from and distorts the ciliary processes, which merge with the retrolental mass, and the persistent hyaloid vasculature spans the vitreous cavity. Metaplasia may result in the presence of fat, smooth muscle and cartilage. The retina may be drawn up behind the retrolental mass and detachment may follow.

Posterior PHPV presents with signs associated with uniocular reduced vision such as strabismus or nystagmus. Pathological features are confined to the posterior segment, where retinal folds result from persistent remnants of the posterior part of the primary vitreous. The retina is often dysplastic in relation to the folds, and detachment is common.

Persistent hyaloid artery

Persistence of the whole artery is rare, but remnants of part of the hyaloid vascular system are not uncommon (Fig. 4.7), particularly in premature infants in whom the anomaly frequently regresses. Insignificant anterior rem-

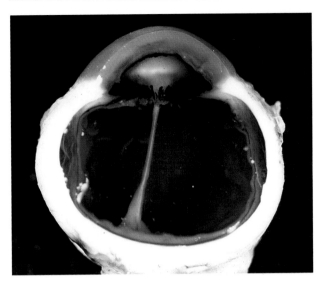

Figure 4.7 Persistent hyaloid artery. The hyaloid artery extends from the optic disc to the posterior surface of the lens.

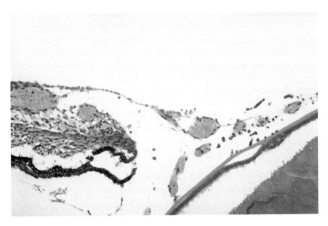

Figure 4.8 Persistent pupillary membrane. Remaining vessels of the anterior tunica vasculosa lentis between the iris (left) and anterior lens capsule.

nants appear as a Mittendorf dot, a small white spot situated usually slightly inferonasally on the posterior lens surface. If the remnant is larger it may disturb normal lens architecture and be associated with a localized lens opacity. Posterior remnants of the hyaloid artery vary in presentation from single strands of tissue emanating from the optic disc (pre-papillary veils) to cystic structures (hyaloid cysts). Bergmeister's papilla is one such anomaly, and consists of the posterior remnant of the hyaloid vascular system with an associated neuroglial sheath. Occasionally only the vascular elements remain as prepapillary vascular loops (most commonly arterial) projecting into the vitreous; posterior detachment of the vitreous may cause these vessels to rupture with resultant vitreous haemorrhage.

Persistent pupillary membrane

Persistent pupillary membranes are remnants of the anterior tunica vasculosa lentis, and are seen as filamentous bands extending from the anterior iris surface (Fig. 4.8). They are common, usually of no significance, and typically adhere to the surface of the lens, to other parts of the anterior iris or, occasionally, to the corneal endothelium. A variant of a persistent pupillary membrane is seen as small, isolated, often stellate pigmented patches of tissue (epicapsular stars) on the anterior lens capsule unattached to the iris.

Retinal vascular anomalies

Congenital absence of the retinal vasculature is exceptionally rare. Many abnormalities of the branching and course of the retinal vasculature have been described, but

most are of little significance. Anomalous vascular branching may be associated with optic nerve drusen. Anomalous retinal vascular tortuosity and dilatation is of more importance because there can be confusion with acquired disease. Vascular dilatation may be inherited as an autosomal dominant and may become symptomatic due to spontaneous haemorrhage. Major retinal vascular anomalies of significance are discussed with vascular disorders and with disorders of postnatal cell and tissue growth.

THE RETINA

Normal development

Retinal development starts at the posterior pole and proceeds to the periphery. By the end of the embryonic period, the retina consists of an outer pigmented layer (the RPE) and a primitive neurosensory layer derived from the outer and inner parts of the optic cup respectively. By the sixth month all layers are well defined and differentiation of the macula, which lags behind that of other areas, begins with thinning in the region of the fovea. This results from lateral movement of neurons in the inner layers, and is associated with elongation and an increased density of foveal cones. Macular differentiation continues for up to 4 months after birth. The neurosensory retina is normally separated from the RPE until the fourth month, but thereafter the two structures lie in apposition.

Anomalies of development

Anomalies of development can affect both the outer and inner layers of the optic vesicle.

Anomalies of development of the outer layer of the optic vesicle

Congenital hypertrophy of the RPE

Congenital hypertrophy of the RPE (CHRPE) presents as well-demarcated, slightly raised, darkly pigmented lesions 1–2 disc diameters in size. Depigmentation within the lesion, or as a halo around it, is common. Three types are described: typical unifocal unilateral lesions, typical multifocal unilateral lesions (congenital grouped pigmentation of the retina) and atypical multifocal bilateral lesions, the latter being associated with systemic neoplasia. CHRPE is asymptomatic and can involve any area of the retina. The RPE is hypertrophic and lies beneath atrophic retina. Some RPE cells contain a large number of abnormal melanosomes, whilst others are depleted of melanin and give rise to the clinically observed areas of depigmentation.

Typical unifocal unilateral lesions are harmless, asymptomatic and are usually identified on routine clinical examination.

Congenital grouped pigmentation of the retina (bear-track pigmentation) is relatively common and asymptomatic. It is characterized by multiple clusters of discrete pigmented spots often distributed throughout the fundus.

Atypical multifocal bilateral lesions (Fig. 4.9) are associated with autosomal dominant colonic adenomatous polyposis/carcinoma syndromes (Gardner's and Turcot's syndromes) and microcephaly.

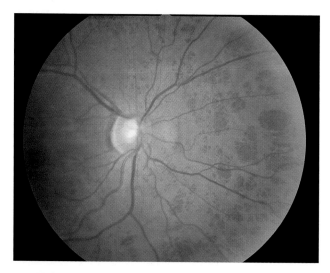

Figure 4.9 Congenital hypertrophy of the RPE (CHRPE). Atypical multifocal bilateral lesions.

Anomalies of development of the inner layer of the optic vesicle

Retinal dysplasia

Retinal dysplasia results from faulty differentiation of the retina in which disordered cellular proliferation, abnormal location and stratification of retinal cellular components leads to the formation of characteristic dysplastic rosettes (Fig. 4.10). Retinal dysplasia is a manifestation of disease rather than a specific disorder. It may be an isolated finding and present as a retinal fold, or may be associated with other ocular and systemic disorders, including Trisomy 13, Norrie's disease and Aicardi's syndrome. Dysplastic retinal rosettes are a cross-section of a tube of one or more layers of primitive cells surrounding a central space lined by a structure analogous to the normal outer limiting membrane. As the RPE is necessary for the normal development of the retina, retinal dysplasia usually only occurs when the developing neurosensory layer is separated from the RPE. Chromosome 13 carries a gene that controls normal retinal development and may also be important.

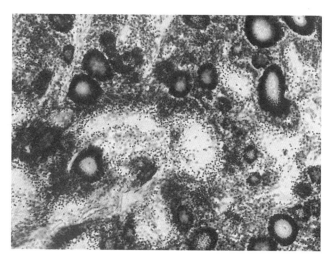

Figure 4.10 Retinal dysplasia. Disordered cellular proliferation with the formation of dysplastic rosettes.

Congenital non-attachment of the retina

The neurosensory retina is normally separated from the RPE until the fourth month of development. After this the two structures lie in apposition and any abnormality preventing this can lead to developmental total or focal non-attachment, which is usually accompanied by retinal dysplasia. Congenital non-attachment of the retina is related to congenital cystic eye due to anomalous invagination of the optic cup. Secondary congenital total retinal detachments may occur as a result of colobomas,

PHPV, retinoblastoma, congenital infections such as toxoplasmosis, and ocular syndromes associated with chromosomal abnormalities.

Retinal folds are a type of congenital non-attachment, and may arise in conjunction with growth anomalies of the neuroectoderm occurring early in development. They are commonly associated with colobomas but may also develop secondary to traction from preretinal lesions such as vitreous haemorrhage, PHPV and the retinopathy of prematurity. A variant, termed a falciform fold (retinal septa), is a narrow well-defined tent-like elevation of the neurosensory retina. Falciform folds are often bilateral, usually occur in the temporal quadrants, and extend anteriorly from the optic disc (Fig. 4.11) sometimes as far as the ciliary body. Contact with the lens may be associated with a localized lens opacity. The fold is formed of poorly differentiated retina that may be dysplastic. Remnants of the hyaloid vasculature may be found in the fold.

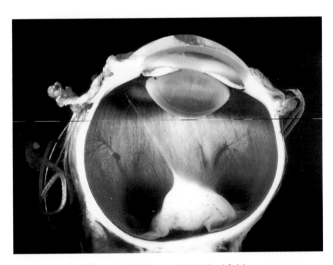

Figure 4.11 Congenital retinal folds.

THE OPTIC DISC AND OPTIC NERVE

Normal development

Following closure of the embryonic fissure, the optic stalk consists of inner and outer layers of undifferentiated cells surrounding the hyaloid vessels. The inner layer of the stalk is directly continuous with the inner layer of the optic cup and acts as a conduit for ganglion cell axons, which extend into it by the beginning of the sixth week and grow posteriorly to the lateral geniculate nucleus. The cells of both layers of the optic stalk either degenerate or differentiate to form the glial tissue of the optic nerve. An excessive number of ganglion cells send their axons along the optic stalk, but when the axons fail to reach their target they undergo retrograde degeneration. Myelination of the optic nerve axons begins late in gestation at the level of the optic chiasm, proceeds distally and ceases at the lamina cribrosa approximately 1 month after birth.

Anomalies of development

Aplasia and hypoplasia of the optic nerve

Aplasia, i.e. complete absence of the optic nerve, is extremely rare and may be associated with other gross malformations such as anencephaly. Hypoplasia of the optic nerve and optic disc is more common, and a significant cause of childhood blindness. Optic nerve hypoplasia (ONH) may be unilateral or bilateral, is non-progressive, and may occur either as an isolated anomaly or in association with other ocular or systemic malformations. Particularly associated with mid-line structural anomalies of the brain, features include variable reduction in visual function, strabismus and nystagmus. Other associated structural abnormalities of the eye and elsewhere include aniridia, microphthalmos, macular hypoplasia and neurological defects. A small grey optic disc is seen on ophthalmoscopy to be surrounded by a concentric yellow ring of visible sclera (double-ring sign). Although the mechanism remains unknown, ONH may arise through excessive retrograde degeneration of the retinal ganglion cells during development; an alternative hypothesis is that ganglion cells fail to differentiate. The optic disc is reduced in diameter, the axons within the nerve are reduced in number or absent, and abnormal glial tissue is sometimes present. Exposure of sclera in the peripapillary area not covered by neurosensory retina and RPE results in the double-ring sign, which may be accentuated by proliferation of RPE at the margin of the ring. Loss of retinal ganglion cells leads to thinning of the nerve fibre layer.

Myelinated retinal nerve fibres

Occasionally myelination of the optic nerve continues into the nerve fibre layer of the peripapillary retina. Oligodendroglia, not normally present in the retina, are associated with such myelination. Myelinated retinal nerve fibres, one of the commonest developmental anomalies of the fundus (1 per cent of the population), are white and irregular with a feathery margin and overlie blood vessels (Fig. 4.12). They are usually of no significance, but are occasionally associated with scotomata, high myopia, amblyopia, the craniofacial dysostoses and the Gorlin–Goltz syndrome.

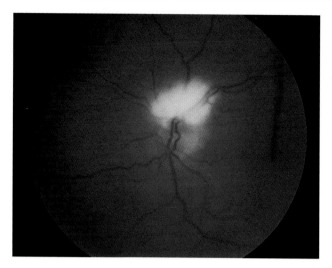

Figure 4.12 Myelinated retinal nerve fibres.

Morning glory syndrome

The Morning glory syndrome is usually unilateral, and comprises a large cup-like defect forming an ectatic cyst lined by retinal tissue and containing residual neuroectodermal elements (Fig. 4.13a). The optic disc is obscured, and anomalous retinal vessels are abnormal in direction and calibre (Fig. 4.13b). The adjacent retina is often abnormal and folded, and the peripapillary fundus hyperpigmented. Anomalous smooth muscle or fat may be present adjacent to the defect due to faulty induction of mesodermal tissue. The pathogenesis of the Morning glory syndrome is not clear, although it may represent an unusual type of coloboma.

Optic disc pits

Optic disc pits are congenital, round, well-circumscribed depressions of the optic disc often occurring within the physiological cup. They are seen in the temporal quadrants, and may be associated with oedema, schisis, degeneration and serous detachment of the macula. A pocket-like depression within the substance of the optic nerve contains rudimentary or degenerate neuroectodermal tissue with neurosensory retinal and RPE elements. The pathogenesis is not understood, although, like the Morning glory syndrome, optic disc pits may be unusual types of colobomas. The pathogenesis of the associated macular abnormalities is similarly unclear.

Optic disc drusen (hyaline bodies)

Optic disc drusen are irregular nodular swellings that may present with an apparently swollen disc. They may be idiopathic, occasionally autosomal dominantly inherited, or associated with other ocular conditions such as the inherited retinal degenerations. The lesions are

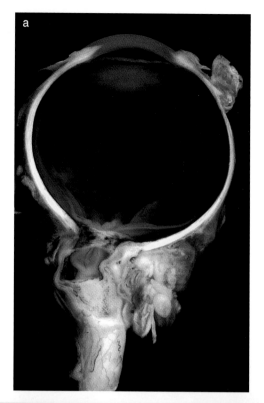

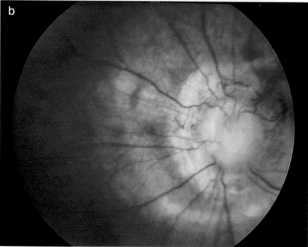

Figure 4.13 Morning glory syndrome. (a) An ectatic lesion at the optic disc. (b) Fundus appearance.

apparently buried within the optic nerve head. They are rarely seen in childhood but become manifest in the late teens, and are present in 2 per cent of the elderly population. Seventy-five per cent are bilateral, and associated features include disc haemorrhage, visual field defects and anomalous retinal vasculature. Disc drusen are concentric laminations of hyaline material, and partial calcification explains their autofluorescence and visibility on CT scanning or ultrasonography. Their pathogenesis is not clear, but they may represent axonal degeneration resulting from a disturbance of axoplasmic transport due to a congenital anomaly of size or vasculature of the disc. The associated calcification may originate from mitochondria within the optic nerve axons.

Anomalies in the appearance of the optic disc

Minor anomalies in the appearance of the optic disc are common, and in the absence of other ocular anomalies are non-progressive and usually of little significance, although associated visual field defects may cause diagnostic confusion.

Tilted optic disc is a relatively common anomaly in which the disc is D-shaped. It is possibly a manifestation of segmental disc hypoplasia, but an alternative hypothesis is that it is colobomatous in nature and results from aberrant closure of the fissure at the junction between the optic cup and optic stalk. The nerve fibre layer of the retina adjacent to the flat part of the D, the RPE and the choroid are thinned. Visual field defects are common and correspond to the affected nerve fibre layer.

Congenital excavation and crowded discs are variations of the normal caused by disproportion in the volume of optic disc neural tissue and the space available in the optic foramen of the sclera. In congenital excavation, the disc is large in proportion to the volume of neural tissue. Congenitally excavated discs are largely determined by genetic factors, and axial myopia may coexist. A crowded disc is the opposite to excavation, and occurs when the optic foramen of the sclera is small compared to the volume of the optic nerve. Crowded discs are found in small hypermetropic eyes.

Congenital crescent (conus)

Congenital crescent is a white semilunar crescent, similar to a myopic crescent, at the margin of the optic disc. The cause is partial failure of development of the peripapillary retina and RPE with secondary thinning or atrophy of the choroid. The lack of RPE and/or choroid in the affected area results in exposure of white sclera.

ABNORMALITIES IN THE SIZE OF THE EYE

Anomalies of development at different stages may result in the eyes being congenitally small (microphthalmos) or large (macrophthalmos).

Microphthalmos

Microphthalmos is one of the commonest ocular developmental anomalies. The net volume of the eye is reduced, and there are often associated proportional changes in ocular structure. The degree of microphthalmos depends on the stage of development at which the cause occurred. Severe microphthalmos results from an insult early in gestation at the time of the formation of the optic cup. Microphthalmos associated with colobomas results from an insult occurring at the time of closure of the embryonic fissure, while lesser degrees of microphthalmos result from causes operating late in gestation. Microphthalmos forms a spectrum of disorders ranging from near anophthalmos to an almost normal eye with a hypermetropic refractive error.

Pure microphthalmos (nanophthalmos) is isolated, idiopathic and without associated ocular or other abnormalities. Pure microphthalmic eyes are hypermetropic, often with shallow anterior chambers, and are prone to develop angle-closure glaucoma and uveal effusion.

Colobomatous microphthalmos results from retardation of ocular growth in association with malclosure of the embryonic fissure. Other associated ocular abnormalities are common.

Microphthalmos associated with other intraocular abnormalities but without colobomas is seen in a number of conditions, including PHPV, retinal dysplasia and sclerocornea.

Microphthalmos associated with ocular and systemic diseases and syndromes may occur in rubella embryopathy, in the toxic syndromes associated with the maternal intake of thalidomide and LSD, in chromosomal abnormalities such as Trisomy 13 and in inherited syndromes such as the oculo–dental–digital syndrome and the CHARGE syndrome (colobomas and microphthalmos, heart defects, choanal atresia, growth retardation, genital and ear abnormalities).

Macrophthalmos

Congenital enlargement of the eye is usually secondary to other ocular abnormalities such as congenital glaucoma. True macrophthalmos is uniform enlargement of the eye in the absence of other ocular defects or raised intraocular pressure, and is extremely rare.

THE OCULAR ADNEXAE

Normal development

Early in the fourth week of intrauterine life, the five facial primordia appear around the stomodeum (primitive mouth). The single frontonasal process lies above the stomodeum and results from proliferation of mesenchyme of neural crest origin situated ventral to the developing brain. The paired maxillary and mandibular prominences, which are derived from the first branchial arch, lie beneath and on either side of the frontonasal process. Bilaterally symmetrical cellular proliferations from the frontonasal process produce medial and lateral nasal prominences. Rapid growth of the maxillary prominences towards the lateral nasal prominences and midline leads to formation of the nasolacrimal groove. The eyes are laterally placed during this period of facial development. Development of other craniofacial structures continues up to approximately 8 weeks. Thereafter, full development of the face, which occurs only slowly, involves changes in the proportions and relative positions of craniofacial components; enlargement of the brain forms a prominent forehead, the eyes move medially and the ears rise. The nasolacrimal duct develops from ectoderm in the floor of the nasolacrimal groove. Proliferation of cells gives rise to a solid cord that separates from the surface and sinks into the mesenchyme to end in the inferior meatus of the lateral wall of the nasal cavity. The lacrimal sac develops as an expansion at the upper end of the cord. The cord usually canalizes later in fetal life, and is normally patent by the sixth month. At 4–5 weeks, the upper and lower lids develop from ectodermal proliferation of the frontonasal process and the maxillary prominences respectively. Over the next few weeks, growth is rapid. The upper and lower lids fuse by the third month and remain fused up to the sixth month of intrauterine life.

Anomalies of development

Lid colobomas

Congenital defects in the lids are relatively common. The inner part of the upper lid and the outer half of the lower lid are the sites most usually affected. Lid colobomas may be isolated or associated with other defects as in Goldenhar's syndrome and mandibulofacial dysostosis (Treacher-Collins syndrome). The pathogenesis is obscure and, since the lids do not develop from the obliteration of a fissure, is unlike that of uveal colobomas. One possible hypothesis is that the defect arises from incomplete development of the blood supply of the lid and ischaemic atrophy in that part furthest from the principal blood supply; another possibility is that neural crest cell migration in the formation of the branchial arches is faulty.

Congenital nasolacrimal stenosis

Canalization of the lower end of the nasolacrimal duct may be delayed until the first year of life and results in congenital nasolacrimal stenosis. The condition is usually isolated, but may be associated with craniofacial abnormalities.

DISORDERS OF POSTNATAL CELL AND TISSUE GROWTH

Disorders of cell and tissue growth can occur at any time after birth. They can affect the lids, the conjunctiva and lacrimal sac, the orbit and the eye. Secondary neoplasms can infiltrate or metastasize to ocular adnexal tissues and the eye.

THE LIDS

Disorders of cell and tissue growth affecting the lids are mainly of cutaneous origin. They are not specific to the lids and occur in skin elsewhere. Lesions arising from fibrous tissue, muscle and fat are rare in the lids. An accurate statistical analysis of the relative incidence of the numerous 'lid lumps' removed is difficult because of the differences in the type of laboratories (i.e. general or specialized, local or regional) to which specimens are referred for histological diagnosis. Nevertheless, some facts are clear and well established:

1. Many lid lumps are not neoplasms but are inflammatory lesions (e.g. chalazions), cysts (e.g. epidermoid, sudoriferous) or histiocytic lesions (e.g. xanthelasmas).
2. Most lid lumps are benign and originate from the epidermis (e.g. basal and squamous cell papillomas), from epidermal-associated structures such as sweat glands (e.g. apocrine cystadenomas, syringomas) and hair follicles (e.g. pilomatricomas, trichilemmomas), and from epidermal melanocytes (melanocytic naevi).
3. Malignant neoplasms, far fewer in number than their benign counterparts, are predominantly basal cell carcinomas. Squamous cell carcinomas, sebaceous carcinomas and melanomas are less common.

The skin of the lids has great elasticity and consists of a thin epidermis overlying a dermis of loose connective tissue containing epidermal-associated structures, namely sebaceous and sweat glands, and lash and other hair follicles, in addition to blood vessels, lymphatics, nerve fibres and striated muscle (orbicularis oculi). A basement membrane lies between the epidermis and dermis.

Epidermis

The epidermis comprises cells (keratinocytes) and keratin, dendritic cells and Merkel cells. Rete ridges (finger-like projections of epithelium toward the dermis) and dermal papillae (upward extensions of dermal connective tissue between the rete ridges) are not as conspicuous as in skin elsewhere.

Keratinocytes and keratin

From the deep to the superficial aspect there are four layers:

1. Basal cell layer: basal cells are the germinative cells of the epidermis. They are relatively tall columnar cells arranged perpendicular to the basement membrane, and have round to oval darkly staining nuclei. Basal cells form a single layer.

2. Squamous cell layer: squamous cells are polygonal in outline, have abundant eosinophilic cytoplasm and oval vesicular nuclei, often with conspicuous nucleoli. They are alternatively referred to as prickle cells because the intercellular bridges (desmosomes) that unite them at their free borders may be seen clearly on microscopy as 'prickles'. The squamous cell layer is approximately five cells thick.

3. Granular cell layer: granular cells are diamond-shaped or flattened. Their cytoplasm is filled with deeply basophilic and irregular keratohyaline granules. The thickness of the granular cell layer relates to the thickness of the keratin layer; in the lids it consists of only one or two layers of cells.

4. Keratin layer: this is eosinophilic and anuclear. It is produced by maturation of the underlying keratinocytes. The keratin layer of the lids is particularly thin.

Dendritic cells

The epidermis contains two types of dendritic cells, namely epidermal melanocytes and Langerhans cells.

Epidermal melanocytes appear as clear cells between the basal cells of the epidermis. They are of neural crest origin and their function is to produce melanin, at least some of which passes to the basal layer of keratinocytes, where it protects the cells from ultraviolet light damage.

Langerhans cells are found within the suprabasal layers of the epidermis but are difficult to identify using standard histological techniques. They act as antigen-presenting cells (APCs).

Merkel cells

Merkel cells lie in the deeper layers of the epidermis adjacent to hair follicles, but cannot be identified in conventionally stained sections. They are mechanoreceptors and mediate the sense of touch.

Epidermal-associated structures

Epidermal-associated structures include sebaceous glands, sweat glands and pilosebaceous units.

Sebaceous glands

Sebaceous glands consist of lobules composed of an outer layer of small cuboidal or flattened basophilic germinative cells, which give rise to the inner zone of lipid-containing vacuolated cells. Sebaceous glands are holocrine glands because their secretion, known as sebum, results from complete degeneration of their cells. Sebaceous glands are associated with and open into the lash and other hair follicles. Meibomian glands are sebaceous glands present in the tarsal plates, and open on to the lid margin.

Sweat glands (sudoriferous glands)

Sweat glands are composed of secretory coils that lie in the dermis, and ducts through which the secretion passes. The two types of sweat glands are apocrine glands and eccrine glands.

Apocrine glands are associated with pilosebaceous units, into which their ducts open. Their secretory coils are lined by cuboidal or columnar cells outside which is a layer of elongated myoepithelial cells. They show 'decapitation' secretion (Fig. 4.32b), where secretory droplets appear to be pinched off from the inner aspect, and although this is a histological artefact it is characteristic of apocrine secretion. Apocrine ducts are composed of a double layer of cuboidal epithelium.

Eccrine glands are located throughout the skin, including the skin of the lids, and their ducts open directly on to the surface. Their secretory coils consist of a single layer of cells, the luminal borders of which are rather irregular. Along the base of these cells there are rather inconspicuous myoepithelial cells. Eccrine ducts have two segments: the intradermal segment is structurally similar to an apocrine duct, i.e. it is composed of a double layer of cuboidal epithelium, while the intraepidermal segment is lined by cells largely derived from the intradermal segment but which may keratinize.

Pilosebaceous units

Pilosebaceous units are hair follicles together with their sebaceous glands. Hair follicles are tubular invaginations of the skin, and comprise inner and outer root sheaths and a central hair shaft. The terminal portion of the follicle is enlarged into the hair bulb, which contains pluripotential germinal matrix cells and scattered melanocytes. The germinal matrix cells give rise to the inner root sheath and hair shaft. At its deepest end the bulb is concave and encloses the hair papilla (analogous to a dermal papilla), which is richly vascularized, contains nerve fibres and is continuous with a vascular sheath that encloses the remainder of the follicle. Superficially the outer root sheath comprises cells analogous to those of the epidermis, but below the entrance of the sebaceous glands it consists only of vacuolated glycogen-containing squamous cells. The internal root sheath has three concentric layers, all of which undergo keratinization; the outer layer is one cell thick, the middle layer is two cells thick and contains eosinophilic trichohyaline granules, while the inner layer consists of flattened scales. The hair shaft is composed of an outer single layer of flattened scales (the cuticle) that interdigitate with the scales of the inner root sheath, a middle layer of cortical cells (their melanin content determines hair colour) and an inner medulla of polyhedral cells (fine hairs lack a medulla).

Lashes are strong and long, their associated sebaceous and apocrine glands are the glands of Zeiss and Moll respectively, and their life duration is about 4 months.

Hair other than the lashes is scanty and fine (eyebrow hair is coarse).

Cysts and choristomas

Epidermoid cyst (keratinous cyst)

Epidermoid cysts are filled with keratin and lined by stratified squamous epithelium (Fig. 4.14). They present as firm cutaneous or subcutaneous nodules. Milia are multiple small epidermoid cysts. Epidermoid cysts may arise in a number of ways:

1. Due to a blocked pilosebaceous follicle where the blockage is in that part of the follicle lined by stratified squamous epithelium. Lesions that develop in this way are usually clinically diagnosed as sebaceous cysts.

2. Following injury or surgery where there has been implantation or inclusion of epidermis into underlying tissues.

3. A developmental lesion along embryonic lines of closure.

Dermoid cyst

Dermoid cysts are choristomas resulting from the sequestration of skin along lines of embryonic closure. They present as subcutaneous nodules, most commonly in the superotemporal quadrant where they may be adherent to the underlying periosteum. On microscopy they are similar to epidermoid cysts but with dermal elements in their wall (Fig. 4.15). Portions of hair shaft may be seen in the cyst cavity (see Fig. 8.3b).

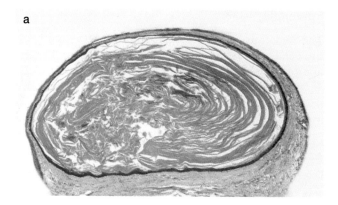

a

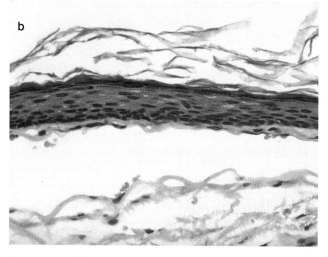

b

Figure 4.14 Epidermoid cyst. (a) Keratin-filled cyst within the dermis. (b) Lining of keratinized stratified squamous epithelium.

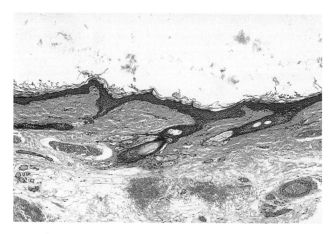

Figure 4.15 Dermoid cyst wall. Lining of keratinized stratified squamous epithelium with pilosebaceous units.

Leaking cysts

If the epithelial lining of an epidermoid or dermoid cyst becomes degenerate, the contents of the cyst may leak into the surrounding tissues and produce a granulomatous inflammatory reaction in which epithelioid histiocytes and foreign body giant cells are present (Fig. 4.16). The cyst may have suddenly enlarged and become inflamed.

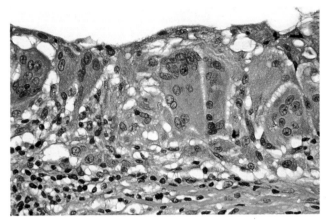

Figure 4.16 Wall of a leaking cyst. The lining is destroyed and replaced by epithelioid histiocytes and foreign body giant cells.

'Meibomian cyst' (chalazion)

'Meibomian cysts' are not cysts but lipogranulomas (see Fig. 2.13), and clinically may simulate a neoplasm.

Sweat gland cyst (sudoriferous cyst)

Sweat gland cysts are retention cysts and in the lids are usually derived from the apocrine glands of Moll. Cysts of Moll appear as translucent vesicles on the lid margin. The cyst cavity contains serous fluid, appears empty in histological sections (Fig. 4.17a) and has a wall of double-layered cuboidal epithelium (Fig. 4.17b). As the intracyst pressure rises this lining becomes flattened and may ultimately appear as a single layer.

Benign proliferations of keratinocytes

Basal cell papilloma (seborrhoeic wart, seborrhoeic keratosis)

Basal cell papillomas are derived from the basal layer of the epidermis and consist mainly, but not exclusively, of basal cells. They commonly involve the lids of the middle-aged and elderly, and appear as brown, greasy, well-demarcated raised lesions with a friable surface. Histologically the epidermis is thickened; this thickening may be fairly uniform, papillomatous (where dermal papillae extend upwards and cause the surface to exhibit irregular undulation) or adenoid (where the proliferating basal cells are seen as elongated or branching strands). The amount of surface keratin is variable, but a characteristic feature is the abrupt transition of basal cells to

a

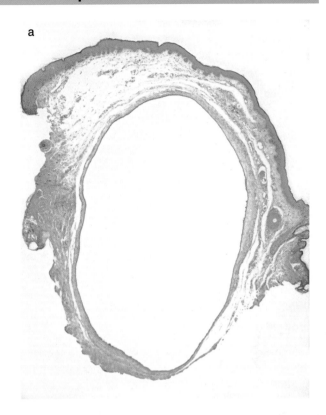

b

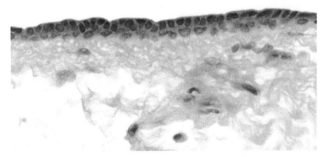

Figure 4.17 Sweat gland cyst. (a) An empty cystic cavity within the dermis. (b) Lining of double layer of cuboidal epithelium.

squamous cells and keratin production in areas throughout the lesion with the development of keratin-filled cysts (horn cysts – Fig. 4.18). The dark colour of basal cell papillomas is due to the presence of melanin, most conspicuously in the basal cells.

Inverted follicular keratosis (irritated seborrhoeic keratosis)

Inverted follicular keratosis is a downward proliferation of keratinocytes, and has a predilection for the lid margin. It is nodular or wart-like, with inflammation and rapid growth being notable features.

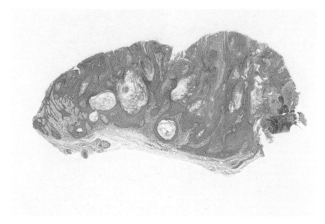

Figure 4.18 Basal cell papilloma. The lesion consists mainly of basal cells, the amount of surface keratin is variable and horn cysts are present.

Squamous cell papilloma (skin tag, fibroepithelial polyp)

Squamous cell papillomas consist predominantly of squamous cells. They are one of the commonest cell proliferations of the skin of the lids, and present as slow growing sessile or pedunculated lesions projecting from the surface. Microscopy (Fig. 4.19) shows a papillomatous configuration with a fibrovascular core and overlying acanthosis (thickened squamous cell layer) and hyperkeratosis (thickened keratin layer).

Keratoacanthoma (molluscum sebaceum)

Keratoacanthoma is a keratotic lesion with a predilection for skin exposed to sunlight. It develops rapidly over a period of 6–8 weeks. It is more common on the lower lid than the upper, and appears as a dome-shaped nodule with a central keratin-filled crater and elevated rolled margins. A viral aetiology has been suspected, and keratoacanthoma can develop in immunocompromised individuals. Microscopy reveals the nodular elevation as being due to irregular thickening of the epidermis. The central keratin-filled crater exhibits well-marked shoulder formation, i.e. there is a sharp transition from the thickened to the adjacent normal epidermis (Fig. 4.20). Downward proliferation may occur but does not extend beyond the dermal appendages, and there is often associated inflammation with the formation of microabscesses within the epidermis. Keratoacanthomas regress spontaneously, but the whole process of evolution and involution may take many months. An important practical point in management is that a diagnostic biopsy is usually unsatisfactory as the histological picture of a small portion of tissue may closely resemble squamous cell carcinoma.

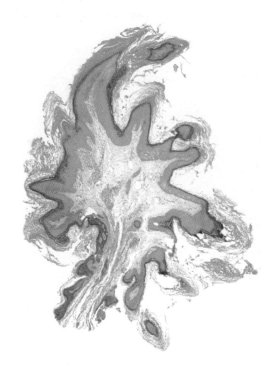

Figure 4.19 Squamous cell papilloma. Pedunculated papillomatous lesion with a fibrovascular core.

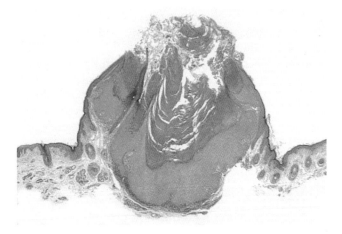

Figure 4.20 Keratoacanthoma. Irregularly thickened epidermis with a keratin-filled crater and shoulder formation.

Molluscum contagiosum

Molluscum contagiosum is a cellular proliferative lesion caused by poxvirus infection (see Fig. 2.42).

Intraepidermal proliferations of keratinocytes

Between the unequivocally benign papillomas and the infiltrating malignant carcinomas there is a spectrum of hyperplastic and dysplastic lesions. Two such clearly defined and designated lesions are actinic keratosis and carcinoma *in situ*.

Actinic keratosis (solar keratosis, senile keratosis)

Actinic keratosis is most often seen in those with fair complexions who burn rather than tan on sun exposure. The lesions are single or multiple, scaly, flat-topped and erythematous, often with a cutaneous horn. Microscopy (Fig. 4.21) reveals acanthosis or atrophy of the epidermis, a degree of dysplasia, elastotic degeneration (basophilic degeneration of collagen) in the underlying dermis and a chronic inflammatory cell infiltrate. Progression to infiltrating malignancy is unusual.

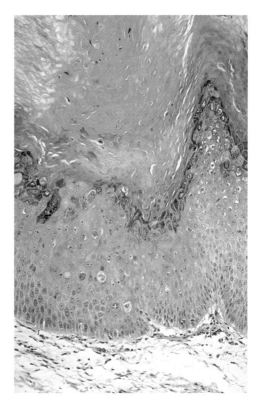

Figure 4.22 Carcinoma *in situ*. Dysplastic changes throughout the thickness of the epidermis and marked hyperkeratosis.

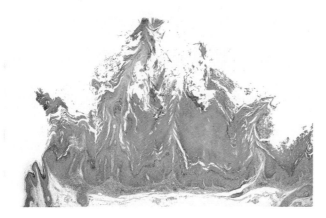

Figure 4.21 Actinic keratosis. Irregular dysplastic epidermis with hyperkeratosis and a developing cutaneous horn.

Carcinoma *in situ* (intraepidermal carcinoma, Bowen's disease)

Carcinoma *in situ* exhibits dysplasia and hyperkeratosis. The dysplastic changes are more marked than those of actinic keratosis and involve the entire thickness of the epidermis (Fig. 4.22). Carcinoma *in situ* occurs predominantly in white males with a fair complexion and presents as erythematous, pigmented, crusty, scaly, fissured keratotic plaques. As with actinic keratosis, progression to infiltrating malignancy is unusual.

Malignant infiltrating proliferations of keratinocytes

Basal cell carcinoma

Basal cell carcinomas arise from the pluripotential germinative cells that form the basal layer of the epidermis.

They comprise nearly 90 per cent of all malignant neoplasms of the lid. Prolonged exposure to sunlight is probably a predisposing factor. The average age of presentation is about 70 years, although recent evidence suggests that younger people are increasingly being affected. Basal cell carcinomas may form part of the Gorlin–Goltz syndrome. Most basal cell carcinomas involve the lower lid, and the inner canthus is more commonly affected than the outer (Fig. 4.23a). There are three clinical categories: nodular, ulcerative and sclerosing. The nodular type usually presents as a firm pearly nodule with small telangiectatic vessels on its surface. The lesion may grow and ulcerate, thereby producing an ulcerative type with rolled everted margins. The sclerosing type appears as a well-defined indurated plaque. Pigmentation due to the presence of melanin or haemosiderin (as a result of previous haemorrhage) may be noticeable, particularly in the nodular type.

Basal cell carcinomas may or may not be differentiated, and the histological appearance frequently varies in different areas. Undifferentiated solid (primordial) basal cell carcinomas (Fig. 4.23b) are composed of lobules of cells exhibiting prominent palisading at the periphery (Fig. 4.23c). Differentiation may occur with the formation of squamous cells (Fig. 4.24a) and keratin resulting in a keratotic type of basal cell carcinoma.

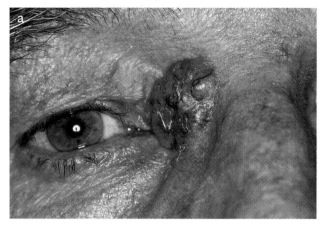

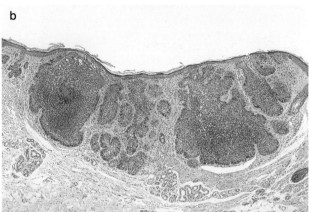

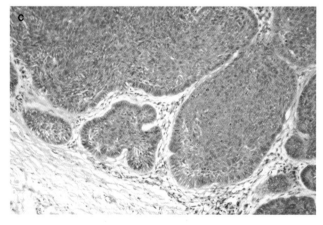

Figure 4.23 Basal cell carcinoma. (a) At inner canthus.
(b) Predominantly undifferentiated type. (c) Palisading of cells at
the periphery of lobules.

Sebaceous (Fig. 4.24b) or adenoid differentiation reflects the embryogenesis of sebaceous and sweat glands. In sclerosing (morpheic) type neoplasms, elongated strands of cells are embedded in a dense fibrous stroma (Fig. 4.24c). A cystic appearance may result from necrosis of centrally situated cells and, in association with adenoid differentiation, produces an adenoid cystic type of basal cell carcinoma (Fig. 4.24d). Basal cell carcinomas only

very rarely metastasize, but can spread into the conjunctiva, orbit, paranasal sinuses and cranial cavity. Some basal cell carcinomas are multicentric in origin. The sclerosing type often extends beyond the margins of clinical involvement, thus making the completeness or otherwise of removal difficult to assess at surgery. In these instances histological examination of frozen sections (Mohs' or modified Mohs' technique) is often useful, particularly if the lesion is situated medially and close to the lacrimal drainage system, where preservation of as much lid tissue as possible is of great importance.

Squamous cell carcinoma

Squamous cell carcinomas are malignant neoplasms in which the vast majority of the cells resemble those of the squamous cell layer. They represent up to about 5 per cent of all malignant neoplasms of the lid, and affect predominantly the older age groups. They arise most often from a pre-existing actinic keratosis, but other precursor lesions include carcinoma *in situ*, radiation dermatosis and xeroderma pigmentosum. Only a small proportion of intraepidermal proliferations, however, give rise to infiltrating malignancy. Squamous cell carcinomas usually present on the lower lid as a single elevated nodule or plaque with irregular borders, and ulceration is frequent. Microscopy shows a markedly dysplastic epithelium with downward proliferation of squamous cells and infiltration through the basement membrane (Fig. 4.25). Metastasis to regional lymph nodes is rare.

Pseudocarcinomatous hyperplasia is an elevated, ulcerated lesion resembling squamous carcinoma, and can occur anywhere on the lids. It is of short duration and may be caused by infection or trauma, or may be idiopathic. Inflammatory cells invariably infiltrate the epidermis.

Benign proliferations of epidermal melanocytes

Melanocytic naevi (moles)

Melanocytic naevi are hamartomas composed of naevus cells (naevocytes). Naevus cells are derived from epidermal melanocytes and form clusters at the epidermal/dermal junction. Epidermal melanocytes lose their dendritic processes and become cuboidal, oval or rounded, and gradually migrate into the underlying dermis. Evolution of melanocytic naevi begins in the young or at adolescence and is usually complete by middle age. There is a higher incidence in those with many freckles (ephelides). Classification of melanocytic naevi is into junctional, compound and intradermal. All are benign, but junctional naevi and compound naevi, because of

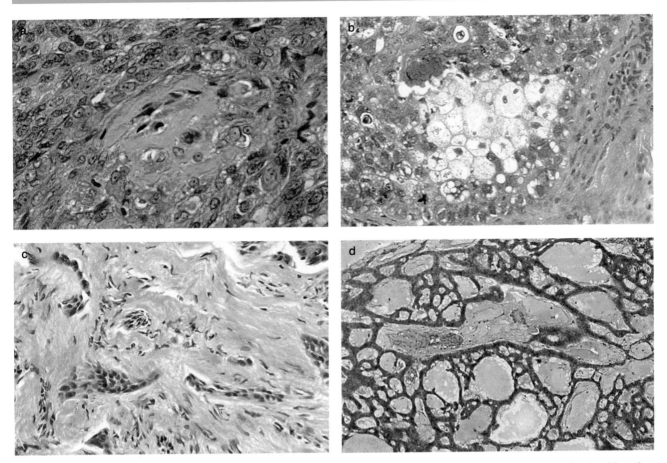

Figure 4.24 Basal cell carcinoma. (a) Squamous cell differentiation. (b) Sebaceous differentiation. (c) Sclerosing type. (d) Adenoid cystic type.

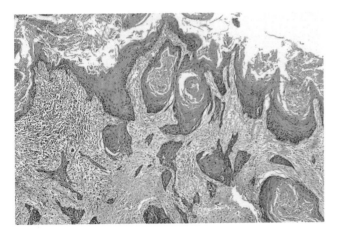

Figure 4.25 Squamous cell carcinoma. Downward proliferation of squamous epithelium with infiltration of dermis.

their junctional component, have malignant potential although transformation to melanoma is rare. The degree of pigmentation is variable, some naevi being virtually amelanotic. Hormonal influence such as occurs at puberty and pregnancy and by the taking of the oral contraceptive pill may increase the pigmentation of naevi, but does not increase the risk of malignant change.

Junctional naevi

These are macular or slightly raised lesions and are usually uniformly light to dark brown in colour. Nests of naevus cells develop at the epidermal/dermal junction (Fig. 4.26a). The cells are cuboidal or oval in shape with a round or oval nucleus and a homogeneous cytoplasm that contains sparse, evenly distributed fine melanin granules.

Compound naevi

These appear as raised pigmented nodules or waxy lesions, occasionally with hairs projecting from the surface. In addition to the junctional component (as seen in junctional naevi), nests and strands of naevus cells lie within the dermis (Fig. 4.26b). The deeper naevus cells are smaller than the superficial cells, and pigmentation is usually marked towards the surface but is lost with pro-

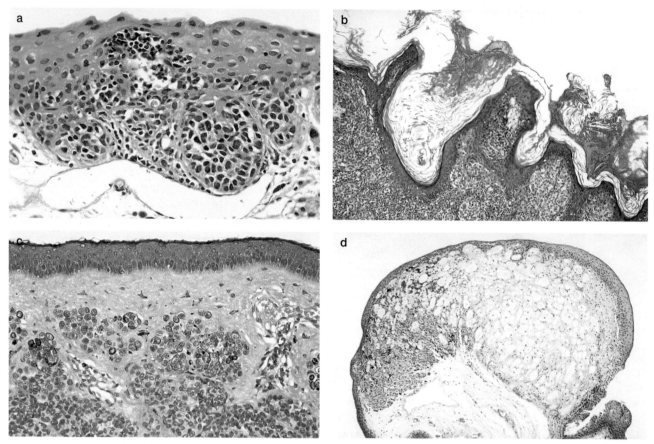

Figure 4.26 Epidermal melanocytic naevi. (a) Junctional naevus; nests of naevus cells at the epidermal/dermal junction. (b) Compound naevus with a papillary configuration; naevus cells are present at the epidermal/dermal junction and also infiltrate the dermis. (c) Intradermal naevus; a clear zone of normal dermis separates the naevus cells from the epidermis. (d) Balloon cell naevus; balloon cells form a large part of the lesion.

gressive depth. Associated acanthosis and papillomatosis account for the warty appearance sometimes seen.

Intradermal naevi

These represent the final stage in the evolution of naevi. They are frequently devoid of pigment, and present as a dome-shaped nodule, a papillomatous lesion or a pedunculated skin tag. They are often excised as 'papillomas'. Naevus cells are present only in the dermis. They are small dark cells with scanty cytoplasm, produce little or no melanin, and a clear zone of normal dermal tissue separates them from the overlying epidermis (Fig. 4.26c).

Variants of naevi

These include balloon cell naevi, Spitz naevi, halo naevi and dysplastic naevi.

Balloon cell naevi are compound or intradermal lesions with no particular clinical distinguishing features. They show a predominance of round or oval variably-sized cells with foamy pale-staining or clear vacuolated cyto-

plasm (balloon cells – Fig. 4.26d). The balloon cells probably result from melanocyte degeneration.

Spitz naevi (juvenile melanomas) are variants of compound naevi that occur in children and young adults. They appear as tiny dome-shaped pinkish nodules. They are benign, although the histological appearance is very disturbing, there being marked junctional activity and cellular pleomorphism with spindle-shaped and epithelioid type cells (cells that resemble epithelial cells), bizarre cell types and multinucleate cells all being present. Pigmentation is usually scanty.

Halo naevi are identified by the striking depigmented halo around a centrally placed melanocytic naevus. The depigmentation is due to the destruction of naevus cells from a local immune response. Such lesions ultimately disappear.

Dysplastic naevi (atypical moles) are irregular in outline and pigmentation, and histologically show cellular atypia and an inflammatory cell infiltrate. Multiple dysplastic naevi constitute the dysplastic naevus syndrome (atypical mole syndrome – AMS). Individuals with AMS are at increased risk of developing conjunctival and uveal naevi and cutaneous, conjunctival and uveal melanomas.

Intraepidermal proliferations of epidermal melanocytes

Lentigo (pl. lentigines)

Lentiginous lesions are benign pigmented macules, commonly seen on the sun-damaged skin of the middle-aged and elderly (senile lentigo). Melanocytes are increased in number and the rete ridges are slightly elongated.

Melanoma *in situ* (intraepidermal melanoma)

There are two types: malignant lentigo and pagetoid melanoma.

Malignant lentigo (Hutchinson's melanotic freckle)

This is relatively uncommon, but can develop in the sun-damaged skin of the elderly. It presents as a slowly spreading macular lesion with an irregular border. Melanocytes proliferate and give rise to pleomorphic melanoma cells that become scattered throughout the epidermis (Fig. 4.27). Pigmentation is variable. Approximately one-third of such lesions exhibit dermal infiltration over a 10–40 year period.

Pagetoid melanoma

This only occasionally involves the lids, and presents in the middle-aged as a small, elevated lesion, which may not be pigmented. Large round melanoma cells are distributed throughout the epidermis, lying as nests in the basal layer. Dermal infiltration usually occurs within a year.

Malignant infiltrating proliferation of epidermal melanocytes

Melanoma

Melanomas of the lid are uncommon, accounting for approximately only 1 per cent of all lid malignancies. Those with a large number of freckles (ephelides), AMS or who experience acute episodes of sunburn are at most risk. Infiltrating melanomas (Fig. 4.28) arise from melanomas *in situ* or, occasionally, from the junctional component of melanocytic naevi. Both malignant lentigo and pagetoid melanoma exhibit a radial *in situ* growth phase before vertical growth and dermal infiltration. The radial growth phase of pagetoid melanoma is more rapid than that of malignant lentigo. The three types of infiltrating melanoma are malignant lentigo melanoma, which arises from malignant lentigo; superficial spreading melanoma, which develops from pagetoid melanoma; and nodular melanoma, which has no *in situ* precursor. Nodular melanoma occurs at all ages but is rare before puberty, and females are more often affected than males.

Melanoma cells are spindle-shaped or epithelioid. Many melanomas show a mixture of cells. Spindle cells predominate in malignant lentigo melanoma, while epithelioid cells occur mainly in superficial spreading and nodular melanoma. Mitotic figures, some of them abnormal, may be seen. Pigmentation is variable, and some melanomas are amelanotic. Unlike uveal melanoma, the cell type does not affect the prognosis. The key factor in determining the outcome of a particular case is the depth of infiltration, and if this is < 0.75 mm the cure rate is nearly 100 per cent, but as the lesion thickens the prognosis worsens. Metastases are rare in malignant lentigo melanoma but common in superficial spreading and nodular melanomas. In nodular melanoma the prognosis is worse if the margin of the lid is

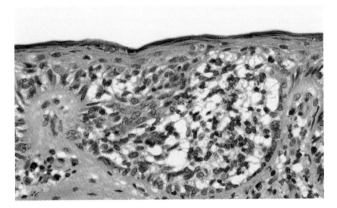

Figure 4.27 Malignant lentigo. Pleomorphic melanoma cells throughout the epidermis.

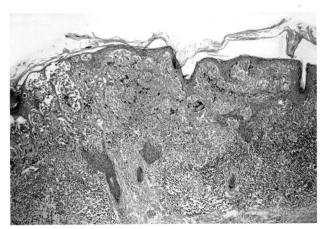

Figure 4.28 Melanoma. Melanoma cells infiltrate the epidermis and dermis.

involved than if only the skin is affected. Melanomas spread by lymphatics to regional lymph nodes and blood-borne metastases occur at distant sites, particularly the skin elsewhere, the brain and viscera.

Proliferation of Merkel cells

Merkel cell carcinoma

Merkel cell carcinomas tend to occur in sun-damaged skin, and can affect the lids of the elderly. They are usually solitary, and present as firm raised non-ulcerated painless nodules with overlying violet or reddish-blue skin. Growth is often rapid and aggressive, metastases are common and the prognosis is poor. Microscopy reveals clusters, anastomosing bands and sheets of cells with scanty cytoplasm, round to oval nuclei and numerous mitotic figures (Fig. 4.29).

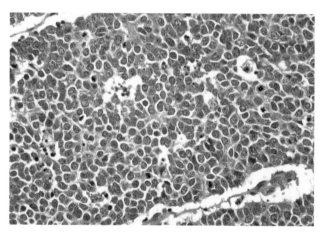

Figure 4.29 Merkel cell carcinoma. A sheet of Merkel cells.

Sebaceous gland proliferations

Sebaceous gland proliferations are hyperplasias, adenomas or carcinomas, and are a feature of the Muir–Torre syndrome.

Sebaceous hyperplasia

Sebaceous hyperplasia affects the skin of the face, scalp and lids in those past middle age, and may be associated with acne rosacea. Cutaneous lesions are often multiple small, yellowish, elevated, slightly umbilicated papules composed of sebaceous gland tissue, with associated telangiectasia. Microscopy reveals multiple mature sebaceous lobules (Fig. 4.30).

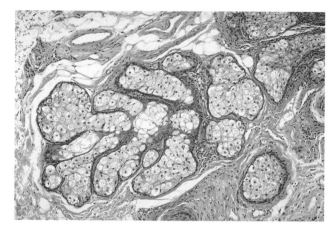

Figure 4.30 Sebaceous hyperplasia. Multiple mature sebaceous lobules.

Sebaceous adenoma

Sebaceous adenomas are benign and similar to sebaceous hyperplasia but more likely to be solitary.

Sebaceous carcinoma

The lid is the commonest site in the body for the development of sebaceous carcinoma, which comprises 1–3 per cent of all malignant lid neoplasms. It occurs most often in elderly women, and when seen in younger age groups has usually followed prior radiotherapy for retinoblastoma or cavernous haemangioma of the face. The upper lid is more frequently involved than the lower, and most sebaceous carcinomas develop from meibomian glands. Presentation is variable; there may be a firm nodule similar to a chalazion (Fig. 4.31a), an atypical or recurring 'chalazion', diffuse thickening of the tarsus, or a papillomatous or fungating growth. Unilateral blepharitis, blepharoconjunctivitis, conjunctivitis, and superficial keratitis with scarring and vascularization may all mask an underlying sebaceous carcinoma, while an orbital mass may represent direct spread.

Microscopy reveals proliferating sebaceous cells in varying degrees of differentiation (Fig. 4.31b). Immature and mature cells are present, mitotic figures are conspicuous and lipid can be demonstrated (Fig. 4.31c). The overall pattern is usually papillary or lobular, with many of the lobules having necrotic centres. Single or small groups of malignant cells infiltrate the epidermis of the skin (Fig. 4.31d) and the epithelium of the conjunctiva and cornea (pagetoid spread); diffuse infiltration may mimic the histological appearance of carcinoma *in situ*. Local spread may occur into the orbit, paranasal sinuses and intracranial cavity. Metastatic spread occurs via the lymphatics into preauricular and cervical lymph

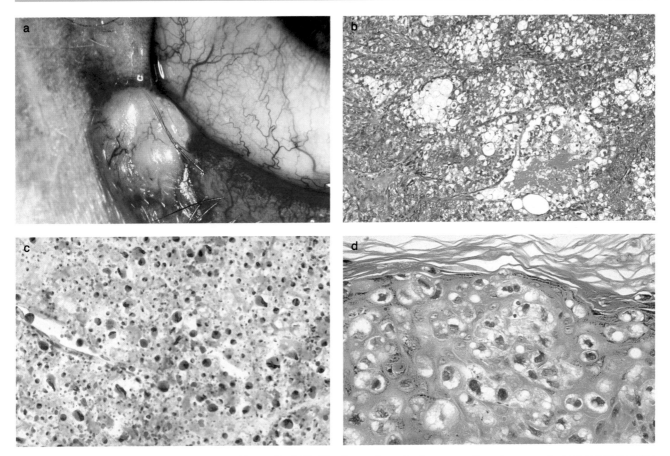

Figure 4.31 Sebaceous carcinoma. (a) Lesion of lower lid. (b) Proliferating malignant sebaceous cells and an area of necrosis below and to the right. (c) Lipid (red globules) within neoplastic cells. Oil red O stain. (d) Malignant sebaceous cells infiltrating the epidermis (pagetoid spread).

nodes, and via the blood stream to the lungs, liver and brain.

Sweat gland proliferations

The range of sweat gland proliferations reflects the distribution of apocrine and eccrine glands. Nomenclature is extensive and confusing because there is no general agreement on terminology. Hidradenoma is a commonly used generic term, while the term syringoma has been used to describe lesions arising from ducts. Many sweat gland proliferations present clinically as nondescript asymptomatic lumps, but a particularly important histological feature is their tendency to maintain a double layer of epithelium.

Apocrine cystadenoma

Apocrine cystadenomas are common benign lesions derived from the secretory coil of apocrine glands. They are revealed on microscopy as irregular cystic spaces lined by a double layer of cells (Fig. 4.32a), an outer layer of myoepithelial cells and an inner layer of columnar cells, which may exhibit artefactual 'decapitation' secretion (Fig. 4.32b).

Cylindroma

Cylindromas are benign lesions of apocrine duct origin. Although they may arise within the lids, they are commonly encountered elsewhere on the face and on the scalp (turban tumours). Varying-sized islands of epithelial cells are enclosed by a hyaline membrane and separated by a fine connective tissue stroma. Ducts are often seen among the proliferating cells.

Papillary syringocystadenoma

Papillary syringocystadenomas are also benign and of apocrine duct origin. They occur in childhood, and appear as warty plaques. Channels and cystic spaces

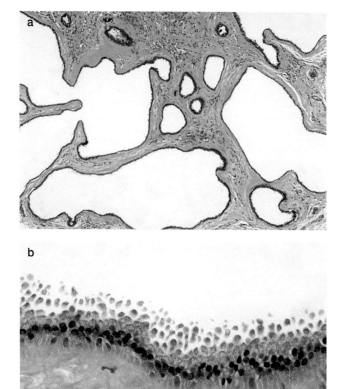

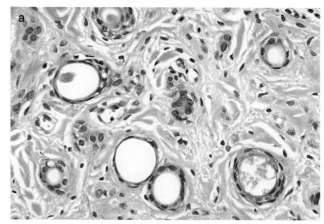

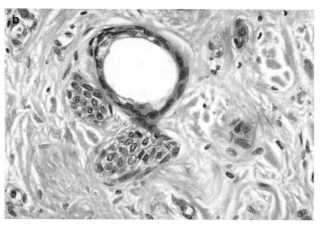

Figure 4.32 Apocrine cystadenoma. (a) Irregular cystic spaces lined by a double layer of epithelial cells. (b) Epithelial lining showing 'decapitation' secretion.

are lined by a double layer of epithelium, and plasma cells are conspicuous in the stroma.

Syringoma

Syringomas are the commonest sweat gland lesions of the lids, show a marked female preponderance and develop as single or multiple waxy nodules. They are benign and arise from the intraepidermal portion of eccrine ducts. Microscopy reveals small ductal elements embedded within a dense fibrous stroma (Fig. 4.33a). Some of the ducts, as seen in cross-section, exhibit comma-shaped cellular tails (Fig. 4.33b), and squamous differentiation may be present with the formation of keratin-filled cysts in the superficial dermis (Fig. 4.33c).

Eccrine poroma

Eccrine poromas, like syringomas, are benign and present as solitary nodules. They arise from intraepidermal ducts, are composed of round deeply basophilic glycogen-containing cells, and exhibit narrow ductal lumina and possibly occasional cystic spaces.

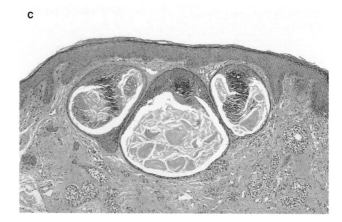

Figure 4.33 Syringoma. (a) Ductal elements within a dense fibrous stroma. (b) Duct with comma-shaped tails. (c) Keratin-filled cysts in the superficial dermis.

Clear cell hidradenoma

Clear cell hidradenomas are benign lesions of eccrine secretory coil and/or ductal origin. They are usually solitary and occur in middle-aged females. Microscopy reveals well-circumscribed dermal nodules composed of lobulated masses of epithelial cells exhibiting small ductal lumina and glycogen-containing clear cells.

Pleomorphic adenoma

Pleomorphic adenomas can arise from apocrine or eccrine glands. They are benign, and are analogous to the same-named lesions that arise in the lacrimal and salivary glands. Tubular structures are lined by two layers of epithelial cells, an inner layer secreting glycosaminoglycans and an outer layer producing a fibrous, myxoid or chondroid stroma.

Sweat gland carcinoma

Carcinomas of sweat gland origin are uncommon and of low-grade malignancy.

Hair follicle proliferations

Trichofolliculoma

Trichofolliculomas are hamartomas, and present as solitary nodular lesions with protruding small white hairs. They open on to the surface and consist of central cystic spaces containing an array of hair follicles in varying stages of development and lined by stratified squamous epithelium.

Trichoepithelioma

Trichoepitheliomas are also hamartomas. They show less follicular differentiation than trichofolliculomas, and histologically resemble basal cell carcinomas of the keratotic type. Trichoepitheliomas may be solitary or multiple. Solitary lesions occur late in life, but multiple lesions begin to appear at or around puberty and can be inherited as an autosomal dominant trait with incomplete penetrance.

Trichilemmoma

Trichilemmomas are benign neoplasms that arise from the outer root sheath. They present as a nodule or a cutaneous horn. They are composed of lobules and anastomosing bands of epidermal glycogen-rich clear cells with palisading at the periphery (Fig. 4.34). Several hair follicles are usually seen within the lesions, and there may be excessive production of keratin. The presence of multiple trichilemmomas is diagnostic of Cowden's disease.

Pilomatricoma (benign calcifying epithelioma of Malherbe)

Pilomatricomas are neoplasms derived from the germinal matrix cells of the hair bulb, and are usually benign. They most often occur in females under 30 years of age, frequently involve the eyebrow or upper lid, and present

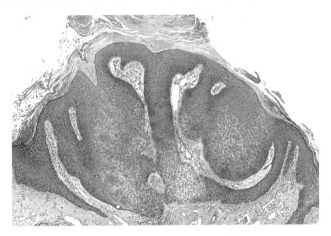

Figure 4.34 Trichilemmoma. Lobules and anastomosing bands of epidermal cells.

as solitary deep dermal nodules that are almost always diagnosed clinically as 'sebaceous cysts'. Microscopy reveals a well-demarcated nodule composed of irregular epithelial islands exhibiting viable basophilic cells at the periphery and degenerate shadow cells more centrally (Fig. 4.35). Pilomatricomas frequently contain calcium. There is often a foreign body giant cell reaction and occasionally ossification.

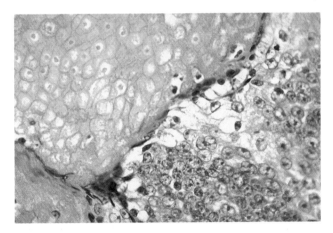

Figure 4.35 Pilomatricoma. Viable basophilic cells to the right, and degenerate shadow cells to the left.

Vascular proliferations

Vascular proliferations in the lid arise within the dermis and are mostly hamartomas.

Capillary haemangioma (strawberry naevus)

Capillary haemangiomas are the commonest vascular lesions of the lid, are apparent at birth or within the first few weeks of life, and rapidly enlarge over a

6-month period. They are elevated and soft, reddish-purple in colour, blanch on pressure and have small surface invaginations (hence the term strawberry naevus). The lesions, however, are not naevi, and microscopy reveals irregular varying-sized capillary channels (Fig. 4.36) extending into the underlying subcutaneous tissue. Capillary haemangiomas of the lids may enlarge to involve the conjunctiva, but most regress by the age of 7 years, regression being associated with progressive fibrosis and wrinkling of the skin ('crêpe paper' change).

Naevus flammeus (port wine stain)

Naevus flammeus is darker than a capillary haemangioma and again is a congenital abnormality of blood vessels and not a naevus. Present at birth, it is flat and does not blanch on pressure. It becomes darker but not larger as age advances and does not regress. Large ectatic vessels of varying calibre are seen in the dermis and probably represent permanent dilatation of existing vessels rather than vasoproliferation. There is a frequent association with the Sturge–Weber syndrome.

Cavernous haemangioma

Cavernous haemangiomas of the lids are composed of large dilated endothelial-lined vascular channels. They are much less common than capillary haemangiomas, and develop in the second to fourth decades of life. Superficial lesions are often dark blue in colour, but more deeply situated lesions cause no change in colour of the overlying skin. Cavernous haemangiomas enlarge slowly and, unlike capillary haemangiomas, show no tendency for spontaneous regression.

Neural proliferations

Neural proliferations, like vascular proliferations, also arise within the dermis.

Neurofibromas and schwannomas

Neurofibromas and schwannomas may occur in the lids as isolated lesions or in association with neurofibromatosis type 1.

Proliferation of dermal melanocytes

Dermal melanocytes are cells that represent arrested melanocytic migration from the neural crest to the epidermis; proliferations are manifest as blue naevi.

Blue naevi

Blue naevi are usually congenital, but may not be apparent until later in life. They appear blue on clinical examination due to the filtering effect of the overlying tissues, and are composed of heavily pigmented branching strap-like melanocytes in the deep dermis (Fig. 4.37).

THE CONJUNCTIVA

The commonest lesions arising within the conjunctiva that necessitate removal are epithelial melanocytic naevi. The majority of disorders of epithelial cell growth are either unequivocally benign or fall into the spectrum of conjunctival intraepithelial proliferations. Lymphoproliferative lesions are also common, most being reactive rather than true lymphomas. The commonest benign proliferations that arise in the car-

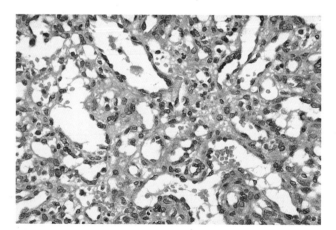

Figure 4.36 Capillary haemangioma. Irregular capillary channels of varying size.

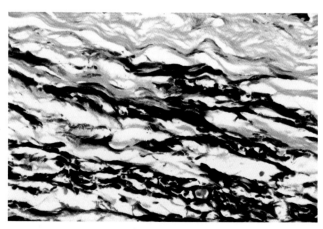

Figure 4.37 Dermal melanocytic naevus. Blue naevus; heavily pigmented branching strap-like melanocytes in the dermis.

uncle are melanocytic naevi, sebaceous adenomas and oncocytomas. The commonest malignant neoplasm of the caruncle is sebaceous carcinoma. Vascular, neural, fibroblastic and histiocytic proliferations involving the conjunctiva are rare. The normal conjunctiva, including the caruncle, consists of epithelium and subepithelial connective tissue.

Epithelium

Most of the conjunctiva is covered by stratified columnar epithelium two to five cells thick, but at the lid margin, at the limbus and covering the caruncle the epithelium is non-keratinized stratified squamous, an appearance that may also be seen elsewhere, particularly in the tarsal conjunctiva. The basal cells throughout lie perpendicular to the thin basement membrane that separates the epithelium from the underlying connective tissue, and their nuclei are deeply staining. The more superficial cells are usually polygonal, but flatten as they approach the surface. Mucin-secreting goblet cells are present in the middle and superficial layers; they are most numerous in the caruncle, semilunar folds and fornices and are usually absent at the limbus. Melanocytes and Langerhans cells are found in the conjunctival epithelium as in the epidermis of the skin.

Subepithelial connective tissue

The subepithelial connective tissue is essentially fibrovascular. Lymphocytes infiltrate shortly after birth, probably in response to antigenic stimuli, and form follicles; this lymphoid tissue is the mucosa-associated lymphoid tissue (MALT). Lymphatic channels are also present as are nerve fibres and accessory lacrimal gland tissue. In the caruncle, pilosebaceous follicles, sweat glands, fat, smooth muscle and cartilage may also be present.

Cysts and choristomas

Conjunctival epithelial inclusion cysts are sometimes seen as are choristomas, which are usually present at birth. Choristomas are generally isolated, although there is an occasional association with Goldenhar's syndrome.

Epithelial cyst

Epithelial-lined inclusion cysts of the conjunctiva are a sequel to inflammation, trauma or surgery. Epithelial cells displaced into the subepithelial stroma proliferate, goblet cells produce mucin, and an inclusion cyst results.

Dermoid

Dermoids usually occur as solitary well-circumscribed elevated nodules of variable size in the inferotemporal limbus (Fig. 4.38a). They are solid and not cystic, being composed of dense collagenous tissue containing dermal elements and are covered by stratified squamous epithelium that may be keratinized (Fig. 4.38b).

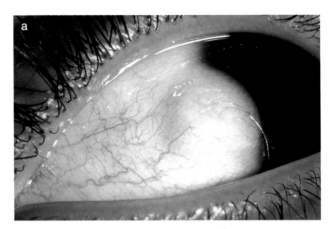

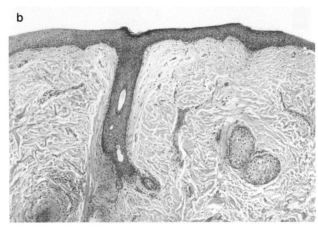

Figure 4.38 Limbal dermoid. (a) Lesion with a protruding hair. (b) A solid mass of collagenous tissue covered by stratified squamous epithelium and containing dermal elements.

Dermolipoma

Dermolipomas are soft pale subconjunctival masses that usually lie beneath the temporal aspect of the conjunctiva towards the lateral canthus. They may extend towards the cornea, or superiorly and posteriorly between the lateral and superior rectus muscles into the orbit. They are composed of fibrofatty tissue and, like dermoids, are covered by stratified squamous epithelium that may be keratinized. Pilosebaceous units are usually absent.

Complex choristoma

Complex choristomas are similar to limbal dermoids and dermolipomas, but in addition contain lacrimal gland elements, cartilage, smooth muscle and nerve fibres.

Epibulbar osseous choristoma

Epibulbar osseous choristomas consist of a nodule of bone lying in the subconjunctival tissues.

Intrascleral nerve loop

An intrascleral nerve loop is a long ciliary nerve that loops through the anterior sclera (Fig. 4.39) and is sometimes seen as a subconjunctival nodule. It can be regarded as a choristoma.

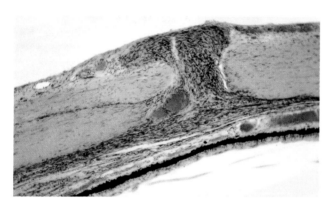

Figure 4.39 Intrascleral nerve loop. A long ciliary nerve looping through the anterior sclera.

Benign proliferation of epithelial cells

Squamous cell papilloma

Squamous cell papillomas appear as soft elevated lesions with an irregular cauliflower-like surface. They may be single or multiple, unilateral or bilateral, pedunculated or sessile. Peduncated lesions usually arise from the inferior fornix of children, while sessile growths affect the bulbar conjunctiva of adults. Squamous cell papillomas are generally asymptomatic, but may occasionally spread to the cornea and interfere with vision. Microscopy reveals fronds of fibrovascular tissue covered by non-keratinized stratified squamous epithelium containing goblet cells (Fig. 4.40). Squamous cell papillomas of the conjunctiva are occasionally inverted (i.e. fold inwards), and histologically resemble similar lesions of the lacrimal sac.

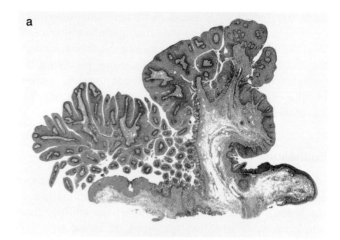

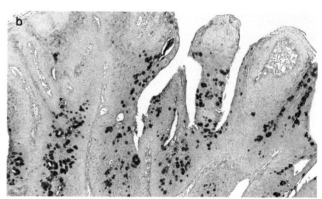

Figure 4.40 Conjunctival papilloma. (a) A pedunculated mass composed of stratified squamous epithelium with a fibrovascular core. (b) Numerous mucin-secreting goblet cells. PAS stain.

Intraepithelial proliferations of epithelial cells

In addition to epithelial hyperplasias, as in the epidermis of the skin, there is a spectrum of proliferations characterized histologically by dysplastic changes. Conditions within this spectrum are analogous to those of other mucous membranes such as the uterine cervix, and are collectively categorized as conjunctival intraepithelial neoplasms (Conj. INs – Fig. 4.41). The lesions can be staged according to the severity of the changes, and in particular on the thickness of the epithelium involved. Progression through the various stages to full thickness involvement (carcinoma *in situ*) may, on rare occasions, lead to infiltrating squamous cell carcinoma. All intraepithelial proliferations of epithelial cells present as thickened conjunctiva, possibly with development into a fleshy elevated mass that may be vascularized or have a gelatinous avascular appearance. The interpalpebral bulbar and limbal conjunctiva is the most usual location for the lesions, which may develop over a pinguecula or pterygium.

a

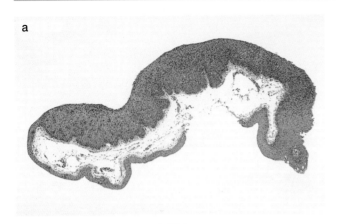

b

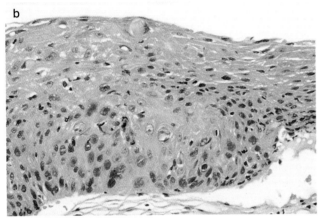

Figure 4.41 Conjunctival intraepithelial neoplasia. (a) Conjunctival biopsy (folded) with thickened dysplastic epithelium above. (b) Marked dysplastic changes throughout the thickened epithelium (carcinoma *in situ*).

Prolonged exposure to sunlight is a predisposing factor and human papilloma viruses (HPVs) are implicated in the pathogenesis, as they are for intraepithelial neoplasms of the uterine cervix (CINs).

Malignant infiltrating proliferations of epithelial cells

Squamous cell carcinoma

Most squamous cell carcinomas of the conjunctiva arise near the limbus in the interpalpebral area, where UV light exposure is greatest. Well-differentiated lesions grow slowly and may have a leukoplakic appearance; other lesions can resemble a pterygium, while less well-differentiated lesions are gelatinous and semitranslucent (Fig. 4.42). Squamous cell carcinomas usually occur in elderly people, but in parts of Asia, Africa and Latin America they are seen in young adults, in Africa there being an epidemic amongst HIV-infected individuals. Squamous cell carcinomas are only superficially invasive and extension into the eye is uncommon, although they

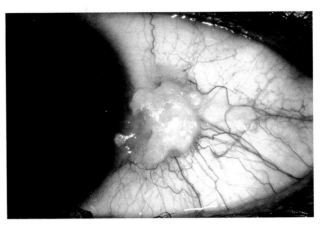

Figure 4.42 Squamous cell carcinoma of conjunctiva.

may spread into the orbit and to regional lymph nodes. Their histological features are essentially similar to squamous cell carcinoma of the lids, but a spindle cell variant is particularly aggressive.

Mucoepidermoid carcinoma

Mucoepidermoid carcinomas consist of varying proportions of mucus-secreting cells and squamous cells, and arise in the limbal conjunctiva of the elderly. They are much less common than squamous cell carcinomas, but are more aggressive and tend to invade the eye.

Benign proliferations of epithelial melanocytes

Melanocytic naevi

Conjunctival naevi (Fig. 4.43a) are similar in type and classification to cutaneous naevi, but there are two important differences:

1. In the conjunctiva there is no dermis, and subepithelial replaces dermal in the nomenclature.
2. Naevus cells migrating from the epithelial/subepithelial junction into the underlying tissue may be accompanied by surface epithelial cells that form cords and islands which, if actively secreting goblet cells are present, develop mucinous cystic inclusions (hence the term cystic naevus). Melanocytic activity may be found within the epithelium of these cystic inclusions.

Most conjunctival naevi are compound (Fig. 4.43b) or subepithelial and possibly cystic (Fig. 4.43c), and are elevated with variable amounts of pigment. Junctional naevi are rarer and flat. Naevi often become larger and more pigmented and inflamed at puberty.

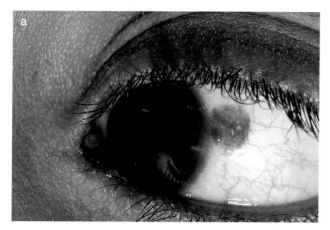

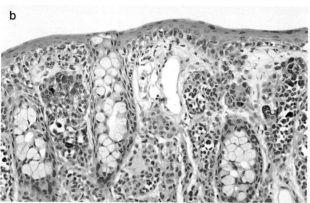

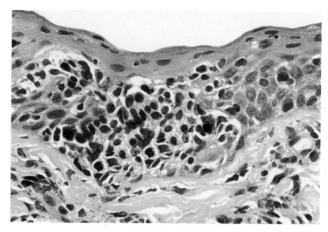

Figure 4.44 Intraepithelial proliferation of conjunctival epithelial melanocytes.

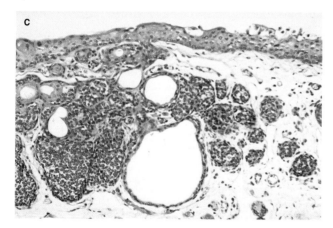

Figure 4.43 Epithelial melanocytic naevi. (a) Lesion of bulbar conjunctiva. (b) Compound naevus with downgrowth of epithelium including goblet cells (vacuolated appearance). (c) A cystic naevus; naevus with subepithelial cyst formation.

Transformation of junctional and compound naevi into melanoma, as in the skin, is possible but unusual.

Intraepithelial proliferations of epithelial melanocytes

Intraepithelial melanocytic proliferations (Fig. 4.44) form a continuum of lesions ranging from benign lentigo to melanoma *in situ*. Nomenclature is confusing, but the term primary acquired melanosis is considered inaccurate because the range of conditions involves cellular proliferation rather than pigment deposition; nevertheless its use continues. The lesions occur most often in Caucasians, and begin to develop at 40–50 years of age as flat indistinct areas of brown pigmentation. The extent of pigmentation is variable, and the lesions may wax and wane but often remain stable for long periods. The key feature to be noted on histological examination of excised specimens is the appearance of the proliferating melanocytes, which show varying degrees of atypia. Apart from lentigo, the microscopical appearance of which is similar to cutaneous lentigo, two main groups are recognized: primary acquired melanosis without atypia (benign acquired melanosis) and primary acquired melanosis with atypia, which can be graded as mild to severe; synonymous terms for the severe types are precancerous melanosis and melanoma *in situ*. Approximately one-third of conjunctival intraepithelial melanocytic proliferations progress to infiltrating melanoma, the risk being greatest with melanoma *in situ*.

Malignant infiltrating proliferation of epithelial melanocytes

Melanoma

Melanomas present in those in their early fifties, usually as solitary pigmented or non-pigmented nodules, most commonly at the limbus, and account for approximately 2 per cent of all ophthalmic malignancies. They develop from intraepithelial melanocytic proliferations, from pre-existing junctional or compound naevi, or arise *de novo* from normal epithelial melanocytes (Fig. 4.45a). Those with AMS are at increased risk. The histological

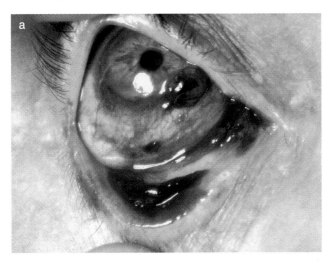

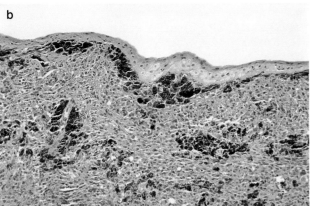

Figure 4.45 Conjunctival melanoma. (a) Melanoma *in situ* with apparent infiltration and the development of nodular lesions. (b) Sheet of melanoma cells within the subepithelial stroma.

features of conjunctival melanomas are similar to those of cutaneous melanomas (Fig. 4.45b). Their behaviour is unpredictable, but in general terms their prognosis depends on their depth of infiltration and their site. Swellings < 1.5 mm in depth have a low risk of metastatic disease, and those on the bulbar conjunctiva carry a more favourable prognosis than those affecting the tarsal conjunctiva.

Vascular proliferations

Telangiectasia

Telangiectasia of the conjunctival blood vessels, when not associated with inflammatory eye disease, occurs in ataxia telangiectasia and in hereditary haemorrhagic telangiectasia (Rendu–Osler–Weber disease, an autosomal dominant generalized vascular dysplasia characterized by multiple telangiectases in the skin, mucous membranes and viscera).

Pyogenic granuloma

A pyogenic granuloma is a round, sessile or pedunculated growth, red to dark brown in colour, that bleeds easily. It may clinically simulate a capillary haemangioma, and histologically resembles inflamed granulation tissue. Pyogenic granulomas occur in the tarsal conjunctiva, often arising on the surface of a chalazion; their precise nature is controversial.

Kaposi sarcoma

Kaposi sarcoma is a vascular proliferative lesion that occurs in the conjunctiva of those with AIDS. It usually develops in the lower fornix as a slowly spreading bright red mass that resembles a subconjunctival haemorrhage. The pathogenesis is related to disordered immunity and infection of vascular endothelium by HHV 8. The histological features of early lesions of short duration (< 4 months) resemble granulation tissue. With advancement, the vascular endothelial cells become plump and later spindle-shaped to produce a lesion consisting of densely packed cells with hyperchromatic nuclei and occasional mitotic figures. Abundant slit-like spaces, often containing erythrocytes, are seen, and chronic inflammatory cells are present in most cases (Fig. 4.46). Advanced cases of Kaposi sarcoma show periodic acid-Schiff (PAS) positive intracellular hyaline globules that are believed to be degenerate erythrocytes.

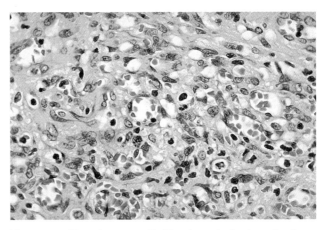

Figure 4.46 Kaposi sarcoma. Proliferating spindle-shaped cells, vascular channels and chronic inflammatory cells.

Lymphatic proliferations

Lymphangioma and lymphangiectasia

Lymphangiomas are hamartomatous malformations of lymphatic channels. The clinical appearance is of transparent dilated vessels, although haemorrhage into their lumen results in a lesion that resembles a haemangioma. Endothelial-lined channels are seen on microscopy to contain eosinophilic proteinaceous material. In lymphangiectasias, the lymphatic channels are somewhat less compact and more dilated.

Accessory lacrimal gland proliferations

Oncocytoma (oxyphil adenoma)

Oncocytomas are benign, and present in individuals over the age of 50 as a slowly enlarging mass in the caruncle. They arise from accessory lacrimal gland tissue and are composed of oncocytes, large cells filled with mitochondria and derived from ductal and acinar cells. The cells are eosinophilic and granular, are arranged in sheets, cords or nests, and exhibit duct-like and cystic glandular formations (Fig. 4.47).

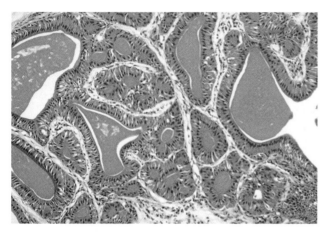

Figure 4.47 Oncocytoma. Proliferating oncocytes exhibiting marked eosinophilic granularity with duct-like and cystic glandular formations.

Non-epithelial melanocytic proliferations

Ocular melanocytosis (melanosis oculi)

Ocular melanocytosis is characterized by an increase in the number, size and pigmentation of melanocytes in the deep subepithelial conjunctiva, episclera, sclera and uvea (Fig. 4.48). It is unilateral, and more common in Caucasians. If only the deep subepithelial conjunctival tissue is affected, the condition can be considered as a blue naevus.

Oculodermal melanocytosis (naevus of Ota)

Oculodermal melanocytosis is ocular melanocytosis accompanied by a dermal naevus (blue naevus) of the

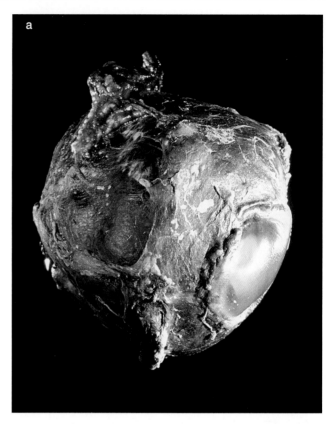

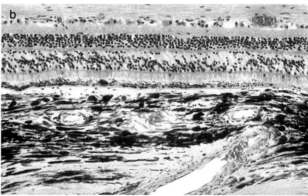

Figure 4.48 Ocular melanocytosis. (a) An enucleated eye with diffuse heavy melanin pigmentation of episclera and sclera. (b) Increased melanocytic activity with heavy melanin pigmentation of inner sclera and choroid.

ipsilateral periorbital and lid skin. The melanocytic proliferation sometimes also involves the nasal and oral mucosa, the orbital tissues and the leptomeninges of the frontal lobe of the brain. Oculodermal melanocytosis, like ocular melanocytosis, is usually unilateral, but unlike ocular melanocytosis is more common in dark-skinned races, particularly Asians.

In both ocular and oculodermal melanocytosis, the affected tissues exhibit a slate blue-grey colour. The lesions are flat, lie beneath the extraocular muscles and stop short of the limbus, leaving a pigment-free circum-corneal band. The conjunctiva moves freely over the pigmented areas. Heavily pigmented branching strap-like melanocytes are present in the affected tissues. Those affected are at increased risk of uveal melanoma, and on rare occasions melanoma may develop in the orbit.

THE LACRIMAL SAC

Proliferative lesions arising within the lacrimal sac are usually neoplasms and present as a localized swelling or with epiphora due to obstruction of tear drainage. Most are papillomas or carcinomas that arise from the pseudostratified columnar (transitional) epithelium containing mucin-secreting goblet cells that lines the sac. They may be associated with similar neoplasms of the upper respiratory mucosa. Papillomas of the lacrimal sac occur in young adults and are exophytic and project into the lumen, or inverted and exhibit infolding into the underlying stroma (Fig. 4.49). They are usually transitional in type but may sometimes be squamous, while occasionally mixed growth patterns are seen. Carcinomas develop in older adults and are equally as common as papillomas. They are locally invasive, metastasize to regional lymph nodes and are classified histologically as transitional, squamous, adenomatous or mucoepidermoid. Melanomas of the lacrimal sac are rare, and arise presumably either from epithelial melanocytes or from the spread of intraepithelial melanocytic proliferations of the conjunctiva.

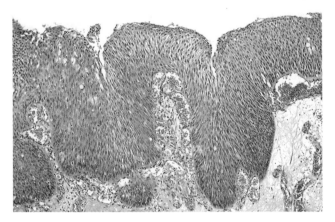

Figure 4.49 Lacrimal sac papilloma (inverted transitional type).

THE ORBIT

The orbit contains many different types of cells and tissues that may proliferate. Apart from proliferations that develop from the lacrimal gland or optic nerve, most proliferations within the orbit are choristomas or originate from blood vessels, nerves, lymphocytes, fibroblasts or histiocytes, or are secondary neoplasms. Space-occupying lesions such as orbital inflammatory conditions may mimic disorders of growth, and the occurrence of such a variety of conditions with their complex pathology has led to the confusing term 'pseudotumour', which is of doubtful value as it gives no indication of the underlying pathological processes. Clinical features such as proptosis, diplopia and visual loss depend upon the site and size of the lesions. Radiological investigations, in particular computer tomography (CT) or magnetic resonance imaging (MRI), are invaluable in locating, delineating and assessing the nature of orbital swellings.

Cysts and choristomas

Dermoid cyst

Dermoid cysts result from the continued growth of congenital rests of ectodermal cells entrapped within the sutures of the orbital bones. The majority develop superiorly at the outer or inner angle, where they form tense ovoid swellings often attached to the underlying bone which may be excavated or absent, thus allowing attachment to the dura. Dermoid cysts comprise about a third of all orbital swellings in children. They are structurally similar to dermoid cysts in the lids (Fig. 4.15). Escape of their contents, possibly following trauma, may lead to an intense inflammatory reaction, and the clinical features in these circumstances resemble an inflammatory or rapidly progressive neoplastic condition. Imaging studies demonstrate the cystic nature and bony involvement.

Epidermoid cyst

Epidermoid cysts are similar to dermoid cysts but have a simple epidermal lining (Fig. 4.14b). They are rare in the orbit but can on occasions be found in the roof beneath the periorbital tissue.

Lymphangioma

Lymphangiomas are classified as choristomas because lymphatic channels are not normally present in the orbit. They usually occur in children and present as an orbital mass, although the lids and conjunctiva may also be involved. Symptoms and signs depend on the extent of the lesion and on associated events, in particular haemorrhage, which may result in fulminant proptosis. Visual disturbance and extraocular muscle dysfunction are common. There are irregular varying-sized endothelial-lined thin-walled channels. Haemorrhage and thrombosis may occur, and lymphoid aggregates may be seen in the interstitial fibrous tissue that separates the channels. Broken-down thrombosed blood can form chocolate cysts.

Teratoma

Teratomas arise from misdirected germ cells and contain tissue derived from all three germ layers. They are rare, always congenital, and produce massive proptosis. Lesions have solid and cystic areas with histological evidence of skin, gut, lung, muscle, cartilage, bone, brain and connective tissue. Malignant change is very unusual.

Other cystic lesions

These include microphthalmos with cyst, mucoceles from the frontal or ethmoid sinuses, and meningoceles, cephaloceles and meningoencephaloceles resulting from herniations through a congenital defect in the orbital wall.

Lacrimal gland proliferations

The lacrimal gland consists of tubules and acini of epithelial cells together with interstitial fibrovascular tissue containing a population of lymphocytes, which is regarded as part of MALT. The tubules are formed by a double layer of cuboidal epithelial cells while the acini are composed of an inner layer of cuboidal or columnar epithelium and an outer layer of spindle-shaped myoepithelial cells. Mucin-secreting goblet cells are present within lacrimal ducts. Neoplasms are similar to those of salivary glands and arise from epithelium but not from the fibrovascular tissue. Neoplasms of the lacrimal epithelium comprise approximately 50 per cent of the expanding lesions of the gland; the remaining 50 per cent are either lymphoproliferative or inflammatory disorders. Epithelial neoplasms may be benign or malignant, over 50 per cent being benign – usually pleomorphic adenomas. Most of the malignant epithelial neoplasms are adenoid cystic carcinomas; pleomorphic carcinomas are less common and other carcinomas are rare.

Pleomorphic adenoma

Pleomorphic adenomas arise most often from the orbital portion of the lacrimal gland and only rarely from the palpebral lobe. Males predominate and all age groups are affected, the mean age of presentation being 40 years. A painless firm smooth round-to-ovoid mass develops in the superotemporal quadrant of the orbit over a fairly long period of time, usually more than 2 years. Proptosis occurs, with downward and inward displacement of the eye. Indentation of bone and sclera adjacent to the growth is revealed by CT scans (Fig. 4.50a). The neoplasm, which may be 2–3 cm in diameter, is encapsulated and often has small projections (bossulations) that are outgrowths of neoplastic cells. The presence of bossulations makes total surgical removal of pleomorphic adenomas a necessity. Microscopy reveals proliferation of epithelium and myoepithelium. The inner layer of cells forms glandular tissue in which there may be squamous differentiation with keratin production (Fig. 4.50b), while the outer cells undergo metaplastic change leading to the formation of myxoid tissue (Fig. 4.50c), fat and cartilage and, on rare occasions, bone. The term pleomorphic refers to this varied histological picture.

Other benign lesions

These include monomorphic adenomas (pure adenomas without the mesenchymal elements that characterize pleomorphic adenomas) and oncocytomas, which are extremely rare.

Adenoid cystic carcinoma

In contrast to pleomorphic adenoma the history of adenoid cystic carcinoma is short, with clinical advancement usually occurring within 6 months. There is no sex predilection, and the mean age of presentation, as for pleomorphic adenoma, is 40 years. Proptosis of rapid onset accompanied by pain, numbness and diplopia is characteristic. The neoplasm forms a mass with irregular and serrated borders, and with destructive or sclerotic bone changes indicative of its infiltrative nature. Microscopy reveals nests of basaloid cells with numerous mitoses and a solid and/or a cribriform pattern (Fig. 4.51a). Solid lesions are either undifferentiated (cylindromatous) or have necrotic centres (comedo), while in cribriform lesions round spaces represent mucin-filled cysts ('swiss cheese' appearance). Perineural (Fig. 4.51b) and bony infiltration (Fig. 4.51c) explain the clinical and radiological features.

Pleomorphic carcinoma

Pleomorphic carcinoma results from malignant transformation of a pre-existing pleomorphic adenoma. Presentation is usually at an older age than with pleomorphic adenoma. Clinical suspicion of malignancy is aroused by the recurrence of a pleomorphic adenoma or by the sudden enlargement of a pre-existing mass.

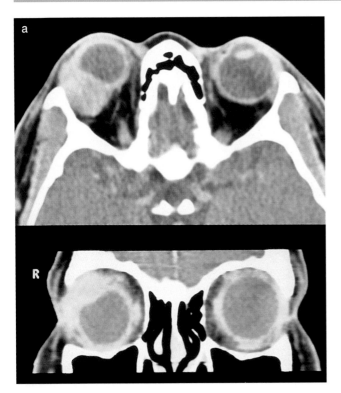

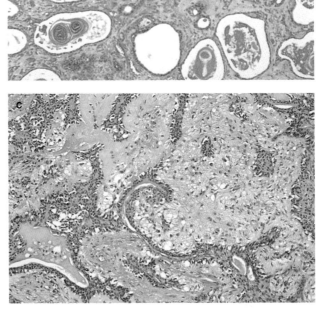

Figure 4.50 Pleomorphic adenoma of lacrimal gland. (a) CT scans showing superotemporal orbital mass indenting the sclera. (b) Glandular tissue and squamous differentiation with formation of keratin. (c) Epithelial and myoepithelial proliferation with the formation of myxoid tissue.

Histology reveals a carcinoma in which a pleomorphic adenoma is identifiable.

Other carcinomas

These are unusual, but include true adenocarcinomas, squamous cell carcinomas and mucoepidermoid carcinomas that may occasionally develop from the ducts. Carcinomas that show sebaceous differentiation are exceptionally rare.

Vascular proliferations

Vascular proliferations are foremost amongst the space-occupying lesions of the orbit developing outside the lacrimal gland. Most are hamartomas, although haemangiopericytomas are true neoplasms.

Cavernous haemangioma

Cavernous haemangiomas are the commonest vascular lesions of the orbit and occur almost exclusively in adults, mostly females. The majority are located posteriorly within the muscle cone, and an axial painless pulsatile proptosis develops slowly over a 4–5-year period. Visual symptoms and signs develop if there is pressure on the optic nerve, while a sudden increase in size can result from haemorrhage, thrombosis or infection. On microscopy, a fibrous capsule is seen to encase congested varying-sized, but mainly large, endothelial-lined vascular channels separated by fibrous septae (Fig. 4.52). Haemosiderin-laden macrophages may be found within the fibrous tissue. The phleboliths sometimes seen on radiological examination are calcified intravascular thrombi.

Capillary haemangioma

Capillary haemangiomas most commonly affect children and are usually noticed within 2 weeks of birth. Their growth is disproportionate to body growth, and symptoms and signs depend on the extent of orbital involvement. Microscopy reveals capillary channels.

Arteriovenous fistulae

Arteriovenous fistulae usually occur as part of the Wyburn–Mason syndrome, and comprise thick-walled

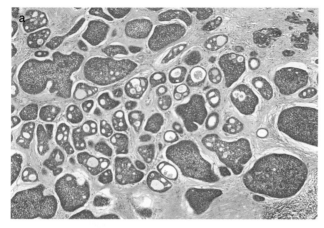

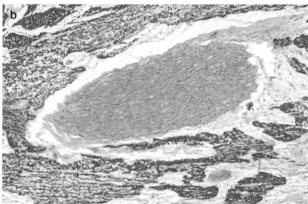

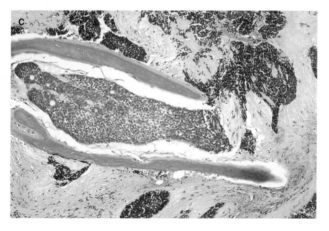

Figure 4.51 Adenoid cystic carcinoma of lacrimal gland. (a) Solid and cribriform areas. (b) Perineural infiltration. (c) Infiltration of bone.

vessels connecting the arterial and venous sides of the circulation with no intervening capillary network.

Racemose haemangioma

Racemose haemangiomas are localized pulsatile masses of convoluted vessels histologically recognizable as arteries.

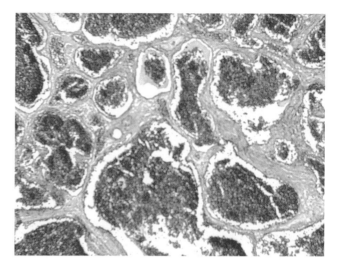

Figure 4.52 Cavernous haemangioma. Congested varying-sized endothelial-lined vascular channels separated by fibrous septae.

Varices

Orbital varices are anomalous abnormally dilated venous channels, and cause intermittent exophthalmos. Smooth muscle is found within their walls, and lymphocytes may infiltrate the intervening connective tissue.

Haemangiopericytoma

Haemangiopericytomas are neoplasms derived from vascular pericytes, and occur principally in the superior aspect of the orbit. Small polyhedral and spindle-shaped cells are tightly packed around blood vessels of varying size. All haemangiopericytomas should be considered malignant, and malignancy is categorized as low- or high-grade based on the histological appearance.

Neural proliferations

Orbital neural proliferations include meningiomas, optic nerve gliomas (juvenile and adult) and peripheral nerve lesions (neurofibromas and schwannomas).

Meningioma

Meningiomas develop from arachnoid cells on the deep surface of the dura or from arachnoid prolongations into the dura (arachnoid granulations). Orbital meningiomas may arise from an intracranial site near the sphenoidal ridge, from where they extend into the orbit. They can also arise from the optic nerve and very rarely from congenital ectopic rests of meningothelial cells in the orbital tissues. Meningiomas are usually seen in females around 40 years of age and have clinical features that vary according to the site of origin, but proptosis, limitation of ocular movements and visual symptoms are characteristic. Disc oedema is common, especially when the meningioma arises anteriorly, while opticociliary shunt vessels (Fig. 4.53) result from expansion of a meningioma of the optic nerve sheath which compromises the circulation of blood through the central retinal vein and induces collateral flow. Diffuse swelling of the optic nerve, irregular excrescences along the nerve, bulbous swelling at the orbital apex, intracranial extension, hyperostosis or erosion of bone, and calcification are other features. Meningiomas are more aggressive in children. The two main histological types are meningothelial and psammomatous. Meningothelial meningiomas are composed of polygonal cells with poorly defined boundaries arranged in varying-sized irregular lobules separated by fibrovascular strands (Fig. 4.54a). Psammomatous meningiomas exhibit whorls and eddies of elongated cells surrounding small blood vessels or hyaline or laminated calcified spherules (psammoma bodies) that probably represent degenerating cells (Fig. 4.54b). Psammoma bodies are identical to the corpora arenacea of the arachnoid of older persons. Other histological types of meningioma are fibroblastic, transitional (exhibiting both meningothelial and fibroblastic features) and angioblastic.

Juvenile optic nerve glioma

Juvenile optic nerve gliomas are probably hamartomas arising from astrocytes, and occur most commonly in infants and young children. There is a significant association (5–15 per cent) with neurofibromatosis type 1. Symptoms and signs develop insidiously, and loss of vision is an early feature; this contrasts with menin-

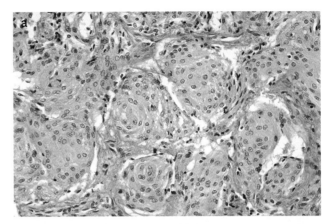
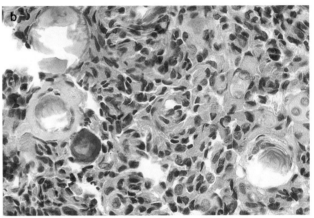

Figure 4.54 Meningioma. (a) Meningothelial type; varying-sized irregular lobules of meningothelial cells separated by fibrovascular strands. (b) Psammomatous type; psammoma bodies among proliferating meningothelial cells.

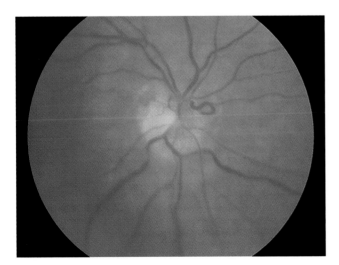

Figure 4.53 Meningioma. Opticociliary shunt vessel in optic nerve sheath meningioma.

gioma, where visual loss usually occurs late. Gliomas that arise from the orbital portion of the optic nerve cause swelling of the disc and possibly occlusion of the central retinal artery or vein, whereas those arising from the intracranial portion of the optic nerve may produce pituitary and hypothalamic dysfunction. Proptosis is often a late sign. Gross examination of an excised specimen reveals fusiform enlargement of the optic nerve (Fig. 4.55a), and large gliomas that extend through the optic canal may have a dumb-bell shape. The limits of the lesion may be ill defined. Microscopy shows proliferating spindle-shaped pilocytic (hair-like) astrocytes (Fig. 4.55b) forming intersecting bundles that distend the pial septae. Glial filaments are demonstrable, and Rosenthal fibres, which are elongated brightly eosinophilic club-like structures derived from astrocytic processes, are occasionally seen. Juvenile gliomas do not transgress the dura, but may grow towards the brain and lamina cribrosa. Associated meningeal hyperplasia is common and can extend beyond the limits of the glioma.

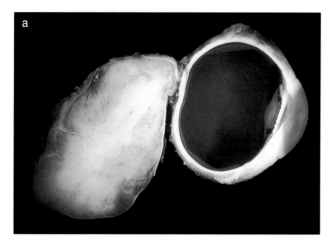

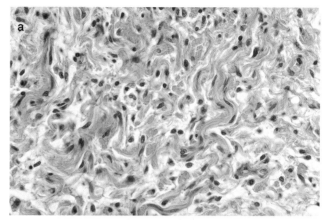

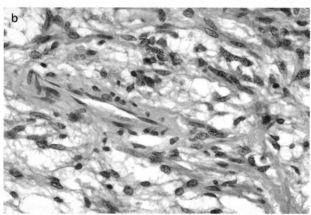

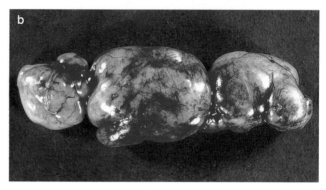

Figure 4.56 Neurofibroma. (a) Proliferation of Schwann cells, fibroblasts and nerve axons with wavy collagen fibres. (b) Plexiform lesion.

Figure 4.55 Optic nerve glioma. (a) A fusiform homogeneous retrobulbar mass. (b) Proliferating spindle-shaped pilocytic astrocytes and glial filaments.

Adult optic nerve glioma

Adult optic nerve gliomas are rare, highly malignant neoplasms that arise from astrocytes and can affect adults of any age. The neoplasms are anaplastic and invasive, with rapid progression to blindness and early death.

Neurofibroma

Neurofibromas are benign, non-encapsulated, and contain Schwann cells, fibroblasts and nerve axons. Microscopy reveals thin elongated cells with comma-shaped nuclei, arranged in cords, whorls or eddies together with wavy collagen fibres (Fig. 4.56a). Plexiform neurofibromas (Fig. 4.56b) occur in children in association with neurofibromatosis type 1. Solitary neurofibromas usually occur in adults and originate most commonly from the first division of the trigeminal nerve, where they are seen as circumscribed masses extending through the superior orbital fissure. Only 25 per cent of isolated neurofibromas are associated with neurofibromatosis type 1.

Schwannoma (neurilemmoma)

Schwannomas are also benign, and originate from Schwann cells. They are often solitary and, like solitary neurofibromas, arise most frequently from the first division of the trigeminal nerve. Pain is a prominent feature, but otherwise schwannomas are clinically indistinguishable from solitary neurofibromas. They have a well-marked capsule (cf. neurofibroma) and histologically two distinct appearances may be seen, often in different areas of the same lesion: one (Antoni type A) is of solid cellular areas which often exhibit regimented nuclei in stripes that sometimes resemble tactile corpuscles, and the other (Antoni type B) is that of stellate or ovoid cells suspended in a loose matrix (Fig. 4.57). Twenty per cent of schwannomas are associated with neurofibromatosis type 1, when they are often multiple.

Other soft tissue proliferations

Other than vascular and neural proliferations, the most important soft tissue proliferation arising within the orbit is embryonal sarcoma. Proliferations that arise from fat

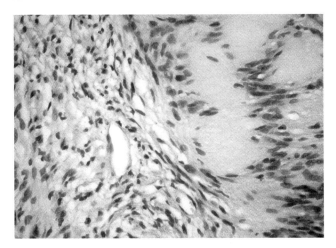

Figure 4.57 Schwannoma. Antoni type A pattern on the right and type B pattern on the left.

(lipoma, pleomorphic liposarcoma, primary myxoliposarcoma), striated muscle (rhabdomyoma, rhabdomyosarcoma), smooth muscle (leiomyoma, leiomyosarcoma), fibrous tissue (fibrosarcoma – there is an association with the retinoblastoma gene) and those of uncertain histogenesis (benign – granular cell myoblastoma; malignant – alveolar soft part sarcoma) are all rare.

Embryonal sarcoma (embryonal rhabdomyosarcoma)

Embryonal sarcomas are malignant neoplasms derived from undifferentiated mesenchymal cell rests, which have the potential to differentiate into striated muscle. They do not arise from striated muscle, and the term rhabdomyosarcoma is appropriate only if there is histological or immunological evidence of differentiation into muscle. Embryonal sarcoma is the commonest primary malignant lesion of the orbit in childhood, and the median age at diagnosis is 7 years. Rapidly progressive proptosis is accompanied by orbital vasocongestion and inflammation. The superonasal quadrant is the most frequently affected location. The neoplasm may occasionally present as a small papillary or nodular lesion in the lids or conjunctiva (botryoid type). Embryonal sarcomas can erode and destroy the bony walls of the orbit and extend into the cranial cavity. Major sites of metastases are the lung, lymph nodes and bone marrow. Microscopy of embryonal sarcomas shows a mass of mesenchymal cells. Undifferentiated neoplasms consist of loosely arranged pleomorphic cells (Fig. 4.58a). In differentiated neoplasms many of the cells are elongated and strap-like (Fig. 4.58b), with some exhibiting a 'tadpole' or 'tennis racket' configuration; such cells are rhabdomyoblasts and are evidence of differentiation into muscle, the most differentiated

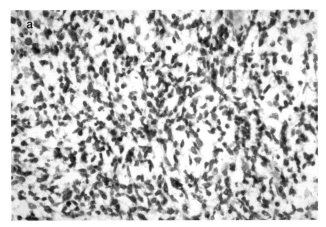

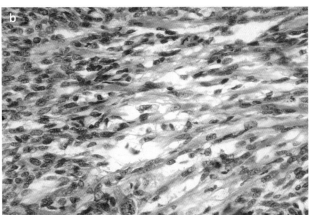

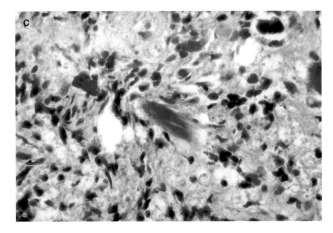

Figure 4.58 Embryonal sarcoma. (a) Undifferentiated; loosely-arranged proliferating mesenchymal cells. (b) Differentiated; many elongated strap-like cells with eosinophilic cytoplasm (rhabdomyoblasts). (c) Differentiated; the rhabdomyoblast in the centre of the field has cross-striations. Masson trichrome stain.

cells exhibiting cross-striations (Fig. 4.58c). Some rhabdomyosarcomas have an alveolar pattern in which fibrous septae form irregular alveolar spaces with polyhedral cells attached in a single layer to the septae. Alveolar rhabdomyosarcomas usually occur in the inferior aspect of the orbit in slightly older children.

Osseous and cartilaginous proliferations

Osseous proliferations are rare, but include osteoma, benign osteoblastoma, aneurysmal bone cyst and fibrous dysplasia, and also osteosarcoma, which is of importance in that it can develop subsequent to radiotherapy and may occur in the survivors of heritable retinoblastoma. Cartilaginous proliferations in the orbit are excessively rare.

THE EYE

Intraocular disorders of cell and tissue growth include cysts, hyperplasias and choristomas, but most intraocular proliferations are of melanocytic or neuroepithelial origin. Less frequently, proliferations arise from blood vessels, nerves or smooth muscle.

Cysts, hyperplasias and choristomas

Iris cysts

Iris cysts lie between the two layers of the pigment epithelium (Fig. 4.59), and can be confused clinically with melanomas.

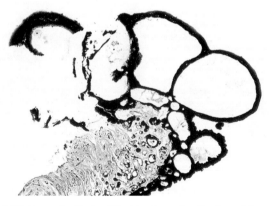

Figure 4.59 Iris cysts. Cysts of the iris pigment epithelium at the pupillary margin.

Fuchs' 'adenoma'

Fuchs' 'adenoma' is an asymptomatic nodular hyperplasia of the ciliary epithelium occasionally noted in enucleated eyes of the elderly (Fig. 4.60). It is not an adenoma.

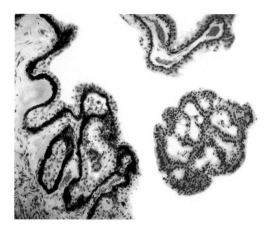

Figure 4.60 Fuchs' 'adenoma'.

Pseudoadenomatous hyperplasia of the ciliary epithelium

Pseudoadenomatous hyperplasia of the ciliary epithelium is sometimes seen on ophthalmoscopy, but more usually on microscopy (Fig. 4.61), in eyes exhibiting low-grade inflammation, particularly following trauma and more often when there is cyclitic membrane formation.

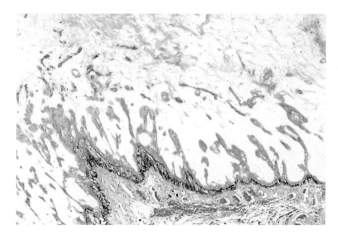

Figure 4.61 Pseudoadenomatous hyperplasia of the ciliary epithelium.

Ringschwiele

Ringschwiele is a proliferation of the ciliary epithelium and peripheral RPE associated with laminar formation of fibrous tissue that possibly contains some blood vessels (Fig. 4.62). It is not evident on clinical examination, but is often seen histologically in enucleated eyes with long-standing retinal detachment.

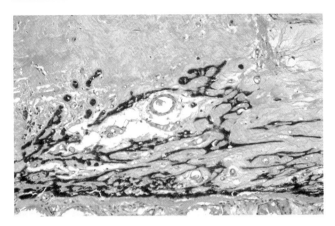

Figure 4.62 Ringschwiele. Hyperplasia of the ciliary epithelium and RPE with laminar formation of vascularized fibrous tissue.

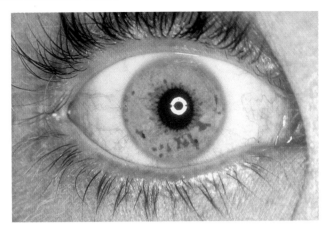

Figure 4.63 Iris naevi.

Congenital hypertrophy of the RPE

Congenital hypertrophy of the RPE (CHRPE) occurs in one of three ways: typical unifocal unilateral lesions, typical multifocal unilateral lesions (congenital grouped pigmentation of the retina), and atypical multifocal bilateral lesions (Fig. 4.9). The commonest presentation is as a solitary dark-pigmented lesion that can involve any area and most often affects young Caucasian females.

Osseous choristoma of the choroid (choroidal osteoma)

Osseous choristoma is the preferred term for this lesion, as there is no pre-existing bone in the normal choroid. Young Caucasian females are most often affected. Ophthalmoscopy reveals an orange/yellow discrete mass with a scalloped border located at the posterior pole and possibly surrounding the optic disc. Histology shows normal cancellous bone with loose vascularized connective tissue filling the intertrabecular spaces.

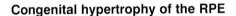

Melanocytic proliferations

Proliferations of uveal melanocytes (neural crest origin) are benign (naevi or melanocytomas – magnocellular naevi) or malignant (melanomas).

Naevi and melanocytomas

Clinical features

Iris naevi are common, and present as flat or slightly elevated pigmented lesions on the anterior surface (Fig. 4.63). They do not distort surrounding tissue unless situated near the pupil, when they can cause ectropion uveae or localized lens opacities.

Ciliary body naevi are rare and usually melanocytomas.

Choroidal naevi are common, occurring in 10 per cent of the population. They are asymptomatic, slate-grey, oval or circular, and flat or minimally elevated (Fig. 4.64). Their maximum diameter is usually < 5 mm and their thickness is rarely > 1.5 mm. Drusen formation and degeneration of the RPE occur with time.

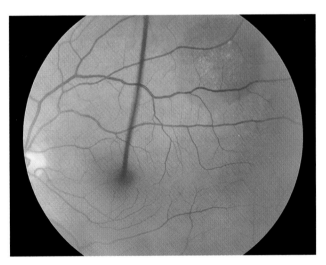

Figure 4.64 Choroidal naevus.

Melanocytomas of the optic nerve head are heavily pigmented (Fig. 4.65), are usually discovered on routine ophthalmoscopy and are seen most often in non-white individuals. Visual loss is rare, and is due to necrosis within the lesion, central retinal vein occlusion, maculopathy or optic atrophy. Melanocytomas are most frequently situated in the lower temporal quadrant of the nerve head and seldom protrude into the vitreous by more than 2 mm. They may extend a few millimetres posteriorly behind the lamina cribrosa and also into

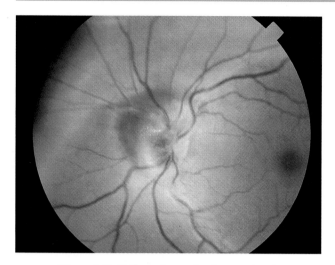

Figure 4.65 Melanocytoma of optic nerve head.

the adjacent retina, when they appear to have a feathery border.

Suspicious lesions and malignant change

All naevi and melanocytomas have malignant potential and can give rise to melanomas. Growth is the main clinical feature that renders a lesion suspicious and indicates that it may be undergoing malignant transformation. Iris lesions that have extended into the filtration angle and produced secondary glaucoma are invariably malignant. Other suspicious features of choroidal naevi include the presence of overlying orange-yellow lipofuscin pigment and associated serous detachment of the retina.

Pathology

Cells specific to naevi are of four types: spindle, dendritic, polyhedral and balloon.

Spindle cells have small nuclei of uniform size exhibiting an even distribution of condensed chromatin.

Dendritic cells have long branching processes, and larger and rounder nuclei with more prominent nucleoli than spindle cells.

Polyhedral cells have small ovoid nuclei with fine chromatin and small nucleoli, and a variable amount of cytoplasm.

Balloon cells are polyhedral with a vacuolated or clear cytoplasm.

Spindle and dendritic cells vary considerably in their degree of pigmentation. Polyhedral cells are heavily pigmented while balloon cells are only lightly pigmented. Iris naevi usually consist of less than five layers of cells on the anterior aspect, and do not infiltrate deeply into the stroma (Fig. 4.66); spindle cells predominate, but dendri-

tic and balloon cells may also be seen. Choroidal naevi are composed of small heavily pigmented spindle cells that may slightly thicken involved tissue, but the choriocapillaris is spared. Lesions that cause gross choroidal thickening or involve the choriocapillaris are regarded as malignant. Melanocytomas are uniformly composed of heavily pigmented polyhedral cells (Fig. 4.67).

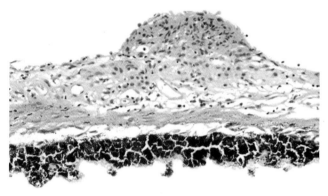

Figure 4.66 Iris naevus. Localized melanocytic proliferation on anterior iris surface.

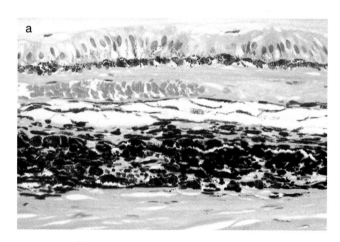

a

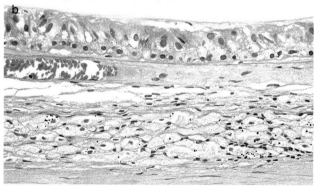

b

Figure 4.67 Melanocytoma of ciliary body. (a) Heavily pigmented melanocytes in the pars plana. (b) Bleached section of the same lesion.

Melanomas

Melanomas are malignant melanocytic neoplasms. The incidence of uveal melanomas is approximately six per million of population per year. Uncommon in Asians and rare in Afro-Caribbeans, there is a probable increased incidence in those with blue or grey irises as compared to those with brown irises. Other significant risk factors include ancestry from northern latitudes, light complexion and the presence of 10 or more cutaneous naevi, especially dysplastic naevi (AMS). Although the role of UV light in the pathogenesis of cutaneous melanoma is well established, its role in the development of uveal melanoma is not clear. Local predisposing lesions include ocular and oculodermal melanocytosis and uveal naevi. The rate of transformation of naevi to melanomas is estimated as 1 : 10–15 000 per year. The median age at which melanomas of the uvea are diagnosed is approximately 55 years; they rarely occur before the age of 20 or after the age of 80.

Genetics

Uveal melanomas are not usually inherited but chromosomal abnormalities have been demonstrated, most notably on chromosomes 3 and 8, and less frequently on chromosomes 9 and 13. It is hypothesized that an anti-oncogene on chromosome 3 is deleted and an oncogene on chromosome 8 is amplified. The association of chromosome 3 abnormalities with melanomas of the ciliary body is especially significant. Predisposition to melanoma may also result from mutations in the p16 gene (CDKN2A) on chromosome 9 (9p13.22) and in the BRCA2 gene on chromosome 13, this gene also being associated with breast and ovarian cancer. Another gene predisposing to uveal melanoma is MC1R, which affects host response to UV radiation. Increased expression of the anti-oncogene p53 on chromosome 17 may also play a role in the pathogenesis.

Clinical features

Iris melanomas constitute 8 per cent of uveal melanomas. They are often noticed by the patient and appear as a localized well-circumscribed mass or as a diffuse irregular thickening; their degree of pigmentation is variable. Although they may appear in any position between the pupillary margin and the drainage angle, they have a predilection for the inferior aspect. Distortion of the pupil, ectropion uveae and hyphaema may occur, and there may be circumferential spread and involvement of the trabecular meshwork with resultant secondary glaucoma.

Ciliary body melanomas constitute 12 per cent of uveal melanomas. They present most commonly with blurred vision due to displacement of the lens or cataract. Invasion of the filtration angle and iris may be visible (Fig. 4.68). Interference with blood flow may result in a dilated episcleral vessel (sentinel vessel) in the same quadrant as the melanoma. Ciliary body melanomas are usually seen as a convex well-circumscribed mass, but may diffusely infiltrate the global circumference (ring melanoma). Extension may be anterior into the iris and anterior chamber, and posterior into the choroid, while centripetal spread can involve scleral and extraocular tissues. Glaucoma may result from displacement of the lens and pupil block, infiltration of the trabecular meshwork by melanoma cells, or necrosis with the release of pigment granules which are taken up by macrophages (melanomalytic glaucoma). Ciliary body melanomas invariably appear black because they are covered by ciliary epithelium, the outer layer of which is heavily pigmented, or, if they have extended posteriorly, by the RPE.

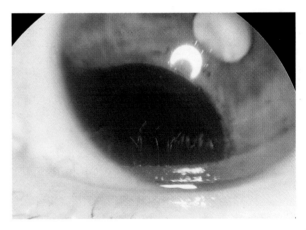

Figure 4.68 Ciliary body melanoma invading the filtration angle and producing cataract.

Choroidal melanomas constitute 80 per cent of uveal melanomas and are the commonest primary intraocular malignant neoplasms. Clinical features depend on their location. Early lesions are often asymptomatic, and even advanced growths may only be discovered on routine ophthalmoscopy. Presenting symptoms include visual loss, field defects and metamorphopsia. Retinal detachment may be solid due to the presence of a mass, or secondary and non-rhegmatogenous consequent upon interference with the fluid-pumping action of the RPE. Choroidal melanomas most often lie at or near the posterior pole and are seen as an elevated, well-circumscribed, variably pigmented mass contained within the uvea (Fig. 4.69). The overlying RPE is frequently atrophic, drusen may be present and deposits of orange-yellow lipofuscin pigment may be seen. If the melanoma has broken through Bruch's membrane, the RPE and possibly the overlying retina, it usually has a mushroom-shaped ('cottage-loaf' or 'collar-stud') configuration. Less frequently, choroidal melanomas may be diffuse and produce extensive flat lesions resembling metastatic carcinoma. Involvement of the drainage angle and trabecular meshwork results in glaucoma.

Extrascleral extension of uveal melanomas can produce a visible subconjunctival mass or proptosis if there is infiltration of the orbit. Necrotic lesions cause inflammation. Blind painful or phthisical eyes may occasionally harbour a clinically unsuspected melanoma, and the diagnosis is only established as the result of histological examination.

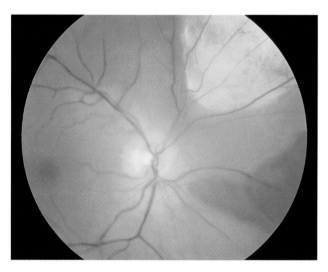

Figure 4.69 Choroidal melanoma in upper nasal quadrant with exudative retinal detachment and subretinal haemorrhage.

Pathology

Iris melanomas are usually seen as iridectomy specimens; they may be nodular or diffuse, and superficial or with varying degrees of stromal infiltration (Fig. 4.70). Ciliary body melanomas < 10 mm in diameter are often seen as cyclectomy or iridocyclectomy specimens, but larger melanomas are seen in enucleated eyes; ciliary body melanomas are usually solid or well-circumscribed. Most choroidal melanomas are seen in enucleated eyes as nodular, ovoid, mushroom-shaped ('cottage-loaf' or 'collar-stud' – Fig. 4.71a) or diffuse lesions.

Iris melanomas may extend into the filtration angle and trabecular meshwork, but rarely outside the eye.

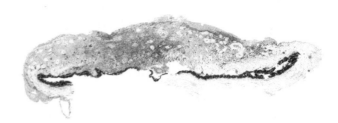

Figure 4.70 Iris melanoma infiltrating the entire thickness of the stroma.

Ciliary body and choroidal melanomas infiltrate inner scleral lamellae, and some extend into neurovascular scleral channels. Choroidal melanomas may involve the retina (Fig. 4.71b), but spread into the vitreous or optic nerve is very unusual. Extraocular extension is sometimes seen, as are emboli of neoplastic cells in blood vessels outside the eye (Fig. 4.71c). The melanin content of melanomas is variable, and, if heavy, histological sections have to be bleached in order to remove the pigment before the cell type can be determined. Some ciliary body and choroidal melanomas exhibit necrosis and/or haemorrhage.

Melanoma cells are spindle or epithelioid. Other cells associated with melanomas are lymphocytes and lipid-containing histiocytes.

Spindle cells are fusiform and usually arranged in tight bundles, their cell membranes are indistinct and their cytoplasm is fibrillar or finely granular. Nuclei vary from slender to plump, and nucleoli may or may not be distinct (Fig. 4.72a).

Epithelioid cells are larger and more pleomorphic than spindle cells, often appearing polyhedral with abundant cytoplasm. Their cell membranes are distinct, and an extracellular space often separates adjacent cells. Epithelioid cells have large nuclei with a coarse chromatin pattern and prominent nucleoli (Fig. 4.72b). Bizarre epithelioid and multinucleate cells are sometimes seen. Mitotic figures are more frequent in epithelioid cells than in spindle cells.

Classification

The classification of uveal melanomas is that issued by the Armed Forces Institute of Pathology (AFIP), Washington, DC (1983). It is a modification of the Callendar classification (1931) and is based on cell type. Two types are recognized:

1. Spindle cell melanomas formed exclusively by spindle cells.

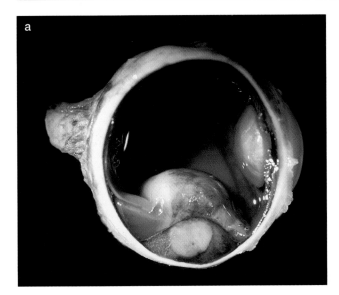

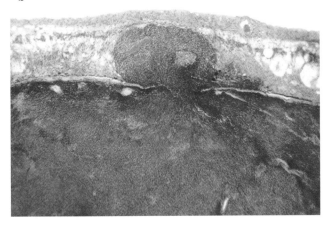

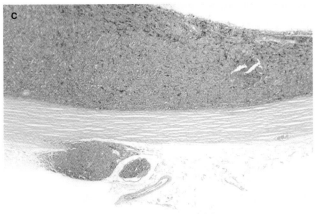

Figure 4.71 Choroidal melanoma. (a) Eye opened anteroposteriorly showing a pigmented mass within the equatorial choroid and associated retinal detachment. (b) The mass has broken through Bruch's membrane and is infiltrating the retina. (c) Extraocular extension and an embolus of neoplastic cells within a blood vessel.

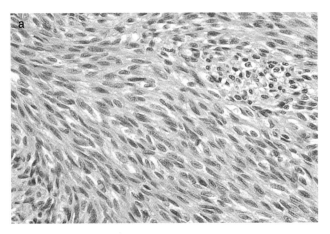

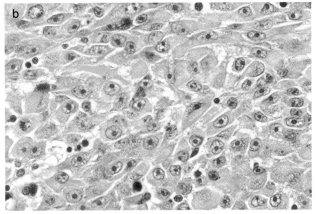

Figure 4.72 Uveal melanoma. (a) Spindle cells. (b) Epithelioid cells.

2. Mixed cell melanomas in which there is a mixture of spindle and epithelioid cells.

In addition to the cell types, melanomas (particularly of the choroid) exhibit other characteristic histological features (fascicular pattern and necrosis) which were originally included in the Callendar classification.

Neoplasms with a fascicular pattern
There are two forms:

1. Vasocentric pattern in which the melanoma cells are arranged perpendicular to a central vessel (Fig. 4.73a).

2. Ribbon pattern in which the melanoma cells are arranged in bundles and form stripes (Fig. 4.73b).

Necrotic neoplasms
Necrosis is so extensive that a classification based on cell type is not possible (Fig. 4.74). Necrosis is due to ischaemia or an immune reaction.

Prognosis

Prognosis is determined by factors in both the melanoma (cell type, nucleolar size and variability, chromosomal

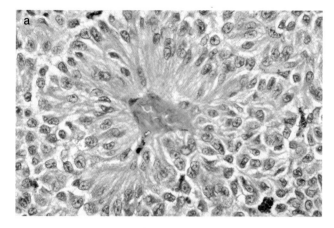

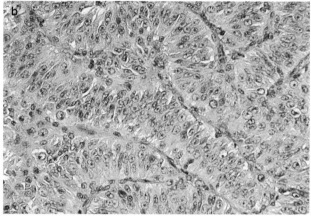

Figure 4.73 Choroidal melanoma: fascicular patterns. (a) Vasocentric pattern of cell growth. (b) Ribbon pattern of cell growth.

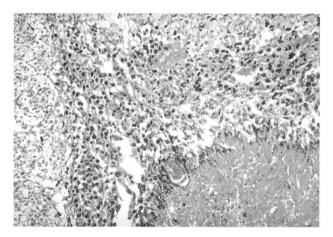

Figure 4.74 Necrotic melanoma. The cell type cannot be determined.

abnormalities, location, size, extraocular extension, vascularity) and the host.

Cell type: epithelioid cells are regarded as more malignant than spindle cells.

Nucleolar size and variability: nuclear pleomorphism: long and wide nuclei and long and multiple nucleoli are probably more important indicators of poor prognosis than cell type. Computerized morphometric analysis is useful in assessing these features, and the standard deviation of the nucleolar area (SDNA) and its inverse (ISDNA) are useful measurements.

Chromosomal abnormalities: monosomy 3 in the melanoma cells carries an unfavourable prognosis.

Location: iris melanomas have a favourable prognosis as they are usually detected early and are composed mainly of spindle cells. Choroidal melanomas situated at the posterior pole produce symptoms early and have a better prognosis than those situated more anteriorly or in the ciliary body.

Size: small melanomas have a more favourable prognosis than large melanomas. Those with a basal diameter < 10 mm are usually associated with good survival rates. Diffuse melanomas, although not of large volume, carry an unfavourable prognosis, probably because they contain many epithelioid cells.

Extraocular extension: extension of melanoma outside the eye adversely affects the prognosis.

Vascularity: the presence of closed vascular loops, particularly when they form networks, is associated with poor survival. Morphological patterns of vessels in tissue sections can be examined using a fluorescein-conjugated vascular endothelial marker.

Host factors: the prognosis is less favourable in those over 60 years of age. The presence of a lymphocytic cellular infiltrate in relation to the melanoma represents an important component of the host's immune response. The majority of the lymphocytes are CD8 + ($T_{C/S}$) cells, which infiltrate in response to the expression of melanocyte lineage peptides. Contrary to expectations, lymphocytic infiltration is associated with an unfavourable prognosis; a possible explanation is that mixed cell melanomas, which are more malignant than spindle cell melanomas, have an abnormal ganglioside profile resulting in conspicuous lymphocytic infiltration.

Metastases

The liver is by far the commonest site of metastatic deposits. This cannot be explained by venous drainage and is indicative of a selection process by disseminating melanoma cells.

Neuroepithelial proliferations

The commonest neuroepithelial proliferations are retinoblastomas. Medulloepitheliomas are less frequent, and other neuroepithelial proliferations are rare.

Retinoblastoma

Retinoblastomas occur in 1 : 20–30 000 live births. They are the commonest malignant intraocular neoplasms in childhood and the second commonest primary intraocular malignancy at any age (choroidal melanomas are more common). Ninety-four per cent of affected children have no family history of retinoblastoma; nevertheless 15 per cent of these have new germinal mutations and therefore can pass the condition to subsequent generations. The remaining 6 per cent of cases have a family history, and in 60–90 per cent of these the inheritance follows an autosomal dominant pattern with incomplete penetrance. Approximately 30 per cent of all cases are bilateral.

The retinoblastoma gene

The retinoblastoma gene (Rb1 gene) is a large 180-kb gene with 27 exons encoding a 94.7-kb RNA transcript. It is located on chromosome 13 (13q14.2). The term 'retinoblastoma gene' is a misnomer as the gene is an antioncogene which, by producing a photoreceptor protein p110Rb1 that binds to DNA, prevents the development of retinoblastoma and possibly other malignant neoplasms such as pinealoblastoma, fibrosarcoma and osteosarcoma. A complex gene locus identified as a retinoblastoma predisposition gene, the function of which is unknown, lies adjacent to the Rb1 gene. Only one normally functioning Rb1 gene (heterozygous) is required to suppress the formation of a retinoblastoma. Two abnormal Rb1 genes (i.e. homozygosity) are required for retinoblastoma development. This is the basis of Knudson's 'two hit' hypothesis, which postulates that two mutational events (one affecting each Rb1 gene) are necessary for a normal retinal cell to develop into a neoplastic cell. Children with a germinal mutation inherit the first 'hit', and only one additional genetic event (somatic mutation) is needed for retinoblastoma to develop.

Identification of the Rb1 gene has been made possible by molecular genetic analysis. Specific mutations are not easy to identify, but molecular genetics information is invaluable in genetic counselling. Mutations are germinal or somatic.

Germinal mutations involve reproductive cells and may be inherited or acquired.

Inherited germinal mutation is when a mutant gene is inherited from a parent.

Acquired germinal mutation occurs early in embryogenesis in those without a family history of retinoblastoma. The defective gene may be passed to subsequent generations.

Somatic mutations occur in cells other than those involved in reproduction, and later in embryogenesis after the major organs have differentiated. Spontaneous Rb1 mutation or a mutation in response to an environmental mutagen occurs in one of the million or more neuroblasts present within the developing retina.

Chromosomal deletion

About 4 per cent of those with retinoblastoma have chromosomal deletion. In these instances, there are additional systemic and mental abnormalities, and a reduced enzyme D esterase level.

Patterns of incidence

The two recognized patterns are familial and sporadic.

Familial
The presence of the germinal mutant gene in all cells throughout the body explains the early onset, the bilateral involvement and the increased risk of developing other malignancies, including pinealoblastoma, fibrosarcoma and osteosarcoma. As reproductive organs are affected, 50 per cent of all sperm and ova contain the germinal mutant gene and transmission to offspring is possible. Incomplete penetrance may be explained by the chance absence of the second mutation in 20 per cent of carrier individuals. The clinical behaviour and the prognosis in the familial type of retinoblastoma can be accurately predicted.

Sporadic
In the presence of one somatic mutation, the chance occurrence of a second mutation (the second 'hit') in the same cell triggers the neoplastic process. Such mutations affect the tissues of one eye only, and the retinoblastomas are usually unilateral and develop later than in those with germinal mutations. Moreover, somatic mutations are not transmitted to subsequent generations and affected individuals are not at increased risk of developing other malignancies. In contrast to those with a family history, sporadic cases overall form a heterogeneous group in which the occurrence of the neoplasm may be due to germinal or somatic mutation; the former is either new or, because of increased penetrance of the inherited condition, was not clinically manifest in previous generations. As the two types cannot be differentiated on clinical grounds, there is some uncertainty as to the prognosis.

Clinical features

Clinical features vary, but most of those affected present before the age of 3 years with leukocoria (Fig. 4.75a), strabismus or visual symptoms. Other presenting features include heterochromia, hyphaema and secondary glaucoma and, in advanced cases, orbital inflammation and proptosis due to extraocular spread. Ophthalmoscopy reveals a white intraocular mass. Small lesions may appear as intraretinal with associated dilated tortuous vessels and sometimes vitreous seeds. Endophytic growths are seen as friable masses that grow into the vitreous with the retinal vessels being lost from view as they enter the mass. Exophytic growths lead to elevation and detachment of the retina with the retinal vessels remaining visible. Growth patterns may be mixed and large retinoblastomas may fill the posterior segment (Fig. 4.75b), with details possibly being obscured by haemorrhage, retinal detachment or other secondary abnormalities. Diffuse infiltrating retinoblastomas occur in older children (6–7 years of age) and often present as a pseudohypopyon. Most retinoblastomas exhibit calcification, which is usually evident on radiological examination. CT scans are of help in determining the size and location of retinoblastomas, and can be used to detect extraocular extension. MRI scans are especially useful for optic nerve evaluation. A spontaneously regressed neoplasm may present as phthisis bulbi. Routine examination of children known to be at risk may reveal subclinical lesions.

Pathology

There is no difference in the pathology between familial and sporadic retinoblastomas. Gross examination reveals five recognizable growth patterns:

1. Endophytic where growth is from the inner surface of the retina into the vitreous. Neoplastic cells are shed and may seed into the vitreous and on to the inner surface of the retina away from the main mass.

2. Exophytic where growth is from the outer surface of the retina towards the choroid, producing elevation and detachment of the retina. Neoplastic cells escape into the subretinal space and seed on to the inner surface of the RPE, which is focally destroyed, and if there is infiltration through Bruch's membrane, cells are deposited within the choroid.

3. Mixed endophytic and exophytic where the growth pattern exhibits features of both types (Fig. 4.76a).

4. Diffuse infiltrating is the least common growth pattern, with diffuse involvement but little thickening of the retina (Fig. 4.76b). Neoplastic cells are discharged into the vitreous and seed into the anterior ocular compartments, often producing a pseudohypopyon.

5. Complete spontaneous regression occurs more commonly in retinoblastoma than in any other intraocular malignant neoplasm, and is probably due to ischaemia. A severe inflammatory response may be associated with subsequent phthisis bulbi.

Microscopic appearance

Retinoblastomas are malignant neuroblastomas that appear on microscopy to arise from any of the nucleated layers of the retina, although immunohistochemical investigations have shown them as being derived from photoreceptor (possibly cone) precursors. The neoplastic cells have large basophilic nuclei exhibiting various

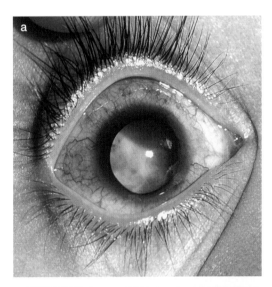

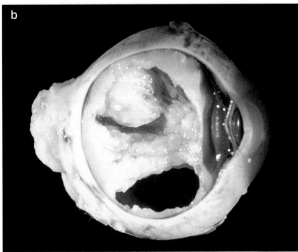

Figure 4.75 Retinoblastoma. (a) Leukocoria. (b) Eye opened anteroposteriorly showing an irregular cream-coloured mass in the posterior segment.

a

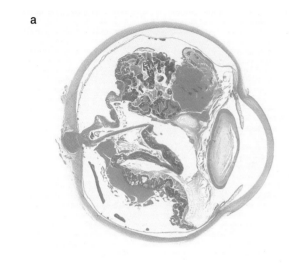

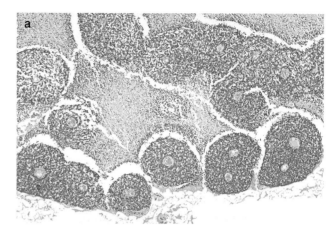

b

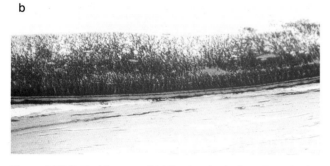

Figure 4.76 Retinoblastoma. (a) Mixed endophytic and exophytic growth patterns with extension into both the vitreous and subretinal space. (b) Diffuse infiltrating type.

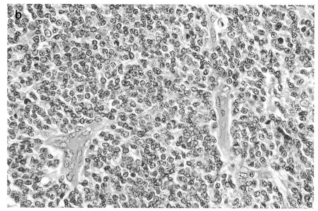

Figure 4.77 Retinoblastoma. (a) Sleeves of viable neoplastic cells arranged around blood vessels with intervening necrotic areas. (b) Undifferentiated.

shapes and numerous mitoses. Sleeves of viable cells may surround blood vessels from which they obtain their metabolic support, the more peripherally placed cells undergoing ischaemic coagulative necrosis (Fig. 4.77a). A contrasting pattern is seen when viable neoplastic cells are shed into the vitreous or subretinal space, where the peripherally placed cells derive their metabolic support from the vitreous and subretinal fluid, and it is the more central cells that undergo necrosis. Viable neoplastic cells in the vitreous and subretinal space can also become attached to the retina or the RPE. In the former case metabolic support is provided by the retinal vessels, and in the latter by the choriocapillaris. Simultaneous with neoplastic growth, a neovascular response is manifest as capillary proliferation in the neoplasm and elsewhere in the eye, particularly on the anterior iris surface. Calcification may occur in the areas of necrosis, and DNA liberated from the neoplastic cells becomes adsorbed, primarily on to the walls of blood vessels and on to the internal limiting membrane of the retina. Inflammation is minimal. Many retinoblastomas are undifferentiated (Fig. 4.77b), but varying degrees of dif-

ferentiation are characterized by the formation of rosettes, of which there are three types:

1. Flexner–Wintersteiner rosettes where a central lumen containing glycosaminoglycans is surrounded by tall cuboidal cells (Fig. 4.78a). The nuclei of these cells lie at the base (away from the lumen); the apical ends (proximal to the lumen) are held together by terminal bars and cytoplasmic processes extend into the lumen. It is considered that Flexner–Wintersteiner rosettes represent an attempt to form photoreceptor cells.

2. Homer Wright rosettes have no lumen, and the central area is occupied by a tangled mass of eosinophilic processes. They are less common than Flexner–Wintersteiner rosettes.

3. Fleurettes are foci of neoplastic cells which exhibit photoreceptor differentiation. Clusters of cells with long cytoplasmic processes project through a fenestrated membrane and assume an appearance resembling a bouquet of flowers (Fig. 4.78b). Fleurettes are seen within cytologically relatively benign areas.

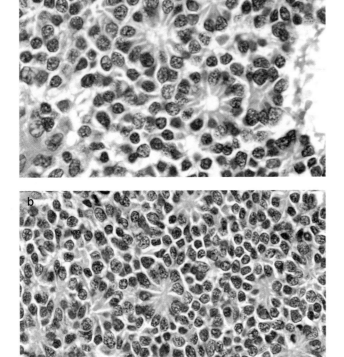

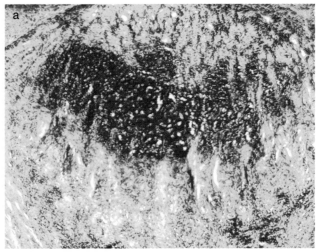

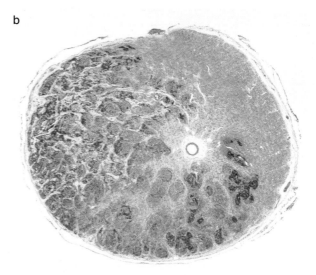

Figure 4.78 Retinoblastoma. (a) Flexner–Wintersteiner rosettes. (b) Fleurettes.

Extraocular dissemination

Direct infiltration along the optic nerve (Fig. 4.79) with extension into the brain is the most usual. If neoplastic cells also invade the soft tissues of the orbit, the orbital bones may be directly infiltrated with subsequent involvement of the paranasal sinuses, nasopharynx and cranial cavity.

Invasion of neoplastic cells into the meninges from the optic nerve with subsequent dispersion into the CSF and consequent involvement of the brain and spinal cord. This may happen even if transverse sections of the surgical cut end of the nerve are seen on histological examination to be free from infiltration.

Haematogenous spread where blood-borne metastases develop in the brain, bone and lungs.

Lymphatic spread is usually associated with conjunctival infiltration from the extraocular extension of an anteriorly situated retinoblastoma.

Figure 4.79 Retinoblastoma. (a) Longitudinal and (b) transverse section of optic nerve showing infiltration with neoplastic cells.

Prognosis

Retinoblastomas are invariably fatal if left untreated, but modern therapy has considerably improved survival. The most important prognostic factors are the extent of infiltration into the optic nerve and through the ocular coats. Choroidal invasion and the degree of differentiation are not significant prognostic factors. Bilaterality carries an unfavourable prognosis. Involvement of the brain may be due to optic nerve invasion and/or the development of an intracranial pinealoblastoma (trilateral retinoblastoma). Although those affected may survive retinoblastoma, those with germ cell mutations have a significant mortality due to other malignancies such as fibrosarcoma and osteosarcoma.

Trilateral retinoblastoma

Trilateral retinoblastoma is the association of bilateral retinoblastoma with a pinealoblastoma, a primary neoplasm of the pineal gland that may exhibit retinoblastomatous differentiation.

Retinocytoma (retinoma)

Retinocytomas are rare benign counterparts of retinoblastomas. They appear in functional eyes with clear media as comparatively small translucent grey slightly elevated retinal masses containing loops of retinal blood vessels; the retina is not detached. Opaque white calcified flecks give a cottage cheese appearance, and pigmentation results from proliferation and migration of RPE. Retinocytomas are composed of uniform cells, fleurettes are conspicuous, but mitotic activity and necrosis are absent. The origin of retinocytomas is controversial, but they are thought to be well-differentiated or benign variants of retinoblastoma. The occurrence of a retinocytoma implies the presence of the Rb1 gene mutation as in retinoblastoma.

Medulloepithelioma

Medulloepitheliomas are rare. They arise from immature neuroepithelium that resembles the medullary epithelium lining the ventricles of the brain. The site of origin is usually where the neurosensory retina transforms into the non-pigmented epithelium of the pars plana of the ciliary body, although occasionally it is at the optic nerve head. Medulloepitheliomas develop almost exclusively in childhood, and present as a unilateral lesion most often of the ciliary body. Clinical features include leukocoria, a mass in the anterior segment, poor vision and pain secondary to neovascular glaucoma. Most medulloepitheliomas are white, grey or yellow, but are sometimes heavily pigmented. They are occasionally cystic, and the cysts can become detached from the main mass and circulate in the aqueous.

Medulloepitheliomas are of two types: non-teratoid and teratoid. Non-teratoid medulloepitheliomas have a myxoid or fibrous stroma in which proliferating neuroepithelial cells form tubules and acini (Fig. 4.80a) with rosette-like structures resembling dysplastic retina in some areas. Teratoid medulloepitheliomas in addition have heterologous elements, usually cartilage (Fig. 4.80b), skeletal muscle or neural tissue, thus reflecting the totipotent capacity of the optic cup. Medulloepitheliomas can be divided into benign and malignant types according to the degree of differentiation. Local invasion with penetration of the corneoscleral coat may occur, but the metastatic death rate is low.

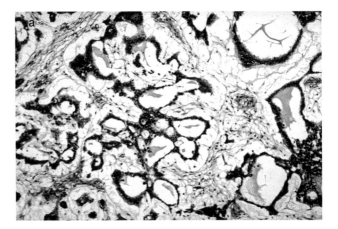

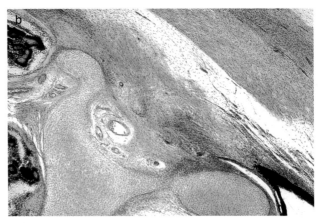

Figure 4.80 Medulloepithelioma. (a) Non-teratoid type with neuroepithelial cells forming tubules and acini. (b) Teratoid type with cartilage.

Other neuroepithelial neoplasms

Neoplasms of the iris epithelium are virtually unknown. Adenomas and adenocarcinomas of the non-pigmented and pigmented ciliary epithelium and of the RPE are extremely rare. Clinically they may all simulate melanomas, but metastases rarely develop even when, on histological grounds, malignancy is diagnosed and there is local extension outside the eye.

Vascular proliferations

Vascular proliferations can arise within the choroid and retina, but their existence in the iris and ciliary body is questionable.

Choroidal haemangioma

Choroidal haemangiomas are either diffuse and associated with the Sturge–Weber syndrome, or localized, when they are clinically often suspected as melanomas. They are composed of large blood vessels (Fig. 4.52), and the diffuse type has less well-defined margins than the localized type. Associated features include RPE atrophy, focal choroidoretinal adhesion and cystic degeneration, gliosis and detachment of the retina.

Retinal haemangioblastoma

Retinal haemangioblastomas are smooth, rounded neoplasms seen most often at the temporal periphery. They are frequently multiple, and conspicuous feeding and draining vessels are present (Fig. 4.81a,b) together with haemorrhages, exudates and retinal detachment. Bilateral involvement occurs in over 50 per cent of cases. Capillary-like vascular channels lie between large foamy cells (Fig. 4.81c) that possibly represent histiocytes, endothelial cells or astrocytes; pericytes are demonstrable, as are fenestrations between the vascular endothelial cells. Large haemangioblastomas lead to cystic degeneration of the retina, and advanced lesions can closely resemble Coats' disease. Retinal haemangioblastomas may occur in isolation, but about 25 per cent of those affected exhibit other manifestations of von Hippel–Lindau disease. VEGF is an important factor in their development.

Retinal cavernous haemangioma

Retinal cavernous haemangiomas are rare congenital vascular malformations manifest as isolated clusters of dilated vessels. They may demonstrate incompletely penetrant autosomal dominant inheritance. There is no association with the Sturge–Weber syndrome.

Retinal racemose haemangioma

Retinal racemose haemangiomas are dilated and tortuous vessels on the optic disc and surrounding retina that may occur in isolation or be part of the Wyburn–Mason syndrome. The abnormal vessels form a direct arteriovenous connection without an intervening capillary bed.

Neural proliferations

Neural proliferations include uveal neurofibromas and schwannomas, and retinal astrocytomas. Uveal neural proliferations can be clinically misdiagnosed as melanomas, while retinal astrocytomas may be mistaken for small retinoblastomas.

Uveal neurofibroma

Diffuse uveal neurofibromas particularly involve the choroid and occur in neurofibromatosis type 1.

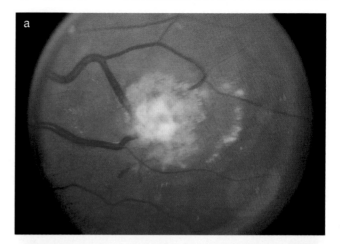

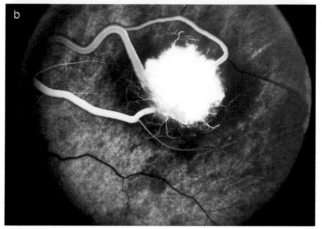

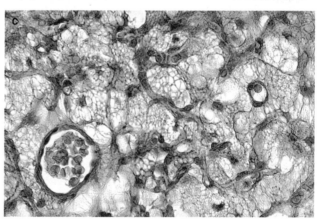

Figure 4.81 Retinal haemangioblastoma. (a) Fundus photograph. (b) Fluorescein fundus angiogram showing feeding and draining vessels. (c) Capillary-like vascular channels between large foamy cells.

Histologically they are similar to solitary neurofibromas (Fig. 4.56a) but some of the proliferating cells resemble sympathetic ganglia (Fig. 4.82). Solitary uveal neurofibromas are rare.

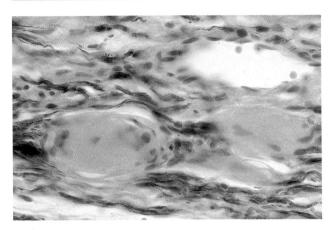

Figure 4.82 Uveal neurofibroma. Cells resembling sympathetic ganglia.

Uveal schwannoma

Uveal schwannomas are well-circumscribed and occur mainly within the ciliary body and choroid.

Retinal astrocytoma

Retinal astrocytomas are benign and, other than in tuberous sclerosis, rare. They are confined to the inner retina and may be single or multiple, but occasionally involve the optic nerve head. Initially flat and translucent, they grow to form elevated refractile yellowish masses (Fig. 4.83); some become multi-nodular or cystic and resemble mulberries. They are composed of elongated fibrous astrocytes with small oval nuclei and cytoplasmic processes that form an interlacing meshwork. Astrocytomas frequently calcify.

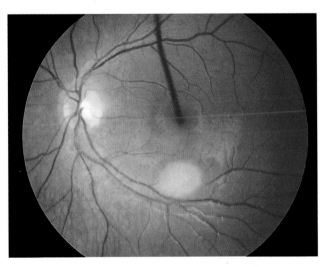

Figure 4.83 Retinal astrocytoma.

Smooth muscle proliferations

Benign smooth muscle proliferations (leiomyomas) arise most often from the ciliary muscle and present as ciliary body masses. Origin from smooth muscle in the iris is also a possibility, although it is now realized that many iris lesions that were in the past described as 'leiomyomas' are probably spindle cell melanocytic proliferations. Leiomyomas can also develop from smooth muscle in the walls of blood vessels. Malignant neoplasms of smooth muscle (leiomyosarcomas) in the eye are extremely rare.

LYMPHOPROLIFERATIVE LESIONS, FIBROBLASTIC AND HISTIOCYTIC PROLIFERATIONS, PLASMA CELL ACCUMULATIONS AND LEUKAEMIC DEPOSITS

Lymphoproliferative lesions

Lymphoproliferative lesions are either lymphomas or reactive lymphoid hyperplasias. Immunochemical investigations to differentiate the various types of cells involved are always necessary. Some lesions are neither obviously neoplastic nor reactive, and are best referred to as lymphocytic lesions of indeterminate type (atypical lymphoid hyperplasia, grey-zone lymphoma).

Lymphoma

Lymphomas are malignant neoplasms of the lymphoreticular system. There are two types: Hodgkin lymphoma and non-Hodgkin lymphoma (NHL). The cell of origin of Hodgkin lymphoma is a B cell. NHLs are derived from T cells, B cells and null cells. Lymphomas form a wide spectrum of disease. Classification is complex and based on the overall appearance (diffuse or nodular) and predominant cell type. The currently used classification is the WHO-REAL (World Health Organization-Revised European/American lymphoma) classification (2000). In general terms, lymphomas are either of low-grade malignancy and indolent (Fig. 4.84a) or of high-grade malignancy and aggressive.

Reactive lymphoid hyperplasia

Reactive lymphoid hyperplasia is a proliferation of both B cells and T cells with germinal follicle formation (immature lymphoid cells are present at the centre of the follicle and mature cells at the periphery ➥ Fig. 4.84b). Other cells such as plasma cells and histiocytes are often seen, and vascular endothelial proliferation is common. Lymphoma may subsequently develop. The

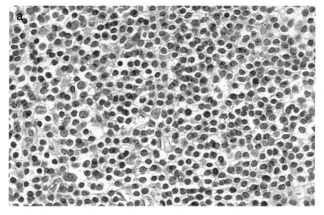

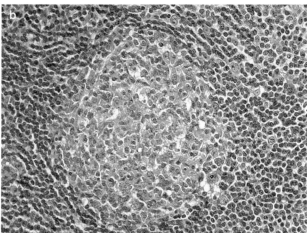

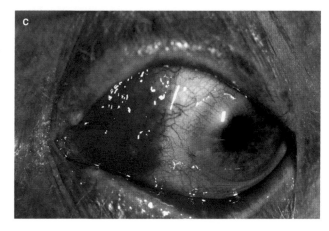

Figure 4.84 Lymphoproliferative lesions. (a) Low-grade non-Hodgkin lymphoma. (b) Reactive lymphoid hyperplasia; centrally situated lymphoid follicle. (c) Conjunctival lesion.

initiating stimulus to reactive lymphoid hyperplasia is not known.

Ophthalmic manifestations of lymphoproliferative lesions

Lymphoproliferative lesions involve the conjunctiva, orbit, uvea and retina.

Conjunctiva

Most lymphoproliferative lesions in the conjunctiva are reactive lymphoid hyperplasias. They appear as smooth salmon-pink swellings (Fig. 4.84c) and, as they occur in the subepithelial connective tissue, they move freely over the surface of the globe. Conjunctival lymphomas are usually B cell lymphomas, and possibly arise from MALT. Conjunctival involvement in systemic lymphoma is unusual.

Orbit

Lymphoproliferative lesions in the orbit are mostly lymphomas and may be a manifestation or the presenting feature of systemic disease, or lesions confined to the orbit. Hodgkin lymphoma rarely if ever presents in the orbit, although the orbit may be involved in systemic disease. Most orbital lymphomas are diffuse NHLs of B cell type and of low-grade malignancy. Those affected are usually over 50 years of age and, other than in parts of Africa where Burkitt's lymphoma is endemic, orbital lymphoma is uncommon in children. The onset is usually insidious, proptosis is moderate, disorders of ocular motility are slight and only occasionally is there loss of vision. The superior orbit is the site most often affected, with some lesions being derived from lacrimal gland-associated MALT. The lesions, which can often be palpated through the lid as firm or rubbery masses, are almost always unifocal, and mould to the orbital bones, the globe and the optic nerve to give the characteristic straight lines, arc-like contours and angulated patterns seen radiologically.

Uvea

Lymphoproliferative lesions in the uvea are usually reactive lymphoid hyperplasias and may be clinically indistinguishable from diffuse melanomas.

Retina

Lymphoproliferative lesions in the retina are associated with primary lymphoma in the CNS. The retinal involvement may be the initial and only manifestation. Uveitis, infiltration of the retina and optic nerve head, mound-like elevations on the RPE and secondary glaucoma – the GUN syndrome (glaucoma–uveitis–neurological signs) – precede CNS symptoms. Haemorrhagic necrosis is extensive, and large neoplastic B lymphocytes infiltrate the retina, vitreous, subretinal space and optic nerve head. T lymphocytes infiltrate the choroid as an inflammatory reaction. Cytological study of vitreous aspirates, CSF and biopsies of retina or brain are helpful in establishing the diagnosis.

Fibroblastic and histiocytic proliferations

Fibroblastic and histiocytic proliferations include fibrous histiocytoma, nodular fasciitis, xanthelasma, juvenile xanthogranuloma, sinus histiocytosis with massive lymphadenopathy, and Langerhans cell histiocytosis.

Fibrous histiocytoma (fibrous xanthoma)

Fibrous histiocytomas arise in soft tissue. Of uncertain histogenesis, they occur in the skin and orbit and can be benign, locally aggressive or frankly malignant. They involve the superior aspect of the orbit, and the symptoms and signs are those of a space-occupying lesion. A well-circumscribed mass is present, and microscopy shows spindle-shaped fibroblasts and lipid-containing histiocytes. A characteristic storiform pattern (collections of cells twisted about a central focus) is seen (Fig. 4.85). Aggression and malignancy are assessed by the degree of mitotic activity, cellular pleomorphism and necrosis. Erdheim–Chester disease is a variant of fibrous histiocytoma in which the histiocytic component predominates and the lung, heart, bones and retroperitoneum are involved.

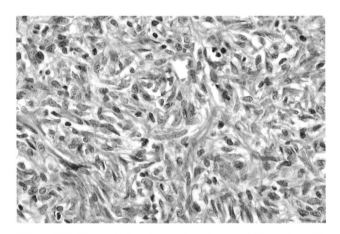

Figure 4.85 Fibrous histiocytoma. Fibroblasts and histiocytes with the suggestion of a storiform pattern.

Nodular fasciitis (pseudosarcomatous fasciitis)

Nodular fasciitis is a well-circumscribed benign proliferation of plump fibroblasts (Fig. 4.86) with the cells and collagen being arranged in a storiform pattern as in fibrous histiocytoma. It may be confused clinically with an embryonal sarcoma.

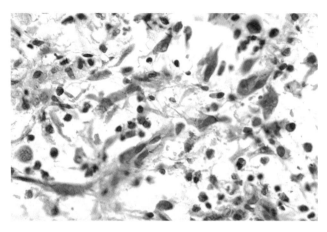

Figure 4.86 Nodular fasciitis. Proliferation of plump fibroblasts accompanied by an inflammatory cell infiltrate.

Xanthelasma

Xanthelasmas are histiocytic lesions that may be manifestations of hyperlipidaemia. They are the commonest xanthoma of the lids and are seen usually in elderly females, where they appear as soft yellow plaques near the inner canthus. The upper lids are initially affected, but eventually all four may be involved (Fig. 4.87a). Microscopy shows lipid-laden histiocytes in the dermis, mainly in relation to blood vessels and epidermal-associated structures (Fig. 4.87b,c).

Juvenile xanthogranuloma

Juvenile xanthogranulomas are histiocytic lesions that occur in infancy. They are characterized by one or more cutaneous nodules and, less often, by lesions in the conjunctiva, orbit and anterior uvea. The head, neck and upper trunk are the sites of predilection, and the lids may be involved. The cutaneous lesions are small, pink and nodular. Involvement of the iris may result in spontaneous hyphaema. Microscopy reveals lipid-containing polygonal and spindle-shaped histiocytes and multinucleate Touton and foreign body giant cells (Fig. 4.88); other inflammatory cells, particularly eosinophils, may also be seen. There is no underlying lipid abnormality.

Sinus histiocytosis with massive lymphadenopathy (Rosai–Dorfman syndrome)

Sinus histiocytosis with massive lymphadenopathy is a proliferation of the sinusoidal cells of lymph nodes. The condition is more common in Africans than in other races, and children are more often affected than adults. The lymph nodes, particularly the cervical chain, are

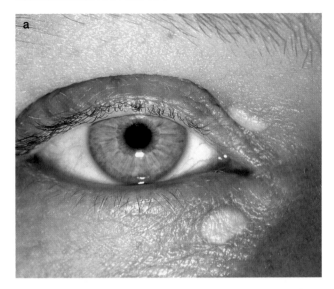

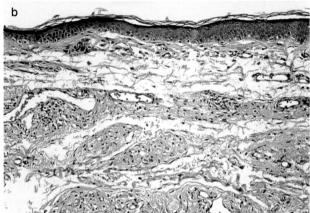

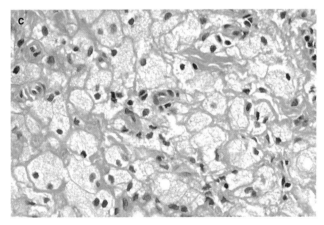

Figure 4.87 Xanthelasma. (a) Lid lesions. (b) Aggregates of lipid-laden histiocytes in the dermis of the skin in relation to blood vessels. (c) A sheet of lipid-laden histiocytes.

usually but not invariably involved, and deposits may be present elsewhere, including one or both orbits with resultant proptosis. Microscopy reveals lymphocytes, plasma cells and histiocytes; the latter have vesicular

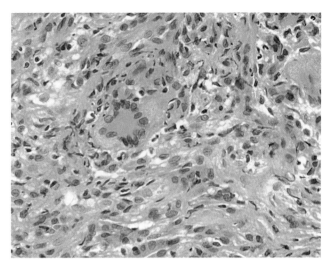

Figure 4.88 Juvenile xanthogranuloma. An infiltrate of inflammatory cells including histiocytes and Touton giant cells.

nuclei and abundant cytoplasm and may contain engulfed lymphocytes and plasma cells (cytophagocytosis – Fig. 4.89).

Langerhans cell histiocytosis

Langerhans cell histiocytosis includes eosinophilic granuloma, Hand–Schüller–Christian disease and Letterer–Siwe disease, which are all proliferations of Langerhans cells. Occurring in children, the skin, viscera and lymph nodes are all affected. Orbital involvement may result in signs similar to those of dacryoadenitis, but there is radiological evidence of irregular lytic lesions of the bones of the superotemporal orbital rim. Biopsy reveals Langerhans cells, histiocytes and multinucleate giant

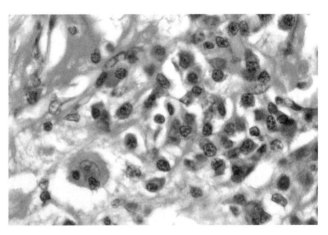

Figure 4.89 Sinus histiocytosis with massive lymphadenopathy. Lymphocytes and a histiocyte (lower left) exhibiting cytophagocytosis.

cells, eosinophils, neutrophils, lymphocytes and plasma cells.

Plasma cell accumulations

Plasmacytoma

Plasmacytomas are accumulations of plasma cells (Fig. 4.90). Solitary lesions may occur in the conjuctiva and orbit and are usually benign. Malignant plasmacytomas are a manifestation of multiple myeloma.

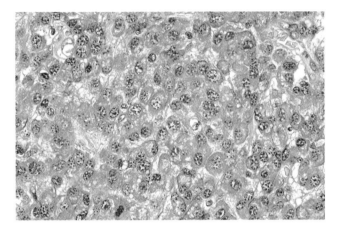

Figure 4.90 Plasmacytoma. A diffuse plasma cell infiltrate.

Leukaemic deposits

Leukaemic deposits may occur throughout the body. Ophthalmic tissues involved include the orbit, uvea and retina.

Orbit

Deposits from granulocytic leukaemias are more common than those from lymphocytic leukaemias and may occur in the absence of blood and bone marrow involvement, possibly being the first sign of the underlying disorder. They are termed granulocytic sarcomas, and their green colour, which led to the traditional term 'chloroma', is due to the presence of myeloperoxidase in the granulocytes.

Uvea and retina

Atypical immature leukocytes may pack the blood vessels of the uvea and retina, and perivascular cellular infiltration may give rise to the formation of a mass.

SYNDROMES ASSOCIATED WITH DISORDERS OF CELL AND TISSUE GROWTH

A number of syndromes are associated with extra- and intraocular disorders of cell and tissue growth. Foremost among them are the phakomatoses, but others include syndromes involving the skin, conjunctiva and RPE.

The phakomatoses

The phakomatoses are a group of disorders characterized by the presence of widespread malformations involving the CNS, eyes and skin. They can be divided into those conditions comprising mainly mesodermal vascular lesions (von Hippel–Lindau disease, Sturge–Weber syndrome, Wyburn–Mason syndrome) and those that are predominantly neuroectodermal dysplasias (neurofibromatosis types 1 and 2, tuberous sclerosis). Other than the Sturge–Weber syndrome, all are autosomal dominant.

von Hippel–Lindau disease

von Hippel–Lindau (VHL) disease is characterized by haemangioblastomas involving the CNS and retina, other neoplasms, and cysts of the viscera. The condition is inherited as a partially penetrant autosomal dominant disorder and the VHL gene, which has been mapped to chromosome 3 (3p25-p24), is an anti-oncogene thought to regulate the production of VEGF. Like other phakomatoses, many cases are sporadic and may represent new mutations or a non-inherited form of the disease.

CNS and ophthalmic lesions

Haemangioblastomas of the CNS and retina are characteristic. In the CNS they usually occur in the cerebellum, and are found less frequently in the medulla, pons and upper spinal cord. The clinical features depend on the site affected, but are usually those of a posterior fossa lesion with or without cerebellar dysfunction.

Visceral lesions

Congenital cysts may be present in the pancreas, suprarenal glands and kidneys. Phaeochromocytomas may arise from the adrenal medulla and sympathetic chain, and there is an increased incidence of renal cell carcinoma.

Sturge–Weber syndrome (encephalotrigeminal angiomatosis)

The Sturge–Weber syndrome is characterized by angiomatous malformations (usually unilateral) involving the face, meninges and eye. This association arises because of the continuity of the embryonic vascular supply of the telencephalon, the eye and overlying skin. The disorder differs from the other phakomatoses in that there is no well-defined pattern of inheritance. Naevus flammeus, contralateral epilepsy, mental retardation and ipsilateral glaucoma are common features.

Naevus flammeus

Naevus flammeus is the characteristic skin lesion, and involves the first and/or second division of the trigeminal nerve (the area supplied by the third division is less frequently affected). Hypertrophy of other tissues may occur in the involved areas.

CNS involvement

The intracranial vascular lesion is an anomaly that takes the form of a capillary or venous malformation confined to the meninges and is most frequently situated over the posterior half of the cerebral hemisphere on the same side as the naevus flammeus. The underlying cerebral cortex may be poorly developed, and calcification may give rise to a tram-line radiological appearance. The clinical features of CNS involvement include mental retardation, epilepsy, hemiparesis and hemianopia. It is said that the CNS is only involved if the naevus flammeus affects the territory of the first division of the trigeminal nerve.

Ophthalmic involvement

Glaucoma develops in 30 per cent of cases and is associated with ipsilateral conjunctival and lid involvement. Although the pathogenesis of the glaucoma is obscure in many cases, in some instances it has been attributed to a congenital anomaly of the drainage angle or elevated episcleral venous pressure caused by the disordered haemodynamics induced by the vascular malformations. In 60 per cent of cases the onset of the glaucoma is early enough in life to result in buphthalmos, although even in the absence of glaucoma the eye may be enlarged.

Choroidal haemangiomas occur in 40 per cent of cases. They are invariably solitary and poorly defined flat lesions that can occupy a large area and give the clinical appearance of a 'tomato ketchup' fundus. They slowly enlarge, and may cause degeneration or serous detachment of the overlying retina.

Other lesions include colobomas, ectopia lentis and iris heterochromia, with the darker iris ipsilateral to the skin lesion.

Wyburn–Mason syndrome

The Wyburn–Mason syndrome comprises malformations of the retinal and ipsilateral middle cerebral vessels. In some instances a continuous skein of vessels extends from the mid-brain to the optic nerve and orbit. The major features are diminished visual acuity and neurological manifestations due to the space-occupying nature of the lesions or haemorrhage therefrom. Orbital involvement may result in proptosis.

Neurofibromatosis type 1 (von Recklinghausen's disease)

Neurofibromatosis type 1 (NF1) is the most usual form of neurofibromatosis and the commonest of the phakomatoses, affecting approximately 1:3500 persons. It is inherited as an autosomal dominant, but there is irregular penetrance and variable expressivity. Approximately half of the cases are sporadic because of the high incidence of mutation in the NF1 gene, which is located in the centromeric region of chromosome 17 (17q11.2). The gene is very large and embedded within it are several smaller genes, one of which encodes for a protein similar to the GTPase-activating protein (GAP). GAP normally interacts with the protein product of the ras oncogene (ras is abbreviated from rat sarcoma, and the ras oncogene has cyclonucleotide binding activity that disrupts intracellular signalling) and dampens growth stimulatory signals. NF1 may result therefore from reduced anti-oncogene function. The genetic influence falls mainly on the sheath tissues of the peripheral nerves, to a lesser extent on the supporting glia of the CNS, and least often on the leptomeninges. The variable expressivity of the NF1 gene results in a variety of manifestations. Clinical diagnosis is based on the presence of multiple cutaneous neurofibromas or more than six café-au-lait spots. Characteristic features are multiple and often disfiguring neurofibromas, other lesions of neural crest origin (schwannomas, meningiomas, cerebral gliomas, juvenile optic nerve gliomas, phaeochromocytomas), and lesions of the skin (café-au-lait spots, axillary freckles), uvea (Lisch nodules) and skeleton (spheno-orbital encephaloceles, congenital bone cysts, cortical thinning of long bones, facial hemiatrophy, acquired scoliosis).

Neurofibromas are multiple and the commonest manifestation of the disease. They may develop anywhere along the course of the peripheral and autonomic nerves, but do not occur on purely motor nerves. Plexiform neuro-fibromas involve the larger peripheral nerves and are diagnostic of NF1. Involvement of the lid gives the characteristic S-shaped deformity, which may be associated with glaucoma in the ipsilateral eye. Elephantiasis nervosa results from an overgrowth of soft tissue around affected nerve trunks, and may cause the skin to hang in thick redundant folds. Neurofibromas of the skin are small soft nodules or pedunculated lesions (mollusca fibrosa) that may be numerous and widespread. Neurofibromas of the choroid are diffuse and seen clinically as areas of thickening and hyperpigmentation. Neurofibromatous involvement of intraosseous nerves may result in the destruction or hypertrophy of bone. Three to five per cent of neurofibromas become malignant.

Café-au-lait spots are ovoid areas of skin pigmentation with their axes in the direction of the dermatome. They are common in normal persons, but occur with increased frequency in those with neurofibromatosis. Histologically they resemble lentigo.

Axillary freckles (ephelides) usually become evident at puberty.

Lisch nodules are iris naevi and are present in nearly all adults with NF1.

Neurofibromatosis type 2

Neurofibromatosis type 2 (NF2) is much less frequent than NF1 and affects only 1 : 50 000 persons. In spite of superficial similarities and being inherited as an autosomal dominant, it is unrelated to NF1. The NF2 gene is located in the middle of chromosome 22 (22q11.21-q11.23). Bilateral acoustic neuromas (schwannomas) are the commonest feature, but NF2 can be diagnosed if a unilateral acoustic neuroma is present together with two of the following: neurofibroma, juvenile glioma of the optic nerve, meningioma, schwannoma or juvenile posterior subcapsular cataract.

Tuberous sclerosis

Tuberous sclerosis is characterized by a triad of epilepsy, mental deficiency and skin lesions. It is inherited as a variably expressed autosomal dominant disorder with low penetrance and, like NF1, new mutations account for half the cases. It is genetically heterogeneous and two loci have been assigned to variants of the condition: one on chromosome 9 (9q33-q34) and the other on chromosome 16 (16p13). Whatever the molecular genetic basis, the lesions result from disordered migration and maturation of neuroectoderm. The condition occurs in 1 : 30–60 000 live births. The commonest presenting feature is epilepsy, which may be diagnosed as infantile spasms. Other features appear later in childhood, and death is common in early to middle adulthood due to CNS involvement. Characteristic findings include lesions of the CNS (astrocytomas), viscera (angiomyolipomas of the kidney, rhabdomyomas of the heart), skin (angiofibromas, ashleaf spots) and eye (retinal astrocytomas, atypical colobomas, hypomelanotic spots of the iris and fundus).

Astrocytomas are the most characteristic lesions of tuberous sclerosis. Cortical and paraventricular astrocytomas account for the epilepsy and mental deficiency, and for other cranial abnormalities such as hydrocephalus. They are discrete firm nodules that resemble a peeled potato (hence tuberous) and consist of large astrocytes and areas of dense gliosis. Retinal astrocytomas develop during the first 2 years of life and are a valuable diagnostic sign.

Angiofibromas are the most characteristic skin lesions. They are slow growing, present as papules on the face and forehead, and usually become evident after 2 years of age. They have been termed 'adenoma sebaceum' because of their superficial resemblance to acne rosacea; this nomenclature is erroneous as they are neither adenomas nor related to sebaceous tissue.

Ashleaf spots are hypopigmented skin lesions. They are present in 80 per cent of cases and involve the trunk, limbs and scalp. Their name is derived from their oval shape. Like the café-au-lait spots of NF1, they are orientated with their long axes in the direction of the dermatome.

Shagreen patches are diffuse thickenings of the skin over the trunk and buttocks seen in adolescence and adult life – shagreen is a rough untanned leather or sharkskin. They occur in 40 per cent of cases, and represent dense plaques of collagen.

Café-au-lait spots and mollusca fibrosa (similar to those of NF1) are common in tuberous sclerosis, and indicate a possible overlap in the pathogenesis of the two conditions.

Other syndromes

Gorlin–Goltz syndrome

The Gorlin–Goltz syndrome is characterized by multiple basal cell carcinomas involving the nose, lids, cheeks, trunk, neck and arms, associated with cysts of the jaw (odontogenic keratocysts), skeletal abnormalities (most commonly bifid ribs), mental retardation and endocrine abnormalities (ovarian cysts, testicular disorders). Other findings include scoliosis, short fourth metacarpals, calcification of the dura and, occasionally, cerebellar medulloblastoma. A variety of ocular and periocular findings include prominence of the supraorbital ridges, hypertelorism, dystopia canthorum, internal strabismus, glaucoma, congenital cataract, colobomas of the choroid and optic nerve, and congenital blindness. Basal cell carcinoma in children may represent a forme fruste of the syndrome, which equally involves males and females and is inherited as an autosomal dominant disorder with high penetrance and varying degrees of expressivity.

Muir–Torre syndrome

The Muir–Torre syndrome is also autosomal dominant, and consists of sebaceous lesions (hyperplasias, adenomas, carcinomas), other cutaneous lesions (keratoacanthomas, basal cell carcinomas with sebaceous differentiation, squamous cell carcinomas), and low-grade visceral carcinomas (especially of the colon but also of the stomach, duodenum, rectum, larynx, bladder, ovary and uterus).

Cowden's disease

Cowden's disease is characterized by multiple trichilemmomas associated in females with a high incidence (50 per cent) of carcinoma of the breast, frequently bilateral. It is inherited as an autosomal dominant trait.

Goldenhar's syndrome

Goldenhar's syndrome is a bilateral condition characterized by epibulbar choristomas, accessory auricular appendages, aural fistulae, vertebral anomalies, and hypoplasia of the soft and bony tissues of the face. The condition occurs in 1 : 3000 live births. It is not inherited, but may occasionally be related to the maternal intake of a teratogenic agent in the first trimester of pregnancy.

Gardner's and Turcot's syndromes

Atypical multifocal bilateral CHRPE (but not typical unifocal unilateral CHRPE) is associated with some familial colonic adenomatous polyposis/carcinoma syndromes. Gardner's syndrome is autosomal dominant and characterized by the presence of CHRPE with colonic adenomatous polyposis, bone cysts and soft tissue hamartomas. Almost all affected individuals eventually develop colonic adenocarcinoma. Turcot's syndrome is Gardner's syndrome with the addition of neuroepithelial neoplasms of the CNS. Gardner's syndrome, Turcot's

syndrome and autosomal dominant colonic adenomatous polyposis without extracolonic features are thought to be phenotypic expressions of different mutations of the same gene with a chromosomal locus of 5q21-q22. The site of mutation within the gene correlates with the presence or absence of CHRPE lesions which, when present (approximately 60 per cent of cases of familial colonic adenomatous polyposis), are useful clinical markers for at-risk individuals.

SECONDARY NEOPLASMS

Secondary neoplasms may involve the lids, conjunctiva, orbit and uvea. They result either from infiltration by a local malignancy or from the spread of a malignant neoplasm from a distal site.

Local infiltration

Neoplasms that locally infiltrate the conjunctiva and orbit include basal cell carcinomas of the lid, intraocular melanomas and retinoblastomas, and malignancies of the nasopharynx and paranasal sinuses.

Metastases

Metastatic deposits of neoplasms occur in the lids, orbit and uvea. They may be the initial manifestation of non-ocular cancer, and in some instances a primary neoplasm is never discovered. By far the commonest primary sites are the lung in men and the breast in women (Fig. 4.91a, 4.91b), but other primary sites include the gastrointestinal and urogenital tracts (Fig. 4.91c) and the thyroid. The manifestations of metastatic neoplasms vary according to the site affected.

Lids

There may be widespread involvement with induration of lid tissues, or alternatively solitary nodules may develop. These nodules can be clinically misdiagnosed as chalazions or other apparently innocent lesions, and the true nature of the underlying pathology is only revealed by histological examination of a biopsy.

Orbit

Proptosis is the usual sign of a secondary orbital neoplasm, but metastatic scirrhous carcinoma of the breast, because of its contractile fibrous component, often results in enophthalmos.

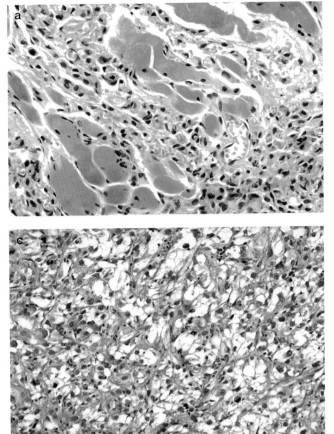

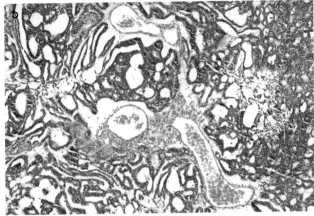

Figure 4.91 Metastatic carcinoma. (a) Undifferentiated neoplasm; polyhedral cells infiltrating musculature of lid (primary breast carcinoma). (b) Adenocarcinoma infiltrating uvea (primary breast carcinoma). (c) Malignant clear cells infiltrating uvea (primary renal carcinoma).

Uvea

Metastatic carcinoma in the uvea is more common than primary melanoma, and the posterior segment is more frequently involved than the anterior. Features include loss of vision and ocular pain due to secondary glaucoma, but the clinical manifestations vary according to the location and size of the lesions and any secondary effects that may develop. Metastatic neoplasms are typically flat, diffuse and often multiple, although on occasions they may be solitary and ovoid.

Chapter 5

Degenerations, dystrophies and deposits

Introduction

Degenerations

Degenerations of the conjunctiva and corneoscleral coat
    Pinguecula and pterygium
    Vogt's white limbal girdle
    Terrien's marginal degeneration
    Spheroidal degeneration
    Salzmann's nodular degeneration
    Corneal keloid
    Cornea guttata
    Senile scleral plaque
Ectasias and staphylomas
    Keratoconus
    Keratoglobus
    Pellucid marginal degeneration
    Myopia
Degenerations of the lens
    Ageing of the lens
    Cataracts
    Abnormalities of lens capsule
    Abnormalities of lens epithelium
    Abnormalities of lens substance
Degenerations of the zonule
Degenerations of the vitreous
    Syneresis
    Asteroid hyalosis
    Synchisis scintillans
Degenerations at the vitreoretinal interface
    Vitreoretinal traction
    Vitreoschisis
    Posterior vitreous detachment
    Lattice degeneration
    Retinal breaks
    Retinal detachment

    Premacular gliosis
    Macular hole
Degenerations of the peripheral retina
    Cystoid degeneration
    Degenerative retinoschisis
Age-related degenerations of the macula and posterior pole
    Photoreceptors and the RPE
    Bruch's membrane
    Sub-RPE deposits
    Age-related macular degeneration
Non-age-related degenerations of the RPE/Bruch's membrane
    Central serous choroidoretinopathy
    Angioid streaks
Age-related peripheral degenerations of the RPE/Bruch's membrane

Dystrophies

Corneal dystrophies
  Anterior dystrophies
    Epithelial basement membrane dystrophy
    Meesmann's juvenile epithelial dystrophy
    Reis–Bückler's dystrophy
  Stromal dystrophies
    Granular dystrophy
    Lattice dystrophy
    Molecular genetics
    Other corneal dystrophies with amyloid deposition
    Macular dystrophy
    Schnyder's central crystalline dystrophy
    Bietti's crystalline corneoretinal dystrophy
  Endothelial dystrophies
    Fuchs' endothelial dystrophy
    Posterior polymorphous dystrophy

Congenital hereditary endothelial dystrophy
Scleral dystrophies
Retinal and choroidal dystrophies
   Genetics
   Classification
   Neurosensory retinal dysfunctions and dystrophies
      Müller cell dystrophy
      Photoreceptor dysfunctions and dystrophies
      Stationary rod dysfunctions
      Stationary cone dysfunctions
      Progressive photoreceptor dystrophies
      Photoreceptor/RPE dystrophies
      RPE/Bruch's membrane dystrophies
      Choroidoretinal dystrophies

Deposits

Metals, metallic salts and related compounds
   Calcium
      Band keratopathy
      Anterior crocodile shagreen
      Diffuse corneal calcification
      Calcium oxalate deposition
   Iron
      Corneal epithelial iron lines
      Siderosis
      Haemochromatosis
   Copper
      Chalcosis
   Silver
   Gold

Corneal tattoo pigment
Mercury
Blood pigments
   Blood staining of the cornea
   Haemosiderosis bulbi
Aromatic amino-acid derivatives
   The melanins
      Ephelis
      Diffuse melanosis of the skin
      Secondary melanosis of the conjunctiva
      Melanin deposition not associated with
         melanocytic activity
   Ochronotic pigment
      Alkaptonuria
      Exogenous ochronosis
Amyloid
   Amyloid fibrillary protein
   Amyloid P
   Physicochemical characteristics of amyloid
      Staining and light microscopy
      Ultrastructure
      Immunohistochemistry
   Amyloidosis
      Ophthalmic amyloidosis
Lipid
      Corneal arcus – senilis and juvenilis
      Lipid keratopathy
Cholesterol, paraproteins, uric acid and cystine
      Crystalline keratopathy
Hexosylceramides and drugs
      Vortex keratopathy

INTRODUCTION

Degenerations, dystrophies and deposits are considered together because of considerable overlap between degenerations and dystrophies, and because deposits are sometimes a feature of both.

DEGENERATIONS

A degenerative disorder is one in which progressive and permanent cellular or tissue dysfunction ultimately results in cell death and loss of specialized function. Degenerative changes may be primary or secondary. Primary degenerations progress in the absence of associated disease processes and are a major cause of morbidity in the elderly. They occur throughout the eye, and the deposition of endogenous substances, as in age-related macular degeneration, is often a feature. Some primary degenerations have an inherited component in their aetiology. Secondary degenerations are associated with other disease processes such as inflammation and neoplasia.

DEGENERATIONS OF THE CONJUNCTIVA AND CORNEOSCLERAL COAT

Conjunctival and corneal degenerations may be unilateral or bilateral. Conjunctival degenerations occur at any age and usually affect the interpalpebral area, while corneal degenerations often present later in life at the periphery and spread to involve central areas. Scleral degenerations comprise increased thickness and rigidity and are frequently age-related.

Pinguecula and pterygium

Pingueculae and pterygia are clinically distinct but have similar histological features and pathogenesis. A pinguecula is a localized elevated yellowish-white lesion of the bulbar conjunctiva in the interpalpebral fissure close to the nasal and/or temporal limbus, while a pterygium is a horizontally orientated triangular sheet of fibrovascular tissue, the apex of which invades the cornea. A pterygium usually occurs on the nasal side with its base originating from the interpalpebral bulbar conjunctiva and appears as an elevated fleshy mass that can be freely moved over the sclera. Unlike a pinguecula, a pterygium is progressive and may cause visual loss due to corneal involvement. Recurrence following surgical excision is not

infrequent. Progressive lesions are richly vascular, but at any stage growth may cease and the lesions become flat and apparently less vascular. Long-standing pterygia may be associated with an arcuate line of iron deposition (Stocker's line) in the superficial cornea at the apex.

The histological features of pingueculae and pterygia are similar. Hyalinization of subepithelial collagen is associated with a variable amount of elastotic degeneration, as evidenced by abnormal curled fibres on light microscopy (Fig. 5.1). Abnormal curled fibres are particularly well demonstrated with elastic stains, although this reaction is not abolished by the enzyme elastase. Some lesions exhibit deposits of amorphous material and calcium. Elastotic degeneration may sometimes be histologically evident in clinically normal conjunctiva. If the cornea is involved, fragmentation and partial destruction of Bowman's layer may be evident. The main histological difference between a pinguecula and a pterygium is that the latter is more vascular. The epithelium overlying pingueculae and pterygia may become atrophic, hypertrophic or hyperplastic, or may even develop dysplastic and *in situ* neoplastic changes (intraepithelial neoplasia), but associated infiltrating

a

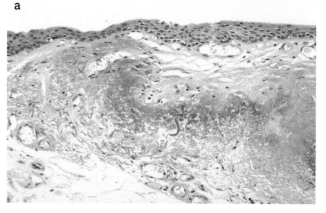

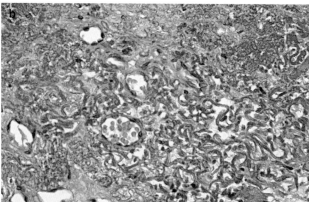

Figure 5.1 Pterygium. Elastotic degeneration of collagen in the vascularized subepithelial conjunctival stroma. (a) Low magnification. (b) High magnification.

malignancy (squamous cell carcinoma) is rare. Conjunctival drying, chronic irritation and the effects of radiation may collectively lead to the degenerative changes which resemble actinic degeneration of the dermis of the skin; pingueculae and pterygia are associated with a warm dry climate, a dusty environment and exposure to UV light.

Pseudopterygium

Pseudopterygia are not degenerations, but are considered here because of their name. They are folds of conjunctiva fixed only by their apices to the cornea, and occur secondary to corneal disease such as peripheral ulceration and degeneration. Subepithelial elastotic degeneration is not a feature.

Vogt's white limbal girdle

Vogt's white limbal girdle is a common harmless age-related peripheral primary corneal degeneration characterized by an opacity consisting of fine crescentic white lines extending irregularly from the medial and temporal limbal regions. Two types are defined according to the presence (Type I) or absence (Type II) of a clear interval between the girdle and the limbus. Type II is the commoner, and exhibits subepithelial elastotic degenerative changes similar to those of pingueculae and pterygia. Type I limbal girdle is possibly early calcific band keratopathy.

Terrien's marginal degeneration

Terrien's marginal degeneration is an uncommon primary corneal degeneration of unknown aetiology. It is usually bilateral but often asymmetric, and is seen mostly in middle-aged or elderly males in whom it slowly progresses over the course of years. Although often asymptomatic, vision may be seriously affected by irregular astigmatism and, rarely, perforation. The condition starts superiorly as a marginal opacification and progresses to stromal thinning, but is separated from the limbus by a clear zone. The epithelium remains intact, but a yellow border of lipid is present at the advancing edge. Circumferential spread is associated with superficial vascularization and occasionally the formation of pseudopterygia. The peripheral corneal thinning and the intact epithelium can be confirmed histologically, and an irregular Bowman's layer is associated with a mild inflammatory cell infiltrate of the superficial stroma. The condition may result from the activity of histiocytes, which appear to phagocytose collagen precursors, stromal ground substances and possibly lipid.

Circulating immune complexes have not been demonstrated.

Spheroidal degeneration (climatic droplet keratopathy, Labrador keratopathy)

Spheroidal degeneration of the cornea is related to climatic conditions, there being a strong association with UV-B light exposure. It occurs usually in men who spend their working life outdoors. Commencing in the periphery and spreading centrally, amber-coloured subepithelial oil-like droplets or spheroidal granules appear in the interpalpebral fissure. These can spread to the conjunctiva and may be associated with pingueculae. Spheroidal degeneration can also occur as a secondary change in absolute glaucoma, phthisis bulbi and in various chronic corneal conditions including post-traumatic scars and lattice dystrophy. Varying-sized deposits are seen on histological examination to replace Bowman's layer and also lie in the anterior stroma (Fig. 5.2). In unstained sections the deposits autofluoresce, but the proteinaceous material of which they are composed has not been identified and its source of origin is unclear. Electron microscopy suggests that the deposits are extracellular and lie in relation to collagen fibrils.

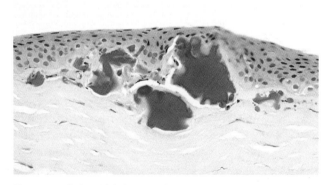

Figure 5.2 Spheroidal degeneration. Irregular proteinaceous deposits (dark red) in the anterior stroma and replacing Bowman's layer.

Salzmann's nodular degeneration

Salzmann's nodular degeneration is manifest as multiple bluish-white superficial nodules, usually in the mid-peripheral cornea (Fig. 5.3). Most of those affected are elderly women and are asymptomatic, although some may develop epithelial erosion or decreased vision. Predisposing factors include inflammatory diseases, epithelial basement membrane dystrophy, contact lens wear, keratoconus and corneal surgery. The nodules

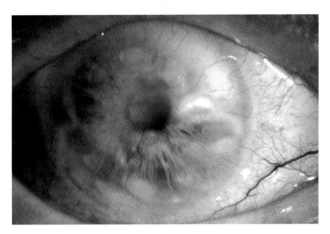

Figure 5.3 Salzmann's nodular degeneration.

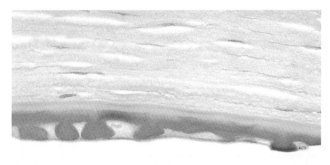

Figure 5.4 Cornea guttata. Multiple wart-like excrescences of Descemet's membrane; endothelial cells are absent. PAS stain.

are areas of hyalinized collagenous tissue lying between the epithelium and Bowman's layer, which is often focally destroyed.

Corneal keloid

Corneal keloid presents as nodules resembling those of Salzmann's nodular degeneration but distributed throughout the cornea. Corneal keloid usually follows injury, inflammation or surgical trauma, but occurs occasionally in children in whom there is no significant history. The nodules comprise exuberant scar tissue and are histologically revealed as broad irregular collagen bundles.

Cornea guttata

Guttata are wart-like excrescences of Descemet's membrane seen on slit-lamp examination as irregularities of the posterior corneal surface. In most cases they are stationary or only slowly progressive. If bilateral and associated with sufficient endothelial dysfunction to cause oedema, the condition is termed Fuchs' endothelial dystrophy. Primary guttata occur in middle to old age and are located in the axial areas. Secondary guttata develop in association with inflammatory, degenerative, dystrophic and traumatic ocular disease. Occasional peripheral guttata of no significance are known as Hassal–Henle warts. Guttata are best seen histologically with periodic acid-Schiff (PAS) stain as wart-like, anvil- or mushroom-shaped excrescences (Fig. 5.4). They are formed by the abnormal production of basement membrane material and fibrillar collagen by distressed or dystrophic endothelial cells. The endothelial cells, which may contain phagocytosed melanin, become atrophic and eventually die, thereby exposing the guttata.

Senile scleral plaque

Senile scleral plaques are well-circumscribed areas of degeneration immediately anterior to the horizontal rectus muscles. Affected areas are translucent and appear blue-grey to dark brown due to transmission of the colour of the underlying choroid. Senile scleral plaques are common in the elderly and sometimes calcify to such an extent as to be visible on radiological examination. The plaques are revealed on microscopy as areas of degenerate collagen, often with calcification.

Ectasias and staphylomas

Ectasias and staphylomas are abnormal protrusions of the corneoscleral coat. Ectasias are differentiated from staphylomas by the absence of a uveal lining; a staphyloma is always lined by uveal tissue. Most corneal ectasias are difficult to classify, as they do not show the characteristic changes of a degeneration or dystrophy. The coexistence of keratoconus, keratoglobus and pellucid marginal degeneration in affected families suggests the possibility of a common element in their pathogenesis. Staphylomas are designated according to their location into corneal, limbal (intercalary) or scleral (ciliary, equatorial or posterior); primary or secondary, they may be either congenital or acquired. Primary staphylomas occur in pathological myopia and in congenital abnormalities, when there may be an association with colobomas, whereas secondary staphylomas can develop in any condition that causes focal weakness of the corneoscleral coat.

Keratoconus

Keratoconus is a common axial ectasia of the cornea presenting at or after puberty with blurred vision due to myopia and irregular astigmatism. It is progressive, and can either advance slowly and stabilize after about 10 years or deteriorate over a number of years and require keratoplasty for visual rehabilitation. In most instances it is bilateral, although asymmetry is common. There is a familial tendency towards keratoconus, but the absence of a clear pattern suggests a multifactorial mode of inheritance. The earliest sign of keratoconus is steepening of the central cornea. Subsequently the contour changes to an irregular conical shape with central or paracentral stromal thinning and protrusion of the apex (Fig. 5.5a). With progression, vertical stress lines (Vogt's striae) appear deep in the affected stroma, the corneal nerves are more conspicuous than normal and a Fleischer's iron ring (intraepithelial deposition of iron) may be seen at the base of the cone (Fig. 5.33a). More advanced cases result in central scarring and occasionally rupture of Descemet's membrane with an acute onset of stromal and epithelial oedema (acute corneal hydrops – Fig. 5.5b) that presents with sudden painful loss of vision; perforation is rare. Keratoconus is frequently associated with an atopic tendency (eczema, asthma, hay fever, allergic eye disease); other associations include genetic disorders (Down's, Turner's, Ehlers–Danlos and Marfan's syndromes) and local ocular disease (aniridia, photoreceptor dystrophies).

Keratoconus results from an undetermined abnormality in the mechanical properties of the cornea. Histological changes have been described in all layers, but many are non-specific. The most consistent findings are thinning of the central stroma with paucity of normal collagen fibres and a reduction in the number of lamellae (Fig. 5.6a). Keratocytes may be surrounded by an abnormal accumulation of fibrillogranular material and, occasionally, amyloid. Focal defects in Bowman's layer are common, and are often filled with collagenous tissue or epithelium. The epithelium is irregular and has an abnormal basement membrane in areas where Bowman's layer is destroyed. Variability in the thickness of Descemet's membrane and non-specific endothelial changes reflect corneal stretching. In acute hydrops, Descemet's membrane is stretched beyond its elastic limit and ruptures (Fig. 5.6b) with the onset of sudden profound stromal and epithelial oedema (Fig. 5.6c). The defect in Descemet's membrane is bridged by endothelium after 6–8 weeks and new basement membrane material is laid down, but a stromal scar remains and the retracted edges of Descemet's membrane assume a scroll-like appearance.

Keratoglobus

Keratoglobus is a rare bilateral disorder in which the cornea is of normal diameter but uniformly thinned and more spherically distorted than in keratoconus. It is present at birth and, although susceptible to traumatic rupture, acute hydrops is unusual. There are no distinctive pathological features.

Pellucid marginal degeneration

Pellucid marginal degeneration is rare and presents in the third and fourth decade with bilateral inferior corneal thinning and consequent severe irregular against-the-rule astigmatism. The normal cornea protrudes above and sags over the inferior thinned area. The morphological changes in the affected area are similar to those of keratoconus.

Myopia

Myopia is most often due to increased axial length of the eye. The main types are stationary myopia, which results from abnormal ocular growth to adolescence but not beyond, and pathological myopia, which progresses far into adult life. Myopia may rarely be congenital, occurring with other malformations such as coloboma.

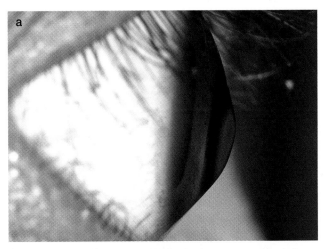

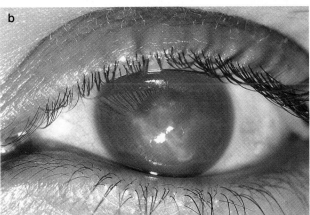

Figure 5.5 Keratoconus. (a) Lateral view. (b) Acute hydrops.

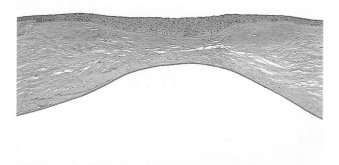

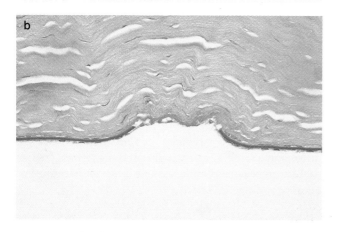

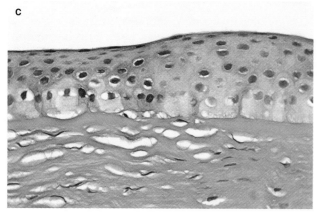

Figure 5.6 Keratoconus. (a) Thinning of central stroma. (b) Acute hydrops; defect in Descemet's membrane. PAS stain. (c) Acute hydrops; oedema of basal epithelial cells and partial loss of Bowman's layer.

Pathological myopia is more common in females and may be associated with ocular albinism, retinal pigmentary dystrophies and Down's syndrome.

A posterior staphyloma may be present in pathological myopia in which the posterior sclera is thinned and becomes progressively thinner. As the posterior segment enlarges the choroid is also thinned and the choriocapillaris is lost. Subsequently the RPE becomes atrophic and photoreceptors are lost. A few of those affected develop splits in Bruch's membrane that either heal to constitute lacquer cracks or are associated with subretinal neovascularization, haemorrhage and the formation of disciform scars. The related RPE may become hyperplastic, and conspicuous melanin pigmentation is seen as Fuchs' spots. Peripheral retinal changes include thinning and lattice degeneration that predispose to retinal tears, thus giving rise to the potential for rhegmatogenous detachment. A white crescent on the temporal side of the optic disc (myopic crescent) is characterized by absence of the RPE and outer retinal cells. Tilting and other anomalies of the optic disc may occur. The retinal axons on the nasal side of the optic disc may be involved in an almost hairpin bend before they reach the lamina cribrosa due to increased angulation of the optic nerve incurred by the lengthening of the eye. This gives rise to an unduly prominent nasal margin of the disc. Posterior segment enlargement is due either to stretching of scleral tissue in which there is an inherent biochemical abnormality or to remodelling of scleral collagen. Genetic factors and environmental influences such as exposure to light and the sharpness of the perceived images on the retina are thought to be important in the pathogenesis of myopia.

DEGENERATIONS OF THE LENS

The normal lens is a transparent semisolid avascular biconvex structure located between the iris and vitreous and held in place by the zonule (suspensory ligament) which passes between the equatorial periphery and the ciliary body. The lens is a component of the refractive system of the eye, and contributes to the formation of a focused image on the retina. Its dynamic function is to vary the depth of focus (accommodation) as a result of its curvature being changed by the action of the ciliary muscle transmitted to the capsule via the zonule. The lens comprises an outer capsule, an anterior epithelium and a bulk of cells (lens fibres) derived from the epithelium. Degenerations of the lens invariably lead to cataract.

Lens capsule

The lens capsule forms the outer envelope and is the basement membrane of the epithelium, by which it is secreted *in utero*. It is the thickest basement membrane in the body, and varies from 3 μm at the posterior pole to 15 μm at the anterior pole. It is relatively amorphous, and consists of up to 40 vaguely defined 40 nm thick lamellae running parallel to its surface. As with other basement membranes, it is composed mainly of Type IV collagen embedded within a matrix of glycoproteins.

The capsule is elastic and, at least in younger eyes, can stretch, thus allowing for the shape of the lens to change with accommodation and for a degree of surgical manipulation without rupture.

Lens epithelium

The lens epithelium is a monolayer of cuboidal cells lying immediately beneath the anterior capsule. It extends to the equator but does not normally continue beneath the posterior capsule. There are central, intermediate and germinative zones.

The central zone is a stable population of polygonal cells with large nuclei that undergo mitosis only in response to injury. Their number slowly declines with age.

The intermediate zone lies peripheral to the central zone and consists of smaller cylindrical cells with central nuclei. The basal surface of the cells is irregular and has complex interdigitations with the capsule.

The germinative zone is located at the periphery immediately anterior to the equator and consists of cells with flattened nuclei lying in the plane of the cell axis. It is the site of cell division and, although mitoses are infrequent in adults, cells migrate posteriorly to form new lens fibres beneath the posterior capsule.

Lens substance

The lens substance is composed of concentric layers of elongated cells (lens fibres) derived from the germinative cells of the epithelium. The layers are arbitrarily subdivided into an outer cortex and an inner nucleus delineated by the junction of the fetal and postnatal fibres. The lens enlarges throughout life due to the continued deposition of fibres in such a way that the outermost are the youngest and those within the nucleus are the oldest. Lens fibres are spindle-shaped cells up to 7 mm in length that arch from the front to the back to form concentric layers. Their anterior and posterior terminations meet those of other fibres to form the anterior and posterior lens sutures. The cell nuclei are lost in older, deeper fibres, and those of younger superficial fibres migrate anteriorly as they become buried by newer generations of cells. Lens fibres are hexagonal in cross-section and are closely packed, there being little intercellular space. They form radial rows in the cortex, but become less regular with increasing depth. Gap junctions, ball-and-socket joints and tongue-and-groove interdigitations link adjacent cells. A complex cytoskeletal matrix within the cytoplasm includes ubiquitous proteins such as actin, vimentin and spectrin, and lens-specific beaded filaments. Superficial lens fibres are rich in ribosomes and rough endoplasmic reticulum, but organelles become less

abundant with increasing depth and deeply situated fibres are homogeneous in appearance. Crystallins are a family of lens-specific proteins contained within the cytoskeletal matrix, and make up over 90 per cent of the total cellular lens protein. There are two broad types of crystallins, α and β/γ, with subtypes of each. The structure and high concentration of the crystallins together with the regular orientation of the fibres accounts for the transparency and high refractive index of the lens.

Ageing of the lens

The lens continues to grow throughout life, with consequent increase in thickness, weight and volume. As successive layers of new fibres are added to the cortex, older fibres are displaced inwards and undergo complex biochemical and structural changes, including loss of nuclei, organelles and cytoskeletal organization. These older fibres form the hard central core or nucleus of the lens. Metabolic activity corresponds to the morphological changes. Protein synthesis and other processes cease in older lens cells, and loss of such activity renders the inner region of the lens incapable of adequate response to metabolic or other insult. The optical and mechanical properties of the lens also change with age, and are manifest as increased light scatter, selective light absorption and increased mechanical rigidity.

With advancing age the physical and chemical properties of the crystallins change. The principal change is in post-synthetic modification, which occurs predominantly in the region of the lens nucleus. Some changes result from protein synthesis in the outer cortex. Changes result in unfolding of the molecular structure of crystallin, and chemical modifications such as protein cross-linkage, non-enzymatic glycation, racemization of constituent amino acids and proteolysis of peptide chains. The concentration of insoluble crystallins increases, and molecules tend to clump and form both soluble and insoluble high molecular weight aggregates.

Lens metabolism decreases with age due to reduced proliferative capacity of the epithelial cells and reduced activity of lens enzymes. Such changes are most marked in the lens nucleus and affect particularly those enzymes involved in glycolytic and oxidative pathways. Lack of these enzymes increases the susceptibility to oxidative stress and the effect of free radicals. Ageing changes of cell membranes include alteration of lipid composition, degradation of gap junction protein and modification of phospholipid content. The consequence is increased permeability to water and low molecular weight solutes, with resultant increased hydration of lens substance. This state may also be due to age-related decline in the efficacy of outwardly directed sodium and potassium activated ATPase and other pumping mechanisms.

Lens transparency depends on many interrelated factors. These include the ordered packing of lens fibres, their homogeneous structure within each generation and the relative lack of extracellular space. The high content of protein (particularly the crystallins) within lens fibres and their molecular structure normally contribute to both the transparency of the lens and its high refractive index. The widespread molecular and cellular changes that occur with advancing age result in gradual reduction in transparency. At birth the lens is colourless, but with advancing age it first becomes yellow and then brown due to the selective absorption of light of shorter wavelengths by pigments (chromophores), some of which may be fluorescent (fluorophores). Chromophores are thought to result from UV-induced photochemical damage of tryptophane and other aromatic amino acids, oxidized β/γ crystallin fragments and glycation of crystallins.

Cataracts

A cataract is any opacity of the lens, and includes opacities of its capsule. Vision may or may not be affected. Cataracts most commonly develop in adult life due to a degenerative process associated with advancing age, but may also be secondary to coexistent ocular or systemic disease. Cataracts may be present at birth (congenital) or develop soon after (infantile). No satisfactory system exists for the classification of cataracts, but those based on morphology or cause are the most frequently used.

Abnormalities of lens capsule

Abnormalities of the lens capsule include exfoliation. Pseudoexfoliation is considered here as its main effects are on the lens capsule and zonule, although it is a systemic disorder and a common cause of secondary glaucoma.

Exfoliation of lens capsule

True exfoliation of the lens capsule is characterized by scroll-like peeling of the anterior lamella. It is associated with heat trauma to the lens, and was previously seen in those with occupations involving exposure to intense heat, such as glass blowers and furnace workers (glass-blowers' cataract).

Pseudoexfoliation syndrome

The pseudoexfoliation syndrome (PXS) is a systemic disorder involving many different tissues, including the skin and visceral organs. Clinical manifestations occur only in the eye, where involvement of the zonule gives rise to lens instability, and the aqueous drainage pathway to secondary open-angle glaucoma. At presentation PXS usually only affects one eye, but in the majority of cases the fellow eye is eventually involved. The condition is rarely diagnosed before the age of 60 years, after when it affects 2–7 per cent of the population in most parts of Europe and the USA. There are marked geographical and racial variations in its prevalence, and its incidence can rise to over 30 per cent in the elderly populations of northern Finland, Lapland, Iceland, parts of Russia and Saudi Arabia. The clinical features are characterized by a fine deposit of grey-white flaky or granular material distributed throughout the anterior segment. The material is seen particularly on the anterior lens surface, which exhibits well demarcated central and peripheral zones separated by a clear ring resulting from abrasion of the anterior capsule by the iris. Other features include iris transillumination, loss of the normal iris vascular pattern, deposits of pigment on the posterior corneal surface, pigmentation of the trabecular meshwork, phacodonesis, lens dislocation and an increased risk of complications during cataract surgery. PXS is associated with secondary open-angle glaucoma in 20 per cent of affected eyes.

Light microscopy reveals fine granular shrub- or Christmas tree-like faintly eosinophilic deposits of pseudoexfoliation material on the anterior and posterior surfaces of the lens, on the zonular fibres and ciliary processes, and on the anterior and posterior surfaces of the iris. These deposits stain weakly positive with periodic acid-Schiff (PAS), but can be well demonstrated with Grocott hexamine (methenamine) silver (Fig. 5.7a) and oxidized aldehyde fuchsin stains (Fig. 5.7b), and by electron microscopy (Fig. 5.7c). Trabecular involvement is evident, and pseudoexfoliation material is found as plaques on the cribriform layer and as a band on the inner surface of the uveal trabecular beams. Melanin lost from the cells of the iris pigment epithelium is seen as phagocytosed granules in trabecular endothelial cells. Degenerative changes in the iris musculature may account for poor reactivity of the pupil. Dissolution of the zonular fibres may be a consequence of lysosomal enzyme activity, the enzymes being present within pseudoexfoliation aggregates. Ultrastructurally, pseudoexfoliation material consists of an irregular meshwork of at least two types of fibre (designated A and B), each of which is composed of fibrillar subunits. The composition of the material is complex, and various carbohydrate and protein components have been identified. Its source is unknown, although it is possibly of basement membrane origin.

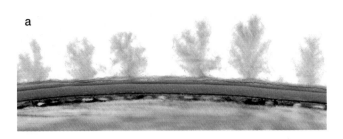

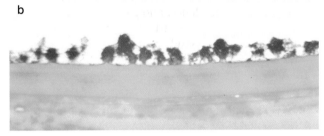

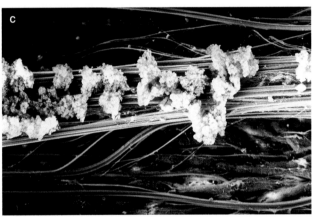

Figure 5.7 Pseudoexfoliation syndrome. (a) Christmas-tree like deposits on lens capsule. Grocott hexamine (methenamine) silver stain. (b) Blue deposits on lens capsule. Oxidized aldehyde fuchsin stain. (c) Deposits on the zonular fibres. SEM.

Pseudoexfoliation material can also be found histologically around posterior ciliary vessels, and in the palpebral and bulbar conjunctiva of the involved eye, in the uninvolved eye, and in skin, orbital tissue, lung, heart, liver, gall bladder, kidney and cerebral meninges.

Abnormalities of lens epithelium

The lens epithelium responds to noxious stimuli by active proliferation. Defects in the anterior capsule such as those produced by perforating trauma lead to proliferation of the anterior epithelium and the production of abnormal lens cells. Focal areas of epithelial necrosis resulting from an acute rise in intraocular pressure present as small, round, white opacities directly beneath the anterior capsule (Glaukomflecken). Dysplastic changes in the epithelium result in posterior subcapsular catar-

acts; equatorial epithelial cells proliferate and become swollen with liquefied cortical material to form bladder cells (Wedl cells) and migrate to the posterior pole, where they degenerate to form a lace-like or granular opacity immediately beneath the capsule. Causes of posterior subcapsular cataract include disorders such as uveitis, retinitis pigmentosa and myopia, physical insult by mechanical trauma or radiation, and the prolonged use of systemic corticosteroids. Dysplastic epithelial changes of a similar nature are an important aetiological component of age-related cataract. Metaplasia of the anterior epithelium results in anterior subcapsular fibrosis.

Abnormalities of lens substance

Abnormalities of the lens substance result from a slow degenerative process and affect both the cortex and nucleus. The abnormalities may be non-opaque or opaque.

Non-opaque abnormalities

Non-opaque abnormalities are common and probable components of cataract formation. They include fibre folds, water clefts and vacuoles.

Fibre folds are seen in the anterior cortex as white lines roughly parallel to the equator but changing in direction at a suture. They represent corrugations of lens fibres due to peripheral breaks with subsequent release of the tension that normally keeps the fibres taut.

Water clefts are radial or wedge-shaped clefts involving the sutures, particularly in the anterior cortex. They arise by either the separation or the absorption of adjacent fibres.

Vacuoles are near-spherical cyst-like spaces in the superficial cortex. They are common in the ageing lens, but also occur as transient abnormalities following trauma or the use of topical corticosteroids.

Opaque abnormalities (cataracts)

Transparency of the lens, as with the cornea, is dependent on the regular arrangement and the relative transparency of its components. Opacification is due to light scatter or light absorption. Light scatter results from changes at the molecular, cellular and extracellular levels. At the molecular level, water entry into lens fibres results in aggregation or separation of molecules and reduction of the ordered packing of crystallins. At the cellular and extracellular level, membrane changes and enlargement of the extracellular space lead to separation of the normally tightly packed cells. Light absorption is due in part to the presence of pigmented substances (chromophores). Opaque fibres form only in congenital cataracts, where the whole lens or a single lamella (*in toto* or in part) may be affected, giving rise to the characteristic morphological appearance. An insult occurring for a limited period during lens development causes a shell-like opacity confined to a particular lamella of lens substance. If lamellae are only partially affected, narrow radial opacities or riders form. More extensive insults result in opacification of the entire nucleus or, in severe cases, the whole lens (as in the congenital rubella syndrome). Superficial young lens fibres are the most susceptible to damage from external sources, whereas the older, deeper fibres undergo degenerative changes. Cataracts that follow mechanical trauma or metabolic disturbance are therefore predominantly superficial, while senile cataracts primarily affect the deeper cortex and nucleus.

Cortical cataracts

Although intrinsically an abnormality of lens fibres, the distribution of cortical opacities may or may not be related to that of the lens fibres (fibre-based and non-fibre-based).

Fibre-based cataracts follow the distribution of lens fibres, and are either sutural or non-sutural. Sutural cataracts follow the anterior and posterior Y-sutures. They may be inherited and congenital, or follow blunt trauma. Cataracts associated with myotonic dystrophy are of this type. Non-sutural cataracts include spoke cataracts, the commonest type of age-related cataracts. They are wedge-shaped and associated with water clefts and fibre folds. They commence in the peripheral anterior cortex and slowly advance centripetally along the course of lens fibres, widening as they proceed until a suture is reached.

Non-fibre-based cataracts do not follow the distribution of lens fibres. They include coronary cataracts, focal dot opacities or retro-dot opacities. Coronary cataracts are developmental opacities in the deep cortical layers where they surround the nucleus. They are more rounded and occur at a deeper level than spoke cataracts, and are often associated with focal dot opacities. Focal dot opacities are bluish dots in the peripheral cortex, and are present in female carriers of Lowe's syndrome (mental retardation, renal rickets, general hypotonia, congenital cataract and glaucoma). Retro-dot opacities are best seen by retroillumination as smooth circular structures in the perinuclear cortex and superficial nucleus. They have a high refractive index, are composed of calcium phosphate and possibly calcium oxalate, and may be the precursors of spheroliths, the crystalline spheroidal opacities found in Morgagnian cataracts.

Nuclear cataracts

As in the cortex, opacities may be developmental, but most nuclear cataracts are the result of age-related degeneration. Diffuse degenerative changes lead to light scatter and the accumulation of intracellular brown pigments. Pigmentation varies from amber to almost black, and is associated with the formation of insoluble cross-linked proteins. Diabetes mellitus, in addition to hastening the ageing process, may promote the formation of chromophores and fluorophores. Changes in the hydration and protein composition of the nucleus result in an increase in refractive index and mechanical hardness (sclerosis).

Christmas tree cataracts

Christmas tree cataracts are uncommon forms of age-related cataracts evident as multiple reflective polychromatic abnormalities in the deep cortex and nucleus. They are composed of multilamellar membranes that reflect light and cause optical interference resulting in the polychromatic effect.

Mature cataracts

Disorganization of the lens fibre system may be sufficiently extensive to render the lens completely opaque or mature.

Hypermature cataracts

Mature cataracts can absorb water and swell to such an extent as to cause narrowing of the anterior chamber angle and angle-closure glaucoma (phacomorphic glaucoma). This swollen or intumescent cataract consists of a distended capsule and liquefied cortex with the more resilient nucleus sinking inferiorly (Morgagnian cataract). Cortical lysis, absorption and dehydration follow, the lens shrinks and the capsule wrinkles. Leakage of lens protein into the anterior ocular compartments may result in phacolytic glaucoma or lens-induced endophthalmitis.

In the development of a hypermature cataract, lens fibres swell and superficial fibres exhibit degeneration of their nuclei. Fibre membranes are convoluted, and the cytoplasm is granular, vesiculated and reduced in density. Termination in the course of fibres results in the formation of isolated bodies of lens material (amorphous bodies) and fibre folds. Water clefts and extracellular vacuoles separate fibres, and eventual degeneration and liquefaction lead to the formation of Morgagnian globules (droplets of liquefied lens protein – Fig. 5.8). In the later stages of cataract formation, small crystalline aggregates of calcium oxalate (spheroliths) are seen and there may be anterior epithelial hypertrophy.

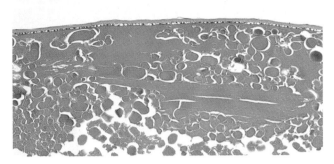

Figure 5.8 Cataract. Conspicuous Morgagnian globules.

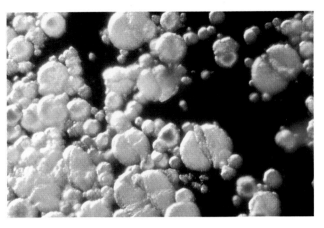

Figure 5.9 Asteroid hyalosis. Asteroid bodies illuminated by oblique light.

DEGENERATIONS OF THE ZONULE

The zonule comprises a series of fibres passing from the ciliary body to the lens. Two sheet-like layers of fibres adhere to the lens capsule, upon which they form brush-like expansions. The anterior layer originates from the sides of the ciliary processes and from the valleys between them, while the posterior layer arises from the bays of the pars plana. Zonular fibres contain fibrillin, a cysteine-rich microfibrillar component of the elastic system, the gene for which maps to chromosome 15 (15q21.1). Degenerations of the zonule can result in dislocation of the lens. At least 75 per cent of non-traumatic lens dislocations are due to Marfan's syndrome, homocystinuria and the Weill–Marchesani syndrome. Unlike Marfan's syndrome and homocystinuria, the Weill–Marchesani syndrome does not exhibit a consistent mode of inheritance and is considered to be a degeneration with similarities to homocystinuria in which changes in the zonular fibres produce a thick periodic acid-Schiff (PAS) positive coating on the ciliary processes with inferior dislocation of the lens. Other ocular abnormalities in the Weill–Marchesani syndrome include myopia, cataract, microspherophakia and secondary glaucoma. Those affected are of short stature and have brachydactyly, hearing defects and decreased flexibility of joints.

DEGENERATIONS OF THE VITREOUS

Syneresis

Syneresis (liquefaction, collapse and condensation) is an age-related degeneration. After the age of 30 liquefaction of the vitreous gel progresses so that by the age of 80 over half of the vitreous is liquid. Syneresis begins centrally and posteriorly, and results from dissolution of the hyaluronic acid collagen complexes that form the vitreous gel. Aggregation of collagen fibrils into matted bundles leads to condensations and the formation of strands and large lacunae containing liquid vitreous. These lacunae appear as optically empty areas.

Asteroid hyalosis

Asteroid hyalosis is a common and asymptomatic degenerative disorder in which small, white or yellow-white particles known as asteroid bodies are suspended like 'stars on a clear night' in an otherwise apparently normal vitreous (Fig. 5.9). The bodies are composed predominantly of calcium-containing phospholipids, and on microscopy appear as birefringent crystalline structures. Their pathogenesis is obscure, but they may result from changes associated with ageing vitreous collagen, or the depolymerization of hyaluronic acid.

Synchisis scintillans

Synchisis scintillans describes the presence of scintillating golden-brown cholesterol crystals freely mobile in a liquefied vitreous. Unlike asteroid bodies, which remain suspended, the crystals settle to the most dependent part when ocular movement ceases. Synchisis scintillans occurs usually in eyes blinded by severe ocular disease in which there has been previous vitreous haemorrhage. The cholesterol crystals are derived from plasma or the degradation products of erythrocytes, and lie either freely or engulfed within foreign body giant cells.

DEGENERATIONS AT THE VITREORETINAL INTERFACE

Vitreoretinal traction

Traction forces at the vitreoretinal interface are caused by eye movement, and partly result from the inertia of the vitreous body and the subsequent movement of the gel once inertia is overcome. These forces are transmitted to the retina at the sites of normal strong vitreoretinal adhesion, i.e. the vitreous base, optic disc and macula, the retinal blood vessels and the sheet-like adhesion at the posterior pole of young persons. Traction forces are also concentrated in areas of abnormal vitreoretinal adhesion, where the retina may be weakened by degenerative processes and is liable to tear. Clinically significant traction may be peripheral, located at blood vessels or occur at the macula.

Peripheral vitreoretinal traction

Focal areas of increased peripheral vitreoretinal adhesion may occur at sites of developmental variations or of degeneration. They account for the majority of retinal breaks resulting from posterior vitreous detachment. Developmental vitreoretinal variations associated with retinal breaks include enclosed ora bays, meridional folds, meridional complexes and cystic retinal tufts.

Enclosed ora bays result from the fusion of adjacent normal bays and morphologically are islands of non-pigmented pars plana epithelium located immediately posterior to the ora serrata.

Meridional folds are ridge-like radially orientated elevations of the peripheral retina, and project into the vitreous. They extend posteriorly from the ora serrata, and are aligned with either a dentate process or the middle of an ora bay. The folded retina is thickened and irregular as a result of cystoid degeneration.

Meridional complexes result from the abnormal alignment of enlarged and possibly continuous dentate and ciliary processes in the same meridian. A meridional fold is usually present, and there may be excavation of the peripheral retina in the corresponding meridian and possibly aberrant zonular bundles.

Cystic retinal tufts are projections of peripheral retina associated with abnormal vitreoretinal adhesion.

Vitreoretinal traction involving blood vessels

Increased vitreoretinal adhesion occurs over blood vessels if the internal limiting membrane of the retina is thinned, so allowing glial cells to migrate and form localized epiretinal membranes. The paravascular retina is also thinned and lacks the stabilizing effect of Müller cell processes, and both it and the retinal blood vessels are susceptible to trauma from vitreoretinal traction. This is the mechanism that explains retinal tear formation and haemorrhages in rhegmatogenous posterior vitreous detachment.

Vitreomacular traction

Vitreomacular traction can cause or contribute to the development of cystoid macular oedema if vitreomacular adhesion is increased.

Vitreoschisis

In vitreoschisis, liquefaction and cavitation cause a split in the vitreous, leaving a posterior layer of cortex attached to the retina. Geographical areas of whiteness may occur in the mid-peripheral and peripheral retina. If only seen during scleral depression these areas are referred to as 'white with pressure', while if they are visible without scleral depression they are termed 'white without pressure'. The white appearance is due to abnormal light reflection from different densities of collagenous material adherent to the retinal surface.

Posterior vitreous detachment

Posterior vitreous detachment (PVD) is a separation of the posterior vitreous cortex from the inner limiting membrane of the retina. It can be localized, partial or total. Rhegmatogenous PVD, like syneresis with which it is associated, is related to age and rises in incidence to 65 per cent in those over 65 years. A higher incidence in females is probably explained by post-menopausal endocrine changes. It occurs earlier, and is more common in myopia and diabetes mellitus. Acute PVD presents with sudden onset of floaters and photopsia. Floaters are an entoptic phenomenon due to condensed vitreous fibres, glial tissue adherent to the posterior vitreous cortex or, occasionally, vitreous haemorrhage. Floaters move with vitreous displacement during eye movement and cast shadows on the retina perceived as hair-like or fly-like images. Photopsia may occur at some time in up to 50 per cent of those with PVD, and is due to persistent vitreoretinal traction or detached vitreous cortex impacting on the retina during eye movement.

PVD results from vitreous syneresis in conjunction with weakening of the adhesion between the vitreous cortex and the inner limiting membrane of the retina. This adhesion is firm in the young, but weakens with age and concomitant ocular disease. Vitreous detachment begins at the macula, where the cortex is less dense and therefore more susceptible to degeneration. Anatomical and degenerative defects in the posterior cortex allow the passage of fluid, while mechanical forces such as rotational eye movements cause liquid vitreous to dissect a plane between the cortex and the inner limiting membrane of the retina. The preretinal or subhyaloid space so formed is bounded anteriorly by the new posterior hyaloid surface. Fluid from the central vitreous drains to this space, and the vitreous collapses to hang like a hammock between its firm attachments at the optic disc and the anterior vitreous base. The development of PVD is rapid and usually complete within days of onset. When vitreous detachment is complete, peripapillary glial tissue may be avulsed to form a ring around the hole in the posterior cortex (Weiss' ring). In most eyes PVD is uncomplicated, but when pre-existing vitreoretinal adhesions are strong, tearing of the retina may proceed to rhegmatogenous retinal detachment.

Lattice degeneration

Lattice degeneration is the commonest vitreoretinal degeneration, and occurs in up to 8 per cent of the general population and in 40 per cent of cases of retinal detachment. It is sharply demarcated and circumferentially oriented, and is characterized by retinal thinning and abnormalities in the adjacent vitreous. The name lattice refers to the appearance of a network of fine lines often continuous with retinal blood vessels and associated with pigmentation consequent upon changes in the RPE. Retinal thinning may be sufficient to form round holes, and the exaggerated vitreoretinal attachments at the margin of the degeneration predispose to the formation of the tears almost always associated with PVD. Atrophy of the retina and its replacement by glial tissue is characteristic. This is initially more marked in the inner layers, but later the entire thickness of the retina is involved. Degeneration and hyperplasia of the RPE give rise to the pigment changes, and sclerosis and occlusion of small blood vessels account for the interlacing white lattice lines. The overlying vitreous is liquefied except at the margins of the involved areas, where it is condensed and reinforced by glial proliferation. Subsequent vitreoretinal traction in the affected areas, combined with retinal fragility, predisposes to retinal tears and detachments.

Retinal breaks

A retinal break is a full-thickness defect in the neurosensory retina. It allows for communication between the vitreous cavity and the potential subretinal space, and therefore predisposes to rhegmatogenous retinal detachment. Retinal breaks are classified according to their appearance and implied pathology into retinal holes, full- and partial-thickness retinal tears, giant retinal tears and retinal dialysis.

Retinal holes may be primary, but are commonly (75 per cent) associated with lattice or other degenerations. Primary retinal holes are round full-thickness breaks without a flap or free operculum. The holes have smooth margins and are usually located anteriorly within the area of the vitreous base. The adjacent retina and vitreous usually appear normal. Many individuals with retinal holes remain asymptomatic, and retinal detachment does not develop.

Full-thickness retinal tears are full-thickness traction-related breaks in the neurosensory retina, and predispose to retinal detachment. Such tears are located posterior to the vitreous base, usually superiorly, and are associated with PVD (which itself may be associated with lattice degeneration) or with abnormal or exaggerated vitreoretinal adhesions. A full-thickness retinal tear is usually U- or V-shaped, with the apex always directed posteriorly. A tapered flap to which condensed vitreous strands are attached extends into the vitreous, and partial or complete avulsion of this flap leads to the formation of a free operculum in the overlying vitreous. Eventually the margins of the tear become smooth or rounded and the flap degenerates. Unlike retinal holes, full-thickness retinal tears exhibit degeneration and gliosis at the margin, and there is a variable degree of retinal detachment with associated degenerative and hyperplastic changes in the underlying RPE.

Partial-thickness retinal tears involve only the inner layers of the retina, but nevertheless result in a flap or free operculum. Like full-thickness tears, with which they are associated, partial-thickness tears are also caused by vitreoretinal traction secondary to PVD. They are usually paravascular or aligned circumferentially along a segment of the posterior border of the vitreous base. The avulsed retinal tissue is degenerate, the vitreous is detached, and the inner limiting membrane of the retina and the inner retinal layers are focally absent.

Giant retinal tears are defined as breaks extending 90° or more around the circumference of the peripheral retina. The posterior flap becomes inverted, and an anterior frill of retina is always present between the tear and the ora serrata. Giant tears may be idiopathic, associated with retinal trauma or occur at the posterior edge of chorioretinal degenerations. Excessive cryotherapy or photocoagulation are other causes. Giant tears fill with vitreous, and are particularly prone to proliferative vitreoretinopathy.

Retinal dialysis (disinsertion) is a linear break at the ora serrata. It occurs particularly in the lower temporal quadrant, and is frequently caused by blunt injury. Unlike giant retinal tears, there is no anterior frill of retina and the vitreous remains attached to the retina posterior to the break and does not become incarcerated in the tear.

Retinal detachment

Retinal detachment is the pathological separation of the neurosensory retina from the RPE. There are two types: rhegmatogenous and non-rhegmatogenous.

Rhegmatogenous retinal detachment

In rhegmatogenous retinal detachment, a break allows fluid derived from degenerate vitreous to gain access to the subretinal space and progressively detach the neurosensory retina from the RPE. It is usually spontaneous and caused by vitreoretinal traction. The initial features are those of PVD, with a sudden onset of floaters and photopsia. Floaters may be particularly pronounced if a retinal blood vessel ruptures and there is vitreous haemorrhage. A progressive curtain-like visual field defect advances over a period of hours from the periphery to involve central vision as the macula detaches. Principal findings include convex retinal elevation, corrugation and mobility of the retina, pigment granules in the anterior vitreous and one or more breaks in the peripheral retina. Without treatment the retina detaches completely and eventually contracts to become funnel-shaped.

Discussion of the pathogenesis of rhegmatogenous retinal detachment necessitates consideration of the factors involved in keeping the retina in place. Less than 2 per cent of eyes with retinal breaks develop a rhegmatogenous detachment, thus implying that strong forces keep the neurosensory retina in apposition with the RPE. Normal attachment of the retina is maintained by:

1. Osmotic pressure differences between the vitreous and choroid, which pull the neurosensory retina on to the RPE.
2. The active pump mechanisms of the RPE responsible for ion transport and water transfer.
3. The hydraulic force resulting from diffusion of fluid across the intact retina due to pressure difference between the vitreous cavity and extraocular tissues.
4. The adhesive effect of glycosaminoglycans between the outer segments of the retina and the RPE.
5. The interdigitation of the cell processes of the RPE and the outer segments of the photoreceptors.

Separation of the neurosensory retina from the RPE occurs when counteracting forces exceed those that normally keep the retina attached. Key elements in the development of rhegmatogenous detachment are the presence of retinal breaks or tears, dynamic vitreoretinal traction and liquefaction of the vitreous. Rhegmatogenous retinal detachment is caused by the combination of traction on the retina and vitreous fluid currents in the presence of a retinal break. Following PVD the subhyaloid space fills with liquid vitreous and during eye movements, because of the inertia of the various vitreous components, this liquid vitreous acts as a wedge in the subhyaloid space and causes further separation of the vitreous from the retina. The combined effect of advancing PVD and vitreoretinal traction produces retinal tears, particularly at sites of increased vitreoretinal adhesion. Once a tear has formed, constant movement of the vitreous cortex causes the tear to gape and thereby allows more liquid vitreous to flow into the subretinal space. This leads to retinal detachment and further weakening of the normal forces that keep the neurosensory retina in apposition with the RPE, so that once a rhegmatogenous detachment is initiated it progresses relentlessly to become total.

Non-rhegmatogenous retinal detachment

In the absence of a retinal break, separation of the neurosensory retina from the RPE may be due to traction or exudation. Non-rhegmatogenous detachments present with chronic visual loss in eyes with pre-existing pathology, and usually in the absence of acute symptoms of PVD. Tractional detachments are immobile, concave in appearance and often localized, while exudative detachments are convex and smooth. The subretinal fluid in non-rhegmatogenous exudative detachments is gravity dependent (shifting fluid).

Traction: retinal detachment occurs when the neurosensory retina is pulled away from the RPE by contracting vitreoretinal membranes. The origin of the subretinal fluid in such cases is not clear. Common causes of tractional detachment are the proliferative retinopathies and penetrating trauma (including surgery). Traction may also cause retinal breaks and so give rise to a superimposed rhegmatogenous component. Conversely, a tractional element in rhegmatogenous detachments may occur in proliferative vitreoretinopathy.

Exudation: a breakdown in the outer blood–retinal barrier results in exudation into the subretinal space and exudative retinal detachment. Causes include choroidal inflammation and tumours, and localized RPE defects associated with central serous choroidoretinopathy.

Pathology of retinal detachment

Intraretinal, subretinal and preretinal changes are found in rhegmatogenous and non-rhegmatogenous detachment.

Intraretinal changes

1. Diffuse intraretinal oedema is the earliest change following detachment. It occurs within a day, and reflects metabolic abnormalities consequent upon the separation of the neurosensory retina from the

RPE. Cystic spaces form after several days, and with time coalesce to form areas of retinoschisis with macrocysts (Fig. 5.10).

2. Photoreceptor degenerative changes develop during the first few days of detachment. The outer segments become irregular in length and contain fragmented saccules and swollen discs, and become surrounded by aggregates of macrophage-like cells probably derived from the RPE. These changes are initially reversible but within a week become permanent, so early reattachment of the retina allows for good photoreceptor (and therefore visual) recovery. Cones are more susceptible to damage than rods.

3. Gliosis is usually associated with atrophy of the photoreceptors. If the detachment is untreated, atrophy proceeds inwards from the photoreceptor cell layer; however, the inner layers, particularly the ganglion cell and nerve fibre layers, remain unaffected for a considerable time. Eventually all the neural elements degenerate, and the retina ultimately assumes the appearance of a glial membrane that forms a rigid funnel detachment. Proliferation of glial and Müller cells may lead to proliferative vitreoretinopathy.

Subretinal changes
Most subretinal changes occur in longstanding retinal detachments.

Subretinal fluid: this has a high protein and hyaluronic acid content, which increases with the duration of the detachment. Subretinal fluid solidifies when fixed, and is amorphous and eosinophilic on microscopy.

Focal proliferation of RPE: this may occur under the area of detachment and at the margin of stable detachments. The latter are seen clinically as pigmented demarcation lines (high water marks).

Bruch's membrane: this is thickened with the formation of hard drusen, which may become calcified (Fig. 5.13c).

Other changes: these include obliteration of the choriocapillaris and Ringschwiele (see Fig. 4.62).

Preretinal changes – proliferative vitreoretinopathy
Cellular proliferation on the inner retinal surface (epiretinal membrane formation) commonly follows retinal detachment. Many such membranes are of no clinical significance, but 10 per cent of eyes with retinal detachment have membranes sufficiently extensive to interfere with surgical reattachment, when the condition is termed proliferative vitreoretinopathy (PVR). Following retinal detachment, vitreous haze and the presence of pigmented macrophages (tobacco dust) herald the onset of PVR

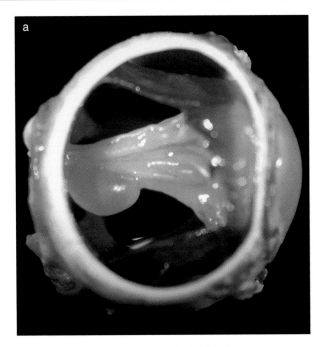

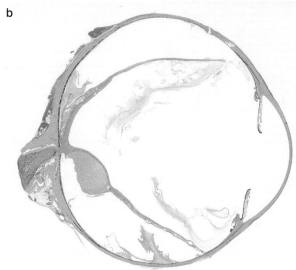

Figure 5.10 Retinal detachment with macrocyst formation. (a) Macroscopic appearance. (b) Histology.

(grade A). Later, rigidity and wrinkling of the inner surface of the retina accompany vascular tortuosity and rolling or irregularity of retinal breaks (grade B). The vitreous progressively condenses into strands, and the retina contracts to form focal (star) folds or diffuse full-thickness folds and subretinal membranes (grade C). Factors that predispose to PVR include previous failed detachment surgery, a fixed posterior edge of retinal tears, a liquefied vitreous gel, incomplete PVD and vitreous haemorrhage.

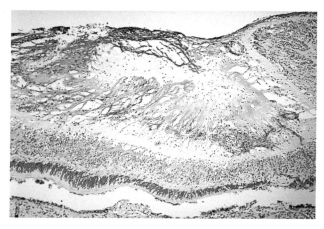

Figure 5.11 Proliferative vitreoretinopathy. A fibroglial epiretinal membrane. GFAP stain.

Epiretinal membranes are essentially fibroglial in nature (Fig. 5.11). Most asymptomatic membranes are composed of glial cells, but membranes that generate traction contain several types of cells and, often, collagenous components. The cellular components of PVR membranes (epiretinal cells) originate from the RPE, glial cells, vascular pericytes and adventitial cells, and occasionally vascular endothelial and inflammatory cells. The extracellular matrix contains glycoproteins, fibronectin, vitronectin and collagen (Types I, III, IV). The cohesion in PVR membranes, at least at an early stage, is due in part to adhesive interactions between extracellular matrix and cell surface receptors of the integrin family.

Full-thickness breaks in the neurosensory retina, displacement of RPE and glial cells to ectopic sites, breakdown of the blood–retinal barrier and an influx of blood-borne inflammatory cells are important factors in the pathogenesis of PVR. Following rhegmatogenous retinal detachment, breakdown of the blood–retinal barriers allows plasma proteins to enter the subretinal space and vitreous. Chemotactic and other factors in subretinal fluid stimulate the RPE and glial cells to migrate via retinal breaks to the surface of the detached retina. Epiretinal cells secrete further factors, including inflammatory mediators and growth factors that induce behaviour similar to the cells of healing wounds elsewhere in the body. Further proliferation of these cells results in the formation of a contractile membrane that generates tension on the inner retinal surface. With time, cellularity of the membrane decreases and the fibrous component becomes more prominent.

Premacular gliosis (macular pucker)

Premacular gliosis is a localized form of PVR affecting the macula. Most cases follow idiopathic PVD or retinal detachment surgery and occur predominantly in the elderly. Twenty per cent of cases are bilateral. The con-

dition is usually asymptomatic and only slowly progressive. The clinical appearance varies from a refractile sheen overlying the macula (cellophane maculopathy) to a definitive white or pigmented membrane that distorts the macula and surrounding blood vessels (macular pucker). Macular oedema, haemorrhages and retinal detachment occasionally develop. A pseudohole (in which contraction of an epiretinal membrane alters the foveal light reflex) may form and results in accentuation of the foveal depression, giving the impression of a full-thickness macular hole.

Macular hole

Full-thickness holes in the neurosensory retina at the macula are relatively common, and result from abnormal vitreomacular interaction. Most are idiopathic, but known causes include trauma, myopia, cystoid macular oedema and inflammation. Idiopathic macular holes occur most frequently in post-menopausal females and are usually unilateral, with less than 10 per cent of those affected having bilateral involvement. Presenting symptoms are blurred central vision, metamorphopsia or a central scotoma. The origin of the forces causing idiopathic macular holes and the precise mechanisms involved are obscure, although the most likely cause is shrinkage of the prefoveal vitreous cortex.

Staging

Macular holes are staged in a way consistent with clinicopathological observations and surgical management:

Stage 1 – macular cysts

Stage 1-A – foveolar detachment: detachment of the foveola from the underlying RPE results in flattening of the normal foveal depression and the appearance of a yellow spot due to the increased visibility of xanthophyll. The vitreous remains adherent to the inner retinal surface.

Stage 1-B – foveal detachment: the foveolar detachment progresses to involve the fovea. The central foveola is stretched and thinned, and xanthophyll is redistributed; the yellow spot enlarges and changes into a ring with a thin reddish centre surrounded by fine superficial radiating striae. At this stage approximately 30 per cent of cases have spontaneous vitreofoveal separation and do not progress further.

Stage 2 – early macular hole: the majority of stage I-B cases progress to a full-thickness macular hole within several months. The initial break is eccentrically placed and enlarges circumferentially to form a crescentic hole and finally a round hole with a central operculum attached to the now separated vitreous cortex.

Stage 3 – fully developed macular hole with vitreofoveal separation:
the stage 2 hole and yellow ring progressively enlarge to form a punched-out defect with a diameter of up to one-third that of the optic disc. The ring becomes grey in appearance and overlies an area of local retinal detachment that may be up to 1 mm in diameter; an operculum or a condensation of vitreous is frequently suspended above the hole. Visual acuity at this stage is about 6/60.

Stage 4 – PVD:
one-third of macular holes are associated with complete PVD, as evidenced by the presence of a peripapillary vitreous condensation ring (Weiss' ring).

DEGENERATIONS OF THE PERIPHERAL RETINA

Cystoid degeneration

There are two types of cystoid degeneration of the peripheral retina: typical cystoid degeneration and reticular cystoid degeneration. They frequently coexist, but have significantly different clinical and pathological features.

Typical cystoid degeneration of the peripheral retina

The formation of cystic spaces (Blessig–Iwanoff cysts) in the peripheral retina is universal in adults. Glycosaminoglycans accumulate in the outer plexiform and inner nuclear layers and form spaces that expand to dissect the two layers, with the formation of interlacing tunnels or local areas of retinoschisis (Fig. 5.12). Delicate vertical columns of Müller cells and other retinal elements deline-

ate the spaces. The condition is seen in the periphery as stippling with multiple small cysts and depressions. The ora serrata is affected first, but as age advances the degeneration spreads to the equatorial region.

Reticular cystoid degeneration of the peripheral retina

This common peripheral degeneration is possibly a variant of typical cystoid degeneration, with which it frequently coexists. Whereas the typical form involves the outer plexiform layer, the reticular form involves predominantly the ganglion cell and nerve fibre layers and is histologically similar to juvenile X-linked retinoschisis. It is seen on clinical examination in the temporal periphery as a fine reticular appearance of the retinal surface often immediately posterior to an area of typical cystoid degeneration.

Degenerative retinoschisis

Retinoschisis is the splitting of the neurosensory retina into two layers. Degenerative retinoschisis is common, and affects 7 per cent of the population over the age of 40 years. It is most often seen in the inferotemporal periphery, and represents the advanced stages of typical and reticular cystoid degeneration with confluence of the cystoid spaces.

Typical degenerative retinoschisis

Typical degenerative retinoschisis occurs as round or ovoid areas of smooth retinal elevation surrounded by typical cystoid degeneration. The condition is usually asymptomatic and found on routine examination in the inferotemporal peripheral retina. On ophthalmoscopy the inner layer is finely textured with variable numbers of glistening white dot opacities (snowflakes). The outer layer is often uneven in appearance and forms the external border of an optically empty cavity. The retinal vessels may be attenuated. Typical degenerative retinoschisis progresses slowly if at all, and does not extend posteriorly to threaten the macula. Only rarely is it associated with breaks in other retinal layers, and it does not predispose to retinal detachment. RPE changes are unusual. The neurosensory retina is split, with the formation of a fusiform intraretinal cavity. The thin inner wall is composed of inner limiting membrane, the nerve fibre layer and blood vessels. The irregular outer wall contains components from the inner nuclear, outer plexiform and outer nuclear layers, the external limiting membrane and the photoreceptor layer. The white dot opacities seen clinically are remnants of Müller cells adherent to the inner limiting membrane. At the margin of the cavity, the retinoschisis blends with typical cystoid degeneration.

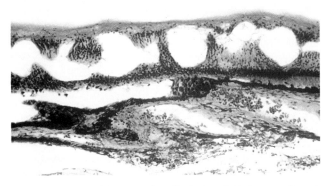

Figure 5.12 Retinal degeneration. Typical cystoid degeneration of the peripheral retina.

Reticular degenerative retinoschisis

Reticular degenerative retinoschisis, unlike its typical counterpart, is often bullous in appearance and may spread posteriorly behind the equator and occasionally threaten the macula. The inner layer of the schisis is thin and fragile, and the reticular pattern results from arborizing blood vessels. The outer layer is irregular and has a pitted or honeycomb appearance with granularity of the underlying RPE. Single or multiple round holes are often present in the outer layer. Both typical and reticular cystoid degenerations are usually present together in the involved eye. The inner layer is very thin, and consists of internal limiting membrane, remnants of the nerve fibre layer and blood vessels. The outer layer is irregular in thickness, and contains elements of the outer plexiform and outer nuclear layers, the external limiting membrane and the photoreceptor layer. Degeneration of the outer layer may give rise to round or ovoid holes.

AGE-RELATED DEGENERATIONS OF THE MACULA AND POSTERIOR POLE

Age-related degenerations of the photoreceptor cells, RPE and Bruch's membrane are universal, but the extent and pattern of degeneration differ widely between individuals. Many of the elderly retain normal vision, whereas others are severely affected by age-related macular degeneration relatively early in life. The macula is predisposed to age-related degenerations. The reasons for this are not entirely clear, but may be related to anatomical differences between the macula and the more peripheral retina or increased metabolic activity and/or environmental factors such as greater exposure to radiant energy. It is uncertain if age-related macular degeneration represents the advanced end of a spectrum of age changes or if it is one or more distinct entities. Its understanding necessitates review of the structures involved.

Photoreceptors and the RPE

Photoreceptors constantly shed their outer segments, which are digested by the RPE. The segments are initially engulfed before being transported as phagosomes to fuse with lysosomal granules. Undigested material remains in the RPE cells as lipofuscin, an autofluorescent pigment probably derived from the peroxidation of polyunsaturated fatty acids that originate mainly from the photoreceptor outer segments. Although the number of photoreceptors declines as age advances, the ability of the RPE to handle the relatively indigestible material is also reduced so that, after the age of 40, the concentration of lipofuscin in the RPE is significantly increased.

This causes the cells to enlarge and reduces the cytoplasmic space available to organelles. After the age of 90 no melanosomes remain, and the melanin in the RPE is either combined with lipofuscin as melanolipofuscin or contained within lysosomes.

Bruch's membrane

Bruch's membrane is a collagenous zone between the RPE and the choriocapillaris. It is appropriate to consider it as trilaminar – inner and outer collagenous layers separated by an elastic layer – and to regard the basement membranes of the RPE and the choriocapillaris as separate structures. Bruch's membrane exhibits a gradual age-related increase in thickness in the macular region, with deposition of calcium and possibly lipid. These changes lead to reduced permeability of the passage of substances between the RPE and choriocapillaris.

Sub-RPE deposits

Sub-RPE deposits are extracellular accumulations of material that probably arise as a consequence of age-related abnormalities in the digestive function of the RPE. The deposits contain lipid, laminin, fibronectin, glycoproteins and ubiquitin (a member of the stress protein family and a key protein for ATP-dependent proteolysis). Sub-RPE deposits are classified as drusen or basement membrane deposit according to their position in relation to the RPE basement membrane.

Drusen

Drusen are distinctive deposits between the basement membrane of the RPE and the inner collagenous layer of Bruch's membrane. They are rare before the age of 45, but increase in number with advancing years. They are often bilaterally symmetrical, and appear as clusters mainly in the macular region. Most affected individuals are asymptomatic or have relatively mild symptoms such as slight metamorphopsia or difficulty with reading. Drusen are a feature of age-related macular degeneration, and vary in size, morphology and distribution.

Hard drusen are small, round, discrete yellowish-white nodules that occur in both the macular region and retinal periphery. The overlying RPE is intact but thinned, and this, together with the absence of a pigmented barrier between them and the choriocapillaris, accounts for the characteristic hyperfluorescent window defects with staining but no leakage visualized by fluorescein angiography. Hard drusen appear on microscopy as discrete compact eosinophilic nodules composed of amorphous debris (Fig. 5.13a). They are often seen in enucleated eyes with long-standing retinal detachment, and may also be inherited as an autosomal dominant.

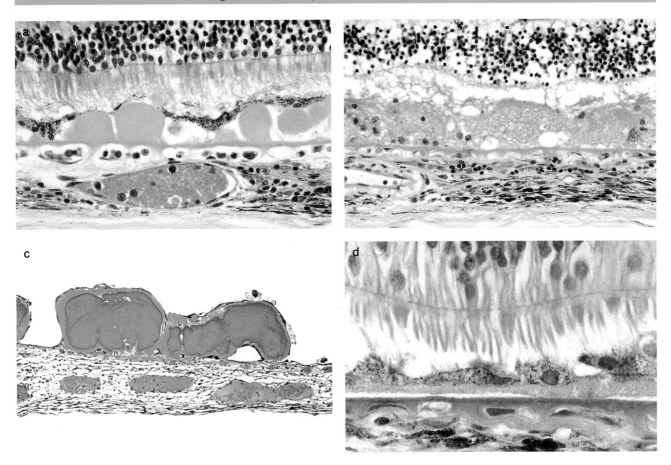

Figure 5.13 Sub-RPE deposits: deposits lying between Bruch's membrane and the RPE. (a) Hard drusen. (b) Soft drusen; the deposits are less homogeneous and their edges less sharply defined than hard drusen. The RPE and photoreceptors are lost. (c) Calcified drusen beneath a detached retina. (d) Basement membrane deposit; purple-blue material beneath the RPE cells. Mallory trichrome stain.

Soft drusen are pale yellow or grey dome-shaped structures with indistinct margins. They are larger than hard drusen and often become confluent. On fluorescein angiography they fluoresce more slowly than hard drusen but remain fluorescent for longer. On microscopy, soft drusen are less homogeneous than hard drusen, their edges are not as sharply defined, they are less eosinophilic and there is significant loss of the overlying RPE and photoreceptors (Fig. 5.13b). They may regress spontaneously, but predispose to choroidal neovascularization.

Calcified drusen (Fig. 5.13c) represent dystrophic calcification of hard or soft drusen.

Basement membrane deposit

Basement membrane deposit (BMD) is located between the RPE cell and its basement membrane, although this can only be appreciated by electron microscopy. The material is obscured by the RPE and cannot be seen clinically. On light microscopy BMD appears as a palisade of fine strands at right angles to Bruch's membrane, and is best demonstrated with Mallory trichrome stain as purple-blue (Fig. 5.13d). It is composed largely of basement membrane material, notably fibrous long-spacing (FLS) collagen. BMD, like soft drusen, is associated with photoreceptor cell loss and choroidal neovascularization.

Age-related macular degeneration

Age-related macular degeneration (AMD) is characterized by the presence of drusen associated with degeneration of the RPE or increased pigmentation in the macular area. Changes may progress to the atrophic ('dry') form of the disorder or the exudative ('wet') form which follows RPE detachment with or without choroidal neovascularization. Visual loss results from secondary degeneration of photoreceptors and other retinal elements. AMD is the commonest cause of blindness in the Western world. Its prevalence increases with age and it occurs in 30 per cent of those over 75 years; advanced disease occurs in about 7 per cent of this group. AMD is probably the manifestation of a number of disorders that are, as yet, impossible to differentiate. The most important risk factor is ageing, but others include gender (female > male), ethnic origin (whites are more commonly affected than blacks), hypermetropia, light ocular pigmentation, tobacco smoking, diet, raised serum LDL-cholesterol, and cardiovascular disease including systemic hypertension. Genetic factors also contribute, although the complex aetiology and the late onset of the disorder have confounded genetic studies. Dystrophies such as Stargardt's disease/fundus flavimaculatus, pigment pattern dystrophies, dominant drusen and Sorsby's fundus dystrophy all resemble AMD, some forms of which may possibly also represent inherited disorders.

Non-exudative (atrophic) macular degeneration

Non-exudative macular degeneration probably represents the advanced end of the spectrum of age-related retinal degenerative changes (Fig. 5.14a). It is the commonest type of AMD, accounting for up to 80–90 per cent of cases. Symptoms gradually progress from initial subtle blurring of vision to later profound central visual loss, depending on the extent of foveal involvement. At a relatively early stage, pre-existing drusen clinically regress and are replaced by patchy areas of RPE atrophy located in the perifoveal area. There may also be a reticular configuration of pigment clumping that spreads away from the fovea. As time passes the atrophic areas of RPE coalesce, and although the fovea is initially spared it later becomes involved, with consequent loss of visual acuity. Ultimately, sharply demarcated areas of atrophic RPE in the macular area are associated with varying degrees of atrophy of the choriocapillaris. Lesions are frequently bilateral and symmetrical. Choroidal neovascularization may develop at the border of an atrophic area but seldom within it because the neovascular response requires the presence of degenerating RPE and an intact choroidal blood supply.

The principal histological feature is loss of the RPE/photoreceptor complex. The outer plexiform layer is thinned and cystic but the inner nuclear layer is less affected. Bruch's membrane may be thickened and basophilic. In less severely affected areas, the RPE is variously hypertrophic, hyperplastic, atrophic and depigmented. In severely affected areas, the outer nuclear layer of the retina comes to lie in direct contact with the basement membrane of the RPE. Choroidal capillaries remain patent for a time, but in advanced disease they end abruptly at the border of the atrophic

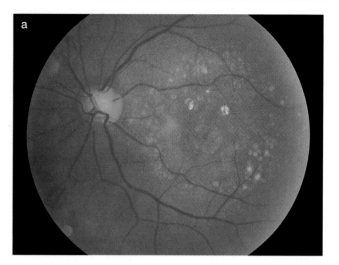

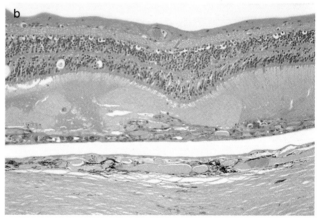

Figure 5.14 Age-related macular degeneration. (a) Non-exudative type with non-calcified and calcified drusen. (b) Exudative type with proteinaceous fluid in the subretinal space.

areas. Atrophy of the choriocapillaris and the middle layer of choroidal vessels reveals the underlying larger choroidal vessels.

Exudative (senile disciform) macular degeneration

The exudative form of AMD is less common than the non-exudative form (10–20 per cent of all AMD), but because of the profound visual loss it accounts for up to 90 per cent of legal blindness in the elderly population. The condition is usually bilateral, and in those with unilateral disease there is a 12–15 per cent per year risk of occurrence in the fellow eye. Other risk factors include soft drusen. The onset of symptoms is sudden, with blurred or distorted vision, micropsia, or a central scotoma. The main feature that differentiates the exudative from the non-exudative form is the presence of proteinaceous fluid exudate in the sub-RPE or subretinal space (Fig. 5.14b). The principal associated components are choroidal neovascularization and RPE detachments and tears.

Choroidal neovascularization

Choroidal neovascularization (CNV) is the process in which new vessels originating from the choroidal circulation grow beneath the neurosensory retina or RPE. CNV is not exclusive to AMD, although this is the most common association, but can develop in any condition that compromises the integrity of the RPE, Bruch's membrane or choriocapillaris. Visual loss results from the tendency of the new vessels to leak fluid or bleed, with the ultimate formation of a fibrovascular disciform scar. The process of CNV results in the formation of a subretinal fibrovascular membrane that is usually difficult to identify in the early stage, although its existence is inferred by the presence of serous or haemorrhagic retinal elevation. Later the subretinal membrane appears as a greyish lesion beneath the retina. There may be accompanying detachment of the overlying neurosensory retina together with cystoid oedema and a pigmented ring that encircles the membrane. Subretinal or sub-RPE haemorrhage is often present, and on rare occasions blood from CNV may dissect through the retina to form a vitreous haemorrhage.

Fluorescein and indocyanine green (ICG) angiography confirm the presence and location of CNV and provide information concerning visual prognosis. On fluorescein angiography the initial appearance is of a discrete, lacy plexus of subretinal vessels with scalloped and irregular edges. Later the dye leaks and pools in the subretinal space, with late staining giving a persistent hyperfluorescence. CNV is often obscured by turbid serous fluid, haemorrhage, RPE detachment or pigment clumping. Such occult CNV has a poorer visual prognosis than that which is easily identified. Occult CNV is more clearly defined by ICG than by fluorescein angiography.

CNV originates from the choriocapillaris. Predisposing factors include defects in Bruch's membrane, soft drusen and BMD. New vessels pass through defects in Bruch's membrane and proliferate initially beneath the RPE, later invading the subretinal space. The defects in Bruch's membrane may pre-exist or result from the neovascular process, either from the effect of the proliferating blood vessels or from macrophage activity. Macrophages are attracted to lipid and occur in increasing numbers in relation to Bruch's membrane as AMD develops. They play a role in the destruction of Bruch's membrane and in angiogenesis. The fragility and high permeability of proliferating vessels can lead to serous or haemorrhagic detachment of the RPE and/or the neurosensory retina. Fibrous tissue proliferation accompanies neovascularization and ultimately becomes the predominant feature, resulting in a disciform scar (Fig.

5.15) involving the choroid, RPE and neurosensory retina and containing soft drusen and BMD. At this stage the RPE may proliferate and, together with pigment-containing macrophages, forms the pigmented ring seen clinically. The RPE may also undergo fibrous metaplasia and contribute to the subretinal fibrosis. The neurosensory retina overlying a disciform scar becomes atrophic following degeneration, with loss of photoreceptors and the formation of cystoid spaces and lamellar or full-thickness macular holes. Blood vessels within a disciform scar may remain excessively permeable, and

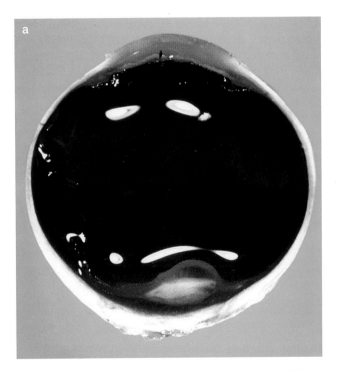

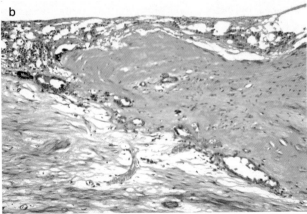

Figure 5.15 Choroidal neovascularization; disciform scar. (a) An eye opened anteroposteriorly showing a raised mass at the posterior pole. (b) Vascularized fibrous tissue beneath atrophic retina. Masson trichrome stain.

extensive exudation can lead to lipid deposition within and beneath the retina.

RPE detachment

As drusen form, the adhesion between the basement membrane of the RPE and the inner collagenous layer of Bruch's membrane weakens, and RPE detachment results when the layers become separated by serous fluid, blood or other deposits. Those affected present with distortion and loss of vision. The lesions are sharply demarcated round-to-oval dome-shaped elevations with a smooth homogeneous surface, possibly associated with pigment clumping or atrophy. Detachment of the neurosensory retina may develop. The basement membrane of the RPE and the overlying structures are seen on microscopy to be separated from the inner collagenous layer of Bruch's membrane by fluid, blood or other deposits. In some instances this fluid or blood results from the excessively permeable vessels of CNV, but in many instances no CNV is evident. In the absence of CNV, pooling of fluid results from age-related changes in the permeability of Bruch's membrane that normally prevents fluid from passing from the RPE to the choriocapillaris.

RPE tear: if an RPE detachment remains taut, the RPE at one edge may tear. Such a tear appears clinically and histologically as a linear rolled edge of RPE. The rolled edge is hypofluorescent on fluorescein angiography, while the exposed area of choroid is hyperfluorescent.

NON-AGE-RELATED DEGENERATIONS OF THE RPE/BRUCH'S MEMBRANE

Central serous choroidoretinopathy

Central serous choroidoretinopathy (CSC) is a permeability disorder of the outer blood–retinal barrier characterized by an accumulation of fluid at the posterior pole causing localized serous retinal detachment. In the majority (95 per cent) of cases fluid collects between the neurosensory retina and RPE (Type I), but occasionally the RPE alone is detached (Type II); alternatively, detachment of the neurosensory retina and RPE is combined (Type III). The disorder is relatively common and typically affects males between the ages of 20 and 50 years, although females may be affected, particularly during pregnancy. An anxious predisposition and similar personality traits are thought to predispose to the condition, which is more common in Caucasians. Presenting features include blurred vision, possibly in association with a scotoma, micropsia and/or metamorphopsia. Visual acuity is often 6/12 or better, and may be improved with a +1D lens. A well-circumscribed round shallow elevation of the neurosensory retina is

seen on ophthalmoscopy. The serous fluid is usually clear, but occasionally it appears turbid and obscures the underlying choroidal vascular pattern. A small RPE detachment may be seen as a grey-yellow well-circumscribed elevation within the area of serous retinal detachment. CSC is self-limiting and the retina spontaneously reattaches in 3–6 months, although recurrences affect 20–30 per cent. Visual recovery usually continues for up to 6 months after the absorption of fluid, but mild symptoms may persist, more commonly following prolonged or recurrent episodes. Chronic cases may be associated with extensive depigmentation of the RPE, lipid retinal exudate, retinal telangiectasis, pigment migration or cystoid macular oedema. There may be clinical or fluorescein angiographic evidence of current or previous involvement of the fellow eye. Fluorescein angiography is characteristic, and identifies the focal breakdown in the outer blood–retinal barrier. During the early stages one or more small areas of hyperfluorescence and points of fluorescein leakage are seen near the margin of the RPE detachment. In most cases the dye diffuses symmetrically within the subretinal fluid from the point of leakage, but occasionally it ascends like smoke and spreads under the influence of convection currents.

The aetiology of CSC is not known, although raised plasma catecholamine levels may play a role and explain the association with stress and males with Type A personalities. Fluorescein angiography indicates a focal breakdown in the outer blood–retinal barrier, resulting in influx of fluid into the subretinal space. The RPE has great ability to remove fluid from the subretinal space, and, for a serous retinal detachment to develop and be maintained, RPE function must be sufficiently disturbed to allow influx of fluid to produce and maintain the lesion. The precise nature of the RPE defect is not known, but hypotheses include focal reversal of the RPE pump mechanism and abnormalities in the choriocapillaris.

Angioid streaks

Angioid streaks (Fig. 5.16) are breaks or dehiscences in a thickened, calcified and abnormally brittle Bruch's membrane. They are relatively common, and may occur in isolation (50 per cent) or in association with a variety of conditions, including pseudoxanthoma elasticum, Ehlers–Danlos syndromes, Paget's disease and the haemoglobinopathies. Angioid streaks may be asymptomatic, but they frequently cause severe visual impairment as a result of rupture or neovascularization from the choroid or because of foveal involvement. They are situated deep to the retina, usually at the posterior pole, and appear as bilateral narrow jagged lines that are either circumferential to or radiating from the peripapil-

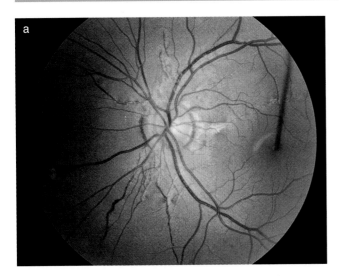

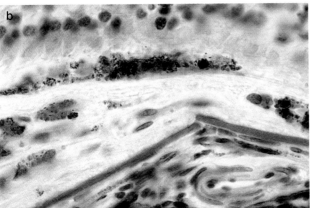

Figure 5.16 Angioid streaks. (a) Fundus appearance. (b) A break in the thickened calcified Bruch's membrane.

lary area. They often intercommunicate, run a convoluted course and end abruptly. Their colour ranges from red to dark brown depending on the degree of fundal pigmentation and RPE atrophy. The adjacent RPE may be abnormal, and gives rise to the 'peau d'orange' (orange-skin) appearance characteristic of the angioid streaks associated with systemic diseases.

The cause of the breaks in Bruch's membrane is unknown. The elastic layer is primarily affected with fraying and degeneration of fibres. In the late stages the choriocapillaris and RPE undergo secondary degeneration, and eventually CNV penetrates to form a disciform scar. The increased fragility of Bruch's membrane may result from an abnormality of elastic tissue, as in pseudoxanthoma elasticum and the Ehlers–Danlos syndromes, or from the abnormal assimilation of metal salts, as in Paget's disease and the haemoglobinopathies. The breaks follow natural lines of stress and result from the ocular muscles acting against the relatively fixed site of the optic nerve.

AGE-RELATED PERIPHERAL DEGENERATIONS OF THE RPE/BRUCH'S MEMBRANE

Paving-stone degeneration is an asymptomatic harmless condition that increases in incidence with advancing age. One or more discrete rounded areas of yellow-white depigmentation and retinal thinning, often with a pigmented margin, are located between the ora serrata and the equator. Sharply defined retinal thinning is due to the loss particularly of the inner retinal layers, including the photoreceptors and external limiting membrane. The RPE is absent apart from hyperplastic areas that form hyperpigmented cuffs and septae within the lesions. The atrophic retina is adherent to Bruch's membrane, and the underlying choriocapillaris is atrophic.

Peripheral drusen are a common finding in the elderly, and are similar to drusen of the posterior pole.

Senile reticular hyperpigmentation is manifest as linear networks of pigmentation in the periphery due to age-related changes of the RPE.

DYSTROPHIES

Dystrophies are degenerations in which disordered structure and function are due to an inherited genetic defect. The defect often resides within the affected tissue, as with most corneal dystrophies, but the changes may be the consequence of primary involvement of adjacent tissue, as in retinitis pigmentosa, or of tissue at a more distant site, as in gyrate atrophy of the choroid and retina. Dystrophies overlap with other inherited disorders, especially those relating to metabolic disease.

CORNEAL DYSTROPHIES

Corneal dystrophies are unrelated to any environmental or systemic factor. They are bilateral and are usually but not exclusively symmetrical. Apart from Fuchs' dystrophy, most present relatively early in life and exhibit variable progression. The primary abnormality is located in one layer of an otherwise normal cornea, thereby allowing an anatomical classification. Clinical features are often characteristic, but definitive diagnosis may only be possible on histological examination. Most dystrophies exhibit autosomal dominant inheritance, exceptions being macular dystrophy (autosomal recessive), autosomal recessive posterior polymorphous dystrophy and isolated cases of Fuchs' endothelial and congenital hereditary endothelial dystrophies. Epithelial basement membrane and Fuchs' endothelial dystrophies are common. Reis–Bückler's, granular, lattice and posterior polymorphous dystrophies are occasionally seen by general ophthalmologists, but the remaining dystrophies are rare. As with dystrophies elsewhere, those of the cornea reflect an underlying metabolic abnormality resulting from a genetic defect, and each type has characteristic histological features.

Anterior dystrophies

The anterior dystrophies occur within the epithelium or its basement membrane and/or Bowman's layer.

Epithelial basement membrane dystrophy (Cogan's microcystic dystrophy, map–dot–fingerprint dystrophy)

Epithelial basement membrane dystrophy is the commonest corneal dystrophy seen in clinical practice, but because of its variable presentation it may be misdiagnosed. The majority of affected individuals are asymptomatic, but recurrent corneal erosions may occur in early adult life. Lesions seen on slit-lamp examination include centrally located intraepithelial microcysts (dots), subepithelial refractile lines and ridges (fingerprints) and grey-white geographic opacities (maps). The condition is bilateral although possibly asymmetric, and the pattern of the lesions changes with time. Some families exhibit autosomal dominant inheritance but, because of the variable symptoms and often subtle signs, in the majority of cases the mode of inheritance cannot be established. The primary defect probably lies in the epithelial cells, and the consequences are intraepithelial extension of basement membrane, intraepithelial microcyst formation, and deposition of fibrillar material between the epithelial basement membrane and Bowman's layer (Fig. 5.17).

Intraepithelial extension of basement membrane follows the misdirected growth of basal cells. Normal desmosomes and anchoring fibrils fail to form, and epithelial instability results. Basement membrane continues to be secreted, and multilaminar intraepithelial basement membrane sheets are seen clinically as maps. Mechanical trauma of the unstable epithelium causes recurrent erosions.

Intraepithelial microcyst formation is due to the sequestration and degeneration of misdirected maturing epithelial cells. The microcysts contain eosinophilic cellular debris and are seen clinically as dots. Migration of the microcysts through the epithelium and their subsequent eruption give rise to ocular irritation.

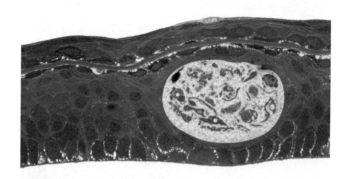

Figure 5.17 Epithelial basement membrane dystrophy. Intraepithelial extension of basement membrane above the intraepithelial microcyst. Toluidine blue stain.

Deposition of fibrillar material between the epithelial basement membrane and Bowman's layer produces ridges, which are thought to be the cause of fingerprints.

Meesmann's juvenile epithelial dystrophy

Meesmann's juvenile epithelial dystrophy is a rare mild autosomal dominant condition appearing in early childhood with the formation of asymptomatic small intraepithelial vesicles. Symptoms in middle age include foreign body sensation and slightly reduced visual acuity. Slit-lamp examination reveals multiple small round or oval bubble-like vesicles of uniform size and shape in the interpalpebral zone. They appear grey-white on focal illumination, and as transparent vesicles on retro-illumination.

The epithelium and its basement membrane are thickened (Fig. 5.18), and the latter may be multilaminar. Intraepithelial cysts contain amorphous material derived from degenerate cells and basement membrane. The underlying lesion is a mutation of one of the genes encoding the cornea specific keratins K3 and K12 located on the long arms of chromosomes 12 and 17 respectively. These proteins, when normal, form the intermediate filament cystoskeleton of corneal epithelial cells, but when abnormal result in cell fragility. A characteristic ultrastructural finding in epithelial cells is a dense intracytoplasmic substance (peculiar substance) that probably represents mutant keratin or related compounds.

Reis–Bückler's dystrophy

Reis–Bückler's dystrophy is relatively common, autosomal dominant, and usually presents in early childhood with painful epithelial erosions. At the time of presentation clinical examination reveals reticular grey-white

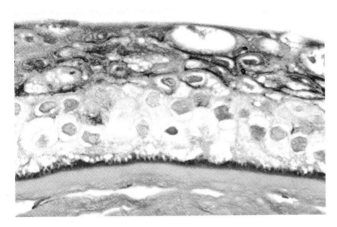

Figure 5.18 Meesman's juvenile epithelial dystrophy. Intraepithelial cysts and thickening of the epithelial basement membrane. PAS stain.

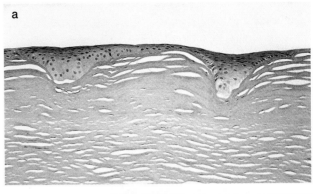

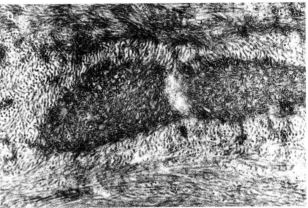

Figure 5.19 Reis–Bückler's dystrophy. (a) Loss of Bowman's layer with fibrous tissue protruding anteriorly to produce an irregular surface epithelium. (b) Fine curled microfilaments. TEM.

subepithelial opacification, which progresses to a characteristic ring-like pattern, giving the central cornea a fishnet or honeycomb appearance. Erosions become less frequent as age advances, but vision decreases because of progressive opacification and irregular astigmatism. Bowman's layer and the epithelial basement membrane are destroyed and replaced by fibrous tissue (Fig. 5.19a) containing abnormal fine curled microfilaments revealed only by electron microscopy (Fig. 5.19b). This tissue protrudes anteriorly into the basal layer of the epithelium, leading to irregularity of the corneal surface, and posteriorly into the anterior stroma, giving rise to the opacification seen clinically. The epithelial cells exhibit loss of desmosomes, and disturbed adhesion accounts for the recurrent erosions. The primary abnormality in Reis–Bückler's dystrophy is probably in Bowman's layer, in which collagen fibrils fragment, although conflicting evidence suggests a primary epithelial disorder with secondary digestion of Bowman's layer.

Stromal dystrophies

Stromal dystrophies are characterized by the deposition of material between stromal collagen fibres or within keratocytes; in macular dystrophy the endothelial cells are also involved. The material may be a normal substance such as cholesterol (central crystalline dystrophy), an abnormal glycosaminoglycan (macular dystrophy), an abnormal protein such as amyloid (lattice, polymorphic stromal and gelatinous drop-like dystrophies), or a protein of unknown composition (granular dystrophy). The most frequently encountered stromal dystrophies are granular and lattice.

Granular dystrophy

Granular dystrophy is autosomal dominant, and presents in adults with blurred vision. Asymptomatic lesions occur in the first decade of life as sharply defined, milky opaque deposits resembling snowflakes or breadcrumbs scattered in an otherwise clear stroma (Fig. 5.20a). They are initially confined to the axial area immediately beneath Bowman's layer and progression is manifest as expansion and posterior extension such that by middle age they become confluent. On occasions they can extend through breaks in Bowman's layer to a subepithelial position. The lesions stain red with Masson trichrome (Fig. 5.20b), and on electron microscopy are seen to consist of extracellular rod-shaped electron-dense crystal-like rhomboidal structures with faintly visible periodicity (Fig. 5.20c). The nature of the material and its pathogenesis are unknown. Visual acuity does not significantly deteriorate, and most of those affected do not require keratoplasty until later life, if at all. If keratoplasty is undertaken, there is a risk of recurrence of the dystrophy in the donor cornea.

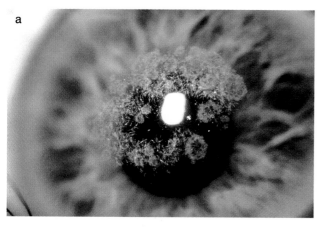

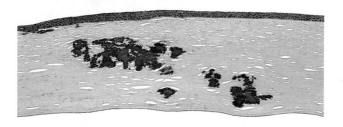

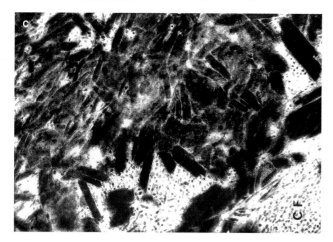

Figure 5.20 Granular dystrophy. (a) Clinical appearance. (b) Irregular stromal deposits of red-staining proteinaceous material. Masson trichrome stain. (c) Rhomboidal structures. TEM.

Variants of granular dystrophy

Superficial variant (Waardenburg Jonker's dystrophy)
Like the classic form, the superficial variant of granular dystrophy is inherited as an autosomal dominant. The granular lesions are present only in the superficial stroma. Recurrent erosions occur in the first decade of life, but by the second decade diffuse stromal haze leads to visual deterioration. Affected corneas exhibit the curly microfilaments of Reis–Bückler's dystrophy and not the characteristic deposits of granular dystrophy.

Avellino dystrophy
Avellino dystrophy is a variant that occurs in individuals tracing their ancestry to Avellino, Italy. The clinical features are similar to granular dystrophy, but also include axial anterior stromal haze and discrete mid-stromal linear opacities. The deposits stain for both granular (Masson trichrome) and lattice (congo red) dystrophies.

Lattice dystrophy

Lattice dystrophy is autosomal dominant with variable expression. Symptoms are progressive and usually begin in the first decade with decreased vision and recurrent erosions. It is bilateral, usually symmetrical, and characterized by refractile lines, white dots and diffuse central opacification. Refractile lines (Fig. 5.21a) are pathognomonic, and vary from small flecks to a dense network of irregular cords. The lines branch dichotomously to form an interlacing lattice predominantly in the centre and not confined to any single layer. White dots are fine, discrete and occur between the lattice lines. Diffuse central opacification occurs in the fourth or fifth decade and eventually extends throughout the stroma with relative sparing of the limbal area.

The three types of lattice dystrophy described are Type 1, Type 2 and Type 3.

Type 1: autosomal dominant without systemic manifestations.

Type 2: autosomal dominant with associated familial systemic amyloidosis (Meretoja's syndrome). The ocular lesions present usually later in life and with milder symptoms than those of Type 1. Fewer lines are seen, they are more superficial than in Type 1, and recurrent erosions are less frequent. Affected families are usually of Dutch, Finnish or Scottish-Dutch descent. Common associations are open-angle glaucoma and/or PXS. Systemic manifestations include progressive cranial and peripheral neuropathy, skin disorders such as lichen amyloidosis and cutis laxa, polycythaemia and ventricular hypertrophy.

Type 3: a rare type with probable autosomal recessive inheritance affecting those of Japanese descent. Recurrent corneal erosions do not occur, visual symptoms develop later in life, and there is no systemic involvement. Stromal deposits are larger than in Types 1 and

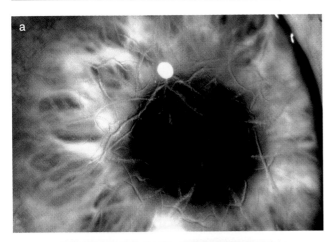

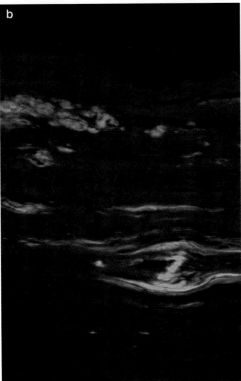

Figure 5.21 Lattice dystrophy. (a) Refractile lines. (b) Fluorescent amyloid deposits. Thioflavine T.

2, subepithelial deposits are not seen, and the epithelium and Bowman's layer are normal.

Microscopic appearance

Microscopy of lattice dystrophy reveals fusiform stromal deposits of amyloid displacing adjacent collagen lamellae (Fig. 5.21b). Other than in Type 3, amyloid can also accumulate under the epithelium and give rise to poor epithelial/stromal adhesion, which accounts for the recurrent erosions. The epithelial basement membrane and Bowman's layer fragment and the overlying epithe-

lium is irregular. Descemet's membrane and the endothelium are not involved. Amyloid deposits are due to the precipitation of an amyloidogenic protein; in the case of lattice dystrophy Type 1, this is an abnormal kerato-epithelin that results from a mutation at 5q31. Penetrating keratoplasty is usually required by the age of 40 years, but recurrence may eventually occur in the graft.

Molecular genetics of Reis–Bückler's, granular, Avellino and lattice Type 1 corneal dystrophies

These four dystrophies overlap in their clinical features and exhibit similarities in their histology. They exhibit disparate mutations of the beta Ig-H3, TGFB1 gene on chromosome 5 (5q31) that encodes for keratoepithelin. In lattice Type 1 and Avellino dystrophies a mutant keratoepithelin forms amyloidogenic intermediates that precipitate in the cornea as amyloid.

Other corneal dystrophies with amyloid deposition

Other corneal dystrophies with amyloid deposition include polymorphic stromal and gelatinous drop-like dystrophies.

Polymorphic stromal dystrophy

This rare dystrophy is characterized by variable posterior stromal features including axial polymorphic star- and snowflake-shaped opacities, grey-white refractile punctate opacities and branching stromal filaments that, by indenting the anterior surface of Descemet's membrane, may cause irregularity of the posterior corneal surface. It is mild, and does not show any clear pattern of inheritance. The corneal deposits exhibit the features of amyloid.

Gelatinous drop-like dystrophy

This is a rare bilateral autosomal recessive condition, and those affected are usually Japanese. It presents in childhood as mulberry-like milky gelatinous elevated lesions of the anterior stroma. The lesions are deposits of amyloid (Fig. 5.22).

Macular dystrophy

Macular dystrophy is autosomal recessive and, like other recessive disorders, is rare and clinically severe. It is bilateral, symmetrical, and presents within the first decade of life with blurred vision. Corneal sensation

a

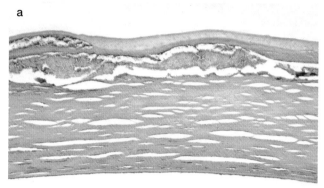

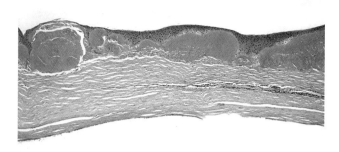

Figure 5.22 Gelatinous drop-like dystrophy. Irregular anterior stromal deposits of amyloid seen as eosinophilic hyaline material.

is reduced, but recurrent erosions do not occur. Characteristic clinical features include a diffuse stromal haze, focal grey-white stromal opacities, and irregularity of Descemet's membrane with cornea guttata. These features are explained by the accumulation of an abnormal keratan sulphate-like glycosaminoglycan within keratinocytes, endothelial cells and stroma. The material deposited is best demonstrated histologically with either colloidal iron (Fig. 5.23a) or alcian blue stains, and is seen on electron microscopy to consist of rounded membrane-bound aggregates of fibrillogranular material (Fig. 5.23b). Macular dystrophy maps to chromosome 16 (16q22) and is thought to be a localized mucopolysaccharidosis resulting from a deficiency of the hydrolytic enzyme, sulphatransferase. Two subtypes are described depending on the absence (Type 1) or presence (Type 2) of antigenic keratan sulphate in the cornea and serum. Penetrating keratoplasty is usually necessary for macular dystrophy by the second or third decade, and recurrence in transplanted corneas is not unusual.

b

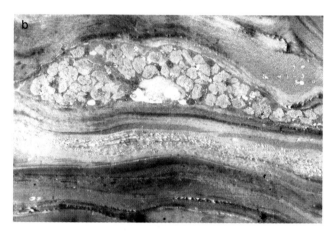

Figure 5.23 Macular dystrophy. (a) Deposits of abnormal keratan sulphate-like glycosaminoglycan staining Prussian blue. Colloidal iron stain. (b) Rounded membrane-bound aggregates of fibrillogranular material. TEM.

Schnyder's central crystalline dystrophy

Schnyder's central crystalline dystrophy is a mild, dominantly inherited dystrophy exhibiting great variation within families. The characteristic feature is bilateral fine polychromatic randomly-orientated crystals, which in early cases are located just beneath Bowman's layer but later form a central disc-, C- or ring-shaped stromal opacity. Late corneal features include the development of arcus, a grey stromal haze and a limbal girdle independent of the arcus. Vision may not be affected until after the third decade, although bilateral crystalline deposits can usually be seen at birth or during the first year of life. The condition is not related to any of the

primary hyperlipidaemias, but elevated serum triglycerides and cholesterol occur in some affected families. Occasional non-ocular associations include genu valgum and chondrodystrophy. Randomly-orientated cholesterol crystals are found among the collagen fibrils in the anterior stroma and Bowman's layer, focal disruption of which may lead to the opacity of advanced cases. Abnormal globular deposits of neutral fats are also present. The lipid deposition of central crystalline dystrophy results from an imbalance in local factors affecting lipid/cholesterol transport or metabolism, and an assignment to chromosome 1 (1p36-p34) has been identified in some affected families.

Bietti's crystalline corneoretinal dystrophy

Bietti's crystalline corneoretinal dystrophy is a rare autosomal recessive disorder in which crystalline deposits are present within the peripheral corneal stroma and retina.

The corneal lesions are subtle and comprise small yellowish-white refractile crystals at the periphery. The crystals have the appearance of cholesterol or cholesterol esters, and are contained within keratocytes and conjunctival fibroblasts. Similar findings within circulating lymphocytes suggest a metabolic abnormality. The onset of symptoms relates to choroidoretinal degeneration, and may vary from loss of central visual field to loss of peripheral vision and night blindness.

Endothelial dystrophies

The endothelial dystrophies have three clinicopathological features in common:

1. The production of collagenous tissue posterior to Descemet's membrane (seen as cornea guttata, polymorphic deposits and/or a uniform grey layer).
2. Disruption of the endothelial cell layer (seen on slit-lamp microscopy as an abnormal specular reflection).
3. Corneal oedema (secondary to endothelial pump dysfunction).

Fuchs' endothelial dystrophy

Fuchs' endothelial 'dystrophy' is classified as a dystrophy, but an autosomal dominant inheritance is rarely demonstrable. Unlike other dystrophies it presents late in life, it usually affects post-menopausal women and is the commonest dystrophy in the Western world but rare in Asian countries. The clinical features reflect endothelial cell dysfunction and are primarily related to oedema. Blurred vision results from stromal and epithelial oedema, the latter being manifest initially as microbullous epithelial elevations that progress to bullous keratopathy (Fig. 5.24). Foreign body sensation and pain result from rupture of bullae. Penetrating keratoplasty is ultimately required for comfort and visual rehabilitation. If untreated, subepithelial vascularized connective tissue forms and the bullous keratopathy resolves, the result being less discomfort but no improvement in vision. In the presymptomatic stage guttata are more extensive than would otherwise be expected for those of similar age. The most striking abnormality is irregular thickening of Descemet's membrane, which bears guttata on its posterior surface (Fig. 5.4). On light microscopy these abnormalities are best demonstrated with periodic acid-Schiff (PAS) stain. The guttata are sometimes buried within the thickened membrane, which is composed of multiple lamellae of newly deposited collagenous material. Endothelial cells are reduced in number, and those that remain are flattened and thinned. The stroma and

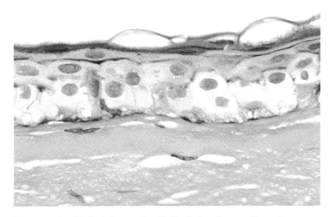

Figure 5.24 Fuchs' dystrophy. Epithelial oedema with surface bullae. PAS stain.

epithelium are oedematous. The epithelial cells initially swell, but later disruption leads to bullae formation. Subepithelial fibrovascular pannus may eventually form, but the epithelial basement membrane and Bowman's layer usually remain intact.

Posterior polymorphous dystrophy

Posterior polymorphous dystrophy (PPD), as its name implies, has a wide range of expression and is usually inherited as an autosomal dominant. It is probably relatively common but, as most cases are asymptomatic, is rarely seen. It may be present at birth, is static or only slowly progressive, and is often asymmetric. Lesions occur at the level of Descemet's membrane; there are small grouped vesicles, larger irregular vesicles or annular lesions, and broad grey bands and sheets. Associated features include cornea guttata, developmental anomalies of the anterior segment, glaucoma and band keratopathy. Normal corneal endothelium is a single layer of cells that lose their mitotic potential when development is complete, but in PPD the endothelium is often multi-layered and exhibits characteristics of epithelium (Fig. 5.25) including the ability to undergo cell division. The Descemet-like membrane secreted by this abnormal endothelium is also abnormal, and consists of multiple layers of immature collagen on the posterior surface. The epithelial-like cells arise through a process in which the phenotype of endothelial cells becomes progressively abnormal. Linkage of the PPD gene to chromosome 20 (20q11) has been identified and is closely linked, and possibly identical, to that of congenital hereditary endothelial dystrophy.

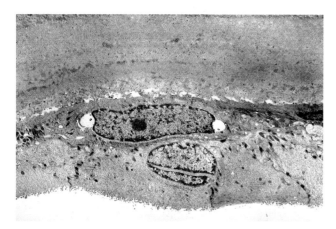

Figure 5.25 Posterior polymorphous dystrophy. Multilayered corneal endothelium with the production of epithelial-like cells. TEM.

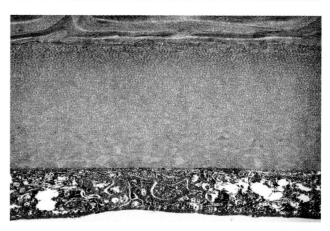

Figure 5.26 Congenital hereditary corneal endothelial dystrophy. A thickened Descemet's membrane. TEM.

Congenital hereditary endothelial dystrophy

Congenital hereditary endothelial dystrophy (CHED) is usually autosomal recessive, although a dominant variant is described. The recessive form is present at birth, and has a relatively stationary clinical course characterized by diffuse bilaterally symmetrical stromal and epithelial oedema. The oedema varies in extent to produce a mild haze or a milky ground-glass opacification with a threefold or more increase in the stromal thickness. Epithelial microbullae may develop. Descemet's membrane is uniformly thinned or thickened, but guttata are absent. Visual loss may be severe with associated nystagmus and amblyopia, but ocular irritation is uncommon. Histological findings are non-specific, with stromal and epithelial changes consistent with endothelial dysfunction and long-standing oedema. The basal cells of the epithelium swell, the epithelial basement membrane is thickened and disrupted, pannus is seen and Bowman's layer is irregular. Descemet's membrane appears histologically as a uniform band that varies in thickness between individuals. The primary abnormality is endothelial cell dysfunction and, as in other endothelial disorders, a posterior corneal layer is formed. In cases where Descemet's membrane is thin, endothelial dysgenesis or failure occurred *in utero* and only the fetal anterior portion was secreted; where Descemet's membrane is thickened (Fig. 5.26), collagen is secreted by dystrophic endothelium.

Dominant variant of CHED

The dominantly inherited form of CHED is classified as a separate disorder. It is not congenital but develops in the first or second year of life with progressive photophobia, lacrimation and corneal oedema. The visual loss is less severe than in the recessive type, and there is no nystagmus. The dominant CHED gene has been linked to chromosome 20 (20q11) and is close to or identical to that of PPD.

SCLERAL DYSTROPHIES

Some inherited disorders of collagen result in abnormal thinning and translucency of the sclera, which appears blue due to visibility of the underlying uvea. Scleral fibres are immature, reduced in thickness and more uniformly distributed than those in normal sclera. In osteogenesis imperfecta at least four types of inherited connective tissue disorders variably affect bones (fractures), ears (deafness), teeth (malformation) and skin (premature ageing). Three of the types are associated with blue sclera, the primary defect being an abnormality in the synthesis of Type I collagen, a major component of sclera and bone. Other conditions associated with blue sclera include lax ligament syndrome (hypermobile joints, blue sclera, bat ears), keratoconus, keratoglobus, chondrodystrophy and hypophosphatasia (band keratopathy, cataract, optic atrophy, craniostenosis, pigmentary dystrophy).

RETINAL AND CHOROIDAL DYSTROPHIES

Dystrophies of the retina (neurosensory retina and RPE) and the choroid (including Bruch's membrane) are a heterogeneous group of inherited conditions forming a spectrum of disorders ranging from congenital stationary abnormalities of function to progressive and blinding degenerations that become manifest later in life. A known or assumed molecular defect resulting from a single gene mutation is fundamental to all. Some of the stationary abnormalities of function are not true dystrophies in that structural changes are not demonstrable, but nevertheless they form part of the group of inherited disorders to which the true dystrophies belong. Some photoreceptor dysfunctions are very common, but the majority of retinal dysfunctions and dystrophies are rare in comparison with acquired retinal disease. Retinitis pigmentosa is probably the commonest 'peripheral' dystrophy, and Stargardt's disease/fundus flavimaculatus the commonest 'macular' dystrophy. X-linked juvenile retinoschisis and Best's vitelliform macular dystrophy occur less frequently, while congenital stationary night blindness, pigment pattern dystrophies of the RPE, dominant drusen of Bruch's membrane and central areolar choroidal dystrophy are much less common. All other dystrophies are rare, and some are limited to single families or isolated case reports.

Genetics

Most of the retinal dystrophies exhibit monogenic inheritance that follows the classical Mendelian modes. Some exhibit considerable genetic heterogeneity, in which different genetic mechanisms result in identical or similar clinical presentations. An example of genetic heterogeneity is retinitis pigmentosa, which can result from a variety of mutations of genes that encode proteins in the rod outer segment or enzymes in the phototransduction pathway, or from a variety of miscellaneous other mutations. Conversely, some disorders display allelic heterogeneity, in which different mutant alleles of the same gene produce different phenotypes; examples include the various phenotypes of the peripherin mutations.

Classification

The term retinal dystrophy is used to describe inherited disorders of the peripheral retina and macula in which there are demonstrable structural abnormalities. The term dysfunction is used for those congenital and stationary conditions in which function is disordered but no structural abnormalities are apparent. Traditionally classified on the basis of clinical findings into peripheral and macular, most of the disorders involve more of the retina than is clinically apparent. The primary lesion may be located within one particular type of cell, and the features depend on the cell involved and on its distribution in the retina; thus a cone dystrophy predominantly affects the macula and a rod dystrophy the mid-peripheral retina. No system of classification is as yet entirely satisfactory. That based on the presumed location of the primary lesion is currently the most valuable in correlating the pathology with the clinical findings, in predicting

the course of the disorder, and in explaining the results of special investigations such as fluorescein angiography and electrophysiology. With advances in the understanding of molecular mechanisms a natural classification will undoubtedly evolve.

Neurosensory retinal dysfunctions and dystrophies

Neurosensory retinal dysfunctions and dystrophies either involve Müller cells (X-linked juvenile retinoschisis) or photoreceptors.

Müller cell dystrophy

X-linked juvenile retinoschisis

X-linked juvenile retinoschisis (XLJR) results from an inherited degeneration of Müller cells. It is probably more common than previously suspected, with an estimated prevalence as high as 1 : 15 000. There are regional variations, and in some parts of Finland XLJR is the commonest cause of visual impairment in young males. Clinical features are probably present at birth, but diagnosis is usually delayed until 4–8 years of age, when visual impairment resulting from foveal dysfunction becomes apparent. At presentation visual acuity is about 6/18. Hypermetropia and astigmatism are usual but, unlike other retinal dystrophies, myopia is rare. Secondary dyschromatopsia occurs with both tritan and red–green deficits. The condition usually remains stable for many years, although there is a tendency to slow progression. Ocular features include foveal schisis, peripheral retinoschisis and vitreous changes.

Foveal schisis is present in almost all cases, the earliest sign being loss of the foveal reflex. Radially arranged perifoveal microcysts, which develop later, are located in the nerve fibre layer and are associated with radiate plications of the overlying internal limiting membrane. Slow progression to macular cyst or hole formation is common. In the elderly, the foveal changes are replaced by a non-specific degeneration of the macula.

Peripheral retinoschisis is present in half of the cases. It is usually bilaterally symmetrical and occurs in the inferotemporal quadrant. The inner layer of the retina is elevated, attached to the vitreous and may exhibit multiple holes. Opaque dendritic vessels may be present.

Vitreous changes include veils (detached portions of superficial retina which may contain branching vessels), syneresis, strands, traction bands and detachment. Apparent improvement in the retinoschisis may result from the release of vitreoretinal traction consequent upon vitreous degeneration. Vitreoretinal changes predispose to haemorrhages and rhegmatogenous retinal detachment.

Other associated features include optic atrophy, macular distortion, anterior chamber angle anomalies, cataracts, neovascularization of the optic disc and peripheral retina, neovascular glaucoma and haemorrhagic retinal cysts.

An abnormal ERG with a reduced b-wave and a persistent or an increased a-wave suggests widespread retinal dysfunction located in the inner layers, leaving the photoreceptors relatively unaffected. The characteristic histological finding is retinoschisis with a split between the nerve fibre layer and the ganglion cell layer due to the disorder of Müller cells. Extracellular filaments, probably derived from defective Müller cells, are seen on electron microscopy within the retina and vitreous. With advancing age, atrophy of the inner and outer layers of the retina progresses and reactive gliosis may appear as vascular sheathing when localized in the region of blood vessels. Vascular defects and degenerative changes in the RPE are secondary phenomena. The gene locus for XLJR is at Xp22.2.

Photoreceptor dysfunctions and dystrophies

Photoreceptor dysfunctions and dystrophies are among the commonest inherited retinal disorders. Classification is based on the predominant photoreceptor involved (rod or cone) and on the clinical presentation and progression (stationary or progressive).

Photoreceptor dysfunctions are congenital non-progressive disorders of cell or neural pathway function. Clinical signs and structural pathological changes are minimal, but primary pathophysiological lesions are evident at the genetic and molecular level. Rod dysfunctions include congenital stationary night blindness, and cone dysfunctions include the dyschromatopsias.

Photoreceptor dystrophies are a large group of disorders associated with progressive visual loss, and form a spectrum of varying degrees of rod and cone involvement. If rod involvement is predominant, presentation is as retinitis pigmentosa, whereas if cone involvement is predominant, presentation is as a cone dystrophy. Intermediate forms are variously described as rod–cone and cone–rod dystrophies. Molecular genetic abnormalities have been identified in many instances, and these dystrophies overlap with those of other retinal layers.

Normal photoreceptors

The photoreceptors are the site of initiation of the transduction of light and are located adjacent to the RPE, upon which they are dependent for metabolic support and the recycling of metabolites. The retina contains two photoreceptor populations, rods and cones.

Rods are sensitive at low level (scotopic) illumination and are saturated by daylight (photopic) illumination. They are monochromatic, and their highest concentration is in the mid-peripheral retina.

Cones are active under photopic conditions and are the basis for colour and central (high acuity) vision. They are most concentrated at the foveola, but are widely distributed throughout the retina. Cones are subdivided according to their spectral sensitivity into long (L), medium (M) and short (S) wavelength sensitive types. More than one type of L and M cone may coexist with slightly different spectral sensitivities.

Photoreceptors are structurally divided into an outer and inner segment by a narrow constriction incorporating a modified cilium. The outer segment in rods is long and tubular and in cones is short and conical except at the fovea, where the cones are longer and more tightly packed. The outer segment has a series of regular disc-like structures that contain the photopigment that interacts with light to initiate the biochemical phototransduction process. The discs of rods are isolated within the cytoplasm, whereas those of cones communicate with the cell membrane. The inner segments of the photoreceptors contain the structures necessary for the synthesis and maintenance of the outer segments. Photoreceptors communicate with the neural circuitry of the retina by an inner rod/cone fibre that ends in a synaptic terminal called a spherule (rods) or pedicle (cones).

Light transduction

The photoreceptor outer segment discs contain a transmembrane protein. In rods this is rhodopsin, while in cones it is one of three categories of cone pigment. Each photoreceptor protein contains a light absorbing component (chromophore) that undergoes a structural change when it absorbs a photon of light. This initiates a series of biochemical cascades that result in hyperpolarization of the photoreceptor membrane potential and inhibition of the release of a neurotransmitter from the respective rod spherule or cone pedicle. The neural circuitry of the retina converts this into a frequency modulated binary action potential that is transmitted along the optic nerve.

Molecular genetics and pathophysiology

Mutation of genes encoding any of a number of key molecules may lead to loss of function and degeneration of photoreceptors. Such mutations have been identified in genes encoding photoreceptor proteins and other proteins involved in transduction. Proteins that merit particular attention are rhodopsin, peripherin/RDS and retinal outer segment membrane protein 1.

Rhodopsin: rhodopsin is a transmembrane protein of the rod outer segment discs. It consists of a convoluted protein chain (opsin) comprising 348 amino acids with seven transmembrane alpha helices forming a cage around a molecule of the Vitamin A derivative retinol. The first stage in the light transduction process is the activation of rhodopsin. Absorption of light quanta by retinol causes a conformational change of the molecule from an 11-cis to an all trans configuration, with a subsequent alteration in the structure of the molecule. Activated rhodopsin reacts with transducin (G-protein) that, when inactive, consists of three units (α, β, γ). Activation of transducin causes the β and γ subunits to dissociate and GTP to replace GDP on the α subunit. The activated GTP α subunit activates the enzyme cyclic GMP phosphodiesterase (PDE) by causing the removal of two inhibitory PDE γ subunits. Activated PDE rapidly hydrolyses cGMP, which, by closing ion channels in the cell membrane, leads to rapid hyperpolarization. To complete the cycle, cGMP is regenerated through the action of increasing calcium concentrations and the enzymes recoverin and guanylate cyclase, and rhodopsin is deactivated by the combined activities of the two proteins, arrestin (S-antigen) and rhodopsin kinase. Rhodopsin is metabolized and recycled via complex biochemical pathways that involve close interaction between the photoreceptor and the RPE cell. Disruption at any level of these pathways leads to rod photoreceptor malfunction. A mutation of the rhodopsin gene, located at 3q21, was the first to be identified as a cause of retinitis pigmentosa. Over 100 mutations at this locus are now known, and all lead to dysfunction and/or degeneration of rods. The mutations thus demonstrate genetic heterogeneity, but the majority are associated with autosomal dominant retinitis pigmentosa. Rhodopsin mutations can also exhibit allelic heterogeneity, as has been found in congenital stationary night blindness.

Peripherin/RDS and retinal outer segment membrane protein 1: peripherin, a glycoprotein in the rod outer segment, is located at the edges of the photoreceptor discs near the plasma membrane. In association with other proteins such as retinal outer segment membrane protein 1 (ROM-1) it maintains the biochemical stability of the discs. The locus of the human peripherin gene (6p21) is homologous to the mouse RDS (retinal degeneration slow) locus. The gene of ROM-1 is situated on chromosome 11 (11q13). Mutations of the peripherin/RDS gene exhibit allelic heterogeneity. Different peripherin gene mutations have been identified in autosomal dominant retinitis pigmentosa, retinitis punctata albescens, pattern macular dystrophy, adult vitelliform macular dystrophy, retinopathy similar to fundus flavimaculatus, adult-onset foveomacular dystrophy with choroidal neovascularization, abnormalities of the choriocapillaris similar to diffuse choroidal atrophy, and central areolar choroidal dystrophy.

Mechanism of cell degeneration and death

Genetic mutation may directly cause photoreceptor dysfunctions and dystrophies. Progressive degeneration occurs in some but not all of these conditions, and is probably secondary to abnormal metabolism of the mutant proteins. Photoreceptors degenerate if normal rhodopsin is over-expressed or if mutant rhodopsins cannot be metabolized. Similarly, a mutation in the β subunit of PDE results in a persistent elevation in intracellular cGMP; the functional effect of this is to prevent closure of sodium channels in the outer segment plasma membrane, thereby keeping the photoreceptor permanently depolarized and preventing the light-induced hyperpolarization vital for photoreceptor transduction. Later, progressive degeneration and cell death result from the toxic effect of sustained elevated intracellular cGMP levels. The particular metabolic abnormality may therefore determine the presence or type of retinal degeneration observed, and could explain the stability of some photoreceptor disorders and the variable progression of others. The photoreceptor dystrophies are remarkable for the number of mutations that can cause them, and for the relatively narrow spectrum of pathological processes involved. It is probable that the various genetic and metabolic abnormalities converge to a final common pathway of cell degeneration and death, and that apoptosis is the most likely mechanism.

Stationary rod dysfunctions – congenital stationary night blindness

Night blindness is the common feature of several rare syndromes of rod dysfunction collectively termed congenital stationary night blindness (CSNB). Uniform classification is not possible, but two broad categories are defined according to the fundal appearance.

CSNB with normal fundi

CSNB with normal fundi is inherited as autosomal dominant, autosomal recessive or X-linked. Rod dark adaptation is absent, but the cone system is unaffected. The ERG is abnormal and has two characteristic patterns.

CSNB 1 (Rigg's type): the photopic response is of normal amplitude but the scotopic response is reduced, with the amplitude of the b-wave being greater than that of the a-wave. CSNB (Rigg's type) is autosomal dominant and the most widely reported variety, most cases being examples of the Nougaret type (so called after the large French pedigree in which the condition was first described). Affected individuals have normal visual acuity, colour vision and photopic visual fields. Absence of dark adaptation is demonstrated on adaptometry. Normal rhodopsin concentration is revealed by fundus reflectometry, and no structural abnormalities have been demonstrated. The autosomal dominant Nougaret type of CSNB is due to abnormal signal coupling between rhodopsin and PDE consequent upon a mutation on chromosome 3 (3p21) in a gene encoding the α subunit of rod transducin. Rods are thus insensitive to light, and those affected are night blind.

CSNB 2 (Schubert–Bornschein type): the photopic response may be normal or subnormal, but the b-wave of the scotopic response is reduced in amplitude compared with the a-wave. This feature is characteristic of an abnormality in the middle layers of the retina, although no structural changes have been demonstrated. Further classification is based on the completeness or incompleteness of rod dysfunction.

Complete: dark adaptation and ERG oscillatory potentials are absent, but the 30-Hz flicker response is normal.

Incomplete: some dark adaptation is present, as are oscillatory potentials, but the 30-Hz flicker response is absent.

In CSNB 2 (Schubert–Bornschein type) inheritance may be autosomal recessive or X-linked. Visual acuity is sufficiently reduced from birth as to be associated with nystagmus. Myopia is mild to moderate in the autosomal recessive type but high in X-linked pedigrees, although the refractive error can vary within affected families. Two loci have been identified for X-linked CSNB (Xp11 – CSNB 1, and Xp21 – CSNB 2). The locus mapped to CSNB 1 is closely linked with two loci for forms of X-linked retinitis pigmentosa and with the locus for Åland Island eye disease. The locus mapped to CSNB 2 is closely linked to the X-linked RP3 locus.

CSNB with abnormal fundi

There are three types of CSNB with abnormal fundi: the flecked retina of Kandori has only been described in Japan, but Oguchi's disease and fundus albipunctatus are less rare.

Oguchi's disease is characterized by prolonged dark adaptation, perhaps over many hours, but finally reaching normal levels. This is the only symptom. Oguchi's disease is autosomal recessive and was originally described in the Japanese. Affected individuals exhibit a characteristic whitish metallic appearance of the light-adapted fundus that returns to normal after prolonged dark adaptation (Mizuo–Nakamura phenomenon). The ERG is normal provided adequate time is given for the eye to dark adapt between stimuli. In several families mutation of the arrestin gene on chromosome 2 (2q37) has been identified. Arrestin (S-antigen) is a protein involved in the deactivation of light-activated rhodopsin, and an abnormality would explain the prolonged dark adaptation. Light and electron microscopy have identified several abnormalities. Lipofuscin is seen to a greater extent than normal both within and external to the RPE. Abnormal interdigitations of the RPE with the outer segments of the photoreceptors form a layer-like structure that may account for the abnormal light reflex, and microvascular or tubular structures replace the normal lamellae of the outer segments of the photoreceptors.

Fundus albipunctatus is also characterized by abnormal dark adaptation. Uniform white dots at the level of the RPE are distributed throughout the fundus, but are most dense in the post-equatorial region. Fundus albipunctatus results from slow rhodopsin regeneration, but the precise defect and the origin of the white dots are not understood. Fundus albipunctatus, like Oguchi's disease, is autosomal recessive.

Stationary cone dysfunctions – dyschromatopsias

The stationary cone dysfunctions are the cone counterparts of the stationary rod dysfunctions. Affected individuals are born with dysfunction of one or all types of cone. They present with degrees of colour blindness and, in the case of monochromatism, with central visual loss. As with the rod dysfunctions, the cone defects are at the molecular level but unlike rod dysfunctions, some cone dysfunctions are very common. Approximately 10 per cent of males and 0.5 per cent of females have defective colour vision resulting in abnormal discrimination of certain colours. Monochromatism, the extreme form of stationary cone dysfunction, is rare (1 : 10 000). The pathophysiology of the dyschromatopsias is complex and results from abnormalities at the molecular genetic level. In most cases, as with some types of CSNB, no fundal abnormality is present and there are no histologically recognizable structural changes.

Molecular genetics of colour vision

Humans have trichromatic vision, whereby any perceived colour can be matched by adjusting the relative intensities of three suitably chosen primaries. Human trichromatic colour vision was at one time thought to result from the presence of three types of cone, each containing a different photopigment, with peak spectral absorbances at approximately 435 nm (blue, short wave or S cones), 534 nm (green, medium wave or M cones) and 560 nm (red, long wave or L cones). It is now realized that colour vision is more complex than this simple model. The gene that encodes S cone pigment is on chromosome 6, and those encoding the L and M cone pigments are on the X chromosome. The L and M pigment genes are similar in sequence and are probably located adjacent to each other in a head-to-tail tandem array, with one or possibly more L pigment genes being followed by one or more M pigment genes. Duplication or even triplication of the M pigment gene can result from unequal crossing over during meiosis, a mechanism that may lead to colour blindness by deletion or the creation of a hybrid gene. In addition to various multiplications, the L and M genes are known to be polymorphic (i.e. different between apparently normal individuals). They each exist in at least two different forms with peak spectral sensitivities 5–7 nm apart, a small number of amino acid substitutions at various positions in the pigment molecules accounting for the differences in their spectral sensitivities. Variability in the expression of the L and M pigment genes results either because of their position within a tandem sequence or because of the presence of hybrid or polymorphic forms. Normal individuals have more than one L and M pigment genes and can express up to five different cone opsins (2 M, 2 L and 1 S). All the variants remain trichromatic, but may show psychophysical differences when subjected to sensitive colour vision tests.

Monochromatism

Monochromatism results from congenital autosomal recessive absence of cones or cone function. There are typical and atypical forms.

Typical: rhodopsin is present in rods and cones, which both respond in the same way.

Atypical/incomplete: typical cone pigments are present and some cone function remains. The defect lies beyond the level of light absorption, and symptoms are less severe than in the typical form.

Blue cone monochromatism is a rare X-linked recessive condition in which rods and S cones are the only functioning photoreceptors. Female carriers may exhibit an abnormal macular appearance and ERG. Blue cone monochromatism is mapped to Xq28, the chromosomal region containing the closely linked genes of L and M cone pigments. Unequal homologous recombination leads to their inactivation because of the genes themselves or because of deletion of a nearby control sequence. The S cone pigment is normal because it is located on a different chromosome (7q31.3-q32), and the L and M cone pigments are not expressed.

Dichromatism

Dichromatism comprises a group of disorders in which two of the three classes of cones are functioning normally. Affected individuals are able to match any colour with two primary colours, but tend to confuse colours easily distinguishable by those with normal vision. As there are three classes of cone pigment, so there are three types of dichromatism: protanopia, deuteranopia and tritanopia.

Protanopia and deuteranopia: in protanopia L cone function is absent, and in deuteranopia M cone function is absent. S cone function is intact in both. The conditions are inherited as X-linked recessives, and affect approximately 1 per cent of Caucasian males. Due to the overlap in the spectral sensitivity curves of the L and S cone pigments, deuteranopes are not green blind, but their perception of colour is different from normal. Protanopes and deuteranopes confuse various shades of red with various shades of green.

Tritanopia: tritanopia is a rare autosomal dominant colour vision defect characterized by functional loss of the S cone pigment. This can result from at least three different point mutations of the S opsin gene located on chromosome 7 (7q31.3-q32). Tritanopes confuse shades of blue with longer wavelengths.

Anomalous trichromatism

Anomalous trichromatism is a less severe form of colour vision defect than dichromatism. Classification, inheritance and clinical features parallel those of dichromatism, but unlike dichromats, in whom only two cone pigments are expressed, anomalous trichromats express all three cone pigments but the spectral characteristics of one are abnormal. Anomalous trichromacy is due to the expression of hybrid genes of the L and M cone pigments or to anomalies of the S cone pigment. Protanomaly and deuteranomaly are common, and affect about 1 per cent and 5 per cent respectively of Caucasian males. The expression of a hybrid gene may lead to abnormal spectral properties of the L cone pigment (protanomaly) or the M cone pigment (deuteranomaly). Alternatively, two polymorphic variants of an L or an M pigment gene may result in two cone pigments with closely related sensitivity curves. Tritanomaly is rare and, if it exists, is probably a partial form of tritanopia.

Progressive photoreceptor dystrophies

Progressive photoreceptor dystrophies comprise a large group of disorders characterized by progressive photoreceptor degeneration. The clinical features fall into two broadly defined pictures identified as retinitis pigmentosa (predominantly rod involvement) and cone dystrophy, although there are intermediate types (rod–cone or cone–rod dystrophies).

Retinitis pigmentosa

Retinitis pigmentosa (RP) is the clinical manifestation of a group of disorders in which an underlying molecular defect leads to malfunction and degeneration of photoreceptors. Rods are preferentially affected but cones are also involved to a variable extent, thereby creating a spectrum of disease ranging from pure rod to pure cone dystrophies. The cone dystrophies differ clinically and are considered separately. An abnormality in the distribution and the amount of pigmentation is associated with and is secondary to the degeneration of the photoreceptors. This is not exclusive to RP and may occur in other inherited and acquired disorders (pseudo-retinitis pigmentosa).

The term retinitis pigmentosa is incorrect in that it implies an inflammatory aetiology. Nevertheless it remains widely used, although other terms such as pigmentary retinal degeneration, photoreceptor dystrophy and rod–cone dystrophy are more precise. The term tapetoretinal degeneration should be disregarded, as there is no tapetum in human eyes. Electrophysiological and psychophysical studies allow classification into rod–cone (diffuse) and cone–rod (regional) types. In a rod–cone degeneration, rods are more severely affected and loss of rod function is diffuse. Conversely, in a cone–rod degeneration, cone function is more severely affected and the disorders tend to have a patchy (regional) loss of both rod and cone function between areas of relatively preserved rod function.

RP is the commonest form of inherited blindness, with a prevalence estimated at about 1 : 4000 but ranging from 1 : 3000 to 1 : 20 000 depending on the population in question. It is estimated that there are over 1.5 million sufferers world-wide. RP can be inherited as autosomal dominant (10–20 per cent) or autosomal recessive (20–40 per cent), or as an X-linked recessive trait (10–25 per cent). Half of the cases of RP occur without a family history (sporadic or simplex RP) and presumably represent autosomal recessive disease, reduced penetrance,

new mutations or phenocopies. A digenic form of RP is recognized in which the disorder is manifest only in individuals with mutations of both peripherin/RDS (6p21.2-cen) and ROM-1 (11q13).

The onset and progression of symptoms in RP vary, and in many cases relate to the mode of inheritance. The X-linked and autosomal recessive types are the most severe, and begin in childhood. The autosomal dominant type is relatively mild. Female carriers of the X-linked type may be asymptomatic or have a relatively mild form of the disease. Symptoms mainly reflect involvement of the rod photoreceptor system but there may also be abnormalities of cone function, including poor central and colour vision and difficulty with bright lights.

Clinical features

The commonest symptoms are night blindness, loss of visual field and loss of visual acuity. Signs seen on ophthalmoscopic examination include retinal pigmentation and changes in the macula, retinal vasculature and optic disc (Fig. 5.27a).

Night blindness: with the exception of the rare congenital onset RP (Leber's congenital amaurosis), poor night vision is the usual presenting symptom although many of those affected have adapted to it without recognizing it as abnormal. Poor scotopic vision is demonstrated by dark adaptometry, which shows a marked elevation of rod threshold throughout.

Loss of visual field: in moderately advanced disease, the mid-peripheral visual field is lost (ring scotoma). In advanced cases, complete loss of the peripheral field leaves only an isolated island of central vision.

Loss of visual acuity: visual acuity is usually relatively unaffected until the late stages unless the RP is severe. Cystoid macular oedema may be present. In most cases where cone involvement is more pronounced (cone–rod dystrophy), central visual loss occurs at an early stage.

Retinal pigmentary changes: early cases exhibit a fine punctate pigment disturbance with depigmentation or atrophy of the RPE. As the disorder progresses, clumps and strands of black pigment form a characteristic bone spicule configuration and less well-defined pigmented clumps and spots. The mid-peripheral retina is most affected, and changes progress circumferentially, anteriorly and posteriorly. Where these pigmentary changes are absent, the retina often has an atrophic moth-eaten appearance or exhibits salt-and-pepper pigmentation.

Macular changes: mild changes at the macula compatible with normal visual acuity include an abnormal light

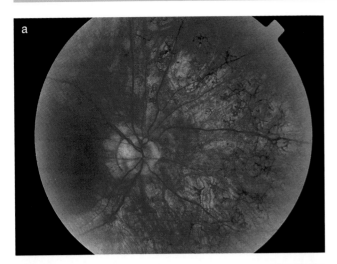

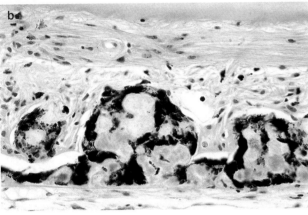

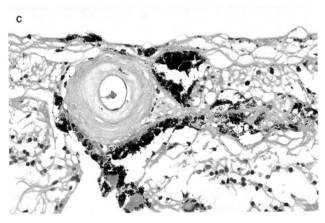

Figure 5.27 Retinitis pigmentosa. (a) Fundus appearance. (b) Photoreceptor degeneration, gliosis and pigment migration. (c) Hyalinized retinal arteriole and pigment migration.

reflex and a cellophane-like maculopathy. Cystic changes, oedema and pigmentation, sometimes in a bull's-eye configuration, are associated with reduced visual acuity.

Retinal vascular changes: in well-established cases vascular attenuation is a secondary phenomenon. The RPE

in the region of the retinal arterioles may be relatively well preserved (preserved para-arteriolar RPE – PPRPE) in a distinct rare and aggressive form of RP.

Optic disc changes: optic atrophy appears in advanced cases as a characteristic waxy optic disc pallor. Other disc abnormalities include a reduced cup : disc ratio and telangiectasis.

Individuals with RP are usually myopic and develop posterior subcapsular cataracts. Syneresis of the vitreous, in which pigment granules occur anteriorly, is also common. The EOG is flat, and an absent or reduced amplitude of the ERG indicates widespread abnormality of photoreceptor function. The predominance of the rod over the cone response allows for an electrodiagnostic classification into rod–cone and cone–rod types of RP which can be related to patterns of visual field loss and psychophysical analysis of cone and rod thresholds. The clinical appearance of RP may vary, and numerous atypical forms have been described. It is speculated that these atypical forms represent specific manifestations of particular mutations.

Systemic associations
RP most commonly occurs without systemic involvement, but there are several important associations with autosomal recessive metabolic, neurological, renal and hepatic disorders. The association of RP with hearing loss is the basis of several related conditions identified as Usher's syndrome. Other rare systemic disorders with RP include Alport's syndrome, Alström's disease, Cockaigne's syndrome, Flynn Aird syndrome, Friedreich's ataxia, Hurler's syndrome (MPS1), Kearns–Sayre syndrome, Marshall's syndrome, osteopetrosis (Albers-Schönberg disease), Refsum's disease and Waardenburg's syndrome.

Usher's syndrome is a relatively common autosomal recessive condition in which congenital neurosensory deafness is associated with RP. In children it accounts for 5 per cent of profound deafness and at least half of all cases of combined deafness and blindness. Four types are distinguished clinically, with further subdivision by genetic analysis. The candidate gene for one of the types encodes for myosin, which is present and presumed to be abnormal in both the photoreceptor cilium and the hair cells of the organ of Corti.

Pathological features
As the retina responds to insults in only a limited number of ways, the pigmentary retinal dystrophies, despite their molecular heterogeneity, have many common pathological features. Photoreceptor degeneration may result from a genetic mutation affecting the photoreceptor directly or support tissue such as the

RPE, and from a metabolic abnormality that causes photoreceptor degeneration by the deprivation of a vital metabolite. Disruption of normal metabolism may result from an abnormal gene product or from shortage of the product of a normal gene. Characteristic pathological features include photoreceptor degeneration, pigmentary changes and vascular changes, epiretinal membranes and optic disc pallor.

Photoreceptors: the fundamental lesion in RP is photoreceptor degeneration. The rods in the mid-periphery are initially affected, and changes include shortening of the outer segments, disorientated and disorganized disc membranes, swelling of the inner segments, loss of both the outer and inner segments, the presence of autophagic vacuoles, and a change in the morphology of the photoreceptor cells, which become spherical. Ultimately, loss of the photoreceptor cells leaves a relatively normal inner retina in contact with the RPE. More advanced cases exhibit complete atrophy and disorganization of the remaining retina, and replacement of neurons by glial tissue (Fig. 5.27b).

Pigmentary changes: secondary changes within the RPE include proliferation, degeneration, depigmentation and atrophy. The characteristic pigment deposition is both extra- and intracellular, and involves Müller cells, macrophages and displaced RPE cells. RPE cells in the mid-periphery migrate to form perivascular clumps, giving rise to the bone spicule configuration. Pigment-laden macrophages come to lie between the inner nuclear layer and the external limiting membrane, approximation of which to the RPE promotes further pigment migration.

Vascular changes, epiretinal membranes and optic disc pallor: the vascular narrowing seen clinically may be an autoregulatory phenomenon whereby perfusion of the retinal arterioles is adjusted to the lower oxygen demands of a thin degenerate retina. In advanced disease the retinal arterioles show hyalinization (Fig. 5.27c). Epiretinal membranes develop in advanced disease, and gliosis of the optic disc accounts for the waxy appearance seen clinically.

Progressive cone and cone–rod dystrophies

Progressive cone and cone–rod photoreceptor dystrophies, like RP, are a heterogeneous group. They probably represent the cone end of the spectrum of photoreceptor dystrophies and degenerations, but as yet are poorly classified. Clinical features mirror the functional and anatomical consequences of the predominant cell lost. A progressive cone deficit results in loss of central and colour vision beginning in the first or second decades of life. Photophobia is present, and the maculo-

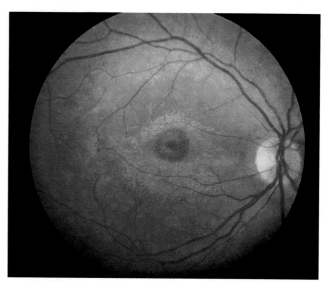

Figure 5.28 Cone–rod photoreceptor dystrophy with bull's eye maculopathy.

pathy varies from a characteristic bull's-eye (Fig. 5.28) to macular atrophy or non-specific granular pigmentation. ERG findings suggest predominantly cone dysfunction and, depending on the demonstration of a normal rod response, allow for classification into a cone or cone–rod dystrophy. In some cone–rod dystrophies, clinical features of rod degeneration may become apparent with mid-peripheral pigmentary changes and arteriolar attenuation. Sporadic forms and all modes of Mendelian inheritance have been described, but little is known of the histological changes.

Photoreceptor/RPE dystrophies

Stargardt's disease/fundus flavimaculatus

Stargardt's disease/fundus flavimaculatus is the commonest inherited macular dystrophy, with an estimated incidence of 1:10 000. Previously classified as separate disorders, Stargardt's disease and fundus flavimaculatus form the opposite ends of a continuum of disorders with similar pathogenesis and pathology, and autosomal recessive inheritance. Stargardt's disease presents in late childhood or early adult life with failing central vision due to a bilaterally symmetrical maculopathy. Fundus flavimaculatus presents in later life with a mid-peripheral retinopathy and slowly failing central vision due to macular involvement. The presence of multiple yellowish-white retinal flecks is common to both and, although these can vary in size and shape, they usually have an angulated or fishtail appearance (Fig. 5.29). The flecks are not fixed in position but fade and reappear elsewhere, sometimes leaving pigmentary retinal changes or choroidal atrophy. A characteristic finding on fluorescein angiography in 85 per cent of those affected is

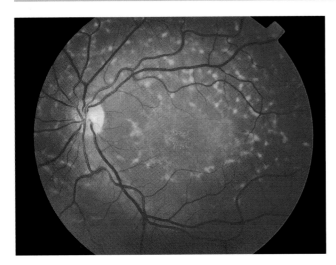

Figure 5.29 Stargardt's disease.

generalized decreased background choroidal fluorescence (dark choroid or choroidal silence) due to diffuse changes in the RPE.

Maculopathy (Stargardt's disease)

Symptoms of macular involvement precede any ophthalmoscopic abnormalities, and occur in children and young adults. A bilaterally symmetrical maculopathy occurs later with progressive loss of central vision due to the formation of central scotomas and acquired red–green dyschromatopsia. The peripheral visual field remains full. Early findings are a beaten bronze appearance in the foveal region and a horizontal oval area of pigment epithelial atrophy. Parafoveal and mid-peripheral yellow-white flecks may appear later. As macular atrophy progresses, the choroid becomes exposed and the fundal appearance ultimately resembles that of central areolar choroidal dystrophy.

Peripheral retinopathy (fundus flavimaculatus)

Peripheral retinopathy presents in adults with failing vision due to macular involvement. If the macula is not involved, the condition is asymptomatic and may only be detected on routine ophthalmoscopic examination. The typical appearance is of yellow flecks at the posterior pole and extending to the equator. In advanced disease, retinal pigmentation and atrophy may resemble that of RP.

In Stargardt's disease/fundus flavimaculatus, lipofuscin-like material accumulates in RPE cells, particularly at the posterior pole where the density of photoreceptors is greatest. Lipofuscin also accumulates in the inner segments of the photoreceptors. Damage to photoreceptors occurs primarily at the macula, and in advanced disease the photoreceptors and the RPE are almost totally lost with only a few degenerate nuclei being visible between Bruch's membrane and the external limiting membrane

of the retina. The yellow flecks are focal accumulations of lipofuscin-like material and glycosaminoglycans within the apices of engorged RPE cells. Since the abnormal pigment absorbs the underlying transmitted choroidal fluorescence, diffuse deposition within the RPE cells explains the dark choroid seen on fluorescein angiography. Genetic linkage analysis confirms that Stargardt's disease and fundus flavimaculatus are different clinical manifestations of a single gene mutation on chromosome 1 (1p22-p21). A candidate gene has been identified that encodes a rod-specific transmembrane protein (retina-specific ATP-binding casette transporter, ABCA4) which is probably involved in the cycling of metabolites between the outer segment of rods and the RPE. Dysfunction of this protein results in the intracellular accumulation of metabolites or their derivatives. Paradoxically, while the disorder is primarily one of rods, clinical manifestations occur at the macula as a result of disturbance at the level of the photoreceptor/RPE interface and the RPE. This macular involvement may reflect regional differences in the susceptibility of photoreceptors or the RPE to metabolic insult. Rare autosomal dominant forms of the disorder have been linked to loci on the long arms of chromosomes 6 and 13.

Best's vitelliform macular dystrophy

Best's vitelliform macular dystrophy is an autosomal dominant disorder of variable penetrance and expressivity. It is the second most common inherited macular dystrophy. The condition may remain asymptomatic, but can be identified on routine examination. More usually it presents with reduced vision in children or young adults. Symptoms are often surprisingly mild considering the extensive maculopathy that can occur. Progressive visual loss is associated with atrophic macular changes or fibrous scarring. A finding of diagnostic importance, even in cases with apparently normal fundi, is a subnormal EOG in the presence of a normal ERG, thus indicating a widespread abnormality relating to the RPE, Bruch's membrane or the intervening potential space. The ophthalmoscopic appearance is variable, and often asymmetrical between the two eyes. The morphology of lesions may change with time, and the classification of Deutman and Mohler suggests a sequential progression:

Stage 0: the macula is relatively normal in appearance but the EOG is abnormal.

Stage I: fine speckled pigmentary changes are seen at the macula.

Stage II (vitelliform or egg-yolk lesion): a discrete round homogeneous opaque yellow cystic lesion, similar in size to the optic disc, is seen at the macula (Fig. 5.30). Vision

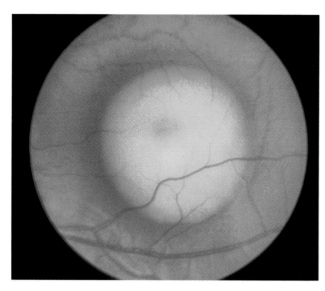

Figure 5.30 Best's vitelliform maculopathy.

is often normal. The lesion may degenerate to give a scrambled egg appearance (stage IIa).

Stage III (pseudohypopyon): the yellow material within the cyst develops a fluid level.

Stage IV: this represents end-stage disease, with macular and RPE atrophy (stage IVa), fibrous scarring (stage IVb), choroidal neovascularization (stage IVc) and macular haemorrhage.

Although these stages suggest an orderly series of events, stages II and III are rarely seen. Occasionally, there are multifocal macular and extramacular lesions (polymorphic macular degeneration of Braley). The massive accumulation of lipofuscin in the RPE cells supports the clinical and electrodiagnostic findings. Lipofuscin is also found between the neurosensory retina and the RPE, within subretinal macrophages, and lying free within the choroid. The gene (VMD2) is located on chromosome 11 (11q13) and encodes a protein (bestrophin) which is thought to be involved in the metabolism/transport of polyunsaturated fatty acids.

Pseudovitelliform lesions are yellowish macular lesions resembling the appearance of true vitelliform dystrophy, and may be differentiated from it by not exhibiting dominant inheritance and by the presence of a normal EOG. Pseudovitelliform lesions occur in a heterogeneous group of acquired macular degenerations, often in association with perifoveal retinal capillary leakage and RPE detachments.

Pigment pattern dystrophies

The pigment pattern dystrophies are a group of related dystrophies of the RPE characterized by granular or reticular patterns of fundal pigmentation and a benign clinical course with normal or near normal vision. Reticular, macroreticular and butterfly-shaped pigment dystrophies are included in the group. Peripherin/RDS mutations have been identified in individuals with butterfly-shaped pigment dystrophies, and in such cases the clinical appearance results from impaired phagocytosis of abnormal photoreceptor outer segments with accumulation of undigested material within the RPE.

RPE/Bruch's membrane dystrophies

Dominant drusen (Doyne's honeycomb choroiditis, Malattia-levantinese)

This autosomal dominant dystrophy of the RPE probably represents a group of disorders in which the synonymously named conditions may exhibit slight variations. Because of the lack of symptoms, the diagnosis may not be made until late in life. Inherited drusen are small, round, yellow to white and usually discrete, although they may occur in clumps or be confluent (Fig. 5.31). The distribution and appearance may show variation, but the condition is bilaterally symmetric and similar within affected family members. Drusen change in size, shape, distribution and consistency over the years and are associated with atrophy of the overlying RPE, which in older individuals may assume a geographic appearance. Symptoms occur late in life from associated exudative or non-exudative retinal and/or RPE detachment. Autosomal dominant dystrophic drusen are similar to acquired degenerative age-related hard drusen. The gene responsible for Malattia-levantinese (EFEMP1) has been localized to the short arm of chromosome 2 (2p21-p16) and encodes EGF-containing fibrillin-like extracellular matrix protein 1.

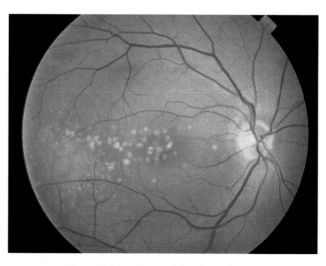

Figure 5.31 Autosomal dominant drusen.

North Carolina macular dystrophy

North Carolina macular dystrophy is autosomal dominantly inherited, and the gene (MCDR1) is mapped to chromosome 6 (6q14-q16.2). Presentation is variable, but features include a crater-like macular staphyloma with a shiny base surrounded by a gliotic rim. Unlike other macular dystrophies, lesions are probably present at birth and are usually non-progressive. The name of the condition refers to the strong founder effect traceable over 200 years and linking many of the North American families. Unrelated families have been identified elsewhere in Europe, Canada and Mexico.

Sorsby's fundus dystrophy

Sorsby's fundus dystrophy (SFD) is a rare and highly penetrant autosomal dominant disorder seen in young individuals and characterized by a tritan colour defect, yellow plaque-like subretinal deposits and RPE atrophy. Associated features include choroidal neovascularization, haemorrhages and exudates, subretinal fibrosis and, later, choroidal atrophy. Ruptures of Bruch's membrane and a maculopathy cause visual loss that starts after the age of 50 years. Progressive atrophy of the retina, RPE and choroid lead to peripheral visual loss by the eighth decade. An abnormal lipid deposit has been identified between the RPE cells and their basement membrane. Degenerative changes include loss of the photoreceptors, discontinuity of the RPE and atrophy of the choriocapillaris. The SFD gene (TIMP3) has been located to chromosome 22 (22q12.1-q13.2) and encodes a tissue inhibitor of metalloproteinase-3.

Choroidoretinal dystrophies

Choroidoretinal dystrophies are a genetically determined group of progressive disorders that, at an early stage, predominantly involve the choroid. The adjacent RPE and retina are also involved, and it may not be possible to determine in which tissue the primary abnormality lies. The dystrophies are divided into regional and diffuse types. The commonest presentation of regional dystrophies is with macular involvement (central areolar choroidal dystrophy), although paramacular (circinate choroidal dystrophy) and peripapillary (peripapillary choroidal dystrophy) forms have been described. Diffuse dystrophies are characterized by night blindness.

Central areolar choroidal dystrophy (central areolar choroidal sclerosis)

Central areolar choroidal dystrophy can be autosomal dominant or recessive, and presents in the third decade with mildly reduced central vision that slowly progresses to severe visual loss. Mild non-specific foveal granularity that may mimic other macular diseases is an early fundus change. The characteristic round or oval macular lesion is due to atrophy of the neurosensory retina, RPE and choriocapillaris, and appears over many years. Several large choroidal vessels may cross the white sclera within the atrophic area. The yellowish appearance of these vessels was previously interpreted as choroidal vascular sclerosis, but this is not supported by microscopy, which demonstrates atrophy rather than sclerosis. A well-demarcated avascular zone consists of atrophic and fibrosed choroidal tissue. Retinal atrophy follows exactly the extent of the underlying choroidal atrophy, but Bruch's membrane is unaffected.

Diffuse atrophy of the choriocapillaris (diffuse choroidal sclerosis)

Diffuse atrophy of the choriocapillaris is a rare disorder inherited as autosomal dominant or recessive. It is characterized by progressive widespread thinning and loss of the choriocapillaris beginning in midlife and resulting in severe loss of vision by later years. Symptoms include night blindness and loss of both central and peripheral vision. Fluorescein angiography reveals widespread loss of the choriocapillaris, with relative preservation of medium-sized and large choroidal vessels. The condition may be related to central areolar choroidal dystrophy, as both may occur in the same family, and it has been associated with mutations of the peripherin/RDS gene.

Gyrate atrophy of the choroid and retina with hyperornithinemia

Gyrate atrophy with hyperornithinemia is an autosomal recessive systemic disorder involving the choroid and retina. Activity of the mitochondrial matrix enzyme ornithine aminotransferase (OAT) is reduced or absent. OAT is pyridoxal phosphate dependent and catalyses the conversion of ornithine to glutamic-γ-semialdehyde, which is metabolized to glutamate or proline. Affected individuals have elevation of plasma and tissue levels of ornithine that may be 20 times above the norm. The disorder is rare, and approximately half of the reported cases are from Finland. Two types of the disorder are identified by their clinical response to pyridoxine treatment. The commonest form is that in which there is little residual enzyme activity and no response to pyridoxine. The OAT gene is located on chromosome 10 (10q26), and two mutations account for the majority of non-pyridoxine-responsive cases. There is a degree of molecular heterogeneity, and loss of gene function may occur from deletions, insertions, splice-site base pair changes and mis-sense mutations. OAT protein immunoreactivity can be demonstrated in most of those affected, indicating that, although the protein is synthesized, it is enzymatically inactive. The OAT gene is expressed throughout the body, and it is not understood why ocular tissues are preferentially involved.

Night blindness occurs in the first or second decade. Irregular round areas of choroidal atrophy develop, enlarge and coalesce to form extensive atrophic areas in the periphery, with consequent constriction of the visual field. The characteristic fundal appearance is of a sharp transition from the normal to marked choroidoretinal atrophy. Central visual loss results from macular involvement, cystoid macular oedema or epiretinal membrane formation. The pathological changes include total loss of all choroidal and retinal elements in affected areas, but structurally normal retina away from the abrupt border that delineates the lesions. Histological abnormalities also occur in muscle (subsarcolemmal deposits), liver and iris (mitochondrial abnormalities). Much is known of the biochemistry of the condition, but the cause of the tissue damage is not understood.

Choroideremia

Choroideremia is an uncommon X-linked progressive bilateral and symmetric choroidoretinal atrophy. Its prevalence varies geographically, and may range from 1 : 40 in certain parts of Finland to approximately 1 : 100 000 elsewhere. The gene for choroideremia (CHM) is localized to Xq21.1-q21.3 and encodes a gene product, Rab escort protein-1 (REP-1). REP-1 (previously termed component A of Rab geranylgeranyl transferase or CHM protein) is involved in the post-translational process of insertion of hydrophobic lipid side chains onto proteins (geranylgeranylation). Such modified proteins more readily attach to membranes, interact with other proteins, and are more readily involved in membrane transport and signal transduction. The mechanism resulting in choroidoretinal degeneration may relate to a defect in membrane transport with disrupted intracellular cycling of proteins between membrane and cytosol. Point mutations or deletions of the CHM gene have been identified in most cases studied.

Night blindness occurs in the first decade of life, and progressive visual loss in the second. Central visual acuity is spared until the third to fourth decade, but most affected males are legally blind by the age of 45 years. Signs of a diffuse atrophic process involving the RPE and choriocapillaris occur with the onset of symptoms, when there is equatorial and paramacular stippling of the RPE, a degree of choroidal atrophy and prominence of choroidal blood vessels. This progresses to more widespread choroidal atrophy with scattered intraretinal pigment clumping in the mid-periphery. Heterozygote female carriers are usually asymptomatic, but may demonstrate fundus changes ranging from diffuse RPE granularity to regional areas of choroidoretinal atrophy. The variable manifestations in a carrier result from random inactivation of one of the two X chromosomes (lyonization), leading to the expression of the defect in a proportion of choroidal and retinal cells. Affected areas exhibit loss of the choriocapillaris, Bruch's membrane and RPE, and degeneration of the outer and middle parts of the retina. Adhesion occurs between the avascular choroid and gliotic retina. The choriocapillaris and RPE are present in areas where photoreceptors remain.

DEPOSITS

Deposits are abnormal tissue accumulations of a substance or substances of exogenous or endogenous origin. Many but by no means all occur in the cornea, and some overlap with degenerations and dystrophies. Substances deposited include metals, metallic salts and related compounds, aromatic amino-acid derivatives, amyloid, lipid, degraded glycosaminoglycans, paraproteins, uric acid, cystine, hexosylceramides, and drugs having a particular affinity for ocular tissue.

METALS, METALLIC SALTS AND RELATED COMPOUNDS

Metals, metallic salts and related compounds include calcium, iron, copper, silver, gold and mercury.

Calcium

The deposition of calcium salts (usually phosphates or carbonates but also oxalates), other than in osteoid and tooth enamel, is heterotopic (occurring in an abnormal location) and classified as dystrophic, metastatic or idiopathic. Calcium salts are basophilic in haematoxylin and eosin stained sections. Small granules appear as stippling and larger granules as irregular and craggy masses. Calcium stains with alizarin red S, but the method of von Kossa is preferred for routine demonstration purposes and stains the phosphate or carbonate radical of the salt black.

Dystrophic calcification

The term dystrophic is used synonymously with degenerative. Dystrophic calcification is due to the persistence of dead or dying tissue and is not inherited. Calcium salts originate from interstitial fluid, and the deposition is extracellular. Serum calcium levels are normal. Lesions associated with dystrophic calcification include arteriosclerosis and calcinosis cutis (subepidermal calcified nodule – the presence of calcific deposits in the dermis of the skin). The main ocular manifestation of dystrophic calcification is band keratopathy due to localized corneal pathology, but other ocular lesions that may become calcified include cataracts, retinoblastomas (Fig. 5.32a), drusen (Fig. 5.13c), degenerate choroidal and retinal tissue, and senile scleral plaques.

Metastatic calcification

The term metastatic in this context means widespread, and does not imply a neoplastic process. The fundamental abnormality is an elevated serum calcium level or, rarely, a high serum phosphate level. Metastatic calcification occurs in hyperparathyroidism, sarcoidosis, vitamin D intoxication, and malignancies with disseminated bone involvement. The ocular manifestation of metastatic calcification, as with dystrophic calcification, is band keratopathy.

Idiopathic calcification

Idiopathic calcification is that in which no predisposing cause can be identified. Again, in the eye, band keratopathy is an example.

Band keratopathy

Band keratopathy is a relatively common condition that presents as a white horizontal band in the interpalpebral superficial cornea (Fig. 5.32b). It exhibits small well-defined clear spaces through which nerve fibres pass, and a clear zone separates its sharp lateral ends from the limbus. The condition is due to the dystrophic, metastatic or idiopathic deposition of a calcium phosphate (hydroxyapatite – $Ca_5(PO_4)_3OH$). An autosomal, usually dominant, form of band keratopathy presents bilaterally in otherwise asymptomatic children. Microscopy reveals the deposits as being extracellular and mainly in Bowman's layer, but also in the epithelial basement membrane and superficial stroma (Fig. 5.32c). With time, fragmentation of Bowman's layer is seen clinically as cracks in the band.

Anterior crocodile shagreen

Anterior crocodile shagreen, so named because of its resemblance to crocodile skin, involves the central cornea and takes the form of a mosaic of subepithelial opacities separated by clear areas. It is associated with band keratopathy and ocular malformations, and is inherited as an autosomal dominant condition. The appearance is

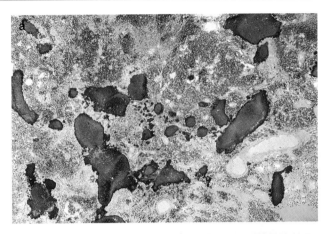

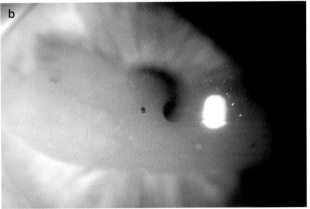

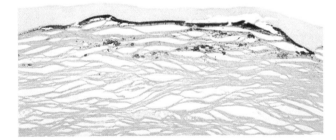

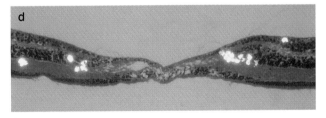

Figure 5.32 Calcium. (a) Irregular basophilic deposits in retinoblastoma. (b) Clinical appearance of band keratopathy. (c) Band keratopathy with fine calcific deposits (black) in disrupted Bowman's layer and superficial stroma. von Kossa stain. (d) Retinal oxalosis; calcium oxalate deposition in the retina. Partially polarized light.

due to the calcification of an undulating Bowman's layer associated with hypotony.

Diffuse corneal calcification

Calcification of the entire cornea may occur rarely in hypercalcaemia.

Calcium oxalate deposition

Calcium oxalate may be deposited as refractile and birefringent crystals in the retina and lens.

Retinal oxalosis (Fig. 5.32d) is associated with primary hyperoxaluria, where circulating blood levels of oxalate are high, or with long-standing retinal detachment, when the calcium oxalate may be derived from precursors in intraocular fluid or RPE.

Lenticular oxalosis is the appearance of calcium oxalate crystals within the nucleus of Morgagnian cataract, possibly due to the presence of increased amounts of ascorbic acid in the aqueous.

Iron

Iron may be deposited in ocular tissues as a result of local disorders (corneal epithelial iron lines, siderosis) and systemic disorders (haemochromatosis). Ferric iron (Fe^{3+}) is demonstrable by the Prussian blue reaction with Perls' stain.

Corneal epithelial iron lines

Corneal epithelial iron lines are asymptomatic delicate brown granular deposits within the corneal epithelium. They are caused by ferritin particles located within cytoplasmic vacuoles and in intercellular spaces, mainly in the basal layers. The iron is of endogenous origin and is demonstrable with Perls' stain. The reason for its deposition is unknown. There are four eponymous types:

1. **Hudson–Stähli line** is a horizontal linear deposition in the inferior third of the cornea, and is a normal ageing phenomenon.

2. **Fleischer's ring** surrounds the base of a keratoconus cone (Fig. 5.33a).

3. **Ferry's line** is situated central to the limbal edge of a filtering trabeculectomy bleb.

4. **Stocker's line** occurs at the advancing edge of a pterygium.

Siderosis

Siderosis is the condition in which exogenous iron compounds are deposited within ocular structures. It may be localized (corneal siderosis) or affect the whole eye (siderosis bulbi).

Corneal siderosis

Iron-containing corneal foreign bodies result in the local deposition of a small pigmented ring (rust ring) in the superficial cornea. Coats' white ring is a white ring-shaped deposit occurring usually in an area of cornea damaged by a foreign body. Originally thought to be lipid, it is composed of an iron and calcium protein complex deposited in Bowman's layer. The iron may be derived from the pre-existing foreign body. Corneal siderosis, like corneal epithelial iron lines, is demonstrable with Perls' stain (Fig. 5.33b).

Siderosis bulbi

Siderosis bulbi results from the presence within the eye of iron compounds derived from a retained intraocular

a

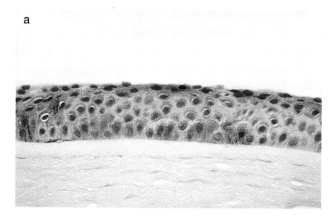

b

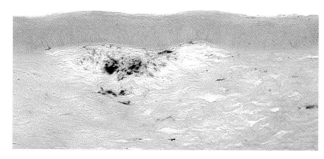

Figure 5.33 Iron. (a) Fleischer's iron ring. Intraepithelial deposition of iron. Perls' stain. (b) Corneal siderosis. Scarred stroma with iron deposition. Perls' stain.

foreign body (IOFB). The effects of intraocular iron deposition are evident in the retina (visual loss and diminished amplitude of the ERG), the iris (heterochromia with the iris of the affected eye appearing darker) and the lens (a characteristic yellow-brown cataract with rust flecks – Fig. 5.34a). Glaucoma may also develop.

Iron is deposited as particles within affected structures, and is demonstrable with Perls' stain as a Prussian blue reaction. Initial deposition in tissues in the adjacent vicinity of the IOFB (Fig. 5.34b) is followed by deposition in tissues for which the iron has a particular affinity, namely epithelial tissues (iris, ciliary epithelium, RPE, lens epithelium) and tissues derived from neuroepithelium (iris muscles, neurosensory retina – Fig. 5.34c). Eventually all ocular tissues may be affected. Although ferrous iron (Fe^{2+}) is said to be more toxic than ferric iron (Fe^{3+}), it is the latter that is demonstrable by Perls' stain. In advanced cases, neurosensory retinal elements are replaced by glial tissue and the trabecular meshwork is sclerosed.

The chemistry of siderosis is not fully understood, but it is likely that electrolytic dissociation of iron and its dissemination in ionic form is brought about by the current that normally passes anteroposteriorly through the eye. On entering cells, these iron ions combine with protein to form insoluble complexes that interfere with cell metabolism. The retinal degenerative changes that result in visual failure are probably due to direct toxic effects. The mechanism of the glaucoma is uncertain, but may be a consequence of degeneration and sclerosis of the trabecular meshwork.

Haemochromatosis

Haemochromatosis is a metabolic disorder in which iron in the form of ferritin and haemosiderin is deposited in cells throughout the body, but particularly in the skin, liver and pancreas. The resulting clinical syndrome comprises a triad of skin pigmentation, hepatic cirrhosis and diabetes mellitus. In the eye, iron may be deposited in the corneal and ciliary epithelium, RPE and sclera, and is demonstrable with Perls' stain. Haemochromatosis may be primary or secondary. The associated diabetes mellitus may lead to retinopathy. Primary haemochromatosis is an autosomal recessive disorder caused by a genetic defect on chromosome 6 that causes iron overload from excessive iron absorption in the small intestine. Secondary haemochromatosis can result from multiple blood transfusions.

Copper

Copper deposition within the eye is termed chalcosis. The cause may be local (IOFBs where the metallic copper

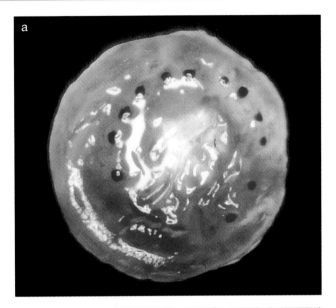

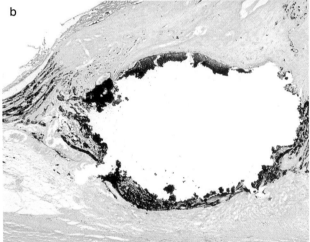

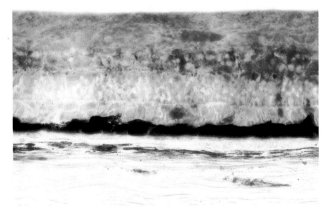

Figure 5.34 Siderosis bulbi. (a) Siderotic deposits in an extracted lens. (b) A large empty cavity in the ciliary region marks the site of an iron-containing foreign body that has been removed. Iron is deposited in the surrounding tissue and in the ciliary epithelium. Perls' stain. (c) Iron deposition in the retina. Perls' stain.

content is < 85 per cent) or systemic (liver failure due to any cause, including Wilson's disease). IOFBs containing >85 per cent copper result in fulminating toxic panophthalmitis.

Chalcosis

In chalcosis, copper (as with iron) diffuses in the eye in ionized form, but (in contrast to iron) it has a particular affinity for basement membranes, in particular Descemet's membrane and the lens capsule. Copper can be demonstrated in tissues by spectrophotometry, by staining with rubeanic acid, which produces a greenish-black colour, and by electron microscopy. The characteristic lesions produced by chalcosis are a Kayser–Fleischer ring and a sunflower cataract, but copper deposits may be found elsewhere.

Kayser–Fleischer ring

A Kayser–Fleischer ring (Fig. 5.35a) is a brown-gold ring at the corneal periphery due to copper deposition in Descemet's membrane. The ring begins as an arc at the upper periphery, and a lower arc develops prior to the formation of a complete ring. The granular deposits tend to be arranged in a linear pattern (Fig. 5.35b), which suggests that the copper has entered the cornea by diffusion from the anterior chamber. The precise nature of the copper is uncertain, but it is possibly in a chelated form related to the proteoglycan content of Descemet's membrane following combination with a sulphur-containing component. A Kayser–Fleischer ring is seen in chalcosis and most of those with untreated Wilson's disease.

Sunflower cataract

The accumulation of copper within the lens capsule results in discoloration of the lens, which becomes dark green or brown, and an opaque central ring with distinctive colourings and tapering extensions suggestive of sunflower petals. This sunflower cataract is due to a myriad of tiny copper granules in the deeper layers of the lens capsule. It is seen in only a relatively small number of those with Wilson's disease.

Other deposits of copper

Brightly reflective particles of copper may be present on the zonular fibres and in the aqueous, vitreous and retina, where the internal limiting membrane, Müller cells, glial cells and vascular endothelium are mainly affected.

Silver

Silver deposition is termed argyrosis. It can occur in the skin, mucous membranes and corneas of individuals

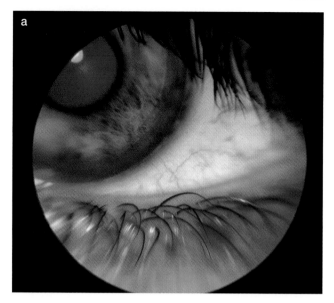

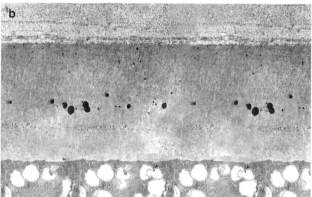

Figure 5.35 Copper: Kayser–Fleischer ring. (a) Clinical appearance. (b) Electron-dense copper granules in Descemet's membrane. TEM.

whose occupations involve long-standing contact with silver salts (silver plating and polishing). It was previously described in association with the use of now obsolete silver-containing eye drops. Affected tissues exhibit a slate-grey discoloration. In skin (including the lids) and mucous membranes (including the conjunctiva) the silver is deposited as fine black granules in the basement membrane of the epidermis/epithelium, in the loose subepidermal/subepithelial connective tissues and in the vascular endothelium. Silver deposition in the cornea occurs primarily in Descemet's membrane.

Gold

Gold deposition is termed chrysiasis. Deposits in the conjunctiva, cornea and lens occur occasionally in individuals taking systemic gold preparations for rheumatoid arthritis. More readily observed clinically in the cornea, it is seen as brownish, golden or red-blue stippling of the deeper stromal layers and Descemet's membrane. Affected conjunctival tissue shows granules within epithelial cells, subepithelial fibroblasts and macrophages.

Corneal tattoo pigment

Carbon, gold, palladium and other noble metal salts have been used for tattooing corneal scars. The deposits appear black and amorphous on microscopy (Fig. 5.36).

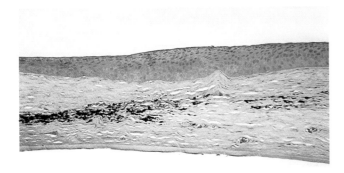

Figure 5.36 Corneal tattoo pigment. Black amorphous deposits in thinned scarred vascularized stroma.

Mercury

Mercury deposition in the cornea and lens (mercurialentis) is rarely seen nowadays. Prolonged topical application of eye drops preserved with phenylmercuric nitrate (PMN) was the most usual cause. As with other heavy and unusual metals, electron probe microanalysis can be used for its identification.

Blood pigments

Blood pigments result from haemoglobin breakdown products, and are characterized as being either in the bilirubin group or in the ferritin/haemosiderin group.

Bilirubin group

Pigments in this group are iron-free and deposited locally or systemically. Bruising due to local trauma in which there is bleeding into the tissues is a manifestation of liberated bilirubin pigments. Excess bilirubin in the bloodstream is due to increased bilirubin production, as in haemolytic anaemia, or to the failure of the liver to excrete it, as in obstruction of the common bile duct. Both entities present as jaundice, in which the serum concentration of bilirubin is raised and bilirubin salts

are deposited in tissues throughout the body. In the eye, the subepithelial conjunctiva, episclera and sclera are all affected.

Ferritin/haemosiderin group

Most iron in the body is ferric and present within red blood cells. Iron in plasma is bound to a β-globulin called transferrin. When red cells break down, ferric compounds are released and seen as yellow-brown intracellular haemosiderin granules. Ferric iron is strikingly demonstrated by Perls' stain, which produces a Prussian blue reaction. Iron deposition in ocular tissues occurs in haemochromatosis, blood staining of the cornea and haemosiderosis bulbi.

Blood staining of the cornea

Blood staining of the cornea can follow hyphaema, particularly if damage of the endothelium is associated with an elevated intraocular pressure. The endothelial cells appear normal, but eosinophilic granular material is seen in the stroma (Fig. 5.37) and a small amount of haemosiderin is contained within keratocytes. The eosinophilic granules are fragments of haemoglobin and do not stain for iron, although the haemosiderin in the keratocytes does. Macrophages eventually infiltrate the cornea to remove the debris. Corneal blood staining appears brown on clinical examination, and clearing takes place from the periphery.

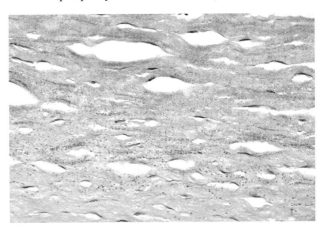

Figure 5.37 Blood staining of cornea. Eosinophilic granular material in stroma.

Haemosiderosis bulbi

Haemosiderosis bulbi is the condition in which iron is deposited in ocular structures following massive intraocular haemorrhage. The clinicopathological features and pathogenesis are the same as for siderosis bulbi following the retention of an iron-containing IOFB.

AROMATIC AMINO-ACID DERIVATIVES

Aromatic amino-acid derivatives include the melanins and melanin-like ochronotic pigment.

The melanins

The melanins are a group of insoluble sulphur-containing light-brown to black pigments found in cutaneous, conjunctival and uveal melanocytes, in intraocular pigmented epithelium, and in naevus and melanoma cells. Melanins are located within intracellular organelles known as melanosomes and are synthesized from tyrosine. The enzyme tyrosinase (DOPA-oxidase) acts on tyrosine to produce dihydroxyphenylalanine (DOPA), which is converted by the same enzyme into an intermediate pigment that polymerizes to form the melanins. The later stages of melanogenesis are largely speculative. Melanins often obscure cytological details, and can be bleached out of tissue sections by oxidizing agents such as potassium permanganate. Submicroscopic particles of melanin are revealed as small black granules by the Masson–Fontana stain. Increased amounts and deposition of melanin may or may not be associated with melanocytic activity. Melanocytes in the epidermis of the skin and epithelium of the conjunctiva can produce melanin, which may be taken up by adjacent cells. This occurs in ephelides, diffuse melanosis of the skin and secondary melanosis of the conjunctiva.

Ephelis (freckle pl. ephelides)

An ephelis is a localized melanosis that may develop in the skin or conjunctiva. Presenting either singly or as clusters of small uniform pigmented macules, ephelides are directly related to sunlight exposure and are particularly common and numerous in the skin of individuals with red hair and blue eyes, where there is probably an autosomal dominant pattern of inheritance. High levels of freckling correlate with a higher frequency of melanocytic naevi, and are indicative of increased susceptibility to the later development of melanoma. The melanin of ephelides is produced by melanocytes and deposited in adjacent cells of the basal layer. Ephelides thus result from increased melanocytic activity, but the number of melanocytes remains normal or is even diminished.

Diffuse melanosis of the skin

In diffuse melanosis of the skin, melanin is deposited in keratinocytes, mainly those of the basal layer. As in ephelides, melanocytic activity is increased but the number of melanocytes is not. The mechanism accounts for racial pigmentation and explains the acquired diffuse increased pigmentation seen in various conditions, including responses to hormonal stimuli and exposure to UV light and ionizing radiation.

Secondary melanosis of the conjunctiva

In secondary melanosis of the conjunctiva, increased production of melanin is also due to increased melanocytic activity. Racial, metabolic and toxic factors contribute to its development. Secondary melanosis is most commonly observed in the limbal and perilimbal conjunctiva of black people, where, although it is considered as a normal aspect of ageing, it is not infrequently observed in relation to scars and tumours.

Melanin deposition not associated with melanocytic activity

Melanin in corneal endothelial cells is usually derived from melanin circulating freely in the aqueous. It is seen in association with diabetes mellitus, myopia, PXS and the pigment dispersion syndrome (Krukenberg spindle), and with cornea guttata as part of the normal ageing process. In advanced disease the retrocorneal cells comprise corneal endothelial cells, iris pigment epithelial cells, iris stromal melanocytes and melanin-containing macrophages. Long-term application of epinephrine-containing eye drops can lead to the accumulation of melanin in the conjunctiva and cornea. Epinephrine is a phenol that, under the influence of naturally occurring phenolic oxidases, is oxidized to the unstable form of adrenochrome and finally to melanin, which comes to lie within the surface epithelium, particularly of the lower palpebral conjunctiva. It is also found within Bowman's layer and within and between stromal keratocytes in the presence of predisposing factors such as corneal epithelial defects or bullous keratopathy. Melanin on the lens capsule may be seen as a fine dusting in the pigment dispersion syndrome, and as a ring-like imprint (Vossius' ring) following blunt trauma.

Ochronotic pigment

Ochronotic pigment is deposited in connective tissue, particularly the cartilage of the nose, ears and joints in alkaptonuria and ochronosis.

Alkaptonuria

Alkaptonuria is a rare autosomal recessive inherited condition in which a deficiency of homogentisic acid oxidase results in a disturbance in tyrosine-phenylalanine metabolism. Homogentisic acid oxidase exists primarily in the liver and kidneys and its deficiency leads to the accumulation of homogentisic acid, which becomes oxidized to byproducts that polymerize to a melanin-like pigment. Serum levels of homogentisic acid are not usually elevated because it is rapidly excreted in the urine, which becomes dark on standing (alkaptonuria).

Ocular ochronosis

In ocular ochronosis the structure mainly affected is the sclera (Fig. 5.38), where triangular patches of brown-black pigmentation develop in both eyes, usually in the third decade. These areas of scleral pigmentation are situated midway between the limbus and the insertions of the horizontal rectus muscles. In the cornea, subepithelial pigmented globules are seen in the periphery of Bowman's layer near the limbus, and lesions resembling pigmented pingueculae lie in the subconjunctiva/episclera. Ochronotic pigment bleaches, as does melanin, and affected areas are revealed as being acellular.

Exogenous ochronosis

Pigment identical to that seen in alkaptonuria may occur as an occupational hazard after prolonged exposure to

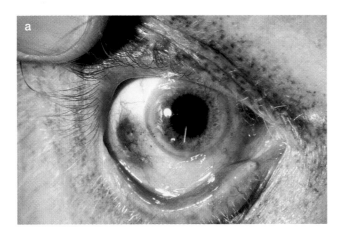

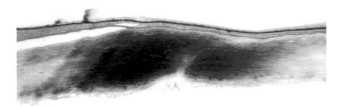

Figure 5.38 Ochronosis. (a) Scleral and skin pigmentation. (b) Brown-black ochronotic pigmentation of sclera.

hydroquinones, after the oral or intramuscular administration of antimalarials such as chloroquine, after the topical treatment of leg ulcers with phenol, or following the application of bleaching creams containing hydroquinone, most often in black women. Exogenous ochronosis due to hydroquinone is thought to be photoactivated.

AMYLOID

Amyloid is the name given to a group of diverse proteins or glycoproteins which appear as extracellular deposits in a variety of conditions. The two basic components of amyloid are amyloid fibrillary protein and amyloid P.

Amyloid fibrillary protein

At least 15 distinct types of amyloid fibrillary protein are recognized, and include:

AL amyloid which consists of the variable region of immunoglobulin light chains (V_L) and is derived from either the kappa (κ) or lambda (λ) moiety. It is deposited in association with plasma cell dyscrasias such as multiple myeloma and B cell lymphomas.

AA amyloid which comprises monomeric fragments and arises from the naturally circulating acute phase protein serum amyloid A (SAA) produced by the liver. The concentration of SAA increases markedly in inflammatory processes, and AA amyloid deposits occur in rheumatoid arthritis, tuberculosis, osteomyelitis and Crohn's disease.

Transthyretin which is a normal constituent of plasma and CSF. It is synthesized predominantly in the liver, but is also produced in the brain by the choroid plexus and in the eye by the RPE. It partakes in the transportation of thyroxine and retinol binding protein.

AE amyloid which is produced from peptide hormone precursors and is associated with endocrine neoplasms (E-endocrine). It is seen in association with medullary carcinoma of the thyroid and islet-secreting neoplasms of the pancreas.

Other amyloid proteins which have been characterized in the skin, joints and brain.

Amyloid P

Amyloid P (AP) is a pentameric glycoprotein identical to the circulating serum P component (SAP), a normal α-1-globulin. AP is a component of nearly all amyloid.

Physicochemical characteristics of amyloid

Amyloid can be identified by light and electron microscopy and by its immune reactions:

Staining and light microscopy

Amyloid is eosinophilic in haematoxylin and eosin stained sections, having a reddish homogeneous (hyaline) appearance no different from many other proteins. Congo red stains amyloid orange-red when viewed in ordinary light (Fig. 5.39a). Polarizing microscopy demonstrates apple-green birefringence and dichroism (Fig. 5.39b). Fluorescence is demonstrable on staining with thioflavine T.

Ultrastructure

Electron microscopy of amyloid fibrillary protein reveals a mass of tangled, randomly-orientated unbranched fibrils (Fig. 5.39c). Each fibril consists of two electron-dense filaments 2.5–3.5 nm in diameter, separated by a 2.5 nm interspace, giving the whole fibril a diameter of 8–10 nm and a variable length that may be up to several millimicrons. The AP component is a series of stacked segments forming a beaded rod 9 nm in diameter and of 4 nm periodicity. In cross-section, the rod has a pentagonal structure surrounding a 2.5 nm electron-dense core. Amyloid fibrils form intertwining strands twisted as a hollow helix, from which stacks of the annular-shaped AP component radiate perpendicularly.

Immunohistochemistry

Antibodies can be used in immunohistochemical techniques to demonstrate AP and AA.

Amyloidosis

Amyloidosis is the clinical condition resulting from the deposition of amyloid. It may be primary or secondary, and systemic or local.

Primary amyloidosis

This occurs spontaneously in the absence of apparent predisposing illness. The substance deposited is AL amyloid. Myeloma-associated amyloidosis is called primary rather than secondary because of the frequent absence of any clinically obvious myeloma. An occult plasma cell lesion may be accompanied by the presence of a monoclonal immunoglobulin band on serum electrophoresis (benign monoclonal gammopathy).

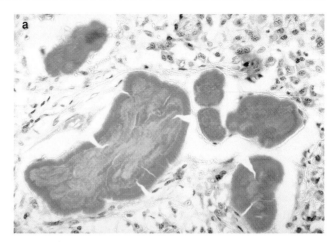

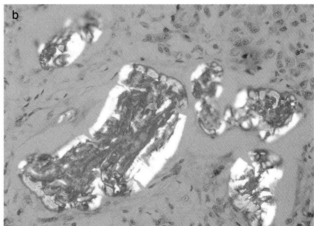

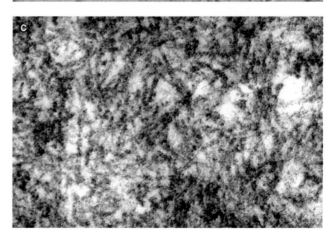

Figure 5.39 Amyloid. (a) Irregular orange-red deposits. Congo red stain: normal light. (b) Apple-green birefringence. Congo red stain: polarized light. (c) Tangled mass of fibrils. TEM.

Secondary amyloidosis

This occurs in association with a wide range of predisposing causes such as chronic inflammatory disorders. The substance deposited is AA amyloid.

Ophthalmic amyloidosis

Both AL and AA amyloid are deposited in ophthalmic tissues.

Primary amyloidosis (AL deposits)

The ophthalmic manifestations of primary systemic amyloidosis include corneal lattice dystrophy Type 2, vitreous amyloid and amyloid deposition in the walls of ocular blood vessels, particularly of the uvea and retina. Primary localized amyloidosis is seen as lid and conjunctival nodules, lattice corneal dystrophies Types 1 and 3 (Fig. 5.21) and polymorphic stromal and gelatinous drop-like corneal dystrophies (Fig. 5.22).

Vitreous amyloid is rare, and may result in progressive visual loss. It is a manifestation of primary systemic amyloidosis, but sometimes occurs years before systemic features. In the early stages, granular opacities with wispy fringes are seen as aggregates on vitreous fibrils and on the posterior vitreous cortex adjacent to blood vessels. The deposits later form strands with a glasswool-like appearance, and involve the anterior vitreous. In about 50 per cent of affected eyes there are characteristic white opacities (footplates) on the posterior lens capsule, from which opaque fibres run posteriorly to join a meshwork of vitreous opacities. Associated features include vascular occlusion and glaucoma.

Secondary amyloidosis (AA deposits)

In secondary systemic amyloidosis due to chronic inflammatory disorders the eye is usually unaffected, but secondary localized amyloidosis may result from chronic inflammation of the lids and conjunctiva.

LIPID

Lipid deposition in the sclera and peripheral bulbar conjunctiva commonly occurs with advancing age. The deposits are seen as microscopic nodules and macroscopically as corneal arcus and lipid keratopathy.

Corneal arcus – senilis and juvenilis

Arcus senilis is the commonest peripheral corneal opacity, and takes the form of a whitish ring with an intervening clear zone between it and the limbus (Fig. 5.40). It occurs in the elderly and is usually an isolated finding, although it may be associated with familial and non-familial dyslipoproteinaemias and rarer conditions such as Schnyder's crystalline dystrophy. Sometimes the area affected is thinned (idiopathic furrow degeneration). Arcus juvenilis (anterior embryotoxon) is a similar opa-

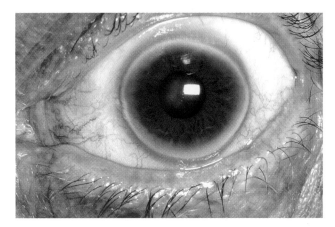

Figure 5.40 Arcus senilis.

city in children and young adults, where it is likely to be associated with hypercholesterolaemia or abnormalities such as blue sclera, megalocornea or aniridia. The histological appearance of arcus senilis and juvenilis is similar and reflects paralimbal stromal accumulations of lipids (cholesterol esters, triglycerides, phospholipids), which form a double triangle with an apex-to-apex configuration, the bases of the triangles being in close relationship and within Bowman's layer and Descemet's membrane.

Lipid keratopathy

In vascularized corneas, plasma lipids (particularly cholesterol) may accumulate in the cytoplasm of capillary cells and extravasate into the stroma. The clinical appearance is of yellow or cream-coloured diffuse deposits of crystalline material (Fig. 5.41a) that, on histological examination, is seen as stromal cholesterol clefts and histiocytes (Fig. 5.41b) possibly with a granulomatous inflammatory reaction.

CHOLESTEROL, PARAPROTEINS, URIC ACID AND CYSTINE

Crystalline keratopathy

Crystalline keratopathy (Fig. 5.42) is the presence of refractile granular deposits in any of the corneal layers, but mainly the stroma and epithelium. Compounds crystallize in the cornea because they have a high affinity for corneal tissue, because they are present in a highly concentrated supersaturated state, or because of an intrinsic metabolic abnormality of corneal tissue. Those that crystallize include cholesterol (Schnyder's central crystalline dystrophy, Bietti's crystalline corneoretinal dystrophy, lipid keratopathy), paraproteins (myeloma,

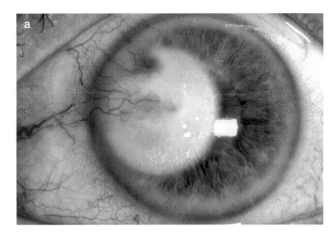

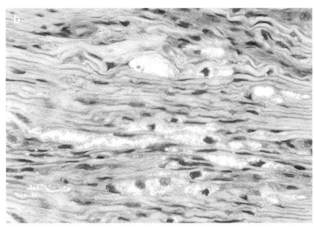

Figure 5.41 Lipid keratopathy. (a) Clinical appearance (b) Lipid-containing histocytes in corneal stroma.

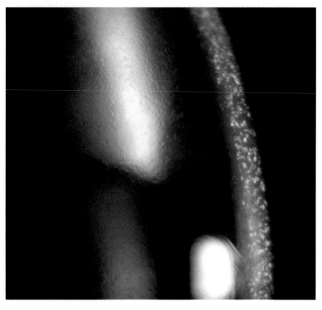

Figure 5.42 Crystalline keratopathy in paraproteinaemia.

HEXOSYLCERAMIDES AND DRUGS

Vortex keratopathy

Vortex keratopathy (cornea verticillata) is characterized by bilateral symmetrical corneal epithelial deposits forming a vortex-like pattern extending from a point below the pupil to the periphery but stopping short of the limbus. It occurs in Fabry's disease (hexosylceramides) and with the use of drugs, most notably amiodarone, chloroquine, chlorpromazine and tamoxifen. Vortex keratopathy is asymptomatic, and the drug-induced form slowly resolves when the medication is withdrawn.

Waldenström's macroglobulinaemia, benign monoclonal gammopathy, chronic lymphatic leukaemia, lymphoma), uric acid (gout) and cystine (cystinosis).

Chapter 6

Vascular, circulatory and blood disorders

The ocular vascular system

The retinal circulation
The uveal circulation
The blood–ocular barriers

Pathophysiological principles and ocular vascular disease

Degenerative changes
    Arteriosclerosis
    Arteriolosclerosis
    Atherosclerosis
Abnormal accumulations of fluid and blood
    Oedema
        Transudates
        Exudates
    Haemorrhage
        Subconjunctival haemorrhage
        Anterior chamber haemorrhage
        Vitreous and subhyaloid haemorrhage
        Retinal haemorrhage
        Subretinal and sub-RPE haemorrhage
        Expulsive haemorrhage
        Optic nerve haemorrhage
Structural abnormalities of blood vessels
    Vascular tortuosity
    Anomalous vascular branching
    Abnormalities of vessel calibre
        Congenital retinal telangiectasia
        Acquired telangiectasia
        Aneurysms
Disorders of perfusion
    Ischaemia
        Retinal ischaemia

Uveal ischaemia
The ocular ischaemic syndrome
Hyperaemia

Specific vascular disorders and their ocular manifestations

Systemic hypertension
Diabetes mellitus
    Mechanisms leading to complications of diabetes mellitus
    Diabetic vascular disease
    Ophthalmic complications of diabetes mellitus
        Diabetic retinopathy
        Other ophthalmic complications of diabetes mellitus
Vasculitis
    Idiopathic retinal vasculitis
    Behçet's disease
    Wegener's granulomatosis
    Hypersensitivity vasculitis
    Polyarteritis nodosa
    Giant cell arteritis/polymyalgia rheumatica
    Takayasu's disease

Blood disorders and their ocular manifestations

The anaemias
Erythrocytosis
The leukaemias
The haemoglobinopathies
    Thalassaemias
    Structural variants of haemoglobin
        Sickle cell haemoglobinopathies

THE OCULAR VASCULAR SYSTEM

The ocular blood vessels arise from the ophthalmic artery, a branch of the internal carotid artery. Within the orbit the ophthalmic artery divides into the central retinal artery, which supplies the retina, and the posterior and anterior ciliary arteries, which supply the uvea. Arteries of all sizes have three anatomical layers. The innermost, the intima, is composed of a single layer of endothelium resting on a collagenous zone in which a few smooth muscle cells and fibroblasts are present. An internal elastic lamina separates the intima from the media. The media consists essentially of smooth muscle. Externally, the adventitia is composed of loose connective tissue. The central retinal vein drains the retina and the vortex veins are the principal routes of venous drainage from the uvea. The eye thus has separate retinal and uveal circulations.

THE RETINAL CIRCULATION

The central retinal artery is a muscular end artery and enters the optic nerve approximately 1 cm behind the globe. At the optic nerve head it shares a common adventitial sheath with the central retinal vein. The continuity of its internal elastic lamina is lost at the lamina cribrosa.

The retinal arterioles lie in the nerve fibre layer and supply all four quadrants of the retina. They contain smooth muscle within their walls, but the internal elastic lamina is not continuous.

The retinal capillaries supply the inner two-thirds of the retina through two plexuses, an inner one in the ganglion cell layer and an outer one in the inner nuclear layer (the outer third of the retina receives metabolic support from the choriocapillaris). Capillary-free zones are present around the retinal arterioles (the periarteriolar capillary-free zone), at the fovea and at the extreme retinal periphery. No smooth muscle is present within capillary walls. Endothelial cells lie as a single layer on an amorphous basement membrane and are linked by tight encircling junctions that are of importance in the relative impermeability of the inner blood–retinal barrier. A second type of cell, the pericyte lies external to the endothelial cells but within an outer connective tissue fibrillar meshwork. Each pericyte has multiple pseudopodial processes that envelop the capillary. Pericytes are contractile cells containing both smooth muscle actin and myosin. They are particularly numerous in the retina, and take part in the autoregulation of the microvascular circulation. External to the pericytes, astrocyte foot processes act as a further physical barrier. Retinal capillaries are best seen anatomically in Indian ink-injected and/or trypsin digest preparations (Fig. 6.1).

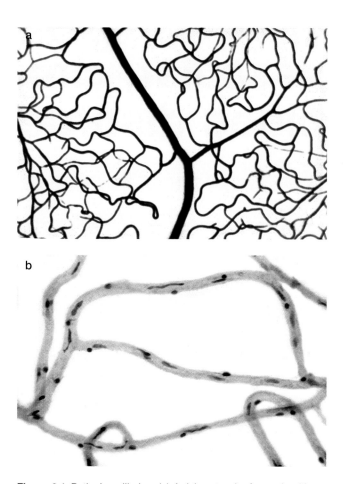

Figure 6.1 Retinal capillaries. (a) A rich network of vessels with a periarteriolar capillary-free zone. Flat preparation of Indian ink injected retina. (b) Endothelial cells with elongated nuclei and pericytes with rounded nuclei. Trypsin digest preparation.

The retinal venules have a larger calibre than capillaries. Small retinal venules are structurally identical to capillaries but functionally different in that they are more permeable, more susceptible to vasoactive amines and more liable to thrombosis. The walls of larger venules contain smooth muscle cells.

The retinal veins are formed by the merging of retinal venules. Reflecting the low pressure of the venous system, they contain very little smooth muscle and elastic tissue, and are relatively distensible. They uniformly and gradually expand in diameter as they pass posteriorly from the periphery to the optic disc and into the central retinal vein, through which blood passes out of the eye.

THE UVEAL CIRCULATION

The uveal circulation comprises the vascular systems of the iris, ciliary body and choroid. It exhibits free anastomoses within itself, but apart from the occasional cilioretinal vessel there is no significant communication with the retinal circulation. The anastomoses allow the choroid to withstand vascular insufficiency more readily than the retina. Occlusion of the choroidal arterial system results in ischaemia of the choroid, RPE and outer third of the retina.

THE BLOOD–OCULAR BARRIERS

The blood–ocular barriers prevent water-soluble substances and macromolecules passing from the circulation into the aqueous and retina. The passage of such substances depends on the presence of pores or specific active transport mechanisms such as pinocytosis. There are three important blood–ocular barriers: one blood–aqueous barrier and two blood–retinal barriers. The integrity of the two blood–retinal barriers can be examined by fundus fluorescein angiography and indocyanine green (ICG) angiography.

The blood–aqueous barrier consists of the tight junctions of the apical portions of the non-pigmented ciliary epithelial cells and the iris vascular endothelium.

The inner blood–retinal barrier is formed by the tight junctions of the vascular endothelial cells of the retinal capillaries. It is the barrier between the retinal circulation and the inner two-thirds of the retina.

The outer blood–retinal barrier is formed by the tight junctions of the RPE and, to a lesser extent, by Bruch's membrane. It is the main barrier between the fenestrated choriocapillaris and the outer third of the retina and the potential subretinal space.

PATHOPHYSIOLOGICAL PRINCIPLES AND OCULAR VASCULAR DISEASE

Degenerative changes, abnormal accumulations of fluid and blood, structural abnormalities of blood vessels and disorders of perfusion can all lead to ocular vascular disease.

DEGENERATIVE CHANGES

Arteriosclerosis

A variety of structural changes in which the strength and elasticity of the arterial walls are reduced occur throughout life and constitute arteriosclerosis, in which the arterial wall is thickened and the lumen is narrowed. These changes are common over the age of 70 but usually insignificant under the age of 40 years. Progressive fibrous thickening of the intima and replacement of the smooth muscle of the media by collagen (Fig. 6.2a) is accompanied by disruption and reduplication of the internal elas-

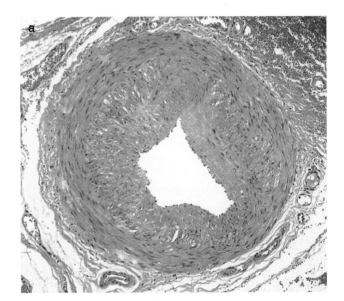

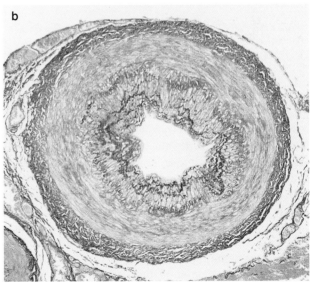

Figure 6.2 Arteriosclerosis. (a) Thickening of arterial wall and narrowing of lumen. (b) Disruption and reduplication of the internal elastic lamina. Verhoeff stain.

tic lamina (Fig. 6.2b). Other changes include the accumulation of glycosaminoglycan-rich ground substances and the deposition of calcium.

Arteriolosclerosis

As with arteries, with advancing age the smooth muscle of the arteriolar wall is replaced by collagen and this results in thickening of the vessel wall and narrowing of the lumen (Fig. 6.3). In addition there is insudation of plasma into the vascular wall and it appears that, even if the blood pressure is only slightly elevated, a degree of systemic hypertension is necessary for the development of arteriolosclerosis. The term hyaline arteriolosclerosis describes the amorphous histological appearance of the vessel wall, and represents mature collagen and plasma protein.

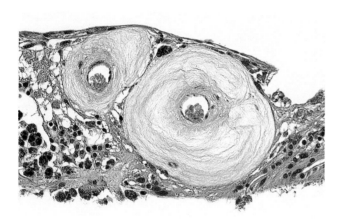

Figure 6.3 Arteriolosclerosis. Hyalinized thickened wall of retinal arterioles with narrowing of the lumen.

Atherosclerosis

Atherosclerosis affects large and medium-sized arteries, and is characterized by the presence of focal intimal thickenings comprising cells of smooth muscle origin, connective tissue and lipid-containing foam cells (Fig. 6.4). Within the orbital vasculature, atherosclerosis affects the ophthalmic artery and its branches outside the eye; intraocular vessels are not affected. The incidence of atherosclerosis increases with age and is accelerated in systemic hypertension, diabetes mellitus and hyperhomocysteinaemia. Other risk factors include raised serum levels of low-density-lipoprotein-cholesterol (LDL-cholesterol), obesity, tobacco smoking, a sedentary lifestyle, low socio-economic status and race.

Atherosclerosis begins in childhood with diffuse thickening of the intima. During teenage years, nodular lesions of fibroelastic tissue and collections of lipid, mainly cholesterol esters, are deposited. These lesions, termed fatty streaks, are assumed to be the precursors of fibrous atheromatous plaques, which consist of myointimal cells, collagen, elastin and lipid-containing foam cells. Myointimal cells are derived from the smooth muscle of the media, while foam cells originate from blood monocytes. Atherosclerotic lesions result in vascular occlusion due to rupture, haemorrhage into the plaque, mural thrombus formation on the plaque surface or calcification.

Systemic hypertension, diabetes mellitus, hyperhomocysteinaemia and turbulent blood flow (as may occur at sites of arterial bifurcation) damage and increase the permeability of vascular endothelium, thus allowing increased concentration of LDL-cholesterol in the intima. It is postulated that this LDL-cholesterol is oxidized and attracts circulating monocytes, which then phagocytose it and become foam cells. Oxidized LDL-cholesterol is subsequently released, possibly because of cell death, and appears to have a direct toxic effect on endothelial cells, which are consequently lost. At this stage, platelet adhesion and aggregation with release of growth factors promotes smooth muscle proliferation and the development of myointimal cells. Nicotine and other components of tobacco smoke increase platelet adhesiveness, fibrinogen levels and blood viscosity, and reduce the production of prostacyclin and anti-aggregating prostaglandin, all factors of importance in thrombus formation.

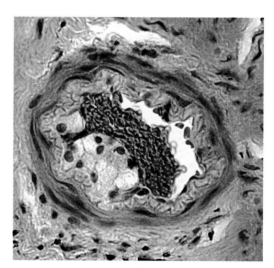

Figure 6.4 Atherosclerosis. Lipid-containing foam cells in the intima of an artery producing localized swelling and narrowing of the lumen.

ABNORMAL ACCUMULATIONS OF FLUID AND BLOOD

Oedema

Oedema is the accumulation of fluid in extravascular tissues, and can be intracellular or extracellular. Intracellular oedema is associated with cell death, while extracellular oedema is either generalized and involves the whole body or localized to an organ or tissue. The fluid balance between the vascular and extravascular tissue compartments is dependent on the hydrostatic pressure differential between the arterial and venous sides of the circulation, on the intravascular oncotic pressure induced by plasma proteins (especially albumin) that keeps the circulating fluid within the vessels, and on capillary permeability. An abnormality in the interaction of these factors results in oedema and, depending on the mechanism involved, this is a transudate or an exudate.

Transudates

Transudative oedema results from an increase in capillary hydrostatic pressure or a reduction in the intravascular oncotic pressure exerted by plasma proteins. Although occurring in hypoproteinaemia, the principal mechanism of relevance to the eye is increased capillary hydrostatic pressure, the extracellular fluid being an ultrafiltrate of the circulating blood. Transudation through the retinal vasculature is a feature of hypertensive retinopathy and retinal vein occlusion.

Exudates

Exudative oedema results from a non-selective increase in vascular permeability. The excess extracellular fluid differs from a transudate in that it has a much higher protein and lipid content. Exudation into the retina results from abnormal or damaged capillary endothelium, and occurs in the congenital retinal telangiectasias, inflammation, and hypertensive, diabetic and other vascular retinopathies.

Retinal exudates

As exudative oedema fluid diffuses from its site of origin, its aqueous component drains across the outer blood–retinal barrier towards the choroid. Protein and lipid are precipitated within retinal tissues to form hard exudates, seen ophthalmoscopically as yellowish deposits with discrete edges. The location of exudates is dependent on the histological structure of the retina. Exuded plasma spreads along paths of least resistance, but tends to remain in the outer plexiform layer where the tissue is

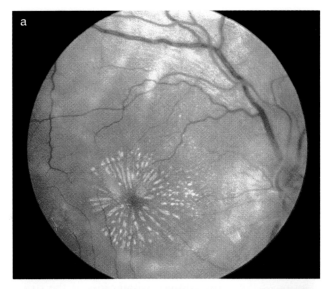

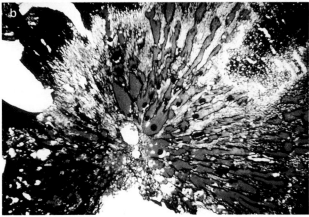

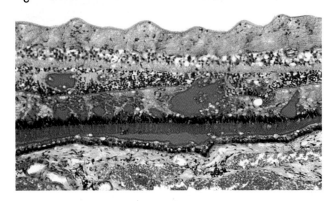

Figure 6.5 Retinal exudates. (a) Macular star; fundus appearance. (b) Macular star; flat preparation of Indian ink injected retina stained for lipid. Oil red O stain. (c) Irregular eosinophilic deposits mainly in the outer plexiform layer.

most lax and where, because of the relative absence of blood vessels, reabsorption is least effective. Retinal oedema diffusing from a point source of leakage is commonly surrounded by exudates arranged in a ring-shaped or circinate pattern. In the foveal region exudates are located between the radially disposed fibres of the axons of the photoreceptors and form a characteristic stellate pattern (macular star – Fig. 6.5a, 6.5b). On microscopy of conventional sections, exudates are seen as eosinophilic masses (Fig. 6.5c) in which lipid-containing foamy macrophages are sometimes present. Resolution of the initial cause results in their eventual dispersion. Factors involved in dispersion include fibrinolysis, phagocytosis by macrophages and dissolution; lipids, particularly cholesterol, often remain longer than proteins, and may persist for many months.

Haemorrhage

Haemorrhage is the loss of blood from the vascular compartment to the extravascular compartment or to the exterior of the body, and necessitates loss of the structural integrity of blood vessels. Trauma, inflammation and ischaemia may damage normal vessels, as may the direct hydrostatic effect of arterial or venous hypertension. The same factors may also damage the abnormal vessels of congenital malformations and vascular and neovascular proliferations, and the diseased vessels of systemic hypertension and diabetes mellitus. Blood clotting abnormalities and haemorrhagic diatheses, particularly where platelets are deficient, can also result in the extravasation of blood.

Subconjunctival haemorrhage

Subconjunctival haemorrhages are common and may occur spontaneously. Trauma and conjunctivitis are local causes, while systemic causes include haemorrhagic diatheses and elevation of the intrathoracic pressure. Bleeding occurs into the loose episcleral connective tissue, but the limbal architecture prevents spread to the cornea. Such haemorrhages usually resolve within a few weeks and, although frequently dramatic in appearance, are of no great importance other than on the rare occasions when they are indicative of an underlying associated disorder.

Anterior chamber haemorrhage

Anterior chamber haemorrhage (hyphaema) is usually the result of trauma. Spontaneous hyphaema may occur in haemorrhagic diatheses and can arise from new vessels or from the vascular component of neoplasms and other disorders of cell growth. The persistent fluidity of a small hyphaema is due to the dilution of clotting factors by the aqueous. Large hyphaemas clot, fibrovascular adhesions may form and, if glaucoma ensues, corneal blood staining often develops.

Vitreous and subhyaloid (preretinal) haemorrhage

Extravasated blood (Fig. 6.6a) may come to lie within the vitreous gel (vitreous haemorrhage) or between the inner limiting membrane of the retina and the posterior hyaloid face (subhyaloid/preretinal haemorrhage). Causes include trauma, when there may be associated retinal tears, and bleeding from new vessels, as in retinal vascular diseases – particularly central retinal vein occlusion and diabetic retinopathy. Subhyaloid haemorrhage may remain fluid, autolyse and completely resolve, organization being unusual possibly because of the absence of collagen. Vitreous haemorrhage usually coagulates, and this may in part explain the protracted clinical course. Absorption of haemoglobin from erythrocytes results in the appearance of ghost cells, which may cause secondary glaucoma if they pass into the trabecular meshwork.

Retinal haemorrhage

Intraretinal haemorrhages can arise from both the inner and outer capillary plexuses. Their configuration is determined by the histology of the adjacent tissue (Fig. 6.6b). The many varied causes of retinal haemorrhages are discussed in the context of the disorders in which they occur. In the retina, as elsewhere, extravasated blood activates the clotting process. Small haemorrhages may disperse spontaneously without sequelae, but larger haemorrhages are invaded by macrophages that remove cellular debris. Subsequent fibroglial and capillary proliferation is followed by scar tissue formation. The lipid content of the extravasated blood, especially cholesterol, is deposited with haemosiderin derived from blood pigments. These deposits may persist for a number of years, and are occasionally the focus of a foreign body giant cell reaction.

Flame-shaped haemorrhages arise from the inner capillary plexus. Blood accumulates within the ganglion cell and nerve fibre layers, and is aligned in the direction of the axons, i.e. in the horizontal plane of the retina. The haemorrhages therefore assume a flame or feather-like shape, with fine striations and indistinct margins. They usually occur at the posterior pole near the optic disc where the nerve fibre layer is thickest.

Dot-blot haemorrhages arise from the outer capillary plexus. Extravasated blood usually remains localized and does not have a specific orientation. The dot-blot description relates to the relative size of the haemorrhages.

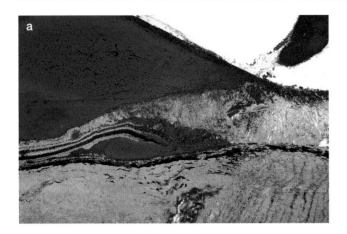

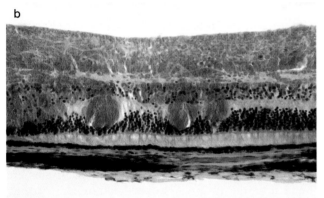

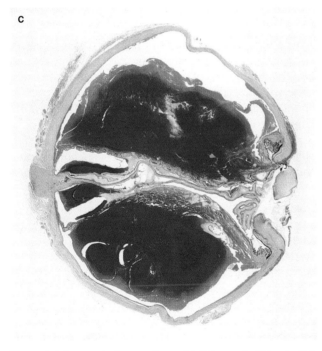

Figure 6.6 Intraocular haemorrhage. (a) Extravasated blood within the vitreous, subhyaloid space, retina and subretinal space. (b) Retinal haemorrhages; extravasated blood lies diffusely in the ganglion cell and nerve fibre layers, and as globules in the outer layers. (c) Massive suprachoroidal haemorrhage secondary to corneal perforation.

Globular haemorrhages result from the confluence of dot-blot haemorrhages.

Massive intraretinal haemorrhages either continue to lie beneath the internal limiting membrane, or rupture the membrane and leak into the subhyaloid space and vitreous.

Roth's spots are intraretinal blot haemorrhages surrounding cotton-wool spots or accumulations of white blood cells such as septic emboli or leukaemic deposits.

Subretinal and sub-RPE haemorrhage

Haemorrhage into the potential spaces between the neurosensory retina and RPE (subretinal), and the RPE and Bruch's membrane (sub-RPE), may occur in association with the choroidal neovascularization of AMD and other maculopathies and trauma. The lesions produced are dome-shaped, and sub-RPE haemorrhages are seen clinically as dark masses that are occasionally confused with choroidal melanomas.

Expulsive haemorrhage

An expulsive haemorrhage is a massive suprachoroidal haemorrhage (Fig. 6.6c) associated with the ocular hypotony that occurs at the time of, or shortly after, perforation of the eye including surgery. Blood extravasates between the choroid and sclera, more particularly anterior to the equator, and especially on the nasal and temporal sides away from the anchorages of the vortex veins. The probable mechanism is that sclerosed and weakened choroidal arterioles rupture due to the lowered intraocular pressure. The inevitable consequence is that the eye fills with blood, and intraocular tissues may prolapse through the wound.

Optic nerve haemorrhage

Haemorrhage into the substance of the optic nerve may result from trauma. Haemorrhage into the optic nerve subarachnoid space may be a consequence of trauma or direct extension from an intracranial subarachnoid bleed. Optic nerve haemorrhage can exert a pressure effect on the central retinal vein and retard the outflow of intraocular blood, leading to swelling of the optic disc and subhyaloid and/or vitreous haemorrhage.

STRUCTURAL ABNORMALITIES OF BLOOD VESSELS

Vascular tortuosity

The tortuosity of normal vessels must be differentiated from that of the abnormal vessels of hamartomatous, neoplastic and neovascular proliferations. Retinal arteriolar tortuosity can be congenital and of no significance, or acquired and associated with arteriolosclerosis and the vascular retinopathies of systemic hypertension and diabetes mellitus. The degree of tortuosity is proportional to the diameter of the vessels and is related to the degree of thickening of the vascular wall. Increased venular tortuosity occurs in many retinal vasculopathies, and is secondary to delayed or obstructed venous outflow.

Anomalous vascular branching

Anomalous retinal vascular branching in the absence of neoplasia or neovascularization is invariably congenital, and may be associated with drusen of the optic disc.

Abnormalities of vessel calibre

Abnormalities of vessel calibre include vascular narrowing and dilatation. Narrowing and straightening of the retinal arterioles is a consequence of arteriolosclerosis, and is conspicuous in hypertension. The optical properties of sclerosed retinal arterioles are changed in such a way that abnormal reflection and refraction of light by the vessel walls alters the ophthalmoscopic appearance and gives rise to copper- and silver-wiring. Thickening is first apparent at arteriolovenous crossings where the sheaths of both vessels merge; A-V nipping is typical of hypertensive retinopathy. As the sclerotic changes advance, although patency is maintained, the entire vessel appears opaque (pipe-stem sheathing). The spectrum of dilatations includes venous dilatation, telangiectasia and aneurysms. Venular dilatation is common in many retinal vasculopathies and usually associated with increased tortuosity. Beading and looping are clinical terms describing extremes of dilatation and tortuosity; beading is an important sign of a sluggish circulation while looping, which frequently occurs adjacent to large areas of capillary non-perfusion, may result from focal vitreous traction. Telangiectasia is the abnormal dilatation of a group of small blood vessels, and can be congenital or acquired.

Congenital retinal telangiectasia

The congenital retinal telangiectasias are a group of anomalies characterized by vascular dilatation and tor-

tuosity, multiple aneurysm formation, and vascular leakage resulting in the deposition of lipid exudate. The underlying defect in the congenital retinal telangiectasias is increased permeability of the telangiectatic vessels. Plasma and, to a lesser extent, whole blood leak into the retinal tissue, with the subsequent formation of exudates composed of lipid and protein. The irregular vascular dilatation and aneurysm formation are secondary to the abnormality in the vessel walls. Macrophages phagocytose the exudates, and many become engorged with lipid to form balloon or bladder cells. As the concentration of non-phagocytosed lipid increases, free cholesterol crystallizes as iridescent particles and foreign body giant cells may be seen. Subretinal exudation and retinal detachment, disorganization and gliosis follow.

Three entities form part of a spectrum: idiopathic juxtafoveal retinal telangiectasia, Leber's miliary aneurysms and Coats' disease. Congenital telangiectasias are also present in the phakomatoses of von Hippel–Lindau and Wyburn–Mason, in ataxia telangiectasia and in hereditary haemorrhagic telangiectasia.

Idiopathic juxtafoveal retinal telangiectasia presents in adults with blurring of central vision. Dilated and anomalous microvascular channels and microaneurysms are found near the fovea. Associated intraretinal oedema and exudate arise from the increased permeability of the anomalous vessels.

Leber's miliary aneurysms are a more severe form of telangiectasia, and also present in adults. Fusiform and saccular dilatations of venules and arterioles are seen together with telangiectasis or varicosity of circumscribed areas of the retinal capillary bed. The temporal retinal periphery is most often involved, and the increased vascular permeability results in intra- and subretinal exudation which may be extensive and lead to a Coats'-type lesion.

Coats' disease presents in childhood with strabismus, leukocoria or visual loss. It is unilateral, predominates in the temporal retina, and the majority of those affected are boys. In the early stages, extensive intra- and subretinal creamy or yellowish exudates and haemorrhages are associated with overlying dilated and tortuous vessels (Fig. 6.7a). Massive subretinal exudation and total retinal detachment with the formation of a retrolental mass occur as the disease progresses (Fig. 6.7b). Secondary cataract, glaucoma, uveitis and iris neovascularization may ensue, and the eye can eventually become phthisical. Coats' disease may result from somatic mutation of a gene (NDP) located on the X chromosome (Xp11.3), germinal mutations of

a

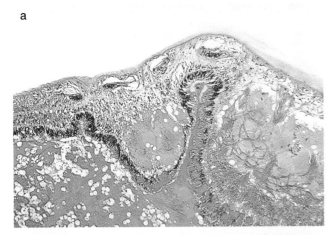

b

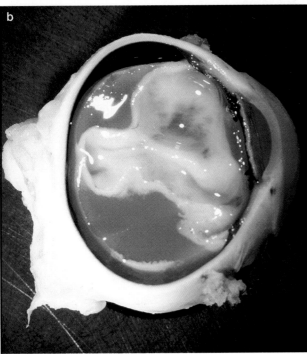

Figure 6.7 Coats' disease. (a) Abnormal telangiectatic vessels in inner retina, protein-containing exudate in thickened folded retina, and exudate and balloon cells in subretinal space. (b) Lipid-containing exudate fills the subretinal space and the retina is detached.

which are associated with Norrie's disease and familial exudative vitreoretinopathy.

Acquired telangiectasia

Acquired retinal telangiectasia occurs in the retinopathies associated with retinal vein occlusion, diabetes mellitus, sickle cell disease, idiopathic retinal vasculitis and prematurity. Conjunctival telangiectasia is seen in ataxia telangiectasia, and may develop secondarily to external ocular disease such as that produced by chemical injuries. Telangiectasia of the skin and lid margin is a feature of chronic blepharitis and acne rosacea.

Aneurysms

An aneurysm is a local dilatation of the lumen of a blood vessel. Aneurysms arise as the result of focal weakness of the vascular wall. They may be fusiform or saccular, and usually affect arteries or capillaries. Intracerebral arterial aneurysms may have ophthalmic manifestations, but aneurysms involving the retinal circulation are of special importance in ophthalmic disease. Retinal aneurysms are classified, according to their size, into micro- or macro-aneurysms.

Retinal microaneurysms are saccular dilatations of retinal capillaries. They are an essential feature of diabetic retinopathy, but are also found in the vascular retinopathies of systemic hypertension, retinal vein occlusion, sickle-cell disease, macroglobulinaemia and HIV infection. Although they occur predominantly on the venous side of the capillary bed, those on the arterial side are particularly associated with systemic hypertension. Microaneurysm formation cannot be satisfactorily explained, although it is thought either to result from fusion of the two arms of a capillary loop (Fig. 6.8a) or to arise as focal dilatations of the capillary wall where pericytes are absent. The walls of microaneurysms are initially thin and commonly rupture, but, with time, increase in thickness is due to the accumulation of plasma residues. The microaneurysms remain freely permeable to water, other components of plasma, including lipid (Fig. 6.8b), and whole blood, resulting in retinal oedema and dot-blot intraretinal haemorrhages. Microaneurysms are small and many measure $< 60\,\mu$m in diameter, which is beyond the resolution of the direct ophthalmoscope. Their presence is inferred by the identification of dot haemorrhages on ophthalmoscopy, or by fluorescein angiography when both microaneurysms and their increased permeability may be identified. Months to years after their appearance, microaneurysms appear to resolve as a result of occlusion by thrombus formation.

Retinal macroaneurysms are outpouchings of the walls of retinal arterioles (Fig. 6.9). They are much less common than microaneurysms, and occur most frequently at the bifurcation of second- or third-order vessels. They may be associated with advancing age or poorly controlled systemic hypertension, and are either asymptomatic or present with visual loss due to macular oedema or haemorrhage. Their occurrence at the branching points of arterioles suggests that mechanical injury related to increased intraluminal pressure may be of

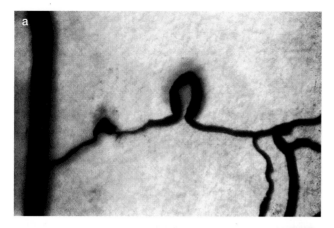

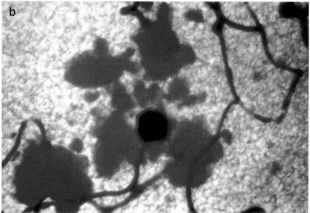

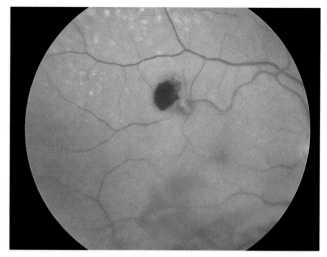

Figure 6.9 Retinal macroaneurysm.

Figure 6.8 Retinal microaneurysms. (a) Formation; the two arms of a capillary loop are not yet fused. Flat preparation of Indian ink injected retina. (b) Saccular dilatation of a capillary and leakage of lipid. Flat preparation of Indian ink injected retina; oil red O stain.

importance in their aetiology. The structural features of retinal macroaneurysms are similar to those of the small intracerebral vessels, and include subendothelial accumulation of hyaline material.

DISORDERS OF PERFUSION

Ischaemia

Ischaemia is a state in which the arterial perfusion of an organ or tissue is insufficient for its requirements. Most of the effects of ocular ischaemic disease involve the retina, which has high metabolic demands. An infarct is an area of tissue necrosis resulting from ischaemia. The extent of ischaemic damage depends on the degree of vascular insufficiency, the availability of an alternative blood supply via anastomotic vessels, and the metabolic needs of the tissues. Although initially reversible, permanent damage is an inevitable consequence of prolonged ischaemia. Retinal ischaemia is usually due to disturbance in the retinal arterioles and

capillaries, but ocular ischaemic disease may also be the consequence of an underlying lesion in large or medium-sized vessels away from the eye. Restriction or obstruction of the arterial blood supply from reduced inflow or impeded outflow is a prerequisite for ischaemia, and the various processes involved can be classified, according to their site of occurrence, as intravascular, intramural or extravascular.

Intravascular

The formation of thrombi or the lodging of emboli in any of the vessels supplying blood to the retina may cause obstruction.

Thrombosis: a thrombus is a solid mass of blood constituents formed within the vascular system. Thrombosis, the process by which a thrombus is formed, is characterized by a series of events involving platelets. Clotting, or the coagulation of blood, differs from thrombosis in that it does not involve platelets but a cascade of biochemical events leading to the conversion of the soluble plasma protein fibrinogen into the insoluble fibrin polymer. Both processes contribute to haemostasis. Once formed, a thrombus may enlarge and occlude the affected vessel; sometimes fragments break away as emboli. Resolution and organization is followed by recanalization. Resolution or dissolution of the thrombus (thrombolysis) depends on the activation of fibrinolysins by plasminogen activators. Organization is a feature of larger thrombi, but may also result from impaired thrombolysis. Both organization and recanalization involve proliferation of fibroblasts and capillaries. Factors predisposing to thrombosis include vascular endothelial damage, abnormal blood flow and increased coagulability of blood.

Vascular endothelial damage: atherosclerosis and vasculitis are foremost among the causes of endothelial damage that allows platelets to adhere to the underlying collagenous tissue. These platelets are then activated and release substances that promote further aggregation.

Abnormal blood flow: turbulence, as may occur over an atheromatous plaque or in the region of localized vascular narrowing, disrupts the normal laminar flow of blood and allows platelets to be exposed to the endothelium. A similar situation arises in sluggish flow that predominates on the venous side of the circulation possibly in association with hyperviscosity states.

Increased coagulability of blood: this can be a complicating feature of a wide range of conditions including infection, neoplasia, severe tissue trauma, liver disease and pregnancy.

Embolism: an embolus is an abnormal mass of material (solid, liquid or gas), transported by the blood stream, which may impact in the lumen of a vessel. The nature of retinal arterial emboli and their source of origin vary considerably (Table 6.1).

Table 6.1 Retinal emboli

Nature	Source
Thrombi, cholesterol and platelets/fibrin	Atheromatous plaques in major arteries
Calcific fragments, thrombi, platelets	Cardiac valves
Lipid	Marrow of fractured bones, damaged adipose tissue
Bacteria, fungi and other organisms	Sites of infection
Amniotic fluid	Amniotic sac
Talc and corn starch particles	Blood of intravenous drug abusers
Silicone, air, mercury, glass beads	Surgical procedures

Intramural

Atherosclerosis, arteriolosclerosis and vasospasm are intramural causes of ischaemia.

Atherosclerosis: a fibrous atheromatous plaque may enlarge, or there may be haemorrhage into the plaque or thrombus formation on its surface. A ruptured plaque or disintegrating thrombus may produce emboli. Atherosclerosis may directly cause central artery occlu-

sion and non-arteritic anterior ischaemic optic neuropathy, and indirectly cause central retinal vein occlusion; in the latter an enlarging plaque in the central retinal artery may result in the expanded vessel impinging on the closely related vein, which becomes obstructed. Ocular involvement can occur secondary to atherosclerosis in arteries away from the eye, particularly the carotids.

Arteriolosclerosis: mural thickening of the retinal arterioles reduces their calibre and constricts branch veins at arteriolovenous crossings.

Vasospasm: the central retinal artery and its principal branches are susceptible to intense focal and usually transient constrictions that do not usually lead to permanent damage. Spasm sufficient to obstruct flow and cause visual loss occasionally occurs in migraine and may follow the ingestion of drugs such as ergot and its derivatives, and possibly quinine. Oxygen causes capillary closure in the immature retina and plays a major role in the pathogenesis of the retinopathy of prematurity.

Extravascular

A raised intraocular pressure exceeding the critical closing pressure of blood vessels, and space-occupying lesions impinging on vessels, can obstruct blood flow and cause ischaemia.

Retinal ischaemia

Retinal ischaemia is the commonest form of ischaemia affecting the eye. Retinal arterial and arteriolar occlusions and capillary obliteration are included here, but other causes of ischaemia such as retinal venous occlusions are discussed under hyperaemia, there being a clear overlap between categories. Retinal ischaemia resulting from reduced inflow may be acute or chronic, diffuse or focal, transient or permanent. Of the conditions considered here, central retinal artery and branch arteriolar occlusions are acute, diffuse and permanent; retinopathy of prematurity is diffuse and transient; hypoperfusion retinopathy is chronic, diffuse and permanent; amaurosis fugax is acute, diffuse and transient; and cotton-wool spots are chronic, focal and transient.

Central retinal artery occlusion

Central retinal artery occlusion (CRAO) is acute, diffuse, permanent and characterized by sudden painless and profound loss of vision. In the early stages ophthalmoscopy reveals a pale opaque retina with a cherry-red spot at the macula. The retinal arterioles are attenuated and irregular, the blood flow in both arterioles and veins is sluggish, and the blood column may be segmented. The fundal changes resolve with time, but the loss of vision is permanent. Occlusion of the central retinal artery is usually secondary to atherosclerosis and often results from haemorrhage within an atheromatous plaque. The occlusion usually occurs at the narrowest part of the artery, at or immediately behind the lamina cribrosa. Embolism, thrombosis, arteritis and hyperlipidaemia are other causes. Arterial occlusion results in intracellular oedema and necrosis of the inner two-thirds of the retina. After approximately 2 hours from the onset of a complete occlusion, the retinal changes are irreversible and improvement is unlikely. As the thickness of the foveal retina is much less than that of the retina elsewhere, the light reflex from the underlying choroid remains visible as the characteristic cherry-red spot. Phagocytosis of necrotic tissue leaves an atrophic retina (Fig. 6.10); there is no glial response because astrocytes are destroyed by the ischaemia. Fibrinolysis and dissolution of any thrombus may lead to at least partial restoration of arterial perfusion. Neovascularization of the retina and iris (possibly resulting in neovascular glaucoma) are rare but recognized complications.

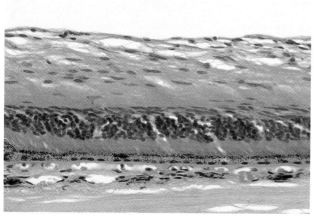

Figure 6.10 Central retinal artery occlusion. The inner two-thirds of the retina are atrophic, with loss of ganglion and bipolar cells.

Branch retinal arteriolar occlusion

A branch retinal arteriolar occlusion (BRAO) causes an acute, profound altitudinal visual field defect. In the acute stage, ophthalmoscopy reveals retinal oedema in the vascular domain of the occluded arteriole. Later, after the vessel has recanalized, ophthalmoscopic findings may be subtle, although notching of the optic disc resulting from anterograde nerve fibre degeneration may be confused with the changes of glaucoma. The commonest cause of BRAO is an embolus from a distant extraocular site, such as a fibrous atheromatous plaque. The involved retina is affected as in CRAO.

Retinopathy of prematurity

Retinopathy of prematurity (ROP) results from diffuse retinal ischaemia due to capillary closure. The condition, which is always bilateral but often to a variable degree, is a vasoproliferative retinopathy occurring mostly in prematurely born infants who are administered oxygen at or following birth.

Normal retinal vascular development
The embryonic retina is initially avascular, and the only intraocular blood supply is provided by the hyaloid vessel. Retinal vascularization commences at the fourth month of intrauterine life with a vasculogenic wave that sweeps through the inner layers. The two principal cellular components are spindle cells and endothelial cells; both are precursors of the retinal vascular system, but spindle cells precede endothelial cells. Vascularization reaches the nasal periphery by the eighth month and the temporal periphery by 1 month postterm. When the vasculogenic wave reaches the periphery, spindle cells disappear. ROP develops at the interface between the vascularized retina and the non-vascularized periphery.

Pathogenesis
Current neonatal medicine allows for the survival of approximately 50 per cent of infants delivered at 25 weeks' gestation or with a minimum birthweight of 700 g. The change in environment from intra- to extrauterine life, particularly the increased oxygen tension associated with neonatal intensive care, has complex and profound effects on the developing vascular bed of the retina. Important factors to be considered are low birthweight, retinal maturity, oxygen and angiogenic growth factors, light and genetics.

Low birthweight: ROP develops in 32 per cent of infants with a birthweight of 1000 g or less, but the incidence falls to 7 per cent if the birthweight is between 1001 g and 1500 g.

Retinal maturity: the extent of vascular development of the retina is of fundamental importance in the pathogenesis of ROP; the less well developed the retinal vasculature, the more severe is the ROP.

Oxygen and angiogenic growth factors: oxygen and angiogenic growth factors, particularly VEGF, play a major role in the pathogenesis of ROP. There are two main theories:

1. The oxygen/hypoxia theory: a high oxygen tension causes capillary obliteration and vascular endothelial cell death in the immature retina. Subsequent exposure to normal levels of oxygen results in only a partial reopening of the vascular network, and the

hypoxic retina is thought to produce growth factors that stimulate endothelial cell proliferation and angiogenesis.

2. The spindle cell theory: a raised oxygen tension may directly affect the spindle cells of the immature retina. These cells then produce growth factors that result in the formation of new vessels from the incompletely developed retinal vasculature.

Light: visible light, particularly of short wavelengths, is known to be toxic to the adult retina, possibly through the synthesis of free radicals, but its role in the pathogenesis of ROP has not been established.

Genetics: ROP occasionally occurs in infants who are full-term, malformed or stillborn, or who have not received oxygen therapy, and it is postulated that it may be caused primarily by in utero injury to the genetic programme controlling vascularization.

Clinicopathological features

According to the International Classification of Retinopathy of Prematurity (ICROP), five stages are recognized:

Stage 1. Demarcation lines A thin tortuous grey-white line running parallel with the ora serrata, particularly at the temporal periphery, develops between the vascularized and non-vascularized retina. The line is formed by spindle and endothelial cells, and acts as a physical barrier to further normal vascularization as well as being a probable source of angiogenic growth factors responsible for the subsequent neovascularization.

Stage 2. Ridge The demarcation line develops into an elevated ridge of tissue that becomes pink due to the formation of capillaries seen as abnormally branched vascular tufts. The ridge is due to the continued proliferation of the cells responsible for the demarcation line.

Stage 3. Ridge with extraretinal fibrovascular proliferation Proliferating fibrovascular tissue breaks through the inner limiting membrane and erupts on to the retinal surface and into the vitreous. Retinal blood vessels posterior to the demarcation line become dilated and tortuous, and there are retinal and vitreous haemorrhages. This stage is divided into mild, moderate and severe, and has a peak incidence at 35 gestational weeks.

Stage 4. Subtotal retinal detachment Further progression of the extraretinal tissue proliferation causes tractional detachment of the underlying retina. This develops at 10 weeks of age, starting in the extreme periphery and spreading centrally. Further expansion into Stages 4a and 4b is recognized depending on foveal involvement.

Stage 5. Total retinal detachment In extreme cases the retina is totally detached and pulled into folds and,

together with extraretinal tissue, is drawn forward and comes to lie against the posterior aspect of the lens (Fig. 6.11). This stage, previously termed retrolental fibroplasia, is the terminal cicatricial stage of ROP.

'Plus' disease A plus sign is added to the ROP stage number when the arterioles are tortuous and the posterior veins dilated; these features result from progressive vascular incompetence and are associated with iris vascular engorgement, pupillary rigidity and vitreous haze.

ROP usually undergoes complete regression if the stage is < 2 +, and only in a small minority of those affected are the advanced stages seen. The first and most reliable sign of regression is the growth of vessels – typically, paired arterioles and venules – peripheral to the ridge. Late complications occur after active proliferation has ceased and continue into adult life; these include abnormal ocular growth, myopia, retinal pigmentation, dragging of the retina, lattice-like vitreoretinal degeneration, retinal folds, retinal holes, retinal detachment and secondary glaucoma.

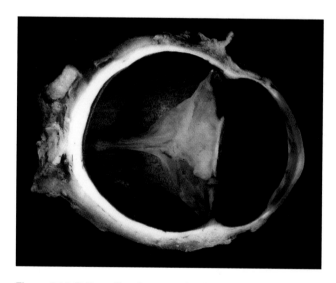

Figure 6.11 Retinopathy of prematurity. An eye opened anteroposteriorly showing total retinal detachment and a retrolental mass.

Hypoperfusion retinopathy

Hypoperfusion retinopathy results from chronic diffuse reduced arterial perfusion consequent upon stenosis of the ipsilateral carotid or ophthalmic artery. Venous engorgement and tortuosity and haemorrhages are seen in the mid-peripheral fundus, but the posterior pole is not usually affected and vision remains normal.

Amaurosis fugax

Amaurosis fugax is transient diffuse ischaemia characterized by sudden painless attacks of visual loss lasting from 2–10 minutes. It is the commonest symptom of carotid artery disease, and most cases are due to emboli from a fibrous atheromatous plaque. Observation of the retina during an attack reveals cholesterol or platelet emboli within the retinal arterioles. Amaurosis fugax sometimes results from transient occlusion of the central retinal artery and is occasionally a feature of peripheral circulatory failure.

Cotton-wool spots

Cotton-wool spots result from focal retinal ischaemia. They are discrete lesions of the nerve fibre layer having a characteristic fluffy whitish elevated appearance, and predominate in the posterior retina where the nerve fibre layer is thickest. They occur in many retinopathies, including the vascular retinopathies of central retinal vein occlusion, systemic hypertension, diabetes mellitus, sickle cell disease and HIV infection. Cotton-wool spots are due to obstruction of the precapillary arterioles, and can be regarded as microinfarcts. Endothelial cells and pericytes are lost from the capillaries, which become empty basement membrane tubes (Fig. 6.12a). Nerve axons are disrupted and swell due to disturbance of the normally bi-directional axoplasmic flow; their swollen ends (cytoid bodies) are seen on light microscopy as globular structures (Fig. 6.12b) and contain degenerate cytoplasmic organelles (Fig. 6.12c). As cotton-wool spots heal, debris is removed by autolysis and phagocytosis. Astrocytes eventually invade to form a glial scar and, although blood flows again through the capillaries, permanent neuronal damage is evident as nerve fibre bundle defects and microscotomata.

Uveal ischaemia

Uveal ischaemic damage can follow accidental or surgical trauma, and may occur in accelerated systemic hypertension, sickle cell disease, and various types of vasculitis. It is less common than retinal ischaemic damage because of the abundant anastomoses in the uveal circulation. Any part of the uvea may be affected.

Iris and ciliary body ischaemia

Acute ischaemia produces oedema and necrosis, which is manifest as pigment dispersion and clumping, and loss of epithelium. Neither oedema nor necrosis occur in chronic ischaemia. Iris ischaemia results in stromal thinning, and the clinical features are segmental iris atrophy with transillumination and a poorly reacting pupil. In

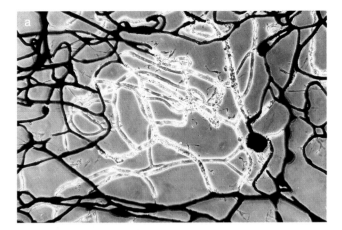

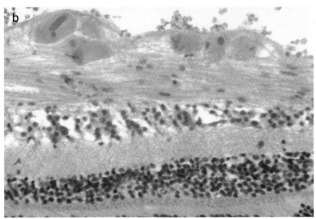

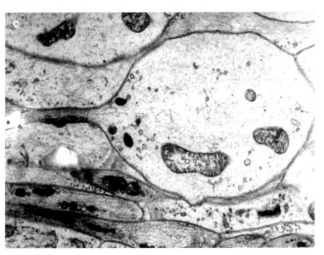

Figure 6.12 Cotton-wool spot. (a) Empty capillaries and adjacent microaneurysms. Flat preparation of Indian ink injected retina. (b) Cytoid bodies in the retinal nerve fibre layer. (c) Cytoid body containing degenerate cytoplasmic organelles. TEM.

ciliary body ischaemia, the ciliary processes become atrophic and the epithelium degenerates. The consequent interference with aqueous production results in ocular hypotony; this is the basis for cyclocryotherapy and similar surgical techniques in the treatment of glaucoma.

Choroidal ischaemia

Arteriolar occlusion in the choroid results in focal degeneration of the RPE. Pigment may aggregate in the centre of these degenerate areas (Elschnig's spots) or along the length of affected vessels (Siegrist's streaks). More extensive choroidal ischaemia results in degeneration of both the RPE and outer layers of the retina.

The ocular ischaemic syndrome

Ischaemia of the whole eye is usually a consequence of carotid artery disease, and presents with severe orbital pain (ocular angina) and signs in both the anterior and posterior segments. In the anterior segment, the iris and ciliary body become atrophic, a neovascular membrane may develop on the anterior iris surface and the lens becomes cataractous. Breakdown of the blood–aqueous barrier leads to the presence of cells and flare in the anterior chamber. In the posterior segment, hypoperfusion retinopathy, panretinal atrophy, retinal neovascularization and choroidal perfusion defects are all apparent, and breakdown of the blood–retinal barriers leads to vitreous exudates.

Hyperaemia

Hyperaemia (vasocongestion) is the presence of a greater amount of blood than normal in a tissue or organ, and results from an increased inflow (active) or a diminished outflow (passive). Active hyperaemia is due to arteriolar dilatation, and occurs in any inflamed tissue containing blood vessels. Passive hyperaemia occurs when the outflow of blood is reduced due to functional or structural obstruction, and causes venous dilatation, vascular damage leading to haemorrhage and exudation, and ischaemia. Ophthalmic examples include retinal vein occlusions, hyperviscosity states, and cranial or orbital arteriovenous malformations. The conditions of major importance causing retinal hyperaemia are central retinal vein occlusion and the hyperviscosity syndromes.

Central retinal vein occlusion

Central retinal vein occlusion (CRVO) is an acute event with variable clinical expression. There are, however, always tortuous congested retinal veins and haemorrhages (Fig. 6.13), and angiographic evidence of venous stasis. The pathophysiology of the condition remains unclear and, while the term 'occlusion' presumes a mechanical obstruction, in most instances this cannot be confirmed histologically. Association with systemic disorders such as arteriosclerosis, hypertension, diabetes mellitus, the anaemias, the haemoglobinopathies, hyperlipidaemia and platelet-coagulant abnormalities is well established, and an important local predisposing cause is glaucoma. The two types of CRVO are non-ischaemic and ischaemic: in the former non-perfusion of capillaries is minimal to moderate, whereas in the latter it is significant (> 50 per cent).

Non-ischaemic CRVO

Non-ischaemic CRVO is thought to represent obstruction of the central retinal venous circulation in the presence of a relatively normal arterial perfusion. It is a relatively mild disorder with variable features, and occurs at an earlier age than the ischaemic form. Blurred vision, often transient, may be the only symptom. Most of those affected have a visual acuity of 6/18 or better at presentation. Ophthalmoscopic findings include tortuosity, dilatation and engorgement of the retinal veins and capillaries. Retinal haemorrhages vary in extent and position, disc oedema may be present but cotton-wool spots are rare. Macular oedema or haemorrhage is the principal cause of the reduced vision. The natural history of non-ischaemic CRVO is resolution over several months, but occasionally cystoid macular oedema, retinal pigmentary changes or microvascular abnormalities persist. Neovascularization is rare, and any remaining abnormality is usually limited to reduced visual acuity in the order of 6/12 and microscotomata.

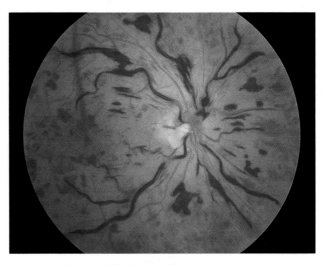

Figure 6.13 Central retinal vein occlusion.

Ischaemic CRVO

Ischaemic CRVO accounts for approximately 30 per cent of all CRVOs, and is much more serious than the non-ischaemic type. The average age of presentation is 68 years. Sudden painless loss of vision is characteristic, with acuity possibly being reduced to hand movements. The ophthalmoscopic features are more marked than in the non-ischaemic type and the signs of hyperaemia, namely vascular engorgement, flame-shaped haemorrhages and oedema, are all seen, as are cotton-wool spots, which are an index of the degree of ischaemia. Many of the features are demonstrable by fluorescein angiography. Obstructed outflow is manifest as delayed filling time of the venous tree or as dilatation of the capillaries and venules; the increased vascular permeability and retinal oedema are seen as leakage of fluorescein, particularly in the macular area; and cotton-wool spots are revealed as areas of capillary non-perfusion. Other sequelae of vascular damage, such as microaneurysms, may not be noted at the time of initial occlusion but are usually manifest shortly after. The retinal oedema away from the macula usually resolves over a period of months to years, but hard exudates, often with a circinate configuration, may form around the macula. Persistent oedema may lead to cystoid macular oedema and hole formation. RPE changes are manifest as clumping or atrophy. The venous tree becomes less dilated and tortuous, and small patent vessels form collateral channels with choroidal or pial capillaries at the optic disc. With resolution of the oedema, the haemorrhages, cotton-wool spots and microaneurysms usually also resolve. Sometimes haemorrhages persist and extend into the vitreous, and areas of capillary non-perfusion can remain. The most serious complication is neovascularization due to the release of angiogenic growth factors, particularly VEGF. Neovascularization may be preretinal, possibly resulting in retinal detachment, or involve the anterior iris surface (rubeosis iridis) where it can lead to neovascular glaucoma, which affects up to 25 per cent of those with ischaemic CRVO.

Pathogenesis
Both structural and haemodynamic factors are involved in the pathogenesis of CRVO, and the predominance of some over others may determine whether the presentation is of the non-ischaemic or the ischaemic type.

Structural factors: sclerotic changes of the central retinal vessels within the optic nerve head are harmful to blood flow as the potential for vascular expansion is limited by the rigidity of the lamina cribrosa and by both artery and vein sharing a common adventitial sheath.

Haemodynamic factors: impaired arterial perfusion predisposes to venous thrombosis particularly when, as in hyperviscosity states, the circulation is sluggish. Turbulence resulting from disturbed laminar flow in the regions of structural vasoconstriction also predisposes to thrombosis. Obstructed outflow of blood may be secondary to a raised intraocular pressure, a raised intracranial pressure, or the mechanical effect of an adjacent space-occupying lesion.

Hemispheric and branch retinal vein occlusion

Occlusion may occur anatomically distal to the central retinal vein. If this is at the initial bifurcation, the lesion is termed a hemispheric retinal vein occlusion and the upper or lower half of the retina is affected. At subsequent bifurcations, branch retinal venous occlusion (BRVO) involves correspondingly smaller areas of retina. BRVO occurs especially at arteriolovenous crossings, where the vessels share a common adventitial sheath and sclerotic changes result in vascular narrowing. Systemic hypertension and arteriolosclerosis are particularly associated with BRVO, the symptoms and signs of which depend on the area of retina affected and the extent to which the macula is involved. The features are essentially similar to those of CRVO, and the two main significant complications are cystoid macular oedema and secondary neovascularization.

SPECIFIC VASCULAR DISORDERS AND THEIR OCULAR MANIFESTATIONS

SYSTEMIC HYPERTENSION

Most authorities regard systemic hypertension as a blood pressure > 140/90 mm Hg. The risk of developing hypertensive related disease is proportional to the increase in blood pressure. Hypertension is either primary or occurs secondary to renal ischaemia, endocrine disorders (Cushing's syndrome, adrenal neoplasms, e.g. phaeochromocytoma), coarctation of the aorta or drug therapy (corticosteroids, some non-steroidal anti-inflammatory agents, the contraceptive pill).

Normal blood pressure

Normal blood pressure is maintained by humoral, neurogenic and local factors affecting arteriolar tone.

Humoral factors: the fundamental control mechanism is the renin–angiotensin system. Renin is a protease formed in the kidney in response to dietary salt intake and renal blood flow. It splits the circulating peptide angiotensinogen. The decapeptide angiotensin I so formed is converted by angiotensin-converting enzyme (ACE) into angiotensin II, which controls arteriolar tone either by direct action or indirectly by promoting aldosterone release from the adrenal cortex.

Neurogenic factors: angiotensin II can activate the sympathetic nervous system, and this affects peripheral vascular resistance.

Local factors: a vasodilator-relaxing factor and a vaso-constrictor peptide are among the vasoactive substances produced locally by vascular endothelium.

Primary systemic hypertension

Most cases of systemic hypertension are primary. The cause is unknown and while there is a familial tendency to develop the condition, no specific genetic defect has yet been found. The most widely held view is that an imbalance between the control mechanisms influences cardiac output, sodium homeostasis, renal function and peripheral vascular resistance. An abnormality in the renin–angiotensin system is the most likely underlying factor. Systemic hypertension has non-accelerated and accelerated phases.

Non-accelerated phase: chronic mild to moderate elevation of blood pressure may result in cardiac (left ventricular) hypertrophy and widespread clinicopathological changes associated with arterio-, arteriolo- and atherosclerosis.

Accelerated phase: severe elevation of blood pressure leads to vascular damage affecting particularly the microvascular systems of the eyes and kidneys. Ocular features include conspicuous retinopathy and optic neuropathy. Renal dysfunction is manifest as proteinuria and microscopic haematuria.

The universal finding in systemic hypertension is constriction of the lumen of small muscular arteries and arterioles. Initially autoregulatory, later sclerotic changes (arterio- and arteriolosclerosis) are similar to those occurring as a natural ageing process. These changes protect against the damage that could be inflicted by a further or sudden rise in blood pressure ('defence by sclerosis'). In the accelerated phase, dramatic changes at the microvascular level are reflected by the severity of the effect on the eyes and renal involvement. The characteristic histological picture is fibrinoid necrosis of small arteries and arterioles (Fig. 6.14a) resulting from damage to the smooth muscle of the vascular wall together with the intramural deposition of plasma proteins following damage to the vascular endothelium. The main ocular manifestations of hypertension result from damage to the small arteries, arterioles and microvascular systems of the retina, optic nerve and uvea. Lesions affecting the eye and visual system may also develop secondary to any associated hypertensive cerebrovascular and carotid artery disease.

Hypertensive retinopathy

Abnormalities include arteriolar narrowing, fibrinoid necrosis and capillary damage (Fig. 6.14b).

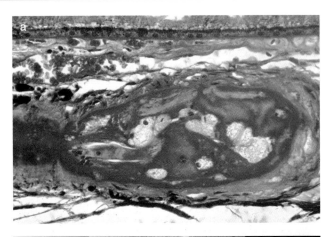

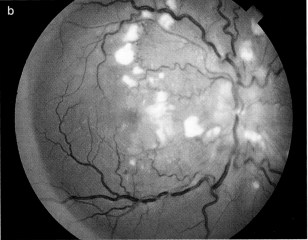

Figure 6.14 Systemic hypertension (accelerated phase). (a) Fibrinoid necrosis in choroidal arteriole. MSB stain. (b) Fundus appearance.

Arteriolar narrowing begins in the non-accelerated phase. At first autoregulatory, it is later due to arteriolosclerosis. Obstruction of the venous return, possibly due to constriction at arteriolovenous crossings, leads to dilatation and tortuosity of retinal veins.

Fibrinoid necrosis develops in the accelerated phase. It affects the precapillary arterioles and results in cotton-wool spots.

Capillary damage is also a feature of the accelerated phase. Permeability is increased and results in oedema and haemorrhages. Microaneurysms develop, particularly on the arterial side of the circulation.

Hypertensive optic neuropathy

Optic disc swelling occurs in the accelerated phase of systemic hypertension, although it is not present in every case. The cause is not clear. Impaired venous outflow due to elevated intracranial pressure is a possible mechanism, but an alternative and more likely explanation is that interference with axonal transport results from damage to the arterioles supplying the optic disc, the mechanism thus being similar to cotton-wool spot formation in the retina.

Hypertensive choroidopathy

An impaired choroidal circulation in the accelerated phase of systemic hypertension is revealed by fluorescein angiography. Ophthalmoscopic findings include serous retinal detachments and RPE changes. Serous retinal detachments are due to focal areas of breakdown of the outer blood–retinal barrier, resulting from ischaemia. RPE lesions (Elschnig's spots, Siegrist's streaks) represent degenerative lesions secondary to choroidal infarction.

Other ophthalmic manifestations of systemic hypertension

These include retinal arterial and arteriolar occlusions, retinal macroaneurysms and anterior ischaemic optic neuropathy.

DIABETES MELLITUS

Diabetes mellitus is a complex disorder of metabolism in which glucose intolerance results from a relative or absolute insufficiency of insulin, the hormone produced by the pancreatic islet cells that controls glucose transport across cell membranes. The predominant features are due to disordered carbohydrate metabolism, but there are secondary effects on fat and protein metabolism. Diabetes mellitus is either primary or occurs secondary to conditions such as other pancreatic disorders (acute and chronic pancreatitis, haemochromatosis, carcinomas) or other endocrine disorders (Cushing's syndrome, phaeochromocytomas, acromegaly, glucagonomas). The primary form is the more common, and affects up to 5 per cent of the population of the Western world. It is broadly categorized into two types, Type I and Type II.

Type I diabetes mellitus: insulin-dependent

Type I diabetes mellitus occurs mostly in children and has a peak incidence at puberty. It usually presents with polyuria and polydipsia due to glycosuria-related diuresis and there may be polyphagia but with weight loss due to inappropriate carbohydrate metabolism. Less commonly it presents with metabolic acidosis, electrolyte imbalance and dehydration or other illnesses, particularly infective disorders. Type I diabetes mellitus is char-

acterized by the loss of β-cells of the pancreatic islets and reduced or absent secretion of insulin. Associated lymphocytic infiltration probably results from an autoimmune process in a genetically susceptible individual. The mode of inheritance is unclear, but the genetic susceptibility is linked to the expression particularly of HLA-DR3, DR4 and DQ on the short arm of chromosome 6.

Type II diabetes mellitus: non-insulin-dependent

Type II diabetes mellitus is more common than Type I and usually, but not invariably, presents in obese middle-aged or elderly adults. It is initially asymptomatic, but manifestations of chronic and progressive hyperglycaemia eventually develop. The pathogenesis is not fully understood, but the hyperglycaemia results from an inability of pancreatic islet β-cells to produce sufficient insulin to meet an increased metabolic demand. Beta cells are not lost as in Type I disease and insulin uptake by peripheral cells is reduced, presumably due to a lack of insulin receptors. Multifactorial inheritance is an important aetiological feature.

Mechanisms leading to complications of diabetes mellitus

The complications of diabetes mellitus relate largely to the chronicity and/or severity of hyperglycaemia, and result from protein glycosylation, the polyol pathway, the DAG–PKC pathway and the production of angiogenic growth factors.

Protein glycosylation: glucose binds to and inactivates proteins approximately in proportion to the degree of hyperglycaemia. Although initially free to dissociate, the glucose moiety becomes covalently bound to the attached protein to form stable glycosylation products (glycosylated haemoglobin is used as an indicator of long-term glycaemic control). Glycosylation is important in the pathogenesis of the basement membrane thickening that is the basis of diabetic capillaropathy. The binding of glycosylated collagens to immunoglobulins and other important compounds such as complement explains the possible mechanism of the damage to the immune system that occurs in diabetes mellitus.

The polyol pathway: in this pathway, aldose reductase catalyses the conversion of intracellular glucose (raised in hyperglycaemia) to sorbitol, which, by increasing cytoplasmic osmolarity, causes cell swelling. This is an important mechanism in the formation of diabetic cataract. Sorbitol or excessive amounts of NADPH produced by the polyol pathway may also damage blood vessels.

The DAG–PKC pathway: hyperglycaemia raises diacylglycerol (DAG) levels and activates protein kinase C (PKC), two important cytokines associated particularly with vascular abnormalities, including those in the retina. DAG–PKC activity is important in regulating vascular permeability and contractility, and in angiogenesis.

Angiogenic growth factors: these include VEGF, IGF-1, angiotensin and pituitary-derived growth hormone.

Diabetic vascular disease

Diabetic vascular disease can be considered as macroangiopathy when it involves large and medium-sized arteries, and as microangiopathy when it involves arterioles and capillaries. Haematological abnormalities also contribute to diabetic vascular disease. The vascular complications of diabetes mellitus are far less responsive to normoglycaemic therapy than the metabolic disorder.

Macroangiopathy

Macroangiopathy is essentially accelerated atherosclerosis. It is the main cause of death in adults with diabetes mellitus, and accounts for considerable morbidity in the form of ischaemic heart disease and cerebrovascular and peripheral vascular disease. Morphologically the atherosclerotic lesions are identical to those seen in non-diabetics, but in diabetes mellitus atherogenesis is accelerated due to a number of factors including hyperlipidaemia, platelet abnormalities, glycosylation of collagen and lipoproteins in the vascular wall, sorbitol damage to the vascular wall, and systemic hypertension secondary to renal disease.

Microangiopathy

Microangiopathy is at the root of the retinopathy, the nephropathy (Kimmelsteil–Wilson lesions) and the neuropathy that develop in diabetes mellitus. It comprises capillaropathy and arteriolosclerosis.

Capillaropathy is characterized by thickening of the endothelial basement membrane by up to five times its normal width. It occurs at an early stage and is widespread throughout the body. Hyperglycaemia has a direct effect on its development, and its progression is delayed by good glycaemic control. The cause of capillary basement membrane thickening is not fully established, but factors involved include protein glycosylation and reduced turnover or increased synthesis of basement membrane material.

Arteriolosclerosis is common in diabetes. The hyalinized vascular wall contains fibrin and lipid derived from the blood, possibly due to alterations in the permeability of the vascular endothelium and in the integrity of the basement membrane.

Haematological abnormalities

Haematological abnormalities in diabetes mellitus contribute to vascular disease. Blood flow through small capillaries may be diminished either because of the reduced deformability of red cells and their increased tendency to aggregate, or because plasma viscosity is increased (hyperlipidaemia, hyperfibrinogenaemia). Platelet abnormalities relate to the activating properties of adenosine diphosphate and epinephrine, and correlate with raised levels of von Willebrand's factor. Increased platelet aggregation and thromboxane formation and decreased release of prostacyclins and anti-aggregating prostaglandins predispose to thrombus formation.

Ophthalmic complications of diabetes mellitus

The principal and most important ophthalmic complication of diabetes mellitus is retinopathy. Other important complications are cataracts (juvenile and adult onset), neovascular glaucoma and cranial neuropathy. Diabetics also have an increased incidence of primary open-angle glaucoma.

Diabetic retinopathy

Retinopathy is the major cause of visual disability in diabetes mellitus. Its overall prevalence is 26 per cent, and it accounts for the 2 per cent of diabetics who are registered blind in the UK. The incidence of diabetic retinopathy rises with the duration of the metabolic defect and the quality of glycaemic control, although some diabetics never develop retinopathy. Additional risk factors include systemic hypertension and raised serum cholesterol. Those with Type I diabetes mellitus are at greatest risk but, because Type II disease is more common than Type I, retinopathy of Type II diabetes mellitus is more frequently encountered. Diabetic retinopathy is divided into preretinopathy, non-proliferative retinopathy, preproliferative retinopathy and proliferative retinopathy.

Preretinopathy

Functional disturbances of the retinal circulation precede clinical manifestations of retinopathy, and are due to breakdown of the inner and outer blood–retinal barriers and to increased retinal blood flow. Blood–retinal barrier breakdown at this stage allows leakage of small molecules only. Structural changes include capillary basement membrane thickening. Increased retinal blood flow occurs because of vasodilatation in response to hyperglycaemia or tissue hypoxia.

Non-proliferative retinopathy

Non-proliferative retinopathy is subdivided into background diabetic retinopathy and maculopathy.

Background diabetic retinopathy

Background diabetic retinopathy (BDR) is common in both types of diabetes mellitus and, in the absence of macular involvement, is asymptomatic. Microaneurysms, exudates and haemorrhages are seen on ophthalmoscopy (Fig. 6.15a), and focal areas of capillary closure on fluorescein angiography. These features are the consequences of abnormalities in arterioles and capillaries.

Arterioles: hyaline arteriolosclerosis is probably due to the insudation of plasma secondary to increased vascular permeability. The arteriolar lumen, especially at bifurcations, is reduced, and gradual occlusion results in foci of

capillary closure. The likely cause of total obstruction is intravascular thrombus formation.

Capillaries: focal areas of closure and microaneurysms are characteristic, and there are changes in endothelial cells, basement membrane and pericytes.

Capillary closure: focal areas of capillary closure in the posterior retina (Fig. 6.15b) are an early feature. The affected vessels are devoid of endothelial cells and pericytes, leaving only a basement membrane tube. Capillary closure probably results from the shunting of blood away from such areas, thrombotic occlusion of feeder vessels or external compression due to tissue oedema. Capillary closure causes scotomata due to ganglion cell and nerve fibre degeneration, and predisposes to the formation of microaneurysms and new vessels.

Endothelial cells: intrinsic endothelial changes are associated with an enhanced risk of thrombotic vascular occlusion. As the retinopathy progresses endothelial

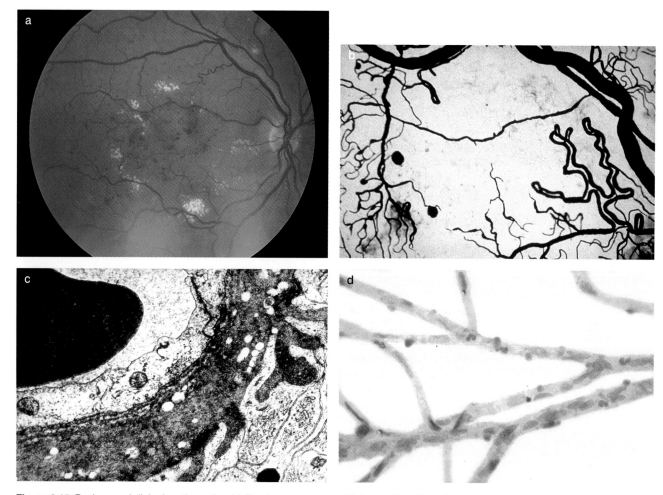

Figure 6.15 Background diabetic retinopathy. (a) Fundus appearance. (b) Areas of capillary closure with capillary loops and microaneurysms. Flat preparation of Indian ink injected retina. (c) Capillary basement membrane thickening with pseudopodia-like extensions into surrounding structures. TEM. (d) The degenerate pericytes are eosinophilic. Trypsin digest preparation.

cell degeneration and loss occur predominantly, but not exclusively, in relation to the focal areas of capillary closure. This leads to intraretinal exudates and haemorrhages. Discrete yellowish waxy hard exudates develop mainly in the outer plexiform layer; these are usually removed by macrophages in 4–6 months, although large exudates take a year or more to resolve. The morphology of haemorrhages depends on their location; most are encountered in the vicinity of microaneurysms, and dot and blot configurations are characteristic.

Basement membrane: the basement membrane of retinal capillaries is thickened and forms pseudopodia-like extensions into adjacent structures (Fig. 6.15c). It incorporates lipid, fibrin, haemosiderin and cellular constituents including degenerate pericytes.

Pericytes: degeneration and loss of pericytes, sometimes in association with endothelial cell degeneration and loss, is an invariable feature of diabetic retinopathy. Pericyte degeneration is not exclusive to diabetes, and occurs to a lesser degree in other vascular retinopathies such as those associated with macroglobulinaemia, multiple myelomatosis and polycythaemia. Pericyte death is thought to be due to apoptosis in response to a high concentration of glucose. Pericyte loss is specific to the retinal capillaries and does not occur outside the eye. It has a putative role in microaneurysm formation and in the initiation of proliferative retinopathy. Degenerate pericytes are eosinophilic and are best demonstrated in trypsin digest preparations (Fig. 6.15d).

Maculopathy

Macular involvement in diabetic retinopathy is the commonest cause of visual impairment. The three clinically recognized types are focal, diffuse and ischaemic. Mixed types may also occur, but macular oedema is the feature common to all. Macular oedema is the result of the capillaropathy that leads to breakdown of the blood–retinal barriers. The clinical picture depends on the severity and distribution of the oedema. Müller cells swell due to absorption of fluid. Although initially reversible, when the intracellular swelling is sufficient, rupture and cell death result in cystoid macular oedema. This is seen microscopically as cystic spaces containing fluid and cell debris in the region of the macula (macular retinoschisis). Tissue damage is located mainly in the outer plexiform layer but may also extend into the inner layers and progress to partial or complete macular hole formation.

Focal (exudative) maculopathy is essentially macular involvement in BDR. It is characterized by the presence of BDR with macular oedema and surrounding exudates. The oedema associated with exudative maculopathy is classified as macular oedema if retinal thickening is evident or if exudates occur within one disc diameter (1500 μm) of the centre of the fovea. Clinically significant macular oedema (CSMO) is defined as the presence of one or other of the following:

1. Retinal oedema within 500 μm of the centre of the fovea.
2. Hard exudates within 500 μm of the foveola if associated with retinal thickening.
3. Retinal oedema of 1 disc diameter or larger, any part of which is within 1 disc diameter of the centre of the fovea.

Diffuse maculopathy is characterized by diffuse retinal thickening, particularly at the macula, in association with haemorrhages and microaneurysms but few exudates. The cause is probably widespread leakage from abnormal blood vessels throughout the posterior pole. Fluorescein angiography demonstrates this abnormality but confirms the presence of relatively good perfusion of the macular blood vessels.

Ischaemic maculopathy is similar to diffuse maculopathy, but fluorescein angiography reveals areas of capillary non-perfusion at the macula. Visual loss is due to retinal ischaemia rather than oedema.

Preproliferative retinopathy

Preproliferative retinopathy increases the risk of progression to proliferative diabetic retinopathy to 50 per cent over 2 years. Features include cotton-wool spots, which are indicative of progressing focal retinal ischaemia, increased intraretinal haemorrhages, venous changes including dilatation, beading, segmentation and looping, and intraretinal microvascular anomalies (Fig. 6.16).

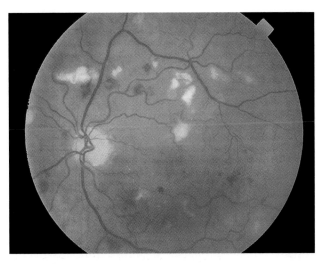

Figure 6.16 Preproliferative diabetic retinopathy.

Intraretinal microvascular abnormalities (IRMAs) are dilated and elongated capillary loops that frequently form bizarre hairpin or corkscrew patterns. They develop adjacent to areas of capillary closure. IRMAs have a larger diameter than new vessels, they do not cross major blood vessels and, being relatively impermeable, are not associated with exudates or haemorrhages. They may arise as the result of re-endothelialization of previously occluded vessels, or alternatively may represent a type of new vessel.

Proliferative diabetic retinopathy

Proliferative diabetic retinopathy (PDR) is characterized by the proliferation of new vessels originating from the optic disc and retina (Fig. 6.17a). It affects about 5 per cent of diabetics and, if untreated, the visual prognosis is poor, with a 30–40 per cent risk of severe visual loss within 2 years. Its incidence 20 years after the diagnosis of diabetes mellitus is 60 per cent. Fragile tortuous new vessels grow at the optic disc (NVD – new vessels at disc) and/or on the surface of the retina (NVE – new vessels elsewhere). At this stage PDR is asymptomatic, but extension of the vessels into the vitreous cavity may result in haemorrhage and sudden painless loss of vision. As PDR progresses, vascularized membranes form and the vitreous may become detached from the inner limiting membrane of the retina. Contraction of these vascularized membranes in areas of vitreoretinal adhesion results in tractional retinal detachment with consequent permanent loss of vision.

The vitreous is extremely important in the development of PDR. New vessels do not extend into formed vitreous, but the detached degenerate vitreous body forms a framework over which neovascular membranes grow. Vitreous degeneration is accelerated in diabetics by non-enzymatic glycosylation and the subsequent aggregation of vitreal collagen. Together with leakage of plasma proteins from the new vessels, this predisposes to posterior vitreous detachment. The mobile detached posterior vitreous causes traction on the fragile new vessels with resultant preretinal or intravitreal haemorrhage, the former being the more common and usual type of 'vitreous haemorrhage' seen in PDR.

The new vessels usually arise either at the periphery of areas of capillary non-perfusion in relation to focal areas of capillary closure, or near the optic disc where the absence of an inner limiting membrane is thought to be a predisposing factor. Neovascularization is initially intraretinal, but proteinases produced by vascular endothelial cells cause local disruption of the internal limiting membrane, thereby allowing new vessels to grow through. Endothelial cells mature, pericytes differentiate, permanent cellular junctions are formed and the new vessels become less fragile. At the same time, fibro-

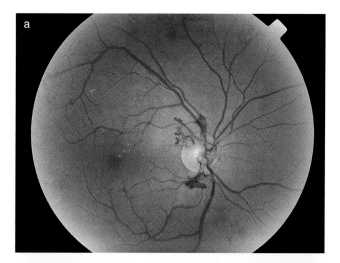

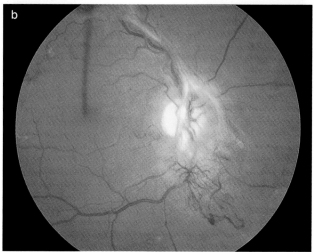

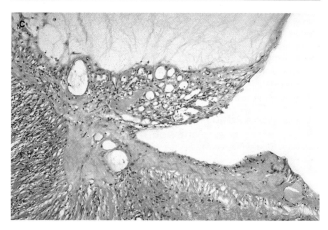

Figure 6.17 Proliferative diabetic retinopathy. (a) Proliferation of new vessels from the optic disc. (b) Vascularized fibroglial tissue extending into the vitreous; fundus appearance. (c) Vascularized fibroglial tissue extending into the vitreous; histology.

glial tissue develops from fibroblasts and glial cells. The result is vascularized fibroglial tissue firmly adherent to both the retina and the vitreous (Fig. 6.17b, 6.17c).

Neovascularization occurs in response to angiogenic growth factors, particularly VEGF secreted as a result of retinal hypoxia due to diabetes-induced vascular insufficiency. In the DAG–PKC pathway, PKC has a role in the mediation of the effect of VEGF. Systemic endocrine factors play a role in angiogenesis and account for the reduced prevalence of PDR following hypophysectomy and the rapid progression sometimes seen in pregnancy. Factors that inhibit neovascularization normally synthesized by pericytes are reduced because of retinal pericyte loss.

Other ophthalmic complications of diabetes mellitus

Structures specifically involved in other ophthalmic complications of diabetes mellitus are the cornea, iris and lens, the optic nerve, and the IIIrd, IVth and VIth cranial nerves.

Cornea

Reduced corneal sensitivity results from abnormalities in the corneal epithelium and its underlying basement membrane. Reduced adhesion of the epithelium to its basement membrane, possibly due to a decreased number of hemidesmosomes, leads to a tendency to develop recurrent erosions. The corneal epithelium of diabetics is therefore easily damaged by procedures that involve the use of a corneal contact lens.

Iris

Diabetic iridopathy is the presence of glycogen-containing vacuoles within lacy degenerate iris pigment epithelium (Fig. 6.18). It may explain the pigment dispersion

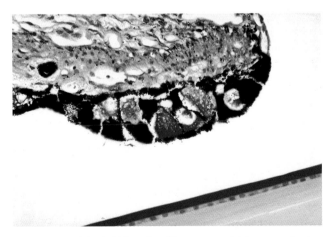

Figure 6.18 Diabetic iridopathy. Glycogen-containing vacuoles in iris pigment epithelium. PAS stain.

encountered during intraocular surgery and the poor response of diabetics to topical mydriatics.

Rubeosis iridis is neovascularization on the anterior iris surface (see Fig. 1.9). It is commonly associated with PDR, and is a response to the angiogenic growth factors derived from ischaemic retinal tissue. Involvement of the drainage angle (see Fig. 1.9a) leads to neovascular glaucoma, and the fragility of the new vessels can result in spontaneous hyphaema. Ectropion uveae (see Fig. 1.9b) develops as a consequence of contraction of the fibrous tissue associated with the neovascularization.

Lens

Diabetics have a predisposition to the formation of cataracts. The lenses of diabetics are larger for age than those of non-diabetics and morphologically appear 15 years older. Transient blurring of vision due to osmotically induced changes in refraction and other physical properties of the lens at the onset of diabetes mellitus are a response to fluctuating and/or high levels of blood glucose.

Juvenile diabetic cataracts develop rapidly in uncontrolled young diabetics. They have a snowflake appearance with dense white anterior and posterior subcapsular opacities, and are thought to result from osmotic changes due to the accumulation of sorbitol.

Adult-onset diabetic cataracts are indistinguishable from age-related cataracts in non-diabetics, but occur at an earlier age and with increased prevalence and a higher female preponderance. They tend to be cortical or posterior subcapsular rather than nuclear. Their pathogenesis is unknown.

Optic nerve

Anterior ischaemic optic neuropathy is identical to that seen in non-diabetics and reflects the microangiopathy within the nerve head.

Diabetic papillopathy differs from anterior ischaemic optic neuropathy in that it is much less severe and has an excellent visual prognosis. It is frequently bilateral. The disc is oedematous but visual acuity is usually better than 6/18.

IIIrd, IVth and VIth cranial nerves

Neuropathy of the IIIrd, IVth and VIth cranial nerves may result in extraocular muscle palsies, sometimes with pain, and may be the presenting feature of undiagnosed diabetes mellitus. The pathology of the neuropathy is segmental demyelination of the affected nerve secondary to ischaemia produced by microangiopathy.

VASCULITIS

Vasculitis is inflammation of any blood vessel, and most often results from a disorder of immunity. Less common causes are infection and injury due to physical agents such as electromagnetic radiation. Ophthalmic involvement is common in systemic vasculitis and, together with retinal vasculitis and anterior ischaemic optic neuropathy, there may be inflammation of the uvea, optic nerve, sclera, cornea, conjunctiva and orbital tissues. Evidence of an immune disorder is common and, while associated findings such as elevated C-reactive protein, autoantibodies and immune complexes are helpful, histological examination of biopsies of affected tissues may be essential for a definitive diagnosis. The association of certain disorders with HLA antigens implies an immunogenetic aetiology in at least some of the conditions. Retinal vasculitis may occur as an apparently idiopathic condition localized to the eye.

Idiopathic retinal vasculitis

Idiopathic retinal vasculitis (Fig. 6.19) may affect any part of the retinal vascular tree, but the venules (periphlebitis) are more commonly involved than the arterioles (arteriolitis). The early stages are asymptomatic but later, symptoms include blurred vision due to macular oedema, floaters due to associated vitritis and sudden visual loss due to vitreous haemorrhage. Fundal examination reveals sheathing of the retinal vessels, and serous exudation and oedema that may involve the macula. Increased vascular permeability is demonstrated by fluorescein angiography. Vascular damage results in aneurysmal and varicose dilatation of retinal venules, and retinal haemorrhages that may break through into

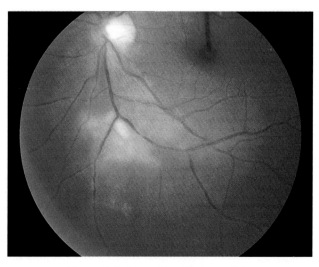

Figure 6.19 Idiopathic retinal vasculitis.

the vitreous. Vascular occlusion due to thrombosis leads to retinal ischaemia, with the formation of cotton-wool spots. More extensive vascular closure may result in ischaemia sufficient to produce neovascularization and associated complications such as glaucoma and tractional retinal detachment. Chronic ischaemia leads to retinal atrophy and scarring with pigment deposition.

Perivascular cuffing by chronic inflammatory cells accounts for the clinical appearance of the vessels; lymphocytes predominate but plasma cells are sometimes present and occasionally there is a sarcoid-like granulomatous reaction. In cases when the vasculitis is no longer active, vascular sheathing is due to mural hyalinization and thickening. Idiopathic retinal vasculitis is presumed to be an autoimmune condition; a T cell-dependent reaction is postulated and the circulating levels of IgA, immune complexes and retinal antibodies may be raised.

Eales' disease

Eales originally described a bilateral retinal vasculitis syndrome in young men, characterized by recurrent retinal and vitreous haemorrhages, epistaxis, constipation and headaches. The condition falls within the definition of idiopathic retinal vasculitis.

Behçet's disease

Behçet's disease is a multisystem disorder, the underlying pathology of which is a vasculitis of unknown aetiology. It is more common in males in their third and fourth decades, and occurs predominantly in those originating from countries around the Mediterranean Sea and in the Middle and Far East. The diagnosis is made clinically. Oral ulceration must be present in association with two of the following: recurrent genital ulceration, skin lesions, ocular involvement and a positive pathergy test (the formation of a pustule following scratching of the skin with a needle – i.e. cutaneous hypersensitivity). Ocular manifestations occur in 70 per cent of cases and, if untreated, frequently lead to blindness. Anterior uveitis is severe, with hypopyon formation. Posterior segment inflammation is manifest as a retinal vasculitis, predominantly a periphlebitis with later involvement of the arterioles. The inflammatory changes give rise to exudates and haemorrhages, and may be sufficiently severe to cause vascular occlusion, retinal ischaemia and a neovascular response. Resolution of the disorder ultimately leads to atrophic changes.

The underlying lesion in Behçet's disease is a destructive vasculitis affecting both large and small vessels. Lymphocytes and plasma cells infiltrate the vascular walls and perivascular tissue, and fibrinoid necrosis is accompanied by thrombosis, aneurysm formation and haemorrhage. The cause of Behçet's disease is unknown, although the strong association with HLA subtypes suggests an immunogenetic basis; HLA-B5 is associated with ocular involvement, HLA-B27 with arthritis and HLA-B12 with mucocutaneous disease. There is no specific laboratory test for Behçet's disease, but immune complexes are found in the acute state together with increased levels of IgG and IgM, and reduced IgG complexes.

Wegener's granulomatosis

Wegener's granulomatosis is a necrotizing granulomatous vasculitis of unknown aetiology affecting the respiratory system, kidneys, eye and orbit. It usually presents in the fourth and fifth decades. A limited form of the disease without renal involvement is thought to be a distinct clinical entity. The eye and orbital tissues are involved in up to 50 per cent of cases, and ophthalmic manifestations are the presenting features in 15 per cent. Progressive marginal corneal ulceration is common, together with scleritis, episcleritis and conjunctivitis. Posterior segment involvement includes retinal vasculitis, uveitis and optic neuropathy. Orbital involvement may be primary or secondary to spread from the upper respiratory system, and results in painful proptosis and limitation of ocular movement.

The necrotizing granulomatous vasculitis involves the small arteries and veins of affected tissues, and the immunological basis of the condition is shown by the response to immunosuppressive therapy and the presence of circulating IgG anti-neutrophil cytoplasmic antibodies (ANCA). Two patterns of ANCA immunofluorescence are identified: cytoplasmic (C-ANCA) results from antibody binding to proteinase 3 and gives rise to a coarsely granular, centrally attenuated immunofluorescence; perinuclear (P-ANCA) results from antibody binding to myeloperoxidase and lactoferrin in granules attached to the nuclear membrane and gives rise to perinuclear immunofluorescence. C-ANCA is a diagnostic marker for Wegener's granulomatosis, but P-ANCA is less specific and may be positive in other autoimmune disorders. It has been suggested that ANCA activates circulating neutrophils to attack blood vessels. Diagnosis is based on the clinical findings, on the histological examination of biopsy material and by the demonstration of C-ANCA and other indicators of an immune disorder, such as elevated C-reactive protein and circulating immune complexes.

Hypersensitivity vasculitis

Type III hypersensitivity is the postulated mechanism for this type of vasculitis, which is seen in many forms of autoimmune vascular diseases, including systemic lupus erythematosus, rheumatoid arthritis, Sjögren's syndrome and Henoch–Schönlein purpura. The retinal changes include inflamed arterioles with relative sparing of the venules. Occlusion of vessels by thrombi or emboli leads to retinal ischaemia and cotton-wool spot formation. Inflammation and ischaemia also occur in the choroid and optic nerve.

Systemic lupus erythematosus (SLE)

This is an autoimmune multisystem disease that affects the skin, kidneys, joints and serous membranes. It is more common in Afro-Caribbean and Asian females, and the peak age of onset is between 20 and 30 years. The retinal vasculitis, which occurs in up to 10 per cent of those affected, is essentially an occlusive arteriolitis with cotton-wool spots, haemorrhages, disc oedema and serous retinal detachment. Other ocular manifestations include punctate epithelial keratopathy, peripheral corneal melt and marginal infiltration, keratoconjunctivitis sicca and scleritis. In SLE a wide range of antibodies is directed against plasma proteins, cell surface antigens, intracellular cytoplasmic components and nuclear components, including DNA, ribonucleoproteins and histones. Small arteries exhibit inflammation and fibrinoid necrosis, the basis of which is deposition of autoimmune complexes, particularly against DNA, and the associated Type III hypersensitivity. Type II hypersensitivity in which cytotoxic antibodies are directed against leukocytes, erythrocytes and platelets may also play a role. The basic cause of SLE is unknown, but infection and certain drugs such as hydralazine, procainamide and isoniazid may precipitate its onset.

Polyarteritis nodosa

Polyarteritis nodosa (PAN) is a rare acute and often fatal necrotizing vasculitis of unknown cause affecting mainly medium-sized and small arteries. Aneurysm formation, thrombosis and infarction are characteristic and lead to the variable presentation that involves predominantly the skin and the gastrointestinal, renal and cardiovascular systems. Immune complexes are deposited in the walls of affected blood vessels, which show patchy fibrinoid necrosis surrounded by a vigorous inflammatory response. The eye is involved in 15 per cent of those affected and, although most ocular tissues can be involved, the commonest manifestation is vascular retinopathy. Features include irregular calibre of retinal vessels, haemorrhages, cotton-wool spots and vascular occlusions. Retinopathy may also be produced by the severe systemic hypertension that results from renal involvement.

Giant cell arteritis/polymyalgia rheumatica

Giant cell arteritis (GCA) and polymyalgia rheumatica (PMR) are disorders at either end of a spectrum of disease that is the commonest form of immune vasculitis.

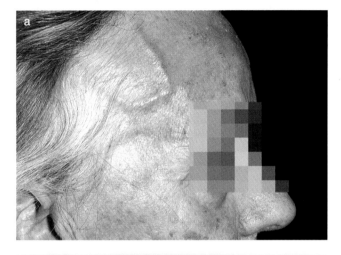

The characteristic pathological finding is a granulomatous arteritis of large and medium-sized vessels. GCA/PMR occurs in the elderly and is rare before the age of 50, thus distinguishing it from other forms of vasculitis. GCA presents with temporal headache and swelling of the temporal arteries (Fig. 6.20a) which are tender and frequently pulseless. Jaw claudication and general features such as malaise, fever or weight loss also occur. A varying degree of myalgia may affect the limb girdles, and when this is the predominant feature the condition is termed polymyalgia rheumatica. The disorder is generally self-limiting, but the ocular complication, anterior ischaemic optic neuropathy, is a medical emergency that if untreated may lead to irreversible bilateral blindness.

The aetiology of GCA/PMR is unknown, but there is a cell-mediated immune response against a substance in the vessel wall, probably elastic tissue or smooth muscle. The distribution of the arteritis corresponds to the amount of elastic tissue within the vessel wall,

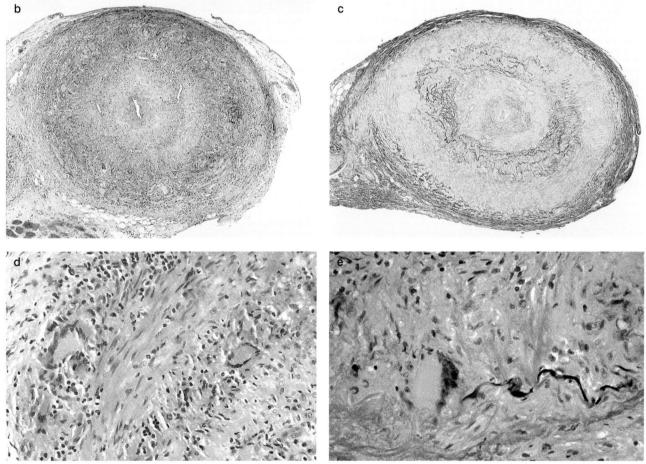

Figure 6.20 Giant cell arteritis. (a) A prominent distended temporal artery. (b) Transmural granulomatous inflammation of temporal artery, the lumen of which is grossly narrowed. (c) The internal elastic lamina of the temporal artery is disrupted. Verhoeff stain. (d) The wall of the temporal artery contains giant cells. (e) Giant cell in relation to disrupted elastic tissue. Verhoeff stain.

so arteries of the head and neck are particularly affected whereas less elastic arteries elsewhere, such as the renal and pulmonary arteries, are uninvolved. As in other forms of vasculitis, histological examination of biopsy material is of diagnostic importance. If clinically indicated, a biopsy of no less than 2 cm of temporal artery should be taken and sectioned at a number of levels. The vessel wall is thickened by transmural granulomatous inflammation (Fig. 6.20b) and the internal elastic lamina is disrupted (Fig. 6.20c). Lymphocytes, plasma cells and eosinophils are seen and giant cells are frequently, but not invariably, present (Fig. 6.20d, 6.20e). The vascular lumen is narrowed or even obliterated by either the mural thickening or thrombus formation. Vessels are not always uniformly affected throughout, and histologically normal skip areas may be present. A negative temporal artery biopsy, which is said to occur in 40 per cent of cases, may represent inadequate lengths of biopsy material, failure to examine the specimen at a sufficient number of levels, or skip areas. Old burnedout GCA is histologically similar to the arteriosclerotic changes of advancing age.

The ESR and PV are often markedly raised, although they are normal in up to 20 per cent of cases. The C-reactive protein level is a sensitive measure of the disorder and is always elevated. The rapid response to corticosteroid medication may also be of diagnostic importance. The effect of corticosteroids on the histological picture of GCA is probably not as marked as might be supposed, and histological evidence of arteritis has been shown after more than 2 weeks of corticosteroid treatment. Nevertheless, if a temporal artery biopsy is to be performed this should ideally be carried out not later than 48 hours after the commencement of therapy.

Takayasu's disease

Takayasu's disease is a rare inflammatory disorder of larger vessels such as the aorta and its proximal branches. It occurs most frequently in young Asian females with symptoms and signs of carotid artery insufficiency, cardiac ischaemia and renal artery involvement with associated systemic hypertension. Severe necrotizing inflammation with loss of elastic tissue is accompanied by lymphocytic cuffing of the vasa vasora in the adventitia. Giant cells may be seen, and the histological appearance is similar to GCA/PMR. Intimal proliferation, narrowing of the vascular lumen and thrombotic occlusion are other features. As with GCA/PMR the cause is unknown, but raised immunoglobulin levels and antinuclear antibodies suggest autoimmunity.

BLOOD DISORDERS AND THEIR OCULAR MANIFESTATIONS

THE ANAEMIAS

Anaemia is defined as a reduction of the haemoglobin concentration, erythrocyte count or packed cell volume to below normal levels. The anaemias are classified according to the underlying cause: the production of erythrocytes may be reduced due to defective proliferation and/or maturation of precursors, erythrocytes may be destroyed at an increased rate as in haemolysis or may be lost from the circulation as in haemorrhage. The most significant ophthalmic manifestation of anaemia is a vascular retinopathy. Usually asymptomatic, features include pallor of the fundal reflex, dilatation and tortuosity of the vasculature, haemorrhages and cotton-wool spots. Other ophthalmic manifestations of anaemia include conjunctival pallor and, rarely, optic neuropathy due to ischaemia or, in the case of pernicious anaemia, to vitamin B_{12} deficiency.

ERYTHROCYTOSIS (POLYCYTHAEMIA)

Erythrocytosis is a general term for several conditions in which the total erythrocyte mass is increased and there is an elevated haematocrit. For haematocrits > 50 per cent the plasma viscosity rises exponentially; with haematocrits > 60 per cent the oxygen-carrying capacity of the blood is no longer able to maintain the supply necessary for most tissues and hypoxia ensues. Erythrocytosis is either relative, as in dehydration, or absolute. Absolute erythrocytosis may be primary or secondary. Primary absolute erythrocytosis is seen in polycythaemia rubra vera, a proliferative disorder of erythrocyte stem cells. Secondary absolute erythrocytosis occurs in arterial hypoxia, which may develop in cardiopulmonary disease, in the haemoglobinopathies and at high altitude, and may also be due to the abnormal or inappropriate secretion of erythropoietin as in renal disease, and in association with neoplasms such as cerebellar haemangioblastomas. The principal ophthalmic manifestation of erythrocytosis is retinopathy. Features include darkening of the fundal reflex, venous dilatation and tortuosity with increased redness or a purplish hue of the blood column, haemorrhages and oedema. Other ophthalmic manifestations of erythrocytosis include optic neuropathy in which hyperaemia precedes disc swelling, cerebrovascular insufficiency that may result in amaurosis fugax, visual field defects and conjunctival congestion.

THE LEUKAEMIAS

The leukaemias are a complex group of neoplastic proliferations of leukocytes. They may be classified according to the cell line of origin into myelocytic and lymphocytic, and each may be acute or chronic depending on the clinical behaviour; further classification of the acute leukaemias is based on cell morphology, but the chronic leukaemias are not further subdivided. In general, the acute types present in childhood and have a rapidly progressive course, although modern treatments have reduced their mortality. The chronic leukaemias occur usually in adults and are frequently asymptomatic, diagnosis often being made on routine blood testing; they are compatible with a long survival even without treatment. Ophthalmic manifestations are common and more frequent in acute leukaemia, with up to 80 per cent of post-mortem eyes and 42 per cent of those with newly diagnosed acute leukaemia being involved. The ophthalmic involvement may take different forms:

Retinopathy may occur due to the associated anaemia, thrombocytopenia and hyperviscosity. Features include venous tortuosity and dilatation, microaneurysms, retinal haemorrhages possibly with Roth's spots, and cotton-wool spots.

Leukaemic infiltration and neoplastic phenomena may involve any ocular or orbital structure, but are relatively rare because of effective treatment of the underlying condition.

Ophthalmic involvement by opportunistic infections results from compromise of an immune system by the disorder and/or its treatment. Such infections include orbital and intraocular fungal infections, and retinal infection due to CMV, HSV and *Toxoplasma gondii*.

THE HAEMOGLOBINOPATHIES

The normal human haemoglobin molecule (HbA) contains two pairs of amino acid chains, each designated α and β; the four chains are folded to form a globular tetramer (globin) around a molecule of haem, an iron-containing pigment that readily combines with oxygen. Inherited abnormalities are either thalassaemias or structural variants of haemoglobin.

Thalassaemias

A mutation reduces the synthesis of either the α or β chain, resulting in a relative excess of one. Precipitation of haemoglobin within the erythrocyte leads to membrane damage and premature haemolysis. The type of thalassaemia produced is designated according to the polypeptide chain affected; thus in α thalassaemia the synthesis of the α chain is reduced and there is an excess of the β chain. Apart from the features of chronic anaemia, the ocular manifestations of pure thalassaemia are of little clinical significance. Thalassaemic haemoglobin is of great ophthalmic importance when combined with HbS.

Structural variants of haemoglobin

A point mutation causes an amino acid substitution in one of the polypeptide chains (usually the β chain) of the globin molecule. Although there are over 200 clinically significant abnormal haemoglobins, the two most common are point mutations that result in the substitution of valine or lysine for glutamic acid at position 6 of the β chain. The former results in the formation of HbS and the latter, HbC.

Sickle cell haemoglobinopathies

The sickle cell haemoglobinopathies are a group of inherited abnormalities of haemoglobin in which erythrocytes, when deoxygenated, transform from their normal biconcave disc shape to a crescentic or sickle shape. These abnormal cells then impact in small blood vessels. The disorders are characterized by the inheritance of at least one allele (S) for HbS that is codominant for other haemoglobin alleles. The homozygous form (SS) causes sickle cell disease (sickle cell anaemia). There are several heterozygous forms where HbS occurs in other combinations; combination with normal haemoglobin A results in the sickle cell trait (AS), combination with haemoglobin C results in sickle cell C disease (SC disease) and combination with thalassaemic haemoglobin results in sickle cell β-thalassaemia (SThal). The prevalence of the HbS gene closely follows the distribution of falciparum malaria, and the heterozygous state conveys some resistance to malarial infection, particularly in children. This may account for the ethnic distribution of the gene, with up to 40 per cent of black Africans being heterozygous for the sickle cell haemoglobinopathies. There is a lower prevalence in Mediterranean countries, in the Middle East and in India. The features depend on the combination of haemoglobins.

SS disease (sickle cell disease, sickle cell anaemia): HbS constitutes 85–90 per cent of the total haemoglobin, and there is severe chronic haemolytic anaemia and vaso-occlusive disease. Many of those affected are asymptomatic for most of the time but develop periodic and potentially fatal crises due to infarction of tissue and haemolysis or sequestration of erythrocytes by the spleen. Features include bone marrow infarcts, aseptic necrosis of the head of the femur, arthralgia, abdominal pain and CNS symptoms. SS disease affects 0.4 per cent of black Americans.

AS disease (sickle cell trait): erythrocytes contain 25–45 per cent of HbS and can be made to sickle only at low, unphysiological oxygen tensions. AS disease affects 10 per cent of black Americans.

SC disease (sickle cell C disease): equal amounts of HbS and HbC are present and increased erythrocyte rigidity results in haemolytic anaemia and infarctive crises that are less severe than in SS disease. SC disease affects 0.2 per cent of black Americans.

SThal disease (sickle cell β-thalassaemia): as much as 60–80 per cent of the haemoglobin may be of the HbS type and, although the anaemia is usually mild, the condition resembles sickle cell disease.

Sickle cell retinopathy

Unlike the systemic manifestations of the disorder, ophthalmic involvement is most severe in SC and SThal disease while those with SS disease are relatively unaffected. The reasons for this are not clear, but possibly the severity of the anaemia, the blood viscosity and the rate of sickling are important factors. Although sickling occurs to a greater extent and at a higher oxygen tension in SS disease, the associated anaemia and therefore low haematocrit means that the effect on blood viscosity is less. In SC and SThal diseases, where the anaemia is less and the haemoglobins exist in higher concentrations, sickling has a more profound effect on blood viscosity and predisposes to vascular occlusion. The extent of the anaemia in SS disease may therefore protect the eye from microvascular occlusion. Apart from its distribution, the retinopathy of the sickle cell haemoglobinopathies is similar to that of diabetes mellitus although diabetic retinopathy is essentially posterior while sickle cell retinopathy is mainly peripheral; maculopathy is common to both. The underlying pathophysiology is vascular occlusion, particularly of the precapillary arterioles. Sickled erythrocytes become impacted in the lumen of small vessels and impede the passage of other erythrocytes, which themselves become hypoxic and begin to sickle, thereby creating a vicious circle. Sickle cell retinopathy can be divided into proliferative and non-proliferative types:

Proliferative retinopathy

Proliferative retinopathy is the most serious ophthalmic complication of the sickle cell haemoglobinopathies, and usually occurs in the third and fourth decades. It is a chronic progressive disorder, and the neovascular growth only occasionally ceases or regresses. There are five clinical stages:

Stage 1: peripheral arteriolar occlusions lead to a failure of perfusion of capillaries and venules. An abrupt interface (junctional zone) is evident between the perfused and non-perfused retina. The cause of this is either thrombus formation or the haemodynamic effect of sickling in the peripheral retina where the oxygen tension is lower than in the central retina.

Stage 2: peripheral arteriolovenular anastomoses arise at the interface of the anterior non-perfused retina and shunt blood to the posterior perfused retina.

Stage 3: peripheral neovascularization originates as capillary budding at the sites of previous arteriolar occlusions and arteriolovenular anastomoses. The superotemporal quadrant is preferentially affected and neovascularization proceeds from perfused to non-perfused retina, i.e. towards the ora serrata, possibly in response to angiogenic growth factors elaborated in the ischaemic area. At an early stage, the new vessels often sprout in a fan-shaped configuration (sea-fan neovascularization) fed initially by a single arteriole and drained by a single venule. As in other proliferative retinopathies, the new vessels are fragile and abnormally permeable and, although initially flat, become adherent to the cortical vitreous. The abnormal permeability results in transudation of plasma proteins. This leads to premature degeneration of the vitreous, which collapses and causes traction, thereby promoting the onset of Stage 4 (vitreous haemorrhage) and Stage 5 (retinal detachment) retinopathy. With time, additional circumferential capillary growth occurs such that a large and complex arborizing neovascular network forms in the peripheral retina. Sea-fan neovascularization occurs most often in those with SC disease and SThal disease, and is uncommon with other haemoglobinopathies.

Stage 4: vitreous haemorrhage is a frequent complication of retinal neovascularization and is the result of vitreous collapse and traction on the adherent neovascular tissue. Small haemorrhages are usually asymptomatic and remain localized to the area surrounding the neovascular tissue, where they organize and are seen as white fibrous plaques.

Stage 5: vitreoretinal traction, together with ischaemic retinal atrophy, leads to tractional retinal detachment and retinal holes that predispose to rhegmatogenous retinal detachment.

Non-proliferative sickle cell retinopathy

Non-proliferative sickle cell retinopathy is characterized by changes involving the retina (vascular changes, haemorrhages) and RPE (black sunbursts).

Retinal vascular changes: venous tortuosity is common in those with SS disease and SC disease but is uncommon in AS disease and SThal disease. Peripheral arteriolar occlusions, seen as silver-wire vessels in the retinal periphery, sometimes herald the onset of neovascularization.

Retinal haemorrhages: peripheral intraretinal haemorrhages result from vascular necrosis near points of occlusion. They usually remain localized and become orange-red in colour (salmon patch haemorrhages), but occasionally leak into the subhyaloid space and vitreous. Localized haemorrhages organize and leave a focal area of retinoschisis sometimes containing haemosiderin-laden macrophages.

Black sunbursts: pigmented ovoid circumscribed fundus lesions resembling choroidoretinal scars are characteristic. Asymptomatic, they occur predominantly in the equatorial region and have stellate or spiculate borders. They probably arise from hyperplasia and dispersion of RPE caused by intraretinal haemorrhage between the photoreceptor outer segments extending into the subretinal space.

Other ophthalmic manifestations of the haemoglobinopathies are seen in the conjunctiva and iris, and in the retina/choroid. The conjunctiva may exhibit vascular abnormalities, including comma- or corkscrew-like configurations. In the iris, circumscribed areas of ischaemic atrophy may extend from the pupillary margin to the colarette. Retinal/choroidal lesions include occlusions of the central retinal artery, the macular arterioles and the choroidal vasculature (particularly in SC and SThal disease), and angioid streaks (see Fig. 5.16), which develop possibly because Bruch's membrane is rendered brittle due to iron deposition secondary to chronic haemolysis.

Chapter 7

Disorders of nerve and muscle

The central nervous system

Cells of the CNS and their response to injury
Neurons
Astrocytes
Oligodendrocytes
Microglia

Clinicopathological features of optic nerve disease

Optic disc oedema
Cerebrospinal fluid and raised intracranial pressure
Idiopathic intracranial hypertension
Optic nerve atrophy

Inherited optic neuropathies

Leber's hereditary optic neuropathy

Acquired optic neuropathies

Inflammatory optic neuropathies
Multiple sclerosis
Vascular optic neuropathies
Anterior ischaemic optic neuropathy
Nutritional and toxic optic neuropathies
Nutritional optic neuropathy
Toxic optic neuropathies
Traumatic, irradiation and compressive optic neuropathies
Traumatic optic neuropathy

Irradiation optic neuropathy
Compressive optic neuropathy
Glaucoma
Primary open-angle glaucoma
Primary angle-closure glaucoma
Secondary glaucoma
Congenital glaucoma

The peripheral nervous system

Axons and their response to injury
Peripheral neuropathies

Striated muscle, the motor unit, the extraocular muscles and their disorders

Striated muscle
The motor unit
The extraocular muscles
Muscle disorders
Neurogenic disorders
Disorders of neuromuscular transmission
Lambert–Eaton myasthenic syndrome
Botulism
Myasthenia gravis
Myopathies
Muscular dystrophies
Myotonic disorders
Inflammatory myopathies

THE CENTRAL NERVOUS SYSTEM

The central nervous system (CNS) consists of the brain and spinal cord. The meninges surround these structures, and are subdivided into the leptomeninges (pia mater and arachnoid mater) and the pachymeninges (dura mater). The optic nerve is also surrounded by meninges as far as the eye, and structurally and functionally is considered as part of the CNS.

CELLS OF THE CNS AND THEIR RESPONSE TO INJURY

Neurons

Neurons are the functional units of the nervous system. They possess a cell body, numerous dendrites and usually one axon. The cell body (perikaryon) has a single, centrally located nucleus with a prominent nucleolus. The cytoplasm contains numerous organelles, in particular conspicuous basophilic granular substance (Nissl substance) composed of rough endoplasmic reticulum. Dendrites and axons project from the cell surface to connect with other neurons and convey electrical impulses to and from the perikaryon. Axons may be of great length and may or may not be ensheathed with myelin. Retinal ganglion cells are neurons, the axons of which pass to the brain via the optic nerve. Neurons respond to injury in a number of ways but once lost are never replaced, and nerve fibres within the CNS, including the optic nerve, do not have regenerative capacity.

Central chromatolysis is the disruption, dispersion and gradual disappearance of the Nissl substance from the cytoplasm surrounding the nucleus, leaving only a narrow rim at the periphery. This pattern of depletion can occur in physiological conditions as the result of excessive electrical stimulation and in a variety of pathological processes. If due to raised physiological activity, the Nissl substance completely recovers after an interval of rest. This structural reconstitution usually starts at the periphery. If due to axonal damage, central chromatolysis is maximal at around 8 days following the insult.

Anterograde degeneration usually accompanied by central chromatolysis follows transection of the axon. The distal part of the axon degenerates and becomes fragmented within about 4 days following separation from the intact perikaryon. If present, a myelin sheath also fragments and both axonal and myelin debris is phagocytosed by macrophages.

Atrophy occurs in slowly progressive degenerative disorders. Atrophic neurons shrivel, appear hyperchromatic and often contain excess lipofuscin pigment. Trans-synaptic atrophy of neurons may follow loss of the main afferent connections; this occurs in neurons of the lateral geniculate body following damage to the retina or optic nerve.

Astrocytes

Astrocytes are glial cells with a star-shaped configuration due to the presence of numerous cytoplasmic processes. They have round or oval vesicular nuclei, and are found in both the white and grey matter of the CNS. Their main function is to provide a supportive framework for other cells. They also have an important role following CNS damage when, being analogous to fibroblasts, they proliferate in a response known as reactive gliosis to form a glial scar (Fig. 7.1).

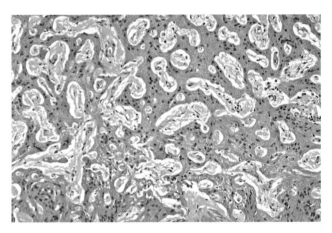

Figure 7.1 Gliosis. Transverse section of an optic nerve in which the normal architecture is destroyed and astrocytic proliferation has led to the formation of a glial scar.

Oligodendrocytes

Oligodendrocytes are the most numerous cells in the CNS. In the grey matter they are frequently satellites of neurons, and in the white matter are arranged longitudinally between myelinated axons. They have round or oval nuclei and a rim of cytoplasm. Their main function is the synthesis of myelin during late gestation and until the age of 2 years, and then its maintenance throughout life. In the eye, other than when there are myelinated retinal nerve fibres, no oligodendrocytes are present anterior to the lamina cribrosa. Myelin is a substance rich in cholesterol and phospholipids. Its function is to protect and insulate neuronal processes and to allow the rapid transmission of electrical impulses. Oligodendrocyte damage leads to demyelination, which may be primary or secondary. Primary demyelination is where destruction of myelin is selective and other neural structures remain intact. Secondary demyelination occurs subsequent to neuronal damage and axonal degeneration. Broken down myelin is phagocytosed, and the cholesterol and phospholipids are transformed into neutral lipids, mainly cholesterol esters. The commonest and most important demyelinating disorder is multiple sclerosis, but others include central pontine myelinosis and progressive multifocal leukoencephalopathy. In the rare inherited leukodystrophies, myelin synthesis fails and this is more correctly referred to as dysmyelination. Remyelination in the CNS is not as efficient as in the peripheral nervous system.

Microglia

Microglial cells are ubiquitous in the CNS. Their nuclei are triangular or elongated but less vesicular than those of astrocytes. The cells have little cytoplasm but they do have cytoplasmic processes, although fewer than astrocytes. The most prominent feature of the cytoplasm is the presence of dense inclusion bodies, mainly lysosomes. In normal neural tissue microglial cells maintain a close functional relationship with neurons, axons and myelin sheaths, and are thought to regulate the ion and fluid balance of the extracellular space. Following CNS damage they become activated, migrate to the site of the lesion, assume different shapes, undergo mitosis and engulf cellular debris. They are thus in effect the macrophages of the CNS; in inflammatory lesions, however, the majority of phagocytic cells are not microglia but macrophages derived from circulating monocytes.

CLINICOPATHOLOGICAL FEATURES OF OPTIC NERVE DISEASE

OPTIC DISC OEDEMA

The causes of optic disc oedema can be classified as prelaminar (intraocular) or retrolaminar (intraorbital, intracranial or within the spinal cord). Prelaminar causes include hypotony, acute glaucoma, intraocular inflammation, and vascular and blood disorders that affect retinal vessels. Retrolaminar causes are mainly inflammatory, demyelination or disturbances of CSF circulation. Papilloedema is specifically defined as disc oedema secondary to raised intracranial pressure.

The earliest manifestation of optic disc oedema is blurring of the disc margins. This is followed by hyperaemia, capillary dilatation, loss of venous pulsation and venous engorgement. The surface of the disc becomes elevated above the plane of the retina and the central optic cup

disappears. Associated signs depend on the cause, but include flame-shaped haemorrhages, cotton-wool spots and circumferential retinal folds on the temporal side of the disc (Paton's concentric lines). Retinal exudates, including macular exudates, may develop. If the disc oedema lasts for a period of several months, the haemorrhages, cotton-wool spots and exudates resolve, and secondary optic atrophy ensues. In disc oedema the volume of tissue confined within the anatomical boundaries at the optic nerve head increases as a result of interference with axoplasmic flow, transudation or exudation – mechanisms that overlap.

Interference with axoplasmic flow: disruption of the normal two-way axoplasmic transport results in the accumulation of intracellular structures within axons. The disruption can be due to a change in the hydrostatic pressure gradient across the lamina cribrosa, or to ischaemia.

Change in the hydrostatic pressure gradient across the lamina cribrosa: under normal circumstances the tissue pressure within the prelaminar portion of the optic nerve is higher than in the retrolaminar. Lowering the pressure in the prelaminar portion or elevating it in the retrolaminar portion disrupts axoplasmic flow gradients.

Ischaemia: impaired vascular perfusion causes local disruption of axonal transport, the mechanism being similar to that of cotton-wool spot formation in the retina.

Transudation: venous obstruction at the lamina cribrosa or anterior or posterior to it results in transudation.

Exudation: inflammation of blood vessels within the optic nerve head causes exudation.

Cerebrospinal fluid and raised intracranial pressure

The cerebrospinal fluid (CSF) is actively secreted by the epithelium of the choroid plexus in the third and lateral ventricles. It flows through the cerebral aqueduct to the fourth ventricle, from where it passes into the subarachnoid space via the foramina of Lushka and Magendie, ultimately draining via the arachnoid villi into the cerebral venous system. An extension of the subarachnoid space ensheaths the optic nerve, and CSF circulates anteriorly as far as the eye. The skull is a rigid, essentially closed structure containing the brain, CSF and intravascular blood, and an increase in their volume leads to a raised intracranial pressure (ICP). Compensatory mechanisms such as a reduction in CSF volume, brain displacement and possibly a reduction in cerebral perfusion are able to buffer the effect, but once these are overcome the elevated ICP is manifest. Raised ICP is most commonly due to an intracranial space-occupying lesion, but may be idiopathic.

Idiopathic intracranial hypertension (benign intracranial hypertension)

Idiopathic intracranial hypertension is a syndrome in which the ICP is raised in the absence of an intracranial space-occupying lesion or other obvious cause. It usually affects obese females between the ages of 18 and 45 years, and can result in optic nerve damage and permanent visual loss – the designation 'benign' is thus misleading. Headache and disc swelling are the usual presenting features but, apart from occasional transient visual obscurations and an enlarged blind spot, visual function is usually normal in the early stages. In chronic cases optic atrophy results in permanent visual loss. Sixth cranial nerve palsy causing horizontal diplopia may occur in up to 30 per cent of those affected. The elevated ICP is thought to result from a defect of CSF absorption by the arachnoid villi in the superior sagittal sinus. Although clinical associations such as predilection for females, obesity, menstrual irregularity and pregnancy suggest an underlying disorder of female endocrinology, no consistent hormonal abnormality has been demonstrated. Other associated conditions include dural venous sinus thrombosis, hypo- and hypervitaminosis A, and drug therapy; tetracyclines, retinoids, nalidixic acid, nitrofurantoin, lithium and corticosteroid withdrawal are noteworthy in this respect.

OPTIC NERVE ATROPHY (OPTIC ATROPHY)

Optic nerve atrophy is the end result of any progressive degenerative or other disorder affecting the retinal ganglion cells and their axons. Axons are irretrievably lost and the optic disc has a characteristic pallor. Optic nerve atrophy is classified as ascending or descending (retrograde).

Ascending: from the primary lesion in the retina or at the optic nerve head, the degenerative process proceeds towards the brain. It involves the axons through the chiasm and optic tract to the primary visual nuclei, including the lateral geniculate nuclei, the pretectum, the superior colliculus and several hypothalamic regions. Subsequent trans-synaptic atrophy may occur in higher order neurons.

Descending: from the primary lesion within the cranial cavity or in the retrobulbar portion of the optic nerve, degeneration proceeds towards the eye. Through trans-synaptic connections, descending degeneration can also follow an insult to the visual cortex.

In optic nerve atrophy, ophthalmoscopic examination reveals a pale or white optic disc with a sharply demarcated rim. The changes may be diffuse or sectorial depending on the extent of nerve damage. Cupping with exposure of the lamina cribrosa may mimic glaucomatous changes (pseudoglaucoma cerebri). Whatever the causes (Table 7.1), the pathological changes are:

1. Loss of retinal ganglion cells and their axons throughout their entire course to the lateral geniculate body.
2. Loss of astrocytes and oligodendrocytes.
3. Demyelination – primary or secondary, depending on the cause of the atrophy.
4. Reactive gliosis that may extend to the optic disc.
5. Shrinkage of the nerve, resulting in widening of the subarachnoid space and subdural spaces.
6. Thickening of the pial septae, which occupy the space left by the loss of parenchyma.

Table 7.1 Optic atrophy

Type	Site of origin	Cause
Ascending	Retina Optic nerve head	Vascular and degenerative disorders Glaucoma, oedema, anterior ischaemic optic neuropathy
Descending	CNS or retrobulbar portion of optic nerve	Demyelinating disorders (e.g. MS), space-occupying lesions (e.g. meningioma, optic nerve glioma), hydrocephalus, and various inherited, infective, toxic and nutritional disorders

INHERITED OPTIC NEUROPATHIES

Inherited optic neuropathies almost invariably present in children (Leber's hereditary optic neuropathy is an exception) with insidious symmetrical bilateral visual loss and optic atrophy (Table 7.2). They may occur in isolation or in association with neurodegenerative syndromes such as Charcot–Marie Tooth disease and Friedreich's ataxia, and despite their genetic aetiology, patterns of inheritance for particular cases may be difficult to establish. The pathological changes of optic neuropathy include loss of ganglion cells in the retina, loss of nerve fibres in the retina, optic nerve and optic tracts, and secondary changes in the visual radiations and cortex. Reactive gliosis follows myelin loss in the optic nerve and other visual pathways. Isolated inherited optic neuropathy is a complex subject with many variants and differing degrees of optic nerve dysfunction.

Table 7.2 Inherited optic neuropathies

Type of inheritance	Condition	Usual age of presentation	Visual deficit	Associated findings	Clinical course
Autosomal dominant	Early infantile	3–4 years	Severe	Nystagmus	Stable
	Juvenile	4–8 years	Mild to moderate	Nil	Stable or slightly progressive
Autosomal recessive	Behr's type	1–9 years	Moderate	Mild mental deficiency, spasticity, hypotonia, ataxia	Stable
	DIDMOAD	6–14 years	Severe	Diabetes insipidus, diabetes mellitus, deafness, ataxia, nystagmus, mental deficiency	Progressive
Mitochondrial	LHON	18–30 years	Moderate to severe	Myopathy and other features mimicking MS	Stable following acute onset

Leber's hereditary optic neuropathy

Leber's hereditary optic neuropathy (LHON) is a rare disorder that can affect both sexes up to the age of 65 years. It generally presents with profound visual loss in males between 18 and 30 years of age. A bilateral condition, an interval of several weeks separates the involvement of each eye. Swelling and mild hyperaemia of the optic disc with irregular telangiectatic dilatation of the disc capillaries are seen in the acute stage. Later, severe optic atrophy develops (Fig. 7.2) and the vascular abnormalities resolve. Visual loss is nearly always permanent and severe, and only occasionally is there any improvement. Non-ocular features of LHON include cardiac conduction defects, demyelinating or other neurological disorders, and skeletal deformities. More than 10 mutations in mtDNA have been found in affected families, and at least four are the cause of the disease. The most common, a nucleotide substitution at position 11778, results in amino acid substitution in subunit 4 of NADH. A single gene defect does not account for features such as the variable expressivity or the male predominance, and heteroplasmy and other genetic or environmental factors are thought to be relevant.

ACQUIRED OPTIC NEUROPATHIES

Acquired optic neuropathies are a heterogeneous group of disorders due to various aetiologies including inflammation, vascular disease, trauma, nutritional deficiencies and toxicity. Within this category may be added the glaucomas, the primary manifestation of which (at least in the chronic glaucomas) is a progressive optic neuropathy.

INFLAMMATORY OPTIC NEUROPATHIES (OPTIC NEURITIS)

Inflammation of the optic nerve may be primary and associated with demyelination, or secondary and contiguous with spread from surrounding structures such as the eye, meninges, orbit or paranasal sinuses. Retrobulbar neuritis is inflammation of the optic nerve posterior to the disc, and is implied on the basis of clinical features and investigations. Papillitis is an inflammatory optic neuropathy manifest at the disc; in neuroretinitis the inflammation extends into the retina. In the absence of a clearly defined cause approximately one-third of all those with optic neuritis develop other evidence of multiple sclerosis, and this is more likely to happen in females 21–40 years of age.

The inflammatory optic neuropathies present more commonly in females between 20 and 50 years of age with rapid, usually monocular, impairment of vision developing over a period of hours or days. Deterioration may continue for several weeks and ocular or orbital discomfort is common, particularly in relation to eye movement. A relative afferent pupillary defect is asso-

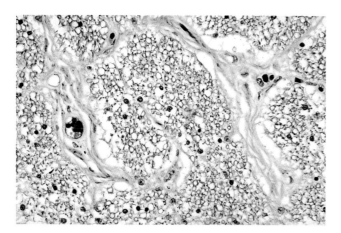

Figure 7.2 Leber's hereditary optic neuropathy. Transverse section of the optic nerve with conspicuous demyelination. Loyez stain.

ciated with disturbed colour vision. The optic disc may appear normal, although in the acute stage papillitis and neuroretinitis may be evident, possibly with associated retinal periphlebitis and vitritis. Spontaneous improvement in visual acuity, often to a normal level, is usual after 6–8 weeks, but other sensory abnormalities such as disturbed contrast sensitivity or colour vision can be permanent. Optic atrophy follows resolution of the acute stage. The specific features and the pattern of inflammation depend on the cause. Involvement of the meninges (perineuritis) and inflammation of the peripheral (periaxial) portions of the nerve are usually caused by the extension of local inflammatory disease. Involvement of the central (axial) portion and complete cross-section (transverse neuritis) of the nerve are associated with demyelination. Changes in the visual evoked cortical potential are helpful in the diagnosis, as they indicate abnormality of optic nerve conduction. Haematological investigations and biochemical and immunological analysis of blood and CSF are usually negative in otherwise asymptomatic individuals.

Multiple sclerosis (disseminated sclerosis)

Multiple sclerosis (MS) is a chronic demyelinating disease of the CNS and is the most common neurological disorder affecting young white adults in the UK and USA, where its prevalence is approximately 1 : 1000. It usually presents between 20 and 40 years of age, and is almost twice as common in females as males. Presenting features include dysfunction of the optic nerve (optic neuritis), brainstem (internuclear ophthalmoplegia – diplopia, vertigo, nystagmus) and spinal cord (limb weakness or paraesthesiae). Thereafter, relapses and remissions are characteristic and associated with progressive deterioration. Complications include chest and urinary tract infections, and survival beyond 20 years after the initial symptoms and signs is uncommon.

The hallmark of MS is the presence of multiple plaques of demyelination throughout the CNS. Discrete plaques, rarely more than 2 cm in diameter, are found in the white matter of the brain (Fig. 7.3a) and spinal cord. The optic nerves, optic chiasma and paraventricular white matter of the corona radiata are preferentially affected. The peripheral nervous system is uninvolved. In the acute stage myelin is lost but axons are preserved and there is perivascular cuffing by CD8 + (T$_{C/S}$) cells and plasma cells, the latter being the cells that synthesize the immunoglobulins found in the CSF. The affected areas are oedematous, and macrophages phagocytose the breakdown products of myelin (Fig. 7.3b). Following the acute stages, astrocytes proliferate with resultant gliosis but oligodendrocytes are lost and remyelination does not occur. Affected axons ultimately degenerate.

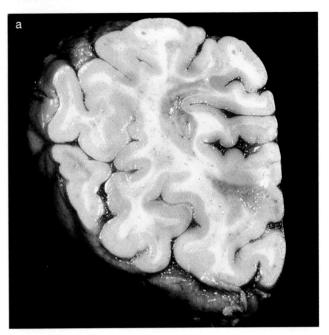

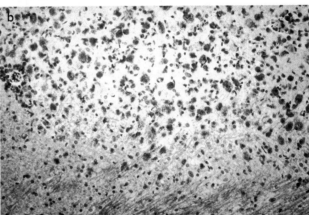

Figure 7.3 Multiple sclerosis. (a) Plaques of demyelination in cerebral white matter. (b) Phagocytosis of myelin by macrophages. Oil red O stain.

The exact cause of MS is unknown but immune mechanisms, possibly in response to a viral infection, with a genetic predisposition are probable aetiological factors.

Immune factors: it is thought that immunoglobulins are synthesized in response to a specific but as yet unknown antigen within the CNS. Oligoclonal IgG bands are revealed by electrophoresis of the CSF in up to 90 per cent of those affected.

Infective agents: although a wide variety of endemic viruses such as measles, mumps and rubella have been implicated, at present there is no definite evidence for any specific infective agent. Epidemiological evidence concerning the geographical distribution of the disease suggests an environmental cause possibly involving infective agents and affecting children. When populations migrate from areas of low prevalence (the tropics) to one of high prevalence (temperate climates), they have the same risk of developing the disease as the indigenous population of the high-risk area.

Genetic predisposition: family members of those affected are at increased risk of developing the disease, and a 25 per cent concordance in identical twins falls to 2 per cent in non-identical twins. In European races MS is associated with certain HLA antigens, particularly DR2 but also A3, B7 and DQ1, thus linking disease susceptibility to the HLA locus on chromosome 6. This suggests that MS is due to involvement of inherited factors affecting the immune system.

Neuromyelitis optica (Devic's disease)

Neuromyelitis optica is considered to be an acute, particularly virulent form of MS that affects children and young adults. It is characterized by rapid bilateral loss of vision due to bilateral optic neuritis, followed days to weeks later by paraplegia secondary to transverse myelitis. The pathology is usually indistinguishable from MS, but on occasions there may be a fulminating intensely destructive necrotic process with demyelination, loss of astrocytes and axons, and possible cavitation.

VASCULAR OPTIC NEUROPATHIES

The commonest optic neuropathy associated with vascular disease is anterior ischaemic optic neuropathy. Rarer forms of vascular optic neuropathy, in which the precise pathophysiology is not understood but in which a vascular component is implicated, occur in diabetes mellitus, migraine and inflammatory conditions such as polyarteritis nodosa and systemic lupus erythematosus. Other diseases associated with a presumed vascular optic neuropathy include syphilis, sickle cell disease, polycythaemia rubra vera, radiation necrosis, acute hypotension (shock) and viral infections. Very occasionally vascular optic neuropathy occurs in ocular hypotension, especially that associated with intraocular surgery.

An understanding of the vascular system of the optic nerve and disc is necessary in order to appreciate the area damaged by vascular insufficiency. The system is complex, but essential features are:

1. The surface capillaries of the optic disc are derived from the retinal circulation.
2. The prelaminar and lamellar portions of the optic nerve are in the main supplied by the short posterior ciliary circulation, with a smaller contribution from the choroidal vessels and the circle of Zinn–Haller.
3. The optic nerve posterior to the lamina cribrosa is supplied peripherally by perforating branches of the pial vessels, which are themselves derived from either the ophthalmic artery or recurrent branches of the posterior ciliary arteries.
4. The anterior part of the retrobulbar optic nerve is supplied by branches of the central retinal artery.
5. The central retinal artery does not supply the optic nerve at or anterior to the lamina cribrosa.
6. Venous drainage of the anterior portion of the optic nerve is predominantly via the central retinal vein, with some prelaminar drainage via the choroid.

Interruption of the short posterior ciliary circulation can cause infarction of the prelaminar and lamellar portions of the optic nerve, and possibly ischaemic damage to the peripheral parts of the retrobulbar portion.

Anterior ischaemic optic neuropathy

Anterior ischaemic optic neuropathy (AION) results from occlusion of the posterior ciliary arteries, and is a cause of sudden profound loss of vision in the elderly. Two forms, non-arteritic and arteritic, are recognized (Table 7.3). The non-arteritic form is either idiopathic or secondary to atherosclerosis, systemic hypertension, possibly diabetes mellitus or rarely migraine; the arteritic form is due to arteritis, most commonly giant cell arteritis. Arteritic AION is initially unilateral but frequently progresses to involve the fellow eye unless prompt corticosteroid medication is administered. A temporal artery biopsy is essential if a positive diagnosis of giant cell arteritis is to be made. Histological features of AION include ischaemic infarction at the optic nerve head, with oedema, necrosis and loss of axons. Ascending and descending degeneration of the nerve fibres subsequently follows.

NUTRITIONAL AND TOXIC OPTIC NEUROPATHIES

Optic neuropathy may be due to abnormalities of nutrition or the action of toxic substances. Characteristically insidious in onset and slowly progressive, bilateral loss of visual acuity is associated with central or centrocaecal scotomas and acquired defects of colour vision. There may be temporal optic disc pallor, but usually no ophthalmoscopic abnormality is seen.

Nutritional optic neuropathy (tobacco–alcohol amblyopia)

Nutritional optic neuropathy may occur particularly in the elderly who have poor diets. Some of those affected are alcoholics and/or heavy smokers, particularly of pipe

Table 7.3 Clinical and pathological features of anterior ischaemic optic neuropathy

	Idiopathic	Arteritic
Age (years)	60–65	70–80
Visual loss	Variable	Usually severe
Second eye involvement	40%	75% (if untreated)
Associated systemic features	Variable, hypertension in 50%	Clinical features of GCA/PMR
Ophthalmoscopic examination	Disc pale and swollen	Disc often swollen but may be normal
ESR/plasma viscosity	Normal	Usually, but not invariably, grossly abnormal
C-reactive protein	Normal	Elevated
Histological features	Arteriosclerotic changes only	Arteritis ± arteriosclerotic changes
Corticosteroid response	Nil	Rapid resolution of arteritis

tobacco. The most likely cause of the neuropathy is a dietary deficiency of B-complex vitamins (predominantly thiamine) rather than the direct toxic effects of tobacco or alcohol. Some of those affected also have defective vitamin B_{12} absorption and develop pernicious anaemia. A possible explanation for the association of alcohol and tobacco is that the deficiency of vitamin B_1 that occurs in chronic alcoholism, and malnutrition prevents transformation of the cyanide normally present in tobacco smoke into a harmless thiocyanate compound, thus allowing the cyanide to exert a toxic effect.

Wernicke's encephalopathy

Wernicke's encephalopathy is characterized by the sudden onset of ocular motility disturbances, ataxia, altered consciousness and abnormal thermoregulation with a chronic progressive optic neuropathy. It affects those with vitamin B_1 deficiency such as alcoholics and the chronically malnourished, and may be associated with psychosis (Wernicke–Korsakoff syndrome). Pathological changes in the region of the fourth ventricle and aqueduct, particularly in the mamillary bodies, and in the pons, mid-brain and thalamus include perivascular haemorrhages accompanied by neuronal cell death and gliosis. The pathogenesis is unknown.

Toxic optic neuropathies

Optic neuropathies may result from exposure to specific toxins, including drugs used in medication. The onset of symptoms may be acute, as in methanol toxicity, but more usually visual loss is only slowly progressive. Numerous substances are potentially toxic (Table 7.4), but because of the severity and frequency of the association with optic neuropathy some, such as the antituberculous drugs ethambutol and isoniazid, are of particular

Table 7.4 Toxic optic neuropathy: common causative substances

Drugs	Barbiturates	Ethambutol
	BCNU (chemotherapy)	Isoniazid
	Cafergot	Quinine
	Chloramphenicol	Sulphonamides
	Chlorpromazine	Tolbutamide
	Digoxin	Vincristine
	Disulfiram	Ethambutol
Industrial chemicals	Analine dyes	Organophosphates
	Carbon tetrachloride	Trichloroethylene
	Ethylene glycol	Toluene
	Methanol	
Heavy metals	Lead	
	Organic arsenicals	

importance. A neurological syndrome that includes optic atrophy (subacute myelo-optic neuropathy) occurs with the halogenated hydroxyquinolines, including clioquinol. Toxic optic neuropathy is also caused by the abuse of solvents such as toluene, carbon tetrachloride and trichloroethylene.

Methanol toxicity

Ingestion of methanol produces symptoms and signs of poisoning within 24 hours. Severe metabolic acidosis, retinal and optic disc oedema with variable visual loss and progressive cerebral dysfunction precede coma and death. The alcohol diffuses throughout the body and is present in the CSF and aqueous. It is oxidized by alcohol dehydrogenase into formic acid and formaldehyde, which cause tissue damage. Necrosis of the retinal ganglion cells is followed by secondary degeneration of their axons and resultant optic atrophy.

TRAUMATIC, IRRADIATION AND COMPRESSIVE OPTIC NEUROPATHIES

Optic neuropathy may follow direct physical injury, ionizing radiation or compression by space-occupying lesions.

Traumatic optic neuropathy

The optic nerve may be injured directly by penetrating wounds of the orbit that result in transection or contusion, or indirectly as a consequence of blunt injury to the eye or orbitofacial and cranial structures. Within the optic canal and at its orbital and cranial openings the nerve is strongly tethered to bone and is not free to move, but as the orbital contents and brain are free, the nerve is at risk from shearing forces. The orbital portion of the optic nerve is not susceptible to indirect injury, as it is mobile and cushioned by orbital fat. The extent of injury varies, but includes contusion necrosis of retrobulbar axons, haemorrhage within both the substance and sheath of the nerve, and possibly avulsion from the eye.

Irradiation optic neuropathy

The optic nerves are subject to direct effects from ionizing radiation, usually as a consequence of radiotherapy administered for lesions of the paranasal sinuses or pituitary neoplasms. Irradiation neuropathy is rare, and may not occur for months or years following initial exposure. Changes in the orbital portion of the optic nerve affect both blood vessels and nerve substance. Vascular changes include endothelial cell proliferation, thickening of the walls with associated fibrinoid necrosis, and obliteration of the vascular lumen. Neural changes include necrosis and reactive gliosis.

Compressive optic neuropathy

Space-occupying lesions may exert a direct compressive effect on the optic nerve. Such lesions include meningiomas and gliomas, secondary neoplasms or masses arising in adjacent structures such as the orbit, the paranasal sinuses, the pituitary gland, parasellar structures and the middle cranial fossa. Aneurysms of the internal carotid artery and inflammatory lesions may also cause compressive optic neuropathy. In addition to a direct compressive effect, space-occupying lesions may interfere with the blood supply of the optic nerve while malignant neoplasms may infiltrate neural tissue. The histological features of compressive optic neuropathy include demyelination and reactive gliosis.

GLAUCOMA

The glaucomas are a group of disorders in which the intraocular pressure (IOP) damages the ocular tissues. The underlying feature in most instances is a characteristic optic neuropathy, but in the acute glaucomas and some congenital glaucomas other ocular tissues are initially more affected. In the majority of glaucomas the IOP is elevated above the accepted upper limit of normal, but in susceptible eyes glaucomatous changes may occur in the presence of a 'normal' IOP (low-tension glaucoma). Conversely, an elevated IOP can occur in an otherwise normal eye with no evidence of tissue damage (ocular hypertension).

Intraocular pressure

The IOP is the result of a dynamic equilibrium between the secretion of aqueous by the ciliary body and its drainage via the trabecular (80 per cent) and uveoscleral (20 per cent) pathways. An elevated IOP results from obstruction of the outflow pathways, either by increased resistance within the drainage channels (open-angle glaucoma) or by closure of the drainage angle consequent upon forward displacement of the peripheral iris (angle-closure glaucoma).

Classification

The glaucomas are classified according to their aetiology (primary or secondary), the anatomy of the anterior chamber (open-angle or angle-closure), their natural history (acute or chronic) and their age of onset (congenital or infantile, juvenile or adult). Both primary and secondary forms may be classified into open-angle and angle-closure types. Infantile or congenital glaucoma is referred to as primary if it results from isolated developmental abnormalities of the drainage pathways, and secondary if these abnormalities are associated with other local or systemic conditions. Absolute glaucoma is the term applied to the condition where a prolonged rise of IOP results in tissue damage to such an extent that the eye is blind and often painful.

Glaucomatous tissue damage

The nature of glaucomatous tissue damage depends upon the type of glaucoma, the age of the individual and the chronicity of the disease. In addition to optic neuropathy, the tissues of all three coats of the eye and the lens can be damaged. In acute forms tissue damage is clinically apparent initially in the anterior segment, with corneal oedema, inflammation, iris ischaemia and cataract formation; optic neuropathy develops later. In the chronic adult forms progressive optic neuropathy is characteristic, but other signs are minimal apart from coexisting ocular disease in the secondary glaucomas. In the infant's eye an elevated IOP causes distension and thinning of the corneoscleral coat (buphthalmos) and associated intraocular tissue damage; optic disc cupping occurs early, but can regress with normalization of the IOP.

Glaucomatous optic neuropathy: the optic neuropathy that characterizes the glaucomas results from destruction of optic nerve axons and blood vessels at the level of the lamina cribrosa. This is usually associated with prolonged elevation of IOP, but may also occur in the presence of apparently normal aqueous dynamics. Acute gross elevation of the IOP causes venous congestion and optic disc swelling. Injury to nerve fibres leads to obstruction of axonal transport, with consequent swelling at the level of the lamina cribrosa. Retrograde degeneration of axons occurs early in the course of the disease, precedes detectable optic disc abnormalities and results in retinal ganglion cell death and atrophy of the inner retinal layers, including the nerve fibre layer (Fig. 7.4a). Atrophy of axons results in a decrease in the

volume occupied by the nerve fibres at the disc, and this is manifest as enlargement of the optic disc cup (glaucomatous cupping – Fig. 7.4b, 7.4c), nasal displacement of the retinal vasculature and visibility of the openings of the lamina cribrosa. Associated vascular damage results in flame-shaped haemorrhages at the disc margin.

Anatomical factors play a role in the distribution of the optic atrophy. Damage is more likely to occur at the upper and lower poles of the disc, where support of axons by the lamina cribrosa is less rigid. This accounts for the characteristic superior and inferior arcuate visual field defects. Small hypermetropic eyes, in which the lamina cribrosa is dense and strong, are less susceptible to damage than large myopic eyes, where structural support for the axons is apparently less. Optic disc damage is manifest as posterior bowing of the lamina cribrosa, atrophic nerve bundles and thickening of the pial septae. In some eyes, cyst-like spaces filled with hyaluronic acid-rich fluid immediately behind the lamina cribrosa (Schnabel's cavernous optic atrophy – Fig. 7.4d) are

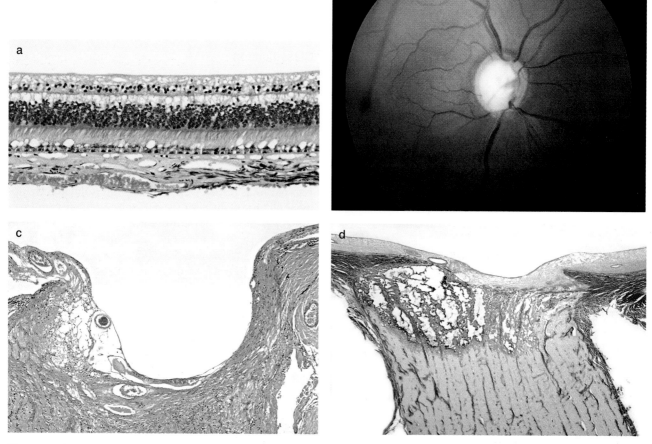

Figure 7.4 Glaucomatous tissue damage. (a) Atrophy of inner retinal layers; the ganglion cells are totally lost and the bipolar cells are reduced in number. (b) Cupping of optic disc: fundus appearance. (c) Cupping of optic disc: histology. (d) Schnabel's cavernous atrophy; hyaluronic acid-rich fluid within cyst-like spaces at the optic nerve head. Colloidal iron stain.

thought to result from infarction of the optic nerve with loss of axons and degeneration of glial cells. Although a distinct histological entity, Schnabel's cavernous optic atrophy does not appear to have a clinical correlate.

The pathogenesis of glaucomatous optic neuropathy is not clear, and vascular and mechanical theories have been proposed.

Vascular theory: this postulates that the changes result from ischaemia due to vascular insufficiency at the optic nerve head. Breakdown in vascular autoregulation is thought to be a contributory factor.

Mechanical theory: this postulates that the elevated IOP compresses the lamina cribrosa, bows it posteriorly and produces shearing forces within the lamina that stretch and buckle structures, including optic nerve axons and associated blood vessels.

Corneoscleral coat: a rapid and dramatic rise of IOP as occurs in acute angle-closure glaucoma leads to failure of the corneal endothelial pump mechanism, with resultant stromal and epithelial oedema. Reversible in the early stages, with prolonged elevation of the IOP permanent endothelial damage leads to intractable oedema. Inter- and intracellular oedema of the epithelium and superficial bullae develop (bullous keratopathy), and ulceration predisposes to infection. If the glaucoma is chronic, band keratopathy and degenerative pannus may develop. In infantile glaucoma, Descemet's membrane is stretched and splits and endothelial cells migrate to cover the breaks; these are seen as curvilinear lesions on the posterior corneal surface (Haab's striae).

Widespread corneal oedema develops later, and corneal opacification may become permanent. A sustained high pressure leads to bulging at points of relative weakness, such as at sites where blood vessels or nerve fibres penetrate the sclera, and, at sites of previous inflammation, corneal, limbal, ciliary, equatorial or posterior staphylomas may result. Posterior bowing of the lamina cribrosa is common, and may be an important factor in the development of glaucomatous optic nerve damage. In buphthalmos expansion is principally at the limbus, thus increasing the corneal diameter and deepening the anterior chamber.

Uvea: an acute rise of IOP that exceeds the critical closing pressure of the iris vasculature results in vasocongestion at the iris root, ischaemic necrosis and inflammation. A more prolonged rise of IOP leads to atrophy of the iris, ciliary body and choroid, the latter being the most resilient.

Lens: in acute glaucoma the capsule and epithelium show localized areas of damage, and necrotic debris accumulates focally in the superficial cortex (Glaukomflecken). In chronic glaucoma the lens often exhibits advanced cataractous changes.

Genetics of glaucoma

The glaucomas are a heterogeneous group of diseases, some of which are inherited or have a genetic component in their aetiology. Some forms of congenital glaucoma, juvenile open-angle glaucoma, some developmental glaucomas associated with aniridia and Rieger's syn-

Table 7.5 Genetics of glaucoma

Glaucoma	Inheritance	Chromosome	Gene	Gene product (if known)
Congenital glaucoma	AR	1p36	GLC3B	
Juvenile onset primary open-angle glaucoma	AD	1q23	GLC1A	TIGR (trabecular meshwork glucocorticoid response protein, myocilin)
Congenital glaucoma	AR	2p21	GLC3A	Cytochrome P4501B1
Primary open-angle glaucoma, adult onset	AD	2qcen-q13	GLC1B	
Primary open-angle glaucoma, adult onset	AD	3q21-q24	GLC1C	
Rieger's syndrome	AD	4q25	RIEG1	Solurshin
Iridodysgenesis	AD	6p25		
Pigment dispersion syndrome and pigmentary glaucoma	AD	7q35-q36		
Rieger's syndrome	AD	13q14	RIEG2	

AD, autosomal dominant; AR, autosomal recessive.

drome, and pigmentary glaucoma show Mendelian inheritance. Primary open-angle glaucoma exhibits multifactorial inheritance. At the time of writing, nine genetic loci associated with glaucoma have been identified (Table 7.5) and some glaucoma-associated genes have been cloned.

Primary open-angle glaucoma

Adult-onset primary open-angle glaucoma (POAG) accounts for 15 per cent of legal blindness in the UK and USA, and affects approximately 1 per cent of the population over 45 years of age. It is characterized by an IOP elevated above 21 mm Hg, an open filtration angle and chronically progressive glaucomatous optic disc cupping with associated visual field loss. Apart from glaucomatous optic neuropathy there are no other clinicopathological features, although in advanced stages the changes are essentially those of long-standing glaucoma due to any cause, namely atrophy of the retina and uvea and a cataractous lens. Despite being one of the commonest blinding conditions in the Western world, little is known of its underlying cause and there has been much speculation concerning its pathogenesis. A familial tendency is well known, with about 10 per cent of first-degree relatives developing the disease. Other indications of the importance of genetic factors in the development of POAG include the increased prevalence of the disease in Afro-Caribbeans, a high concordance between monozygotic twins with the condition, and the association of POAG with the Duffy blood group and the ability to taste phenothiocarbamide. POAG is also associated with the inherited trait of developing an elevated intraocular pressure in response to topical corticosteroids. It is likely that POAG is not a single disease but a common manifestation of several or many disorders, and whilst several single genetic loci have been reported (e.g. GLC1B mapped to 2qcen-q13 and GLC1C mapped to 3q21-q24), clinical and epidemiological evidence suggests multifactorial inheritance in most cases.

Elevated IOP is strongly associated with optic neuropathy in POAG although it is not clear, at least in some cases, if it is the cause of the neuropathy. The raised IOP results from an increased resistance to the outflow of aqueous in the trabecular meshwork. The cause of this increased resistance is unclear, but currently the generally accepted view is that it is due to either a structural alteration or an abnormal accumulation of material in the extracellular matrix of the endothelial part of the meshwork. An increase in the quantity of extracellular matrix collagens can follow the administration of corticosteroids, and this may be associated with corticosteroid-induced glaucoma. An alternative possibility is exaggeration of the normal age changes, which include thickening of the trabeculae due to excessive collagen deposition, fusion of trabeculae and loss of trabecular cells. Closure of Schlemm's canal has been proposed as another alternative mechanism.

Primary angle-closure glaucoma

Primary angle-closure glaucoma (PACG) is much less common than POAG, and affects approximately 0.1 per cent of the population over 40 years of age. It presents at an older age than POAG, and females are more commonly affected (F : M = 4 :1). It usually presents acutely with an intensely painful red eye and loss of vision, but latent, intermittent (subacute) and chronic stages can occur. In PACG, peripheral iridotrabecular contact compromises the outflow of aqueous. Anatomical and physiological factors are involved.

Anatomical: a narrow drainage angle associated with a relatively anterior convex iris–lens diaphragm predisposes to PACG. This configuration is found in hypermetropic eyes with short axial lengths and small corneal diameters. The ageing lens also plays an important role, with anterior displacement of the iris—lens diaphragm resulting from both axial (anteroposterior) growth and slackening of the zonule due to equatorial growth.

Physiological: physiological factors precipitate an acute attack. Resistance to aqueous flow through the pupil results from contact between the iris and anterior lens capsule (relative pupil block). As a consequence the hydrostatic pressure of aqueous in the posterior chamber is greater than in the anterior chamber, resulting in anterior bowing of the peripheral iris (iris bombé). Relative pupil block is increased by anatomical factors, and at a certain critical point the iris bombé is sufficient to occlude the drainage angle and produce a catastrophic rise of IOP. Acute anterior segment ischaemia results, and the consequent tissue swelling further compounds the situation. If left untreated for any length of time, adhesions develop between the iris root and the angle structures. Physiological mechanisms predisposing to an increase in relative pupil block involve both pupillary dilatation and constriction.

Dilatation of the pupil: iris–lens contact (and therefore relative pupil block) is maximal in mid-dilatation, and this, combined with the relative laxity and increased thickness of the peripheral iris, may precipitate angle-closure. Causes of dilatation include darkness, emotion and medication.

Constriction of the pupil: although miotics are used in the treatment of PACG, they may occasionally precipitate an attack in predisposed eyes. Relative pupil block may be increased by the added iris–lens contact resulting from miosis, and by the forward movement of the lens produced by ciliary muscle contraction and zonular relaxation.

Predisposed eyes may develop intermittent subacute episodes of self-limiting angle-closure before developing an acute attack. Chronic progressive elevation of the IOP may be a consequence of gradual occlusion of the drainage angle with associated development of peripheral iridocorneal adhesions. An acute attack of PACG results in the characteristic features of a rapid rise in IOP, namely corneal oedema, damage to the uvea and lens, and later to the optic nerve. In untreated end-stage PACG advanced atrophic changes are identical with those of end-stage glaucoma due to other causes.

Secondary glaucoma

The secondary glaucomas result from coexisting eye disease, the principal causes of which are intraocular inflammation, iris neovascularization (neovascular glaucoma), haemorrhage and neoplasia. A further group comprises ocular specific processes, and includes those related to lens disorders and those associated with the pseudoexfoliation, pigment dispersion and iridocorneal endothelial syndromes. Secondary glaucoma may also result from trauma (accidental or surgical) or may be iatrogenic (corticosteroid-induced glaucoma). Rarely, a raised episcleral venous pressure such as that due to an orbital vascular lesion or mediastinal obstruction is associated with glaucoma. Classification into open-angle and angle-closure types is useful in understanding the basic pathophysiology, but more than one mechanism may be involved, and the secondary glaucomas are classified according to the major cause rather than the putative mechanism.

Intraocular inflammation and glaucoma

Most inflammatory conditions involving the anterior segment can result in glaucoma (Fig. 7.5a). Although the outflow pathway may be compromised in the inflamed eye, an elevated IOP may not occur because of a coexisting reduction in aqueous secretion. The IOP may become raised during resolution of the inflammation, when aqueous secretion returns to normal. An additional factor is that glaucoma can result from corticosteroid medication rather than the inflammation itself. Secondary glaucoma in anterior segment inflammation may result from angle-closure with or without pupil block, trabecular obstruction with an open angle, or damage to the post-trabecular drainage pathways and episcleral venous system. Chronic uveitis is associated

with proliferation of new capillaries, which can result in permanent changes leading to glaucoma.

Angle-closure with pupil block occurs in anterior segment inflammation. An annular adhesion forms between the pupillary margin of the iris and underlying structures, i.e. the anterior lens capsule in phakic eyes, the intraocular lens implant in pseudophakia, or the posterior lens capsule or the anterior vitreous face in aphakia. Adhesion and pupil block lead to iris bombé (Fig. 7.5b), angle-closure and peripheral iridocorneal adhesions.

Angle-closure without pupil block occurs when inflammatory exudate between the peripheral iris and trabecular meshwork organizes, or when neovascularization develops on the anterior iris surface.

Trabecular obstruction with open angle may develop in one of three ways:

1. In active inflammation, inflammatory cells and exudate are present within the anterior chamber. Aqueous outflow may be compromised by the increased viscosity of protein-rich aqueous or blockage of the trabecular meshwork by inflamma-

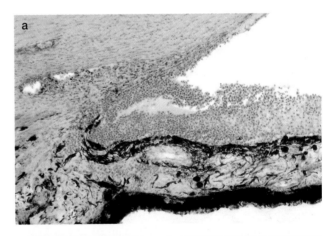

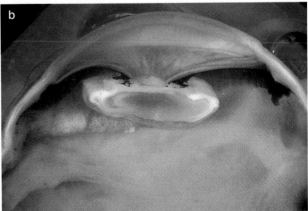

Figure 7.5 Inflammatory glaucoma. (a) Inflammatory cells in the anterior chamber and filtration angle leading to trabecular obstruction. (b) Iridolenticular adhesion and iris bombé.

tory cells and exudate. Resolution of the inflammation results in restoration of normal drainage in most instances, but occasionally structural damage leads to permanent impairment of outflow.

2. Acute or chronic trabecular inflammation (trabeculitis) is a possible mechanism for the raised IOP encountered in certain forms of uveitis (e.g. herpetic eye disease).

3. Inflammatory mediators (e.g. some prostaglandins) cause a raised IOP by their action on the trabecular meshwork or by increasing the production of aqueous. This mechanism occurs particularly in acute inflammation, and may be important in the development of glaucomatocyclitic crisis (Posner–Schlossman syndrome).

Damage to the post-trabecular drainage pathways and episcleral venous system can result from scleritis and orbital inflammatory lesions.

Cellular proliferation and glaucoma

The non-neoplastic proliferation of cells and tissues within the anterior segment can cause glaucoma by open- or closed-angle mechanisms. The cells may originate from vascular, corneal and conjunctival tissues.

Neovascular glaucoma results from the formation and proliferation of new vessels on the anterior surface of the iris (rubeosis iridis – see Fig. 1.9). The commonest causes are retinal ischaemia due to central retinal vein occlusion (CRVO) and diabetes mellitus. The neovascular glaucoma secondary to CRVO is also termed thrombotic glaucoma. Other rarer causes include uveitis and intraocular neoplasms, notably retinoblastoma.

New vessels are formed by the proliferation of endothelial cells from existing vessels in response to hypoxia and circulating angiogenic growth factors. Neovascularization originates from capillary tufts at the pupil margin, and later from capillaries and venules in the central and peripheral parts of the iris. It continues radially to the angle where new vessels join the circumferential ciliary artery and arborize over the trabecular meshwork, thereby obstructing aqueous drainage. Fibroblasts migrate together with the new vessels, leading to fibrovascular membrane formation that may extend across the trabecular meshwork, resulting in peripheral iridocorneal adhesions, and occasionally across the pupil to form a pupillary membrane. Corneal endothelial cells and a Descemet-like membrane may extend over the occluded angle and on to the iris.

Iridocorneal endothelial (ICE) syndrome is a rare sporadic unilateral disorder that most commonly affects white females in their third to fifth decade. Features include corneal and iris abnormalities. The underlying pathology of ICE is the proliferation of corneal endothelial cells on to the trabecular meshwork and iris surface, and the deposition of a Descemet-like basement membrane. The cause is unknown, but the distribution and extent of the proliferation account for the variation in features. Contraction of the membrane results in peripheral iridocorneal adhesion and characteristic iris changes. Glaucoma results from proliferation of the membrane over the trabecular meshwork and progressive iridocorneal adhesion. Three clinical syndromes represent the spectrum of disorder:

1. Essential iris atrophy: peripheral iridocorneal adhesion results in distortion of the pupil and ectropion uveae. Atrophy of the iris is eventually full thickness with hole formation. Corneal involvement is not a prominent feature.

2. Chandler's syndrome: corneal oedema often develops in the absence of a raised IOP. Iris changes are not prominent.

3. Iris naevus (Cogan–Rees) syndrome: the features are pigmented nodular naevus-like iris lesions, loss of normal iris surface detail, ectropion uveae and other structural iris defects. Peripheral iridocorneal adhesions, corneal oedema and glaucoma are characteristic. The nodular iris lesions are not true naevi but are thought to be islands of iris tissue encircled and constricted by the cellular membrane.

Epithelial and fibrous displacement are uncommon and serious complications of traumatic or surgical ocular penetration or perforation. Both present either as a membrane on the posterior corneal surface or as a cystic mass in the anterior segment. The corneal stroma may become oedematous and vascularized before an intractable glaucoma develops. Corneal and/or conjunctival epithelial cells or connective tissue may either migrate into the eye through a poorly constructed wound (epithelial or fibrous downgrowth) or cells become implanted into the anterior chamber at the time of injury or surgery (implantation). Glaucoma results from occlusion of the trabecular meshwork by desquamated epithelial cells, by growth of a membrane of epithelial cells (see Fig. 1.2) and/or connective tissue over the drainage angle, or from pupil block produced by growth of a similar membrane over the pupil.

Acellular material and glaucoma

Acellular particulate material causes physical obstruction of the intertrabecular spaces. Swollen trabecular endothelial cells containing phagocytosed debris further narrow the intertrabecular spaces. Particulate material may arise from the lens, intraocular haemorrhage or injected silicone oil. Rarely, following trauma to the peripheral retina, photoreceptor debris blocks the trabecular outflow system (Schwartz–Matsuo syndrome). The pseudoexfoliation and pigment dispersion syndromes are characterized by the deposition throughout the anterior chamber of proteinaceous material and of melanin particles respectively. A significant proportion of those affected develop secondary glaucoma.

Pseudoexfoliation syndrome (PXS) is a systemic disorder in which proteinaceous material is deposited throughout the anterior segment (see Fig. 5.7) and elsewhere. The trabecular meshwork is involved, and open-angle glaucoma occurs in up to 60 per cent of affected eyes.

Pigment dispersion syndrome (PDS) is a disorder of unknown aetiology, like PXS, in which 10 per cent of affected individuals have open-angle glaucoma (pigmentary glaucoma). The characteristic clinical features include a vertical accumulation of pigment on the corneal endothelium (Krukenberg's spindle), midperipheral iris transillumination, loss of iris contour, deposition of pigment on the anterior iris surface that may lead to heterochromia, and pigment deposition on the zonule, lens surface and extreme retinal periphery. PDS affects predominantly white myopic males in their third and fourth decades. Autosomal dominant inheritance has been demonstrated at least in some cases, and one locus has been identified on 7q35-q36 near to the gene (PHTC) responsible for phenothiocarbamide tasting. It is thought that PDS results from the mechanical abrasion of an abnormal iris pigment epithelium by the constant motion of the iris over the peripheral lens capsule and anteriorly placed zonular fibres. The released pigment is distributed throughout the anterior segment, where it either settles or is phagocytosed by corneal endothelial cells or iris stromal macrophages. Pigment trapped in the trabecular meshwork is phagocytosed by trabecular endothelial cells, which are damaged as a result, and it is thought that structural changes ensue, with narrowing or occlusion of the intertrabecular spaces resulting in increased resistance to aqueous outflow. Focal defects of the iris pigment epithelium are associated with many pigment-laden macrophages in the adjacent iris stroma. The dilator pupillae muscle may be hypertrophic, dysplastic, atrophic or absent.

Intraocular haemorrhage and glaucoma

Glaucoma secondary to intraocular haemorrhage (Fig. 7.6) may result from blockage of the trabecular meshwork by blood or its derivatives. This occurs in hyphaema, haemolytic glaucoma and ghost cell glaucoma.

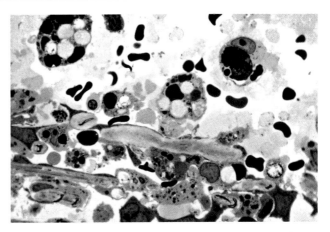

Figure 7.6 Haemorrhagic glaucoma. Red cell debris, macrophages and ghost cells (pale cells in background) entering the outflow system. Toluidine blue stain.

Hyphaema: blood in the anterior chamber is most commonly caused by blunt trauma, but in conditions such as rubeosis iridis or bleeding disorders, haemorrhage may result from minimal trauma or occur spontaneously. Neoplasms may also cause anterior chamber haemorrhage, while in children hyphaemas may be due to the presence of a juvenile xanthogranuloma of the iris. In small hyphaemas the blood does not clot but erythrocytes may obstruct the trabecular meshwork, while in larger hyphaemas aqueous outflow is obstructed by clot formation that causes pupil block or transient angle-closure. A particularly severe form of secondary glaucoma may occur following hyphaema in those with sickle cell trait or disease, where the environment of the anterior chamber causes the erythrocytes to sickle and become rigid. The removal of erythrocytes via the trabecular meshwork depends on their deformability, so that the rigid sickled cells cause a more persistent and profound occlusion than normal erythrocytes.

Haemolytic glaucoma: haemolysed erythrocytes and macrophages may block the filtration angle. The associated presence of iron salts can lead to degeneration and sclerosis of the trabecular fibres, thereby permanently compromising the aqueous drainage (the same mechanism can occur in siderosis and haemosiderosis). Organization of haemorrhagic exudate may result in peripheral iridocorneal adhesions.

Ghost cell glaucoma: ghost cells (erythroclasts) are erythrocytes that have lost their haemoglobin, their biconcave shape and their deformability, and usually form 2 or more weeks after a vitreous haemorrhage. If they leak into the anterior chamber because of a communication between the posterior and anterior segments, as in aphakia, they may obstruct the trabecular meshwork.

The lens and glaucoma

Glaucoma can result from open-angle or angle-closure mechanisms caused by displacement of the lens, swelling of the lens (phacomorphic glaucoma), dissolution of the lens (phacolytic glaucoma) or lens-associated inflammation (lens-induced endophthalmitis).

Displacement of the lens results from many causes, and a number of possible mechanisms account for the glaucoma. Pupil block may occur if the lens is displaced into the anterior chamber or becomes incarcerated in the pupil (e.g. microspherophakia and partial zonular disruption of Weill–Marchesani syndrome). With posterior displacement of the lens, herniation of vitreous into the anterior chamber may cause pupil block. A displaced intumescent cataractous lens may lead to phacolytic glaucoma if the capsule is attenuated or ruptured. Congenital displacement of the lens (ectopia lentis) may be associated with congenital glaucoma due to a developmental angle anomaly.

Phacomorphic glaucoma is an angle-closure glaucoma secondary to intumescence of a cataractous lens. It is distinct from acute PACG, where normal lens growth accounts for the anterior displacement of the iris–lens diaphragm and consequent pupil block in a predisposed eye.

Phacolytic glaucoma presents most commonly with acute onset of pain and congestion in an eye in which vision has been lost over a period of time due to cataract. It may also occur after traumatic rupture of the lens capsule. The IOP is often elevated sufficiently to cause corneal oedema. When anterior chamber detail is visible, a heavy flare, a cellular response and white flocculent material are sometimes seen in association with a mature or hypermature cataract. The lens capsule is attenuated and occasionally ruptured, and the lens cortex is liquefied. Free lens material may be seen in the anterior chamber, and numerous macrophages, engorged with phagocytosed lens material, infiltrate the trabecular meshwork (Fig. 7.7). No other inflammatory cells are present, and the clinical appearance of inflammation results from the raised IOP produced by lens material and lens-filled macrophages compromising the outflow of aqueous.

Lens-associated intraocular inflammation can cause glaucoma by the mechanisms described under inflammation and glaucoma, namely obstruction of outflow channels by inflammatory debris, pupil block and the formation of peripheral iridocorneal adhesions.

Intraocular neoplasia and glaucoma

Both benign and malignant intraocular neoplasms may produce secondary glaucoma due usually to angle-

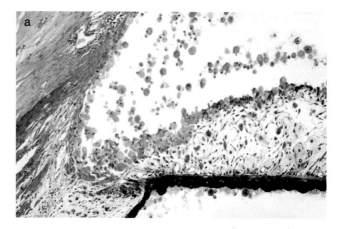

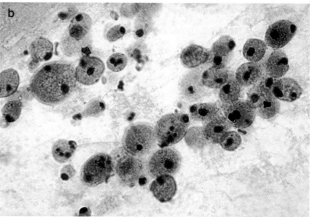

Figure 7.7 Phacolytic glaucoma. (a) Lens-containing macrophages in the anterior chamber and filtration angle. (b) Lens-containing macrophages. High magnification.

closure or iris neovascularization. Intraocular neoplasms, most commonly melanomas, particularly of the iris or ciliary body, may cause anterior displacement of the iris–lens diaphragm and may also shed cells that become entrapped in the aqueous outflow pathway (Fig. 7.8). Necrosis of melanomas may cause melanomalytic glaucoma, in which trabecular obstruction is by free melanin granules or macrophages containing necrotic debris. Ocular inflammation associated with neoplasms may also lead to angle-closure. Iris neovascularization and neovascular glaucoma occur particularly with retinoblastoma.

Accidental trauma and glaucoma

Mechanical trauma and chemical injuries are the commonest causes of accidental traumatic glaucoma.

Mechanical trauma: may be non-perforating or perforating. Elevated IOP following non-perforating injury is most commonly due to hyphaema. Other traumatic causes of secondary glaucoma include traumatic uveitis

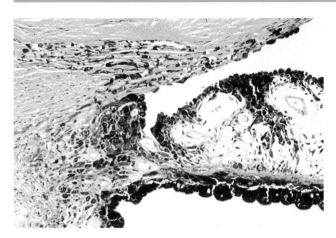

Figure 7.8 Melanoma-induced glaucoma. Melanoma cells entrapped in the aqueous outflow pathway.

or its treatment with corticosteroids, lens subluxation or dislocation, and vitreous haemorrhage. A rarer secondary glaucoma of late onset is associated with traumatic angle recession. Although less than 20 per cent of cases of angle recession develop glaucoma, it may not occur until many years after the injury. The cause of the glaucoma is obscure but, particularly in children, may be associated with endothelial cell proliferation from the posterior corneal surface. If the eye is perforated or penetrated, other causes of secondary glaucoma arise. Hypotonic collapse of the anterior chamber may result in iridocorneal adhesion and possible angle-closure, while displacement and damage to the lens can also lead to an elevated IOP. Occasionally, epithelium from the conjunctiva or cornea extends through a healing wound or is implanted into the eye and intractable glaucoma may ensue. The intraocular retention of an iron-containing foreign body causes siderosis and possibly secondary glaucoma.

Chemical injuries: alkali burns damage the post-trabecular aqueous outflow pathway, and the ensuing secondary glaucoma may be compounded by any intraocular damage due to absorption of the chemical and associated uveitis.

Surgical trauma, medication and glaucoma

The same mechanisms that cause secondary glaucoma following accidental trauma can occur following surgery. In addition, excessive cautery and limbal incisions can damage the aqueous drainage channels, and there are also several specific types of glaucoma with established pathophysiology.

Malignant glaucoma is a serious but rare complication that can follow surgery for angle-closure glaucoma. A persistent flat anterior chamber is associated with an ele-

vated IOP that does not respond to conventional treatment. The most accepted hypothesis concerning its pathogenesis is that posterior misdirection of aqueous into the vitreous leads to anterior chamber collapse, pupil block and obstruction of aqueous outflow.

Cyclocongestive angle-closure glaucoma presents in a similar way to malignant glaucoma. Its pathogenesis, however, is quite different. Several surgical procedures (including scleral buckling for retinal detachment and panretinal photocoagulation) can result in vasocongestion of the choroid, which produces anterior rotation of the ciliary body, resulting in closure of the drainage angle. Cyclocongestive angle-closure glaucoma may also occur in expulsive haemorrhage.

Injected intraocular substances that cause secondary glaucoma include viscoelastics, alpha chymotrypsin, silicone oil and intraocular gases.

Viscoelastic substances such as hyaluronic acid, hydroxypropyl methylcellulose and chondroitin sulphate have high viscosities which probably account for the transient rise in IOP associated with their use.

Alpha chymotrypsin used in intracapsular cataract surgery can lead to a transient rise in IOP due to trabecular block by zonular fragments.

Silicone oil used in the treatment of retinal detachments can lead to glaucoma (Fig. 7.9). Angle-closure may occur as a result of pupil block from overfilling an aphakic eye, while at a later stage the trabecular meshwork may be obstructed by microscopic droplets of emulsified oil, by silicone- or pigment-laden macrophages, or by fibrosis induced by the oil.

Intraocular gases including sulphur hexafluoride (SF_6) and perfluoropropane (C_3F_8) or mixtures of these gases with air are frequently injected into the eye during vitreoretinal surgery. Elevation of the IOP may result both from open-angle or angle-closure mechanisms. An elevated IOP may develop initially through over-filling or, if SF_6 or C_3F_8 are used, at a later stage when the bubble expands. In air travel, expansion of the bubble induced by reduction in atmospheric pressure can cause an acute rise in IOP with the development of acute glaucoma.

Corticosteroid-induced glaucoma may result from the use of topical corticosteroids. When administered for several weeks, they induce an elevation of IOP in 40 per cent of the general population. This proportion is considerably higher in those with POAG. The pathogenesis is obscure, but the raised IOP probably results from obstruction of the trabecular outflow pathway. Fibrillar material (Fig. 7.10) is seen on electron microscopic examination, the glycosaminoglycan concentration in the tra-

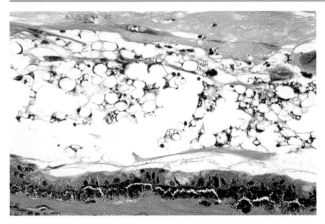

Figure 7.9 Silicone oil-induced glaucoma. Silicone oil globules (empty spaces) in the region of the pars plana.

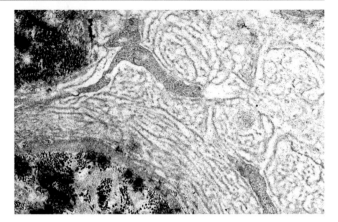

Figure 7.10 Corticosteroid-induced glaucoma. Fibrillar material in the trabecular meshwork. TEM.

becular meshwork is increased and the trabecular endothelial cells may show an increase in the number of mitochondria and rough endoplasmic reticulum content.

Congenital glaucoma

The term congenital glaucoma describes a diverse group of rare disorders that present in the neonate or infant. Different classifications have led to confusion, but that indicated in Table 7.6 is generally accepted. Congenital glaucoma is primary if it is caused by an intrinsic disorder of aqueous outflow, or secondary if it results from a disease process in other parts of the eye or body. The characteristic feature of the primary congenital glaucomas and of the glaucomas associated with other congenital abnormalities is abnormal development of the drainage angle (goniodysgenesis). Very little is known of the pathology of the congenital glaucomas, and only the primary form will be detailed here.

Primary infantile (congenital) glaucoma

This is the commonest form of congenital glaucoma, and affects approximately 1 : 10 000 live births. The underlying disorder is present at birth, but the presenting fea-

tures depend on the severity and the age of onset of the elevated IOP. In the majority of cases an enlarged globe is found during the first year of life; other features include lacrimation, photophobia, corneal oedema with breaks in Descemet's membrane, and optic disc cupping that may be reversible with prompt treatment. Several different abnormalities can account for the development of primary infantile glaucoma, the mechanisms and the severity of the condition depending on the time at which disturbance to angle development occurred in utero. Most commonly there is aberrant insertion of the iris into the trabeculum at or anterior to the scleral spur, and this may be associated with abnormal development of the peripheral iris stroma. A membrane (Barkan's membrane) may appear to overlie the trabecular meshwork on clinical examination, although there is no histological evidence for this. The histological features of

Table 7.6 Congenital glaucoma

Primary	Isolated	Infantile (congenital) Juvenile Late juvenile
	Associated with other congenital abnormalities of eye or body	Anterior chamber dysgenesis, aniridia, congenital ectropion uveae, phakomatoses
Secondary		Inflammatory, neoplastic, haemorrhagic, traumatic, retinopathy of prematurity

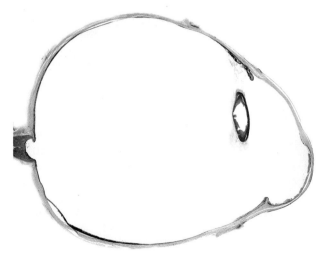

Figure 7.11 Buphthalmos. Section of an enlarged eye with a thinned corneoscleral coat, an anterior staphyloma and a cupped optic disc.

primary congenital glaucoma are common to all types of congenital glaucoma. Elevation of the IOP in children under 3 years of age causes buphthalmos (Fig. 7.11); the limbal region is particularly affected, and there may be staphyloma formation. Haab's striae and corneal oedema develop, and there may eventually be permanent opacification. Late findings in congenital glaucoma include fibrosis of the trabecular meshwork and iris root, occlusion or loss of Schlemm's canal, atrophy of the ciliary body and choroid, and glaucomatous optic neuropathy.

THE PERIPHERAL NERVOUS SYSTEM

The peripheral nervous system (PNS) consists of the peripheral nerves (spinal nerves and cranial nerves III to XII) and their ganglia. Its principal function is to act as a line of communication, bringing information from sensory receptors to the CNS and conveying motor commands from the CNS to striated muscle and effector organs controlled by the autonomic nervous system.

AXONS AND THEIR RESPONSE TO INJURY

The axons of peripheral nerves lie within a compartment known as the endoneurium, which is enclosed by a perineural sheath consisting of a number of sheets of flattened cells continuous with the leptomeninges of the CNS. External to this, connective tissue and lymphatics comprise the epineurium. Peripheral nerves receive their blood supply from local small arteries and the presence of many collateral channels prevents ischaemia unless a major vessel is occluded or many small vessels are affected by disease. The axons are ensheathed by Schwann cells, the compact cell membranes of which form the myelin of myelinated fibres. The nodes of Ranvier are where adjacent Schwann cells meet and the otherwise continuous myelin sheath is interrupted. The length between two nodes is an internode. The nodes are the only points where the axons are directly exposed to the endoneurium. Non-myelinated fibres are much smaller in diameter than myelinated fibres, and are surrounded only by Schwann cell cytoplasm. Peripheral nerves exhibit a limited number of reactions to injury, with axonal debris and myelin being removed by macrophages.

Axonal degeneration (Wallerian degeneration) follows degeneration of the neuronal cell body, and results in degeneration of the axon throughout its length (neuro-

nopathy). As the neuronal cell body is responsible for the maintenance of the axon, when neuronal metabolism is disturbed (as in metabolic diseases) degeneration may be restricted to the distal ends of longer peripheral axons (distal axonopathy). Damage to the nerve itself results in axonal degeneration distal to the site of injury.

Retrograde axonal changes occur up to 4 mm from the site of injury, with degeneration back to at least one node of Ranvier.

Segmental demyelination is due to Schwann cell dysfunction, which causes loss of myelin from one or more internodes with accompanying degeneration of the underlying axon.

Regeneration and remyelination

The PNS differs from the CNS in that the axons have the capability to regenerate and remyelination frequently occurs. In neuronopathy there is little potential for recovery, but in distal axonopathy axonal regeneration is possible if the cause is removed and no significant retrograde degeneration is present. Interruption of axons elsewhere results in sprouting from nearby nodes of Ranvier on the proximal side of the damage. If the basement membrane of the Schwann cells is not damaged, newly sprouted axons find their way into appropriate channels that will guide them back to their end organs. Complete transection of a nerve may result in recovering axons wandering aimlessly into adjacent connective tissue unless careful suturing of the damaged nerve is carried out (traumatic or amputation neuroma). When nerve fibres entering muscles are lost, the newly sprouted axons from the terminal and subterminal regions directly reinnervate motor end plates. Schwann cell proliferation following myelin loss results in remyelination.

PERIPHERAL NEUROPATHIES

Peripheral neuropathies are a diverse group of conditions affecting all ages, and may be inherited or acquired. They may occur in isolation or as a manifestation of a systemic disorder. The major clinical features reflect disturbance of sensory, motor or autonomic function, and may be acute, subacute or chronic. A disorder may involve one nerve (mononeuropathy) or several nerves (mononeuropathy multiplex), or there may be diffuse and symmetrical involvement (polyneuropathy). The peripheral neuropathies of ophthalmic importance are mononeuropathies of the cranial nerves, particularly III, IV and VI; they are usually of vascular aetiology, diabetes mellitus being the major cause.

STRIATED MUSCLE, THE MOTOR UNIT, THE EXTRAOCULAR MUSCLES AND THEIR DISORDERS

STRIATED MUSCLE

The functional unit of striated muscle is the muscle fibre, which is surrounded by a delicate fibrous sheath (endomysium) in which the feeding capillaries lie. Up to several hundred muscle fibres are grouped into varying-sized fascicles enclosed by a thin fibrous capsule (perimysium). The muscle comprises groups of fascicles, and is surrounded by fibrofatty tissue (epimysium) that contains arteries, veins and lymphatics. Muscle fibres are surrounded by a smooth sarcolemma that comprises the plasma membrane and a basement membrane. The sarcolemma is thrown into complicated folds in the region of motor end plates. Satellite cells are present between the plasma membrane and basement membrane, and are important in the response to cell injury. The sarcoplasm is the muscular cytoplasm that, apart from the usual organelles, contains an intricate interconnecting network of tubules known as the sarcoplasmic reticulum. Muscle fibre nuclei are usually situated at the periphery in a subsarcolemmal position, while the slightly larger endomysial nuclei are less conspicuous and lie transversely across longitudinally sectioned fibres. The bulk of the muscle fibre is composed of myofibrils that are approximately 1 μm in diameter and composed of even smaller contractile units, the myofilaments. Myofilaments are composed predominantly of two proteins, actin and myosin, with at least six other proteins of structural and functional importance (tropomyosin, troponin, α- and β-actinin, M protein, C protein). The arrangement of myofibrils gives the muscle the characteristic striated appearance on light microscopy; on electron microscopy this appears as a complex arrangement of overlapping myofilaments that form repeating units or sarcomeres.

THE MOTOR UNIT

The motor unit consists of a motor neuron, its axon and the muscle fibres that it innervates. Motor end plates are specialized portions of the muscle fibres that are the postsynaptic terminals of the motor neuron. From the smallest nerve bundles, single subterminal myelinated axons fan out to the motor end-plate zone and each subterminal fibre forms one end plate. The number of subterminal nerve and muscle fibres comprising the motor unit varies with the size and function of the muscle.

THE EXTRAOCULAR MUSCLES

The specialized function of the extraocular muscles is reflected in their structure. They have a rich vascular and sensory nerve supply and small motor units. An unusually large amount of perimysium is present, but the endomysium is very thin by comparison with other muscles. Peripherally, the muscle fibres are rounded or oval in shape with the larger fibres and their nuclei being more centrally situated; in addition, a mild mononuclear cell infiltrate is seen. In skeletal muscle elsewhere these changes are usually associated with myopathies.

MUSCLE DISORDERS

The three main groups of muscle disorders are neurogenic disorders, disorders of neuromuscular transmission and myopathies.

Neurogenic disorders

Neurogenic muscle disorders result from damage to the muscle innervation as a consequence of lesions affecting the motor neurons in the brainstem, spinal cord, motor nerve roots or peripheral nerves. The function of the motor unit is lost. The affected subterminal nerve fibres fragment and neighbouring healthy fibres sprout and reinnervate the recently denervated end plates. This is known as collateral reinnervation, and it persists indefinitely or until the nerve supply is ultimately lost due to neuronal or axonal degeneration. Three or four weeks after the muscle fibres are permanently denervated they atrophy, eventually to neonatal size. Striations persist and most nuclei retain their normal peripheral position, but eventually atrophy is complete (neurogenic atrophy) and the few intact fibres that remain are scattered within large areas of fibrous tissue and fat.

Disorders of neuromuscular transmission

Neuromuscular transmission is disrupted by the inhibition or the reduced release of neurotransmitter from the presynaptic nerve terminals, as in the Lambert–Eaton myasthenic syndrome and botulism, or by insensitivity of the postsynaptic motor end plate, as in myasthenia gravis.

Lambert–Eaton myasthenic syndrome

The Lambert–Eaton myasthenic syndrome (LEMS) is an autoimmune disorder of the presynaptic nerve terminal.

It occurs in late life, more often in males than females. The presenting symptom is usually a gradual progressive difficulty with walking because of leg muscle weakness. Autonomic symptoms such as dry mouth, constipation and sexual dysfunction in males are accompanied by ptosis and diplopia, but the extraocular and intraocular muscles are not significantly affected. Augmentation of strength during the first few seconds of a maximal muscular effort is characteristic. The amount of acetylcholine released by the nerve action potential at the neuromuscular junction and autonomic synapse is reduced due to a decrease in the number of voltage-gated calcium channels at the nerve terminals. IgG anticalcium channel antibodies bind to and disturb the normal function of the channels, but the mechanism of sensitization is unknown.

About two-thirds of those affected with LEMS have associated small-cell lung cancer (SCLC), a neoplasm of presumed neuroectodermal origin that shares antigenic determinants with the nervous system. It is thought that membrane voltage-gated calcium channel antigens expressed by SCLC cells provoke synthesis of anti-calcium-channel antibodies. The clinical features of LEMS may precede radiological evidence of the neoplasm by up to 2 years or more.

Botulism

Botulism is an acute symmetrical descending paralysis affecting predominantly cranial and autonomic nerves and, to a lesser extent, peripheral nerves. It is produced by the neurotoxins of *Clostridium botulinum*, a Gram-positive anaerobic bacillus widely distributed in soil. Intoxication usually results from the ingestion of contaminated canned, smoked or fermented foods, following which blurred vision and diplopia herald the onset of a persistent flaccid paralysis. Symptoms and signs reflect involvement of the autonomic and motor nervous systems. The mouth is dry and paralysis of accommodation is associated with fixed dilated pupils, ptosis and lateral rectus weakness, and dysfunction of other motor cranial nerves. Progressive lower motor neuron weakness of the limbs is accompanied by rapid onset of respiratory paralysis. Evidence of widespread autonomic dysfunction includes hypotension without compensatory tachycardia, intestinal ileus and urinary retention. Most cases are fatal if untreated, and recovery takes weeks or months.

Botulinum toxin

Clostridium botulinum produces a heat-labile water-soluble neurotoxin that exists as one of seven serotypes (A–G). The toxin is one of the most lethal substances known; for botulinum toxin type A, the LD50 for humans is 40 units/kg which, depending on the preparation, is 1–15 mg/kg of toxin. Botulinum toxin is absorbed directly across mucous membranes. It enters the blood stream from the proximal small intestine and circulates to reach cholinergic nerve endings at neuromuscular junctions, autonomic ganglia and parasympathetic nerve terminals. The toxin binds irreversibly to gangliosides on the presynaptic nerve terminal, where it acts to prevent release of acetylcholine. The resulting flaccid paralysis and autonomic dysfunction is long-lasting, and recovery only occurs when nerve terminals sprout from the axon to form new end plates or synapses. Once bound to the nerve terminal, the toxin cannot be displaced by antitoxin or other medication. Botulinum toxin type A is easily crystallized to a stable form, and a commercially available preparation is used for the induction of temporary muscle paralysis such as that required in the diagnosis and treatment of strabismus, corneal disease (induction of a temporary ptosis), blepharospasm and other dyskinesias. Once injected into the body of the appropriate muscle the toxin rapidly and strongly binds to the presynaptic nerve terminal of cholinergic axons, where it inhibits the release of acetylcholine. The low dose injected and the strength of tissue binding minimizes systemic absorption. The clinical effect peaks at approximately 5–7 days, after which time the muscle exhibits denervation and atrophy. Muscle function slowly returns after 3–4 months, when the axon terminals sprout and form new synaptic contacts on adjacent muscle fibres.

Myasthenia gravis

Myasthenia gravis is an autoimmune disorder of the postsynaptic motor end plate. The condition typically occurs in the 20–40 years age group, and is more common in females than males (2:1). Varying degrees of weakness of skeletal muscle that worsen with exercise, i.e. exhibit fatigability, are early symptoms. Diplopia and ptosis are present in 90 per cent of those affected and are the presenting features in 60 per cent. Clinical features may be confined to the extraocular muscles (ocular myasthenia) although it is more usual for the disease to involve other muscle groups, such as those of the limbs and trunk and those associated with swallowing. The primary abnormality is loss of acetylcholine receptors (AChRs) at the motor end plate, which results in inhibition of neuromuscular transmission. The loss of AChRs is an autoimmune phenomenon caused by the presence of heterogeneous anti-AChR IgG antibodies. These antibodies may be detected in the serum of approximately 85 per cent of those affected, and their demonstration is diagnostic for the disorder. The antibodies cause AChR loss by complement-mediated lysis or direct agonist block.

Complement-mediated lysis is the most important mechanism. The antigen–antibody complex binds complement and stimulates endocytosis and destruction of the receptor protein at a rate that exceeds its synthesis. Structural changes, identifiable by electron microscopy, include evidence of a destructive process, with marked simplification of the postsynaptic folds and widening of the synaptic cleft.

Direct agonist block is when antibodies bind to receptors and prevent the action of acetylcholine in a way similar to non-depolarizing muscle relaxants such as curare derivatives.

Thymus involvement

The thymus is often abnormal in myasthenia gravis and plays an important role in its pathogenesis. Up to 75 per cent of those affected with early onset disease have thymic hyperplasia in which many lymphoid follicles with germinal centres are present in the medulla. AChRs are present on the surface of some thymic cells, and it is likely that thymic T lymphocytes activate B lymphocytes to produce AChR antibodies. Ten per cent of those with myasthenia gravis have a thymoma, a neoplasm arising in the anterior mediastinum in which proliferating epithelial cells are intermingled with immature lymphocytes. Thymomas rarely metastasize, although they may be locally invasive and seed in the pleural cavity.

Myopathies

The term myopathy defines any disorder in which the clinical features are attributable to pathological changes, including biochemical and electrophysiological abnormalities, that involve the muscle fibres or the muscular interstitial tissue. Many are genetically determined or are disorders of inflammatory, immune or metabolic origin. Most are rare, but some have important ophthalmic manifestations either due to the myopathy or because of associated features such as cataract in myotonic dystrophy or pigmentary retinopathy in the mitochondrial myopathies.

Muscular dystrophies

Involvement of the extraocular muscles is uncommon in most types of muscular dystrophy. A few dystrophies, however, involve specifically the oculomotor system, and those affected develop ptosis and progressive limitation of ocular movements. Such conditions may be inherited, and mitochondrial myopathy is responsible for many cases of external ophthalmoplegia.

Ocular myopathies

Ocular myopathies are a rare group of disorders. The main types are ocular myopathy with progressive external ophthalmoplegia, oculopharyngeal muscular dystrophy, and mitochondrial ocular myopathy.

Ocular myopathy with progressive external ophthalmoplegia usually presents after the age of 20 years with ptosis and weakness of the extraocular muscles. Most cases are sporadic, but occasionally they are autosomal dominant. Muscle study at autopsy shows the atrophic changes of end-stage myopathic disease, which are similar to those of neurogenic atrophy.

Oculopharyngeal muscular dystrophy also presents with ptosis and weakness of the extraocular muscles, but usually after the age of 50 years. The dystrophy spreads in a caudal direction to involve the pharyngeal muscles and the proximal muscles of the upper and lower limbs. A biopsy of the deltoid, even if it is clinically unaffected, is likely to show mild myopathic features as evidenced by necrosis of some muscle fibres, others of which have a moth-eaten appearance due to partial or complete loss of muscle fibre substance.

Mitochondrial ocular myopathy is exemplified by chronic progressive external ophthalmoplegia and heart block. If associated with pigmentary retinopathy, the disorder is termed Kearns–Sayre syndrome. Other systemic manifestations include short stature, neurosensory deafness, mental handicap, myopathy and delayed puberty. A progressive ptosis with late development of diplopia is the most common presenting feature, and the onset usually occurs before the age of 20 years. The pigmentary retinopathy has a salt and pepper appearance and involves the peripapillary region. Visual symptoms result primarily from the ophthalmoplegia and the retinopathy. Histological examination of extraocular muscles reveals ragged-red fibres typical of other myopathies, an appearance due to the intramuscular accumulation of abnormal mitochondria (Fig. 7.12). The RPE cells also contain abnormal mitochondria, resulting in their widespread degeneration, loss of photoreceptors and pigmentary retinopathy. The condition is due to large deletions (13–42 per cent) of the mitochondrial genome, thereby disrupting oxidative phosphorylation. Metabolically active tissues such as those of the eye, CNS and musculoskeletal system have little tolerance to abnormalities of respiratory processes and are those predominantly affected.

Myotonic disorders

Myotonia is the continued active contraction of a muscle after the cessation of voluntary effort or stimulation. The

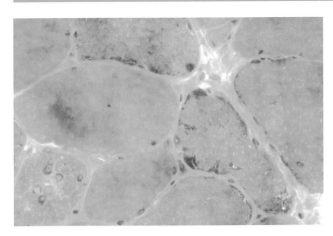

Figure 7.12 Mitochondrial myopathy. Ragged red fibres exhibiting peripheral red staining due to the accumulation of abnormal mitochondria. Modified Gomori stain.

myotonias are inherited mainly as autosomal dominant conditions, and comprise congenital myotonia, myotonic dystrophy and paramyotonia; myotonic dystrophy is of ophthalmic importance.

Myotonic dystrophy

Myotonic dystrophy is a systemic disorder usually presenting in adults between 20 and 30 years of age with weakness and wasting of the facial and limb girdle muscles. Associated features include abnormalities of the endocrine and immune systems, cataracts, ptosis, frontal baldness in the male, gonadal atrophy, cardiomyopathy, impaired pulmonary ventilation and dementia. It has autosomal dominant inheritance, with the responsible gene located on chromosome 19 (19q13.1). A large number of fibres with internally displaced nuclei are accompanied by other cytoskeletal abnormalities, e.g. sarcoplasmic masses in which fibrillar material collects near the periphery of the fibre and separates the sarcolemma from the myofibrils.

Inflammatory myopathies

Most inflammatory myopathies are probably autoimmune and are often associated with other autoimmune diseases (e.g. systemic lupus erythematosus, polyarteritis nodosa). They include polymyositis, dermatomyositis, inclusion-body myositis and ocular myositis. Although no target antigen has yet been identified, the damage to the muscle is mediated by CD8 + ($T_{C/S}$) cells or results from immune microangiopathy. Myositis attributable to known infective causes such as viruses (e.g. coxsackie B, influenza), bacteria (e.g. staphylococci, streptococci, clostridia) and other organisms (e.g. *Toxoplasma gondii*, *Trichinella spiralis*, *Taenia solium*) are in the minority.

Ocular myositis (orbital myositis)

Inflammation of the extraocular muscles may occur in association with, or overlap with, idiopathic orbital inflammatory disease. It can also develop in isolation with involvement of one or more of the extraocular muscles. Acute onset of usually bilateral painful and limited ocular movements is characteristic. Enlargement of the affected muscles is seen on CT scans. Histology shows lymphocytes within the endomysium and around blood vessels (Fig. 7.13), muscle fibre necrosis, phagocytosis by macrophages and evidence of muscle fibre regeneration.

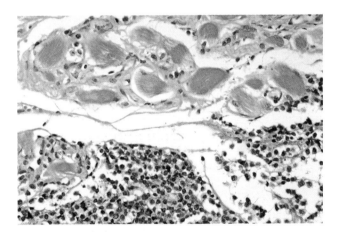

Figure 7.13 Myositis. A chronic inflammatory cell infiltrate in relation to muscle fibres.

Chapter 8

The clinician and the laboratory

Introduction

Histology
Fixation and processing
Frozen sections
Electron microscopy
Polarizing microscopy
Retinal digest preparations
Injection techniques

Cytology
Fine needle biopsies and intraocular aspirates
Conjunctival scrapings
Conjunctival impression cytology

Stains

The examination of eye and tissue specimens
Museum specimens
Histological sections
Macrophotographs and photomicrographs

Microbiology
Specimens from the lids and outer eye
Anterior chamber and vitreous aspirates

Immunochemistry

Molecular methods

INTRODUCTION

Close liaison between clinical ophthalmologists, pathologists and biomedical scientists concerning the investigation of patients is paramount. This chapter incorporates information about the taking and submission of specimens for laboratory investigation. It is imperative that patient details and full clinical information are given with any specimens submitted. A number of laboratory procedures are outlined, and there are explanatory protocols for the examination of museum specimens and histological sections.

HISTOLOGY

Enucleated and eviscerated eyes, exenterated orbits and all other tissues removed, apart from emulsified lens material and non-diagnostic vitrectomy specimens, should be submitted for histological examination. In order to assist with orientation it is often helpful if the relevant sides of tissue specimens are marked with Indian ink or by the insertion of a suture, but this must never intrude on the lesion to be examined.

FIXATION AND PROCESSING

Specimens must be fixed immediately in 10 per cent neutral buffered formalin (formal saline). Twenty-four hours' fixation is necessary for most specimens, but enucleated eyes and exenterated orbits require at least 48 hours. Fixation is followed by gross examination with the naked eye and with a dissecting microscope. Specimens are then processed through alcohol and xylene (this accounts for the leaching out of lipid) and embedded in paraffin wax. Sections are cut at a thickness of 4–5 μm. Certain specimens need special attention.

Wedge resections of lid margins

Wedge resections of lid margins must be orientated so that the initial sections can be cut at right angles to the margin. Subsequent sections are cut either parallel or at right angles to the initial section so as to allow the totality or otherwise of removal of the lesion to be judged. It is useful to keep a portion of a lid margin lesion unprocessed until other sections are examined so that, if necessary, frozen sections can be cut and lipid demonstrated, this being especially helpful in the diagnosing of sebaceous carcinoma.

Conjunctival specimens and corneal discs

Conjunctival specimens, and lamellar and full-thickness corneal discs must be orientated so that sections are cut perpendicular to the surface. In the case of corneal discs, half the specimen should be kept unprocessed lest frozen sections and lipid stains are required for the visualization of lipid keratopathy.

Temporal artery biopsies

Temporal artery specimens should be as long as possible and the pathologist will orientate them in such a way as to produce serial cross-sections.

Muscle biopsies

It is essential for the clinician to contact the laboratory staff prior to the taking of a muscle biopsy. Muscle specimens should be divided into three portions: one portion, for light microscopy, is fixed in 10 per cent neutral buffered formalin; a second portion, for electron microscopy, is fixed in glutaraldehyde; and a third portion, for enzyme histochemistry, is rapidly frozen.

Trabeculectomies

Orientation during processing is especially important with trabeculectomy specimens, so that the meshwork can be visualized on microscopy.

Iridectomies and iridocyclectomies

Iridectomy and iridocyclectomy specimens need to be orientated in such a way as to allow for sections to be cut at right angles to the pupil margin.

Cyclectomies and choroidectomies

Cyclectomy and choroidectomy specimens are unusual, but orientation is necessary so that the lesion to be examined is visualized as lying between the sclera and the overlying ciliary epithelium or RPE.

Eviscerations

Orientation of eviscerated ocular contents is not possible, and sections are best cut so as to include as much tissue as possible. Eviscerations performed because of intraocular infection should always be referred for microbiological studies prior to fixation.

Enucleations

Enucleated eyes, like other tissues, are best fixed in 10 per cent neutral buffered formalin. Eyes must not be opened prior to fixation, fixative must not be injected into the vitreous and the specimen must not be frozen. Delay in fixation results in autolysis, which is manifest initially in the retina as folding and detachment together with degeneration of the photoreceptors. After fixation the specimen is washed in tap water, which removes the formalin and lessens the risk of artefactual retinal detachment. In order to restore the natural colour prior to macroscopical examination, the specimen is placed in 70 per cent alcohol. External examination must be carried out before opening, and internal examination of the eye is necessary before processing.

External examination

The eye is first identified as right or left by locating the positions of the superior and inferior oblique muscles. The diameters of the eye and cornea are measured and recorded, and variations from the normal are noted. The length of the optic nerve should be measured, especially if there is a suspected retinoblastoma. Palpation of the sclera and transillumination of the eye are helpful in identifying the position of an intraocular tumour, and transillumination may also be of value in revealing iris atrophy. Special features to look for on external examination include corneal ulcers and opacities, tumours and evidence of inflammation, previous trauma or surgery.

Radiological examination

X-ray examination is necessary if there is reason to suspect the presence of a radio-opaque intraocular foreign body.

Opening

The eye is opened anteroposteriorly through the limbus, preferably with a long razor blade. Normally this is done in the horizontal plane unless there is a reason (such as the presence of a wound or a tumour) why sectioning in another plane would be advantageous. The portion removed is referred to as the calotte (because it resembles a priest's skullcap), and it should contain a portion of any tumour that may be present. If a retinoblastoma is suspected, transverse sections of the surgical cut end of the optic nerve must be taken for processing.

Internal examination

It should be noted if the architecture is preserved or whether the intraocular structures are disorganized. Tumours, cataract, calcification, bone formation, haemorrhages, exudates, and retinal and choroidal detachment can all be clearly seen, as, in most instances, can the appearance of the optic disc. Subretinal exudate that existed as a fluid during life is gelatinous in fixed specimens. Following internal examination, a symmetrical calotte is removed from the opposite side.

Processing

The main specimen to be processed is the central portion of the eye remaining after removal of the two calottes. In the case of an intraocular tumour, the first removed calotte is processed without delay to enable a rapid diagnosis to be made. Following this, the eye can be sectioned at a number of different levels to assess the possibility of extraocular extension of a neoplasm.

Exenterations

Exenterated specimens invariably contain a primary, infiltrating or metastatic orbital neoplasm. Examination with the naked eye and the dissecting microscope is carried out as for other specimens, and a long razor blade is used so that the eye, which is always included unless it has previously been enucleated, is opened anteroposteriorly through the limbus in a plane that maximizes the amount of relevant orbital material in the eventual sections.

FROZEN SECTIONS

Frozen sections on fixed but unprocessed material are of value in the demonstration of lipid (as in sebaceous carcinoma and lipid keratopathy). In Mohs' or modified Mohs' technique for assessing the totality or otherwise of removal of a lid neoplasm, tissue is fixed by freezing before being cut; in such cases the lesion must have been previously diagnosed by the microscopical examination of a paraffin-wax embedded biopsy.

ELECTRON MICROSCOPY

If it is envisaged that transmission electron microscopy (TEM) or scanning electron microscopy (SEM) will be required the pathologist should be consulted, as special fixative such as glutaraldehyde or osmium tetroxide may be necessary. Thin toluidine blue-stained sections are helpful prior to TEM.

POLARIZING MICROSCOPY

Polarizing microscopy is helpful in the identification of substances such as amyloid, and for the demonstration of refractile foreign particles. Two polarizing filters are used; one, always referred to as the polarizer, is placed beneath the substage condenser where it can be rotated, while the other, called the analyser, is placed between the objective and the eyepiece. Rotation of the polarizer ensures that light waves in one plane only pass through the section being examined, and the analyser partially or completely absorbs all the light transmitted. Birefringence is exhibited by a substance, often crystalline, whose molecular structure is asymmetrical or laminated so that the two rays of light vibrating in perpendicular planes will travel at different velocities through the substance. Birefringent substances normally appear colourless (white) against a dark background under polarizers crossed at right angles to each other. Partial recombination results in the appearance of interference colours. Dichroism is due to light-absorbing differences along different planes of an asymmetrically structured substance, and can be studied in tissue sections using one polarizer only.

RETINAL DIGEST PREPARATIONS

Retinal digest preparations are made on formalin-fixed material. The retina is removed and, by digestion with pepsin and trypsin or trypsin alone, the retinal vasculature can be left intact and stained and examined as a flat preparation. Capillary endothelial cells, pericytes and microaneurysm formation can be clearly observed.

INJECTION TECHNIQUES

Injection techniques can be carried out on unfixed enucleated eyes. The central retinal vessels in the optic nerve are cannulated and the retinal vasculature irrigated with normal saline. Following this, Indian ink or latex suspensions can be injected. The eye is then fixed in formalin. Subsequently, the retina is dissected off and studied as a flat preparation, the pattern of the retinal vasculature being readily observed.

CYTOLOGY

FINE NEEDLE BIOPSIES AND INTRAOCULAR ASPIRATES

For fine needle biopsies and intraocular aspirates, precise localization of lesions is required. In the orbit, CT and ultrasound are helpful, while in the eye the use of a contact lens and a dissecting microscope may allow direct visualization. Samples are drawn through a needle into a syringe, and both needle and syringe should be sent without delay to the laboratory for processing. If a delay is inevitable, laboratory staff should be contacted about alternative procedures. When appropriate, the laboratory staff will split samples for microbiological as well as cytological investigations.

CONJUNCTIVAL SCRAPINGS

The conjunctival epithelium can be scraped with a fine-tipped plastic swab and smeared onto a microscope slide. The specimen is air-dried and fixed in methanol (15–30 minutes). Cytology is assessed on Giemsa-stained preparations, and is helpful in the diagnosing of viral and chlamydial infections, and allergic reactions.

CONJUNCTIVAL IMPRESSION CYTOLOGY

Impression cytology of the conjunctiva is carried out by pressing cellulose acetate paper against the bulbar conjunctiva. Air-drying and methanol fixation is used as for conjunctival scrapings. The technique is helpful in the study of conjunctival surface cells.

STAINS

Haematoxylin and eosin (H & E) are the most widely used stains. Cell nuclei stain blue-black and reveal good intranuclear detail; cell cytoplasm, keratin and most connective tissues stain varying shades and intensities of pink and red (H & E staining has been used on all histological sections illustrated in this book unless otherwise indicated). Special stains are used for specific structures, substances and selected pathogenic organisms (Tables 8.1, 8.2 and 8.3).

Table 8.1 Special stains for specific structures

Structure	Stain	Colour
Collagen	Masson trichrome	Blue/green
	Gomori trichrome	Green
	Mallory trichrome	Purple-blue
	van Gieson	Red
Reticulin	Gordon & Sweets'	Black
Elastic	Verhoeff	Black
Muscle	van Gieson	Yellow
	Masson trichrome	Red
	Gomori trichrome	Red
	Mallory trichrome	Red
Nerve axons	Marsland, Glees and Erikson	Dark brown-black
Neuroglia	Mallory phosphotungstic acid haematoxylin	Dark blue

Table 8.2 Special stains for specific substances

Substance	Stain	Colour
Amyloid	Congo red	Orange-red; apple-green birefringence and dichroism
	Thioflavine T	Fluorescence
Calcium	Alizarin red S[1]	Orange-red
Copper	Rubeanic acid	Greenish-black
Ferric iron	Perls'	Prussian blue
Fibrin	MSB (Martius yellow, scarlet and blue)	Red, yellow or blue – depending on the age of the fibrin
Glycogen	PAS (Periodic acid-Schiff)[2]	Magenta
Glycosaminoglycans (GAGs)	Alcian blue	Acid GAGs – blue
	PAS	Neutral GAGs – magenta
	Colloidal iron	Acid GAGs – Prussian blue
Lipids[3]	Oil red O	Red
	Sudan black	Black
Melanin[4]	Masson–Fontana	Black
Myelin	Loyez	Black
	Luxol fast blue	Blue
Pseudoexfoliation material	Grocott hexamine (methenamine) silver	Grey-black
	Oxidized aldehyde fuchsin	Blue

[1] von Kossa is usually used to demonstrate calcium but it stains the base of the salt and not the calcium, and the colour produced is black.
[2] In diastase-treated sections glycogen will not stain.
[3] Lipid stains are usually carried out on frozen sections.
[4] Melanin bleaches with strong oxidizing agents, e.g. potassium permanganate.

Table 8.3 Special stains for selected pathogens

Pathogens	Stain	Colour
Chlamydial inclusions	Giemsa	Blue-purple
	Iodine	Brown
Bacteria		
Cocci and rods	Gram	Positive – blue-black
		Negative – red
M. tuberculosis	Ziehl–Neelsen (ZN)	Red
M. leprae	Wade–Fite	Red
Atypical mycobacteria	Wade–Fite and/or ZN	Red
A. israelii	Gram	Blue-black
Nocardia spp.	Gram	Blue-black
	Modified ZN	Red
T. pallidum	Warthin and Starry	Black
Fungi	Grocott hexamine (methenamine) silver	Black
	PAS	Magenta
Protozoa		
Acanthanamoeba spp cysts	PAS	Magenta
	Grocott hexamine (methenamine) silver	Black
	Calcofluor white	Apple-green fluorescence

THE EXAMINATION OF EYE AND TISSUE SPECIMENS

MUSEUM SPECIMENS

Museum specimens in ophthalmology are enucleated eyes, exenterated orbits or excised lid, conjunctival or orbital tissues mounted in rectangular transparent containers filled with preservative fluid.

Enucleations and exenterations

Enucleated and exenterated specimens are invariably prepared in such a way that the eye (exenterated orbits usually contain an eye) is opened anteroposteriorly; in an exenterated specimen, other than when the lids are present, it is not possible to determine if this is horizontal or vertical. Exenterated specimens almost always contain a neoplasm. Measurements of intraocular lesions are impractical and examination is, of necessity, with the naked eye. Some enucleated and exenterated specimens are illustrated (Figs 8.1, 8.2). Features to be noted are:

Size and shape of the eye: buphthalmos; megalocornea; pathological myopia; microphthalmos; phthisis; scleral

a

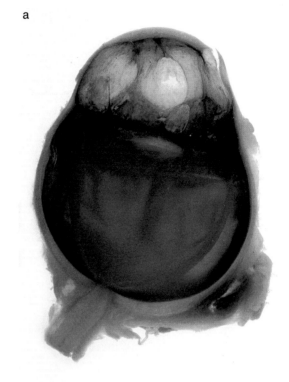

b

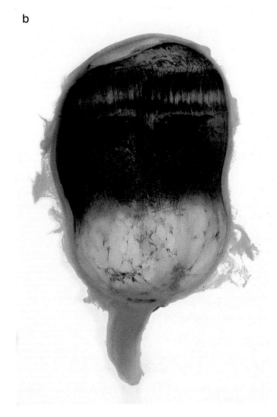

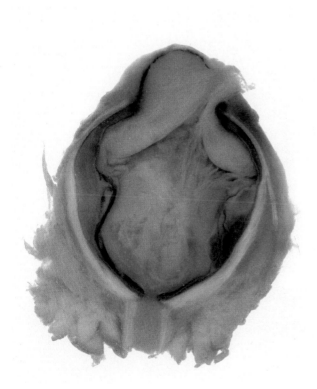

Figure 8.1 Panophthalmitis. There is a corneolimbal perforation and the eye is filled with purulent exudate.

Figure 8.2 Staphylomas. (a) Anterior; the cornea is bulging and lined by atrophic degenerate iris remnants. (b) Posterior; the posterior sclera is bulging and lined by atrophic degenerate choroidal and retinal remnants.

infoldings; ectasias; staphylomas; thickness of the corneoscleral coat.

Presence of a tumour:

Extraocular: position; relationship to the eye and optic nerve; size; shape; consistency; pigmentation (black pigment in a museum specimen may represent altered blood).

Intraocular: position; size; shape; consistency; pigmentation; site of origin; direction of growth and extension.

General intraocular architecture: position, size and shape of the lens; retinal and/or choroidal detachment – real or artefactual; choroidoretinal atrophy; pigment disturbance; haemorrhages; exudates; calcium; bone.

Lid, conjunctival and orbital specimens

Excised tissues from these sites are often tumours, and examination entails noting their size, shape and consistency, and their relationship to any normal structures. Three orbital specimens are illustrated (Fig. 8.3).

HISTOLOGICAL SECTIONS

For practical purposes, the examination of histological sections is considered under two headings: eye sections and tissue sections. The ability to recognize normal structures is an essential requirement for histological examination.

Eye sections

Macroscopical examination is carried out with the naked eye and by the use of a hand lens. As with museum specimens, the features to be noted are the size and shape of the eye, the presence of a tumour, extra- or intraocular, and the general intraocular architecture.

Microscopy must always begin with the low power objective, high power microscopy being subsequently used to confirm earlier observations and to establish details of the specific lesion being examined. Observations made at an early stage may reveal an inflammatory process or a tumour, and these must be analysed.

a

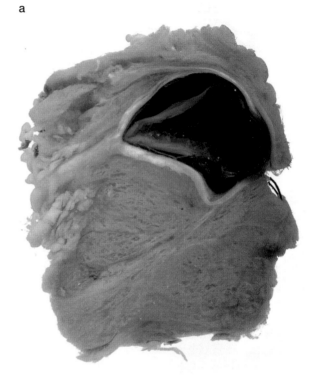

b

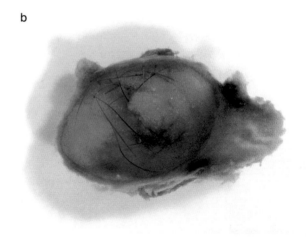

c

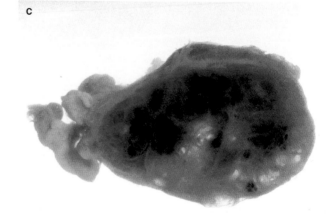

Figure 8.3 Orbital lesions (a) The orbital contents have been exenterated and the eye is surrounded by a homogeneous mass, the nature of which can only be ascertained by microscopy (e.g. see Fig. 4.58). (b) Dermoid cyst; the cyst has been opened and contains a number of hairs (see Fig. 4.15). (c) Cavernous haemangioma; the encapsulated circumscribed lesion comprises a honeycomb-like pattern of spaces (see Fig 4.52); the dark pigment is altered blood.

Analysing inflammation

1. Is the inflammation acute or chronic, localized or diffuse, and which structure is primarily involved?
2. If chronic, is it non-granulomatous or granulomatous?
3. Is it infective or non-infective?

Analysing a tumour

1. Is the tumour a neoplasm, or does it result from some other disorder of cell and tissue growth?
2. If a neoplasm, is it benign or malignant?
3. If malignant, is it primary or secondary?

Even when there is an obvious inflammatory disorder or tumour, the corneoscleral coat, the uvea, the retina and optic nerve and the intraocular compartments must all be examined in a systematic way. Important features to be noted include:

Cornea

Epithelium: number of layers of cells; oedema; bullae; subepithelial fibrovascular pannus.

Bowman's layer: breaks; deposits.

Stroma: thickness; scarring; vascularization; deposits.

Descemet's membrane: thickness; breaks; excrescences on posterior surface; deposits.

Endothelium: density of cell population; deposits.

Sclera

Thickness; scarring; deposits.

Iris

Atrophy; neovascular, fibrous or Descemet-like membrane on anterior surface; deposits.

Ciliary body

Atrophy; deposits.

Choroid

Atrophy; vascular changes; thickness of Bruch's membrane; breaks in Bruch's membrane; drusen and other deposits.

Retina

Detachment – real or artefactual; atrophy – ganglion cells or photoreceptors; pigment disturbance; vascular changes; haemorrhages; exudates; deposits.

Optic nerve

Cupping of nerve head; atrophy; vascular changes; haemorrhages; deposits.

Lens

Integrity of capsule; cataract; subepithelial fibrosis; deposits.

Anterior chamber

Depth; filtration angle; iridocorneal and iridolenticular adhesions; haemorrhage; exudate; deposits.

Posterior chamber

Haemorrhage; exudate; deposits (including those on the zonular fibres).

Vitreous

New vessels; bands; haemorrhage; exudate; deposits.

Artefacts and irrelevant features

Artefacts and irrelevant features involve a number of structures and include:

Corneal epithelium: artefactual separation or absence of the corneal epithelium is frequently observed. In an artefact the edge of the remaining epithelium is seen as a sharply demarcated step, but in true ulceration there is gradual shelving from the intact epithelium to the ulcerated area.

Corneal stroma: in the absence of any extracellular material, clefts between the corneal lamellae are usually meaningless.

Lens capsule: pigment on the anterior lens capsule is usually artefactual unless accompanied by other evidence of iridolenticular adhesion.

Lens cortex/nucleus: large clefts and splits in the lens are usually the result of processing. True cataractous changes take the form of definite globules and vacuoles, or fibrosis and/or calcification.

Retinal detachment: the neurosensory retina is firmly attached to the RPE only at the optic nerve head and ora serrata, and artefactual detachment is common. In the absence of a tumour or subretinal exudate, detachment probably occurred after enucleation. Also, in artefactual detachment, very fine granules of melanin from the RPE are present on the outer limbs of the photoreceptors.

Retinal breaks: artefactual breaks in the retina have sharp irregular margins.

Microcystic changes in retina: microcystic appearances are often a sequel to processing.

'Pseudohyphae' in retina: following intraocular haemorrhage, blood degradation products are adsorbed onto the walls of retinal capillaries which, when stained with H & E, can easily be misinterpreted as fungal elements.

Myelin extrusion: extrusion of myelin (a granular basophilic substance) from the nerve fibres is not infrequently seen at the optic disc if the optic nerve was crushed during enucleation. Myelin extrusion may also extend peripherally beneath the retina and even into retinal blood vessels.

Tissue sections

Tissue sections include lid, conjunctival and orbital specimens, and corneal discs. Their examination involves the use of a hand lens and microscopy. Analysis of inflammation and tumours is as described for eye sections. Corneal discs are revealed as full thickness or lamellar by the presence or absence of Descemet's membrane. Detailed observation of the corneal layers is as described for eye sections.

MACROPHOTOGRAPHS AND PHOTOMICROGRAPHS

Macrophotographs and photomicrographs are examined and analysed in the same way as described for museum specmens and microscope slides.

MICROBIOLOGY

SPECIMENS FROM THE LIDS AND OUTER EYE

Before sampling infected lesions involving the lids and/or outer eye, it is essential that all scales, crusts and superficial slough be removed as specimens must be taken from the epidermal/epithelial surface or the base of an ulcer. If topical anaesthesia is required, preservative-free eye drops must be used.

Specimens for viruses

Investigations for viral infections include culture and nucleic acid detection. Viral cultures are taken from affected areas with a sterile fine-tipped plastic swab. The end is cut off into a tube containing viral transport medium, which is sent as soon as possible to the laboratory. If there is an unavoidable delay of not more than 24 hours, then the specimen should be stored in a refrigerator ($+4°C$); longer delays require a lower temperature ($-70°C$).

Specimens for chlamydiae

Enzyme immunoassay to detect chlamydial antigen is currently the most widely used test. As far as possible, commercial kits are utilized for the collection of specimens and there must be strict compliance with the accompanying instructions. In the laboratory, confirmatory immunofluorescence is carried out on specimens with positive or doubtful results. Other tests for chlamydial disease include direct immunofluorescence (DIF), culture using a sterile fine-tipped plastic swab and chlamydial transport medium (not viral transport medium), and nucleic acid detection. For DIF in suspected trachoma, material should be scraped with a dry sterile swab from the upper tarsal conjunctiva, while in oculogenital disease and neonatal conjunctivitis, material can be swabbed from the lower tarsal conjunctiva. Material for DIF should be rubbed in small concentrated circles on a microscope slide and not laid as linear streaks (this allows for it to be more readily seen by laboratory workers). As with viral cultures, delay in sending chlamydial cultures to the laboratory necessitates storage at low temperatures ($+4°C$ for 24 hours; and $-70°C$ if longer). Where immunofluorescence, culture and methods for nucleic acid detection are unavailable, conjunctival scrapings stained with Giemsa or iodine may prove helpful.

Specimens for bacteria and fungi

Lid cultures

Lid cultures are taken with a sterile cotton-wool swab moistened with phosphate-buffered normal saline or tryptic digest broth. These are then either inoculated directly on to a blood agar plate or placed in transport medium and sent without delay to the laboratory. For the culture of meibomian secretion it may be necessary to press the lid against suitable firm support until secretion oozes from the gland orifices.

Conjunctival cultures

Conjunctival cultures are best taken with a wire (e.g. nichrome) or disposable plastic loop and inoculated directly on to a culture plate. A blood agar plate must always be inoculated, and if there is clinical suspicion of infection with *Neisseria* spp. or *Haemophilus* spp., a chocolate agar plate should also be inoculated. Inoculated plates must be incubated ($+37°C$) without delay.

Corneal scrapings

Corneal scrapings, to provide material for examination of smears and culture, are preferably taken with a 1–1½″ 21 gauge needle or a surgical blade using slit-lamp microscopy. Smears for microscopy should be air-dried and methanol- (15–30 minutes) or heat-fixed (using a Bunsen burner). Ideally three thin smears should be made, but one good preparation is often adequate. Stains to be used, in order of priority, are:

1. Gram – for bacteria, yeasts and some filamentous fungi.
2. Periodic acid-Schiff (PAS) – for fungi and amoebae.

Additional stains depend on the number of smears made and on the clinical situation, but may include those for acid-fast organisms and amoebae. If the amount of material available from corneal scrapings is limited, preference should be given to solid and liquid phase cultures rather than to smears.

Both solid and liquid phase media are necessary for culture:

Solid phase media: blood agar for most bacteria, chocolate agar for *Neisseria* spp., *Haemophilus* spp. and other fastidious organisms, and Sabouraud agar for fungi.

Liquid phase media: advisable for fastidious organisms or if antibiotics have been previously administered and organisms are likely to be few in number. Those used are Robertson's cooked meat and thioglycollate broth for microaerophilic and anaerobic bacteria, and brain–heart infusion for aerobic bacteria and fungi.

Corneal biopsy

Corneal biopsy is performed with a disposable skin punch or small corneal trephine. The excised material is divided and placed in two separate sterile containers. The first, containing either Ringer's solution or balanced salt solution (normal saline), is sent for microbiological investigations (culture and smears). The second, containing 10 per cent neutral buffered formalin (formal saline), is referred for histological study. If there is a delay in sending the specimens to the laboratory, the one for microbiological investigation should be placed in a refrigerator ($+4°C$).

Material from the canaliculi and lacrimal sac

Pressure over the canaliculi and lacrimal sac may be required to obtain material, which is then crushed onto a microscope slide and stained with Gram, PAS and/or Grocott hexamine (methenamine) silver.

Specimens for acanthamoebae

The investigations for acanthamoebic keratitis involve culture, microscopy and immunological methods.

Culture: a non-nutrient agar plate must be inoculated directly and sent to the laboratory where it is seeded with *E. coli*, which serves as a food source for the amoebae.

Microscopy: wet-mount preparations may reveal the amoebae. In fixed material, stains used to identify amoebae include PAS, Grocott hexamine (methenamine) silver and calcofluor white. Electron microscopy can also be helpful.

Immunological methods: enzyme histochemistry (immunoperoxidase) and immunofluorescence can also be used to identify the amoebae.

ANTERIOR CHAMBER AND VITREOUS ASPIRATES

Aspirates from the anterior chamber and vitreous for microbiological examination are dealt with in the same way as material from corneal scrapings. Fluid should be sent to the laboratory in a capped syringe for full and accurate analysis, which will include cultures and smears and, when appropriate, nucleic acid detection. If there is a delay in despatching the syringe to the laboratory, it should be stored in a refrigerator ($+4°C$).

IMMUNOCHEMISTRY

Immunochemistry identifies specific antigens produced by cells (e.g. epithelial cells, lymphocytes) and extracellular matrix (e.g. collagen, amyloid). If the investigation is carried out on tissue samples the term immunohistochemistry is used; if on cytology specimens the term immunocytochemistry is more appropriate. Antibodies suitably labelled with enzymes, fluorochromes, heavy metals or radio-isotopes are used to produce immune complexes, the presence of which can then be identified by light, fluorescence or electron microscopy, or by autoradiography. Immunoenzymatic staining and immunofluorescence are the most widely used methods.

Immunoenzymatic staining

Immunoenzymatic staining involves enzyme substrate reactions that convert colourless chromogens into coloured end-products which can be seen by the use of the light microscope. Techniques used include immunoperoxidase, peroxidase-antiperoxidase (PAP), avidin–biotin complex (ABC) and alkaline phosphatase–anti-alkaline phosphatase (APAAP). Many different types of cells can be identified (Table 8.4); this is of value in the histological diagnosis of lymphoproliferative lesions and other tumours. An ever-increasing number of antibodies (cell markers) is becoming available. Many reactions are not specific, and not infrequently there is cross-reactivity with other types of cells; an example of this is seen with S100 protein, which is expressed not only by melanoma cells but also by other cells of neural crest lineage and by totally unrelated cells such as lipocytes, chondrocytes, muscle cells, and epithelial cells of the breast, and of salivary and sweat glands. Most immunoenzymatic staining can be carried out on formalin-fixed paraffin-wax embedded material.

Table 8.4 Cells and their identification by immunoenzymatic staining

Cells	Antibodies (cell markers)
All epithelial cells Glandular epithelial cells	Cytokeratins Epithelial membrane antigen (EMA) Human milk factor globulin (HMFG)
Muscle cells	Desmin Smooth muscle actin
Vascular endothelial cells	von Willebrand (Factor VIII)
Melanoma cells	S100, NKIC3, HMB45
Glial cells	Glial fibrillary acidic protein (GFAP)
Neuroendocrine cells	Neuron specific enolase (NSE) Chromogranin

All lymphocytes
    T lymphocytes
    T_H lymphocytes
    $T_{C/S}$ lymphocytes
    B lymphocytes
	CD45 (leukocyte common antigen – LCA)
	CD3
	CD4
	CD8
	CD20, CD79a

Plasma cells	CD79a
Macrophages and histiocytes	CD68

Immunofluorescence

Immunofluorescence involves the use of a fluorochrome such as fluorescein or rhodamine. Immunofluorescent methods are invaluable when the quantity of immune complex being sought is small, as is the case in chlamydial ocular infections and in autoimmune disorders such as ocular cicatricial pemphigoid (OCP). Tissue samples removed for immunofluorescence in suspected cases of OCP are best snap-frozen in liquid nitrogen and stored at $-70°$ C; it is usually best, however, to contact the laboratory prior to taking the specimen, as practices vary and sometimes special transport media are preferred. If immunofluorescence antibody studies are required on conjunctival or corneal specimens, it is important that fluorescein is not instilled into the patient's eye before submitting the specimen for examination.

Enzyme immunoassay (enzyme linked immunosorbent assay – ELISA)

In enzyme immunoassay (EIA), antigen or antibody is detected by the binding of an enzyme coupled to antibody specific for the antigen or anti-immunoglobulin. Widely used enzymes are peroxidase and alkaline phosphatase. The intensity of the colour produced is measured spectrophotometrically, and is proportional to the concentration of antigen or antibody being measured.

MOLECULAR METHODS

A detailed description of molecular methods is beyond the scope of this book, but it is important for the reader to understand the increasing importance of these techniques. Close liaison with the molecular biologist is essential whenever the clinician considers that molecular methods would be helpful.

Techniques including the polymerase chain reaction (PCR) and in-situ hybridization (ISH) are used to detect specific nucleic acids, and are currently valuable in microbiology and genetics. PCR is a method of amplifying predetermined segments of DNA from a small sample. Techniques based on PCR, because of their sensitivity and speed, are important diagnostic tools frequently used in microbiology, particularly in viral and chlamydial infections. Trace amounts of RNA can be amplified and detected in a similar way by first converting them to DNA by using the enzyme reverse transcriptase (RT-PCR). ISH techniques demonstrate sequences of DNA and RNA in tissue sections. The application of molecular methods to genetics and inherited disorders (molecular genetics) allows for diagnosis, and for the identification of candidate genes and their mutations. It also allows for a detailed understanding of the link between mutation and the expression of disease by establishing the intervening molecular processes.

Glossary of abbreviations

A

AA	amyloid protein A
AAFB	acid and alcohol-fast bacilli
AAU	acute anterior uveitis
ABC	avidin–biotin complex
ACAID	anterior chamber-associated immune deviation
ACE	angiotensin-converting enzyme
AChR	acetylcholine receptor
ADCC	antibody-dependent cell-mediated cytotoxicity
AFB	acid-fast bacilli
AFIP	Armed Forces Institute of Pathology
AIDS	acquired immunodeficiency syndrome
AION	anterior ischaemic optic neuropathy
AKC	acute keratoconjunctivitis
AL	amyloid protein L
AMD	age-related macular degeneration
AMS	atypical mole syndrome
α-MSH	alpha-melanocyte stimulating hormone
ANA	antinuclear antibody
ANCA	antineutrophil cytoplasmic antibody
AP	amyloid protein P
APAAP	alkaline phosphatase–antialkaline phosphatase
APC	antigen-presenting cell
APMPPE	acute posterior multifocal placoid pigment epitheliopathy
ARN	acute retinal necrosis
AS	ankylosing spondylitis
ATP	adenosine triphosphate

B

B cell	B lymphocyte
BARN	bilateral acute retinal necrosis
BDR	background diabetic retinopathy
BMD	basement membrane deposit
bp	base pairs
BRAO	branch retinal arteriolar occlusion
BRVO	branch retinal vein occlusion
BSE	bovine spongiform encephalopathy

C

C1–C9	components of complement
CALT	conjunctiva-associated lymphoid tissue
CAR	cancer-associated retinopathy
CD	cluster designation/cluster of differentiation
CDC	Centres for Disease Control
CGD	chronic granulomatous disease
cGMP	cyclic guanosine monophosphate
CGRP	calcitonin gene-related peptide
CHARGE	colobomas and microphthalmos, heart defects, choanal atresia, growth retardation, genital and ear abnormalities
CHED	congenital hereditary endothelial dystrophy
CHRPE	congenital hypertrophy of the retinal pigment epithelium
CIN	cervical intraepithelial neoplasia
CJD	Creutzfeldt–Jakob disease
CMC	chronic mucocutaneous candidiasis

CMI	cell-mediated immunity
CMO	cystoid macular oedema
CMV	cytomegalovirus
CNS	central nervous system
CNV	choroidal neovascularization
Conj. IN	conjunctival intraepithelial neoplasia
CRAO	central retinal artery occlusion
CRVO	central retinal vein occlusion
CSF	cerebrospinal fluid or colony stimulating factor
CSMO	clinically significant macular oedema (in diabetes mellitus)
CSNB	congenital stationary night blindness
CSR	central serous retinopathy
CT	computerized tomography

D

DAG	diacylglycerol
DIDMOAD	diabetes insipidus, diabetes mellitus, optic atrophy and deafness
DIF	direct immunofluorescence
DNA	deoxyribonucleic acid
DOPA	dihydroxyphenylalanine

E

EA	Early antigen
EBNA	Epstein–Barr nuclear antigen
EBV	Epstein–Barr virus
ECAF	endothelial cell angiogenic factor
ECF-A	eosinophilic chemotactic factor of anaphylaxis
ECG	electrocardiogram
EDTA	ethylenediamine tetra-acetic acid
EGF	epidermal growth factor
EIA	enzyme immunoassay
EKC	epidemic keratoconjunctivitis
ELISA	enzyme-linked immunosorbent assay
EM	electron microscopy
EMA	epithelial membrane antigen
EMBP	eosinophilic major basic protein
EOG	electro-oculogram
ERG	electroretinogram
ESR	erythrocyte sedimentation rate

F

Fab	fragment antigen binding (of immunoglobulin)
Fas L	Fas ligand
Fc	fragment crystallizable (of immunoglobulin)
Fe^{2+}	ferrous iron
Fe^{3+}	ferric iron

FGF	fibroblast growth factor
FLS	fibrous long-spacing (collagen)
FTA-Abs	fluorescent treponemal antibody absorption

G

GAG	glycosaminoglycan
GAP	GTPase-activating protein
GCA	giant cell arteritis
GCA/PMR	giant cell arteritis/polymyalgia rheumatica
GDP	guanosine diphosphate
GFAP	glial fibrillary acidic protein
GK	galactokinase
GM-CSF	granulocyte-macrophage colony stimulating factor
GMP	guanosine monophosphate
gp	glycoprotein
GPC	giant papillary conjunctivitis
GPUT	galactose-1-phosphatase uridyltransferase
GTP	guanosine triphosphate
GUN	glaucoma, uveitis and neurological signs
GVHD	graft-versus-host disease

H

Hb	haemoglobin
HEV	high endothelial venule
HHV	human herpes virus
HIV	human immunodeficiency virus
HLA	human leukocyte antigen
HMFG	human milk factor globulin
HPV	human papilloma virus
hRNA	heterogeneous RNA
HSV	herpes simplex virus
HTLV	human T-lymphotrophic virus
HZO	herpes zoster ophthalmicus

I

ICAM	intercellular adhesion molecule
ICG	indocyanine green
ICP	intracranial pressure
ICROP	International Classification of Retinopathy of Prematurity
IFA	indirect fluorescein antibody
IFN	interferon
Ig	immunoglobulin
IGF	insulin-like growth factor
IL	interleukin
ILAR	International League of Associations for Rheumatology

IOFB	intraocular foreign body
IOI	intraocular inflammation
IOL	intraocular lens
IOP	intraocular pressure
IR	infrared
IRBP	interphotoreceptor cell binding protein
IRMA	intraretinal microvascular anomaly
ISAGA	immunosorbent agglutination assay
ISDNA	inverse standard deviation of nucleolar area
ISH	*in situ* hybridization

J

JCA	juvenile chronic arthritis

K

kb	kilobase
KCS	keratoconjunctivitis sicca
KGF	keratinocyte growth factor
KID	keratitis, ichthyosis and deafness
KSV	Kaposi sarcoma virus

L

LASIK	laser-assisted *in situ* keratomileusis
LAT	latency-associated transcript
LCA	leukocyte common antigen
LDL	low-density-lipoprotein
LEMS	Lambert–Eaton myasthenic syndrome
LFA	lymphocyte function associated antigen
LGL	large granular lymphocyte
LHON	Leber's hereditary optic neuropathy
LSD	lysergic acid diethylamide

M

MAdCAM	mucin-like cell adhesion molecule
MALT	mucosa-associated lymphoid tissue
MAR	melanoma-associated retinopathy
Mb	megabase
MEWDS	multiple evanescent white dot syndrome
MHC	major histocompatibility complex
MOMP	major outer membrane protein
MPS	mucopolysaccharidoses
MRI	magnetic resonance imaging
mRNA	messenger RNA
MS	multiple sclerosis
mtDNA	mitochondrial DNA

N

NADPH	nicotinamide adenine dinucleotide phosphate (reduced form)
NCL	neuronal ceroid lipofuscinoses

Nd:YAG	neodymium:yttrium aluminium garnet
NF	neurofibromatosis
NKcell	natural killer cell
NSE	neuron-specific elonase
NVD	new vessels at disc
NVE	new vessels elsewhere

O

OA	ocular albinism
OAT	ornithine aminotransferase
OCA	oculocutaneous albinism
OCA1-MP	minimal pigment albinism
OCA1-TP	temperature-dependent albinism
OCP	ocular cicatricial pemphigoid
ONH	optic nerve hypoplasia

P

p	short arm of a chromosome
PACG	primary angle-closure glaucoma
PAF	platelet activating factor
PAN	polyarteritis nodosa
PAP	peroxidase–antiperoxidase
PAS	periodic acid-Schiff
PCR	polymerase chain reaction
PDE	phosphodiesterase
PDGF	platelet-derived growth factor
PDR	proliferative diabetic retinopathy
PDS	pigment dispersion syndrome
PEE	punctate epithelial erosions
PEK	punctate epithelial keratitis
PGL	persistent generalized lymphadenopathy
PHPV	persistent hyperplastic primary vitreous
PIC	punctate inner choroidopathy
PKC	protein kinase C
PMR	polymyalgia rheumatica
PMMA	polymethylmethacrylate
PMR	polymyalgia rheumatica
PNS	peripheral nervous system
POAG	primary open-angle glaucoma
PORN	progressive outer retinal necrosis
PPD	purified protein derivative or posterior polymorphous dystrophy
PPRPE	preserved para-arteriolar retinal pigment epithelium
PRK	photorefractive keratectomy
PrP	prion protein
PV	plasma viscosity
PVD	posterior vitreous detachment
PVR	proliferative vitreoretinopathy
PXS	pseudoexfoliation syndrome

Q

q	long arm of a chromosome

R

Rb	retinoblastoma gene
RBC	red blood cell
RDS	retinal degeneration slow locus
RNA	ribonucleic acid
ROCA	rufous oculocutaneous albinism
ROM	retinal outer segment membrane protein
ROP	retinopathy of prematurity
RP	retinitis pigmentosa
RPE	retinal pigment epithelium
rRNA	ribosomal RNA
RT-PCR	reverse transcriptase polymerase chain reaction

S

SAA	serum amyloid protein A
SAP	serum amyloid protein P
SCID	severe combined immunodeficiency
SCLC	small cell lung cancer
SDNA	standard deviation of the nucleolar area
SEM	scanning electron microscopy
SFD	Sorsby's fundus dystrophy
SLE	systemic lupus erythematosus
SRF	subretinal fluid

T

TBIA	thyroid binding inhibiting antibody
TBII	thyroid binding inhibiting immunoglobulin
TFBUT	tear film break-up time
T cell	T lymphocyte
TCR	T cell receptor
TEM	transmission electron microscopy
TGF	transforming growth factor
TIGR	trabecular meshwork glucocorticoid response protein
TNF	tumour necrosis factor
TNFR	tumour necrosis factor receptor
TPI	*Treponema pallidum* immobilization
TRAb	thyrotropin receptor antibody
tRNA	transfer RNA
TSAb	thyroid stimulating antibody
TSH	thyroid stimulating hormone
TSI	thyroid stimulating immunoglobulin

U

UDP	uridine diphosphate
UV	ultraviolet

V

VCA	viral capsid antigen
VDRL	Venereal Disease Research Laboratory
VEGF	vascular endothelial growth factor
VEP	visual evoked potential
VHL	von Hippel–Lindau disease
VIP	vasoactive intestinal peptide
VKC	vernal keratoconjunctivitis
VKH	Vogt–Koyanagi–Harada syndrome
VZV	varicella zoster virus
VLM	visceral larva migrans

W

WAGR	Wilms' tumour, aniridia, genitourinary abnormalities and mental retardation
WBC	white blood cell
WHO-REAL	World Health Organization – Revised European/American lymphoma classification

X

X	X sex chromosome
XLJR	X-linked juvenile retinoschisis

Y

Y	Y sex chromosome

Z

ZN	Ziehl–Neelsen

Further reading

Albert, D. M. and Jakobiec, F. A. (1999). *Principles and Practice of Ophthalmology*, 2nd edn. W. B. Saunders.

American Academy of Ophthalmology (1997–1998). *Ophthalmic Pathology and Intraocular Tumours.* AAO.

Apple, D. J. and Rabb, M. F. (1998). *Ocular Pathology: Clinical Applications and Self Assessment*, 5th edn. Mosby.

Bancroft, J. D. and Stevens, A. (eds) (1996). *Theory and Practice of Histological Techniques*, 4th edn. Churchill Livingstone.

Bron, A. J. and Seal, D. V. (1998). *Ocular Infections: Management and Treatment in Practice.* Martin Dunitz.

Brown, N. P. and Bron, A. J. (1996). *Lens Disorders: A Clinical Manual of Cataract Diagnosis.* Butterworth-Heinemann.

Campbell, J. and Sobin, L. H. (1998). *Histological Typing of Tumours of the Eye and its Adnexa*, 2nd edn. Springer-Verlag.

Crocker, J. G. and Burnett, D. (1998). *The Science of Laboratory Diagnosis.* Isis Medical Media.

Eagle, R. C. (1999). *Eye Pathology. An Atlas and Basic Text.* W. B. Saunders.

Easty, D. L. and Sparrow, J. M. (eds) (1999). *Oxford Textbook of Ophthalmology.* Oxford University Press.

Forrester, J., Dick, A., McMenamin, P. and Lee, W. (1996). *The Eye: Basic Sciences in Practice.* W. B. Saunders.

Garner, A. and Klintworth, G. K. (1994). *Pathology of Ocular Disease*, 2nd edn. Marcel Dekker Inc.

Janeway, J. J. and Travers, P. (2000). *Immunobiology: The Immune System in Health and Disease*, 5th edn. Garland Publishing Inc.

Kanski, J. J. (1999). *Clinical Ophthalmology*, 4th edn. Butterworth-Heinemann.

Koevary, S. B. (1999). *Ocular Immunology in Health and Disease.* Butterworth-Heinemann.

Lee, W. R. (1993). *Ophthalmic Histopathology.* Springer-Verlag.

McLean, I. W., Burnier, M. N., Zimmerman, L. E. and Jakobiec, F. A. (1995). *Atlas of Tumour Pathology: Tumours of the Eye and Ocular Adnexa.* Armed Forces Institute of Pathology, Washington DC.

Mims, C., Playfair, J., Roitt, I. *et al.* (1998). *Medical Microbiology*, 2nd edn. Mosby.

Murray, P. R., Rosenthal, K. S., Kobayashin, G. and Pfaller, M. A. (1998). *Medical Microbiology*, 3rd edn. Mosby.

Pepose, J. S., Holland, G. N. and Wilhelmus, K. R. (1996). *Ocular Infection and Immunity.* Mosby.

Rao, N. A. (1996). *Biopsy Pathology of the Eye and Ocular Adnexa.* Chapman & Hall.

Roitt, I. M., Brostoff, J., Male, D. K. (1998). *Immunology*, 5th edn. Mosby.

Rubin, E. and Farber, J. L. (1999). *Pathology*, 3rd edn. J. B. Lippincott Company.

Sassani, J. W. (ed.) (1997). *Ophthalmic Pathology with Clinical Correlations.* Lippincott-Raven.

Spalton, D. J., Hitchings, R. A. and Hunter, P. A. (eds) (1994). *Atlas of Clinical Ophthalmology*, 2nd edn. Wolfe.

Spencer, W. H. (ed.) (1996). *Ophthalmic Pathology: An Atlas and Textbook.* W. B. Saunders.

Tabarra, K. F. and Hyndiuk, R. A. (1996). *Infections of the Eye*, 2nd edn. Little, Brown and Company.

Traboulsi, E. P. (ed.) (1999). *Genetic Diseases of the Eye.* Oxford University Press.

Underwood, J. C. E. (2000). *General and Systematic Pathology*, 3rd edn. Churchill Livingstone.

Wright, A. F. and Jay, B. (eds) (1995). *Molecular Genetics of Inherited Eye Disorders*. Harwood Academic Publications.

Yanoff, M. and Duker, J. (1999). *Ophthalmology*. Mosby-Wolfe.

Yanoff, M. and Fine, B. S. (1996). *Ocular Pathology*, 4th edn. Mosby-Wolfe.

Index

Page numbers in **bold** refer to illustrations, tables or illustrated text

A

AA amyloid, 261, 262, 263
ABCA4, 251
ABO antigens
  corneal allograft rejection, 75
  transplanted tissue compatibility, 74
Abrasion, 3
  corneal epithelial, 16
  regeneration processes, 15
Abscess formation, **45**
Absidia, 101
ACAID *see* Anterior chamber associated
    immune deviation
Acanthamoeba, 22, 104, 107, **108**
Acanthamoebic keratitis, **107–8**
  investigations, 108, 327
Accessory lacrimal gland proliferations,
    182
Accommodation, 218
Acid burns, 12
Acidic fibroblast growth factor (aFGF),
    14–15
Acidic lipids, acute inflammation, 44
Acinetobacter, 92
  keratitis, 93
Acne rosacea, 50
Acquired immune deficiency syndrome
    (AIDS) *see* HIV infection/AIDS
Acrylic intraocular lenses, 27
Actinic keratosis (solar keratosis; senile
    keratosis), 141, **167**
Actinomyces, 64, 91
Actinomyces israeli, **91**
  canaliculitis/dacryocystitis, 93
Acute phase response, 45

Adaptive immune system, 32, 39–41
  afferent limb, 40
  antigen processing, 40
  efferent limb, 40–1
  eyes/associated structures, 42–3
Adenocarcinoma
  lacrimal gland, 185
  metastatic, **211**
Adenoid cystic carcinoma, 184, **186**
  perineural infiltration, 144
Adenoma, **142**
  monomorphic, 184
  oxyphil (oncocytoma), **182**
  pleomorphic, 141, 175, 184, **185**
  sebaceous, 172
Adenoma sebaceum *see* Angiofibroma
Adenoviruses, **77–8**
  chronic conjunctivitis, 78
  epidemic keratoconjunctivitis, 78
  investigations, 78
  pharyngoconjunctival fever, 78
Adherent leukoma, 5, **6**
Adhesins, 89
Adhesion molecules, 38
Adhesions, inflammation sequelae, **53,
  54**
Adipose tissue healing, 18
Adnexae, ocular
  developmental anomalies, 162
  normal development, 161–2
Adult vitelliform macular dystrophy,
    245
Adult-onset foveomacular dystrophy
    with choroidal neovascularization,
    245
AE amyloid, 261

Aerobic micro-organisms, 88
African eyeworm (*Loa loa*), **111**
Age-related changes, 214
  Bruch's membrane, 230, 235
  chromosomal nondisjunction, 117
  crystallins, 219, 220
  degenerations, 230–4
    see also Age-related macular
        degeneration
  drusen, **230–1**
  lens, 219–20
  photoreceptors, 230
  posterior vitreous detachment, 224
  retinal pigment epithelium (RPE),
    230, 235
  sub-RPE deposits, **230–1**
    basement membrane, **231**
  syneresis, 223
  wound healing, 16
Age-related macular degeneration, 13,
    214, 230, 231–4
  choroidal neovascularization, 232,
    233–4
  exudative (senile disciform) macular
      degeneration, **232–3**
  non-exudative (atrophic) macular
      degeneration, **232**
  retinal pigment epithelium (RPE)
      tears/detachment, 234
Agenesis *see* Aplasia
Aggressins, 89
Aicardi's syndrome, 132, 133, 158
AIDS *see* HIV infection/AIDS
AIDS dementia complex, 59
AL amyloid, 261, 263
Åland Island eye disease, 246

Albers–Schönberg disease
(osteopetrosis), 249
Albinism, 123, 126
Alcoholism, 302
Alkali burns, 11–12
secondary glaucoma, 311
Alkaptonuria, 125, 127, 260–1
see also Ochronosis
Alleles, 116
Allelic heterogeneity, 117, 243, 245
Allergic conjunctivitis
acute, 61
contact lens wear-related, 22
Allergic granulomatous nodule, **61**
Allergic microbial
blepharoconjunctivitis, 64
Allergic reactions, 34, 59
contact, 60–1
contact lens related, 21, 22
ophthalmic disorders, 61–5
Allergic rhinoconjunctivitis, acute, 61
Allografts, 74
Alpha chymotrypsin-induced glaucoma,
311
Alpha particles, 8, 11
Alpha-fetoprotein, 145
Alpha-melanocyte-stimulating hormone
(α-MSH), 43
Alport's syndrome, 155, 249
Alström's disease, 249
Alveolar soft part sarcoma, 189
Amaurosis fugax, 278
Amblyopia
nutritional, 13
tobacco–alcohol (nutritional optic
neuropathy), 301–2
Amino acid disorders, 123, 126–7
Amiodarone, 17, 264
Amputation neuroma, 18
Amsler's sign, 70
Amyloid
AA amyloid, 261, 262, 263
AE amyloid, 261
AL amyloid, 261, 263
deposits, 261–3
gelatinous drop-like dystrophy, 239
lattice dystrophy, 239, 263
microscopy, **262**
ophthalmic tissues, 263
P amyloid, 261–2
polymorphic stromal dystrophy, 239
primary amyloidosis, 262, 263
secondary amyloidosis, 262, 263
serum components, 45
Amyloid fibrillary protein, 261
Amyloid P, 261–2
Anaemias, 291
Anaerobic micro-organisms, 88
Anaphylaxis *see* Hypersensitivity Type I
reactions
Anencephaly, 140
Aneuploidy, 117, 143
Aneurysmal bone cyst, 190
Aneurysms, retinal, 273–4
Leber's miliary, 272

macroaneurysms, **273–4**
microaneurysms, **273**
Angina, ocular, 279
Angiofibroma, 209
Angiogenesis, 18
see also Neovascularization
Angiogenic growth factors, 14
diabetic retinopathy, 283, 287
retinopathy of prematurity, 276
Angioid streaks, **234–5**
Angiokeratoma diffusum (Fabry's
disease; galactosidase deficiency),
17, 133–4, 264
Angiotensin, 280, 283
Aniridia, 148, **153–4**
associated disorders, 217, 305
Ankylosing spondylitis, 65
acute anterior uveitis (AAU)
association, 68, 69
HLA associations, 68, 69
Anogenital carcinoma, AIDS-related,
58
Anomalous trichromatism, 247–8
Anophthalmos, 140, 148
degenerative, 149
primary, 149
secondary, 149
Anorexia of neoplastic disease, 145
Anterior capsulotomy, 27
Anterior chamber
angle recession, 4
battered child, 5
aspirates for microbiology, 327
dysgenesis, 140, 148, 152–3
haemorrhage, 270
see also Hyphaema
histological sections examination,
325
Anterior chamber-associated immune
deviation (ACAID), 43
corneal allograft survival, 75
Anterior ciliary artery, 266
Anterior crocodile shagreen, 255–6
Anterior intraocular inflammation, 52
Anterior ischaemic optic neuropathy,
288, 301, **302**
diabetes mellitus, 287
Anterior segment
developmental anomalies, 152–4
inflammation, secondary glaucoma,
307
normal development, 151–2
surgical complications
endothelialization, 25
epithelialization, 25
ischaemic necrosis, 28
Anterior subcapsular fibrosis, 4
Anterior uveitis, 52, 68–70
acute (AAU), 68–9
HLA associations, 68, 69
isolated, 68
molecular mechanisms, 69
seronegative spondyloarthropathies-
related, 68
chronic, 69–70

see also Uveitis, autoimmune
Anterograde degeneration, neuronal
injury response, 296
Antibiotics, 55
Antibody (immunoglobulin), 32
antigen binding site (hypervariable
regions), 40
antigen interaction, 40, 41
B cell production, 37, 41
corneal allograft rejection, 75
isotype switching, 41
isotypes (classes), 40, 41
primary/secondary response, 39
structural aspects, 40, 41
Antibody-dependent cell-mediated
cytotoxicity (ADCC), 37, 41, 45, 60
Antibody-mediated (humoral) immunity,
40–1
Antigen, 32
antibody binding site (hypervariable
regions), 40
antibody interaction, 40, 41
lymphocyte activation, 39
presentation, 40
B cell activation, 37
processing, 40, 42
T cell subset interactions, 36
tolerance to self, 41–2
uveitogenic, 43
Antigen–antibody complexes *see*
Immune complexes
Antigen-presenting cells, 32, 36, 40, 42,
163
acute inflammation, 45
antigen processing, 40
dendritic cells, 35
lymphoid organs, 35
macrophages, 34
Antimetabolites, 16, 28
Anti-oncogenes (tumour-suppressor
genes), 147
Antioxidant vitamins, 13
Aphakia, congenital, 154
Aplasia (agenesis), 3, 140
optic nerve, 159
Apocrine cystadenoma, 173, **174**
Apocrine glands, 163
Apoptosis, 2–3
Fas ligand (Fas L)-mediated, 43
neoplastic cells, 143
pathological, 3
physiological, 2–3
Aqueous
cells, 52
flare, 52
immunosuppressive factors, 43
response to injury, 18
Arachnida, 112
Arcus juvenilis, 263
Arcus senilis, **263**
Argon laser, 10
cyclophotocoagulation, 27
trabeculoplasty, 27
Argyll–Robertson pupil, 99
Argyrosis (silver deposits), 258

Aromatic amino-acid derivative deposits, 260–1
Arrestin gene mutations, 246
Arterial structure, 266
Arteriolosclerosis, **268**, 272, 275
  diabetes mellitus, 284
Arteriosclerosis, **267–8**
Arteriovenous (A–V) nipping, 272
Arteriovenous fistulae, 185–6
Arthritis
  childhood, ILAR classification, 69
  juvenile chronic, 69
  juvenile idiopathic, 69
  psoriatic, 68
  reactive, 68, 69, 94
  rheumatoid, 60, 66, 67, 72–3, 261, 289
Arthropods, 76, 112
Arthus reaction, 60
Ascomycetes, 102
Ascorbic acid (vitamin C) deficiency, 13, 16
Ashleaf spots, 209
Aspergillosis, 104
Aspergillus, **102**
  keratitis, 103
  orbital cellulitis, 104
Aspergillus flavus, **102**
Aspergillus fumigatus, **102**
Asphyxia, intraocular haemorrhages, 5
Asteroid hyalosis, **223**
Astrocytes, 296
Astrocytoma, **203**
Ataxia telangiectasia (Louis–Bar syndrome), 55, 56, 125, **132**, 147, 272, 273
Atherosclerosis, **268**, 275
Atopic keratoconjunctivitis, 64–5
Atopy, 59, 217
Atresia, 140
Atrophia bulbi, 54
Atrophy, 2, 3, 139
  denervated muscle, 314
  iris, 308
  neurons, 296
  optic (optic nerve), 18, **298**, 300
Atropine, 63
Atypical coloboma, 151
Atypical mole (dysplastic naevus) and syndrome, 170–1
Atypical mycobacteria, 95
  AIDS opportunistic infection, 59
Autografts, 74
Autoimmune disorders, 54, 60, 65–74
  conjunctiva, 66
  corneoscleral coat, 66–7
  genetic aspects, 65
  lens, 72
  orbit, 72–4
  uvea, 67–71
Autolysis, 2
Autosomal dominant disorders, **120–3**
  congenital cataract, **155–6**
  connective tissue, 122–3
  key features, 121–2

Autosomal recessive disorders, 121, **123–5**
  amino acid metabolism, 126–7
  carbohydrate metabolism, 127–8
  DNA repair, 132
  key features, 123
  lipid metabolism, 128
  lysosomal storage diseases, 129–32
  metabolic disorders, 125
  mineral metabolism, 129
Autosomes, 115
  homologues, 116
Avellino corneal dystrophy, 238
  molecular genetics, 239
Axenfeld's anomaly *and* syndrome, 153
Axial cataract, congenital, 155
Axons, 313
  degeneration (Wallerian degeneration), 18, 313
  glaucomatous optic neuropathy, 304
  regeneration/remyelination, 296, 313
  response to injury, 313

B

B cell deficiencies, primary, 56
  combined T cell deficiencies, 56
B cell lymphoma, 261
  AIDS-related, 57–8
  immunodeficiency-related, 55
  Sjögren's syndrome-related, 73
B cells, 36–7
  activation, 39
  antibody production, 40, 41
  antigen presentation, 40
  differentiation, 35
  lymphoid organs, 35
  memory cells, 39
Bacilli, 88–9, 91–2
  classification, 89
  genetic processes, 88
  Gram reaction, 88–9
  Gram-negative, **91–2**
    autoimmune uveitis/arthritis association, 94
  Gram-positive, **91**
  growth/culture, 88
  harmful host immune responses, 89
  metabolism, 88
  ophthalmic infections, 92–4
    canaliculitis/dacryocystitis, 93
    conjunctivitis, 92–3
    endophthalmitis/panophthalmitis, **94**
    keratitis, 93–4
    orbital cellulitis, 94
  pathogenicity, 89
  spore formation, 88
  structural aspects, 88
Bacillus, 64, 91, 94
Bacillus anthracis, 91
Bacillus cereus, 91
Bacillus subtilis, 91
Bacteria, 76, 85–100

microbiological specimens, 326–7
normal flora, 42
  see also Bacilli, Cocci and individual species
Bacterial defences
  barriers to infection, 42
  cellular, 33
  tears, 42
Bacteroides, 92
Balanced translocation, 118
Balloon cell naevus, **170**
Bancroftian filariasis, 111
Band keratopathy, **255**
  glaucoma, 305
  sarcoidosis, 48
  vitamin D (calciferol) excess, 13
Barkan's membrane, 312
Barriers to infection, 42
Bartonella, 92
Bartonella henselae, 92
Basal cell carcinoma, **167–8**, **169**
  local invasion, 144
Basal cell layer, 163
Basal cell papilloma (seborrhoeic wart; seborrhoeic keratosis), 165, **166**
Basement membrane
  autoantibodies, 60
    ocular cicatricial pemphigoid, 66
  deposit, sub-retinal pigment epithelium, **231**
  lysis, neovascularization, 18
  thickening in diabetes mellitus, 282, **284**, 285
Basic fibroblast growth factor (bFGF), 14–15
Basidiomycetes, 102
Basophils, **34**
  degranulation, 59
  inflammatory mediators, 44
Batten's disease *see* Neuronal ceroid lipofuscinosis
Battered child, 5
Behçet's disease, 65, 288–9
  HLA associations, 289
  posterior/panuveitis, 70
  retinal vasculitis, 60
Benign calcifying epithelioma of Malherbe (pilomatricoma), **175**
Benign (idiopathic) intracranial hypertension, 298
Benign monoclonal gammopathy, 264
Benign mucous membrane pemphigoid *see* Pemphigoid, ocular cicatricial
Benign neoplasms, **143**
Bergmeister's papilla, 157
Beri beri, 13
Berlin's oedema (commotio retinae), 4
Bestrophin, 252
Best's vitelliform macular dystrophy, 243, **251–2**
Beta particles, 8, 11
Bietti's crystalline corneoretinal dystrophy, 240–1, 263
Bilirubin pigment deposits, 259
Biological carcinogens, 146–7

Birbeck granules, **35**
Birdshot retinochoroidopathy, 71
Bitot's spots, 13
Black sunbursts, 294
Blepharitis, 49–50
    anterior (staphylococcal infection),
        50
    posterior, 50
    sequelae, 49
Blepharoconjunctivitis, allergic
        microbial, 64
Blepharoptosis, contact lens wear-
        related, 23
Blessig–Iwanoff cysts, 229
Blink reflex, 42
Blood disorders, 291–4
Blood dyscrasias, 5
Blood pigment deposits, 259, 270
Blood pressure regulation, 280–1
Blood vessel structural abnormalities,
        272–4
Blood–aqueous barrier, 267
Blood–ocular barrier, 267
    immune privilege, 42–3
Blood–retinal barriers, inner/outer, 267
Blue cone monochromatism, 247
Blue naevus, **176**
Blue sclera, 242
Bone healing, 18
Bone marrow, 35, 36
    primary failure (reticular dysgenesis),
        56
Borrelia burgdoferi, 98, 100
Botulinum toxin, 315
Botulism, 315
Bovine spongiform encephalopathy
        (BSE), 76
Bowen's disease (carcinoma *in situ*;
        intraepidermal carcinoma), 141,
        167
Bowman's layer healing, 17
Branch retinal arteriolar occlusion, 276
Branch retinal vein occlusion, 19, 280
Branhamella catarrhalis, 90
BRCA2, 193
Brucella, 68
    autoimmune uveitis/arthritis
        association, 94
Bruch's membrane
    ageing changes, 230
    degenerations
        age-related, 235
        non-age-related, 234–5
    dystrophies, 252–3
    retinal detachment-related changes,
        227
Brushfield's spots, 119, 154
Bullous keratopathy, 305
Buphthalmos, 304, 305, **312**, 313
Burkitt's lymphoma, 81, 146, 204
Burns
    acid, 12
    alkali, 11–12
    macular, 10
    thermal, 7

Bursa of Fabricius, 36
Busacca nodules, 52

C

C3 receptors, 41
C-reactive protein, 45
Cachexia of neoplastic disease, 145
Café au lait spots, 209
Calabar swellings, 111
Calciferol (vitamin D) excess, 13
Calcification
    diffuse corneal, 256
    dystrophic, 254–5
    idiopathic, 255
    metastatic, 255
Calcitonin gene-related peptide (CGRP),
        43, 44
Calcium oxalate deposition, 256
Calcium salt deposits, **254–6**
Callus, 18
Campylobacter, 68
    autoimmune uveitis/arthritis
        association, 94
Canaliculitis, bacterial, 93
Canaliculus, microbiological specimens,
        327
Cancer-associated retinopathy, 145–6
Candida, 55, 63, 102, 103
    AIDS opportunistic infection, 57, 59
    endophthalmitis, 104
    keratitis, 103
Candida albicans, **103**, 104
Capillaropathy, diabetes mellitus, 282,
        283, 284
Capillary haemangioma (strawberry
        naevus), **175–6**
    orbit, 185
Capsid, 77
Capsomere, 77
Capsulotomy anterior, 27
Carbohydrate metabolism disorders,
        125, 127–8
Carcinoembryonic antigen, 145
Carcinogenesis, 146–7
    host factors, 147
Carcinogens, 146–7
Carcinoma
    anogenital, AIDS-related, 58
    basal cell, 167–8, **169**
        local invasion, 144
    conjunctival, AIDS-related, 58, 59
    intraepidermal (carcinoma *in situ*;
        Bowen's disease), 141, **167**
    lacrimal sac, 183
    Merkel cell, **172**
    mucoepidermoid, 179, 185
    nasopharyngeal, 146
    pleomorphic, 184–5
    sebaceous, **172–3**
    squamous cell 59, 168, **169**, **179**,
        185
    sweat gland, 175
    thyroid, 73

Carcinoma *in situ* (intraepidermal
        carcinoma; Bowen's disease), 141, **167**
Carcinomatosis, 144
Carotid artery disease, 278, 279
Cartilaginous proliferations, 190
Caruncle, 177
Caseous necrosis, 2
Cat-scratch disease, 92
Cataract, 220, 221–2
    alkali burns, 12
    axial, 155
    calcification, 255
    cerulean, 156
    Christmas tree, 222
    congenital, 155–6
        autosomal dominant, **155–6**
        types, 155
    Coppock, 156
    cortical, 222
    diabetes mellitus, 282, 287
    fibre-based/non-fibre-based, 222
    galactosaemia, **128**
    glassblowers', 9, 220
    hypermature, 222
    inflammation-related, 53
    infrared radiation exposure-related, 9
    lamellar, 155
    lightning, 8
    mature, 222
    microwave exposure-related, 9
    Morgagnian, 222, **223**, 256
    nuclear, 155, 222
    polar, 155
    posterior capsule, 221
    radiation exposure related (radiation
        cataract), 11
    sunflower, 258
    sutural, 155
    trauma-related, 4, 18
Cataract surgery
    complications, 26–7
    intraocular lenses, 27
    lens/lens capsule manipulation, 27
Catarrhal infiltrates/keratitis (marginal
        keratitis), 64
Cavernous haemangioma, 176
    choroid, 201–2
    orbit, 185, **186**
    retina, 202
CD (cluster designation/cluster of
        differentiation) classification, 32
CD3, 36
CD4, 36, 38
    T cells *see* Helper T cells (T$_H$)
CD8, 36, 38
    T cells *see* Cytotoxic/suppressor T
        cells (T$_{C/S}$)
CD19, 38
CD20, 36
CD45, 32
CD68, 34
CD79a, 36, 37
CDKN2A (p16), 193
Cell
    adhesion, 17

injury, 2–14
migration, 17
proliferation, 17, 139
Cell cycle, 139
Cell-mediated hypersensitivity reactions
see Hypersensitivity Type IV
reactions
Cell-mediated immunity, 40
bacterial pathogenicity, 89
response to malignant neoplasms, 145
Cellophane maculopathy, 228
Cellular oedema, acute (hydropic
change; cloudy swelling), 2
Cellular phase of wound healing, 16
Cellulitis, orbital, 49, 51, 94, 104
Central areolar choroidal dystrophy
(central areolar choroidal sclerosis),
243, 245, 253
Central nervous system, 296
cells/cellular response to injury, 296–7
Central retinal artery, 266
Central retinal artery occlusion, **275–6**
Central retinal vein, 266
Central retinal vein occlusion, 278,
279–80
ischaemic, 279–80
neovascular (thrombotic) glaucoma,
308
non-ischaemic, 279
pathogenesis, 280
Central serous choroidoretinopathy, 234
Cephalocele, 184
Cerebrospinal fluid, 297–8
Cerulean cataract, 156
Cestodes (tapeworms), 108, 111–12
Chalazion ('meibomian cyst'), 46–7, **48**,
165
Chalcosis, 6, 258
Chandler's syndrome, 308
Charcot–Leyden crystals, 61, 62
Charcot–Marie Tooth disease, 298
CHARGE syndrome, 161
Chédiak–Higashi syndrome, 55, 126
Chemical carcinogens, 146
Chemical injury, 11–12
secondary glaucoma, 311
Chemical mediators
acute inflammation, 44
Type I hypersensitivity reactions, 59
Chemical warfare, 12
Chemokines, 39, 44
Chemotaxis, 39
Chickenpox (varicella), 80, 81
Childhood arthritis, ILAR classification,
69
Children, non-accidental injury, 4–5
Chlamydia pectorum, 86
Chlamydia pneumoniae, 86
Chlamydia psittaci, 86
Chlamydia trachomatis, 86, 87, 93
biovars, 86
Chlamydial infection, 68, 69, **86–7**
inclusion bodies, 86, **87**
investigations, **87**
microbiological specimens, 326

oculogenital disease, 86
adult conjunctivitis, 86
neonatal conjunctivitis, 86, 87, 93
'Chloroma' (granulocytic sarcoma), 207
Chloroquine, 261, 264
Chlorpromazine, 264
CHM, 254
Cholesterol
deposits, 263–4
granuloma, 46, **47**
low-density-lipoprotein (LDL), 268
Chondrodystrophy, 242
Choristoma, 140–1
complex, 178
conjunctiva, 178
intraocular, 191
lids, 164–5
orbit, 183–4
osseous, choroidal (choroidal
osteoma), 191
osseous, epibulbar, 178
Choroid
circulation, immune function, 42
electromagnetic radiation protection,
8
histological sections examination, 325
hypertensive damage, 282
mechanical trauma, 4
posterior intraocular inflammation,
53
response to injury, 18
Choroidal dystrophies, 242–54
central areolar (central areolar
choroidal sclerosis), 243, 245,
253
Choroidal haemangioma, 201–2
Choroidal ischaemia, 279
Choroidal melanoma, 193–4, **195**, **196**
see also Melanoma, uvea
Choroidal naevus, **191**, 192
Choroidal neovascularization, 20
age-related macula degeneration, 232,
233–4
Choroidal osteoma (osseous
choristoma), 191
Choroidal sclerosis
central areolar, 243, 245, 253
diffuse, 253
Choroidectomy specimens, 319
Choroideremia, 254
Choroiditis, 52
Choroidoretinal adhesions, **54**
Choroidoretinal dystrophies, 253–4
Choroidoretinal scarring, 54
Choroidoretinitis, 53
Christmas tree cataract, 222
Chromate sensitivity, 63
Chromatolysis, central, 296
Chromophores, 220, 222
Chromosomal abnormalities, 117–19
biological effects, 118
congenital malformations, 140
mosaicism, 118
neoplasia, 143, 147
numerical, 117

syndromic associations, 118–19
structural, 117–18
syndromic associations, 119
Chromosomal nondisjunction, 117
Chromosomes, 115
homologues, 116
Philadelphia, 147
replication, 139
ring, 118
Chronic granulomatous disease (CGD),
55
Chronic mucocutaneous candidiasis
(CMC), 55–6
Chrysiasis (gold deposits), 258–9
Cicatricial entropion, 16
Ciliary body
coloboma, 150
histological sections examination, 325
inflammation sequelae, 53
ischaemia, 278
mechanical trauma, 4
melanoma, **193**, 194, 196
naevus, 191
response to injury, 18
Ciliary epithelium
pseudoadenomatous hyperplasia, 53,
139, **190**
response to injury, 18
Clear cell hidradenoma, 174
Climatic droplet keratopathy (spheroidal
degeneration; Labrador
keratopathy), **215**
Clonal deletion, 41
Cloquet's canal, 156
Clostridium, 2, 91
orbital cellulitis, 94
Clostridium botulinum, 91, 315
Clostridium perfringens, 91
Clostridium tetani, 91
Clotting cascade, 44
Cloudy swelling (acute cellular oedema;
hydropic change), 2
Coagulase, 89
Coagulative necrosis, 2
Coats' disease, **272–3**
Cocci, 88–90
classification, 89
genetic processes, 88
Gram reaction, 88–9
Gram-negative, **90**
Gram-positive, **89–90**
growth/culture, 88
harmful host immune responses, 89
metabolism, 88
ophthalmic infections, 92–4
canaliculitis/dacryocystitis, 93
conjunctivitis, 92–3
endophthalmitis/panophthalmitis,
94
keratitis, 93–4
orbital cellulitis, 94
pathogenicity, 89
spore formation, 88
structural aspects, 88
Coccidioides immitis, 63, 102, 103

Cockaigne's syndrome, 249
Codons, 116
Cogan–Rees (iris naevus) syndrome, 308
Cogan's microcystic corneal dystrophy
(epithelial basement membrane
dystrophy; map-dot-fingerprint
dystrophy), **236**
Cogan's syndrome, 67
Collagen
scar tissue formation, 15
wound healing, 17
Colliquative necrosis (liquefaction), 2
Coloboma, 148, **150–1**
atypical, 151
chromosomal abnormalities, 118
ciliary body, 150
fundus, 150–1
iris, **150**
lens, 155
lid, 162
macula, 151
optic disc/nerve, **151**
Colobomatous microphthalmos, 161
Colony stimulating factors (CSFs), 39,
44
Colour vision
defects, 246, 247–8
molecular genetics, 247
Commensalism, 76
Commotio retinae (Berlin's oedema), 4
Complement activation, 39
acute inflammation, 44, 45
alternative pathway, 39, 41
classical pathway, 39, 41
immunoglobulins, 41
lectin pathway, 39
Type II (cytotoxic) hypersensitivity
reactions, 59–60
Complement deficiencies, 55
Complement system, 39
Complex choristoma, 178
Compound naevus, 168, **169–70**
conjunctiva, 179, **180**
Compressive optic neuropathy, 303
Concussion, 3, 4
Cone–rod dystrophies, progressive, **250**
Cones, 244
absence/absent function, 247
light transduction, 244
pigments, 244
molecular genetics, 247
progressive dystrophies, 250
stationary dysfunctions
(dyschromatopsias), 244, 246–8
Congenital malformations, 140–1
embryonic period, 148
fetal period, 148
pre-embryonic period, 148
see also Developmental anomalies
Congenital stationary night blindness
(CSNB), 243, 244, 245–6
abnormal fundi, 246
complete, 246
incomplete, 246
normal fundi, 245–6

Rigg's Type (CSNB 1), 246
Schubert–Bornschein Type (CSNB 2),
246
Conidial fungi, 102–3
Conjunctiva
accessory lacrimal gland
proliferations, 182
allergic disease, 61–5
autoimmune disorders, 66
bacterial flora, 42
chemical burns-related scarring, 12
contact lens wear-related injury, 22–3
degenerations, 214–18
epithelium, 177
epithelial cell proliferations, 178–9
melanocyte proliferations, 179–81
growth disorders (proliferations),
176–83
impression cytology, 321
lymphatic proliferations, 181–2
lymphatics, 35
lymphoproliferative lesions, **204**
mechanical trauma, 3
microbial barrier function, 42
microbiological specimens, 326
non-epithelial melanocyte
proliferations, 182–3
scrapings, 321
specimens, 319
subepithelial connective tissue, 177
thermal burns, 7
ultraviolet light absorption, 10
vascular proliferations, 181
wound healing, 16
Conjunctiva-associated lymphoid tissue
(CALT), 35
Conjunctival carcinoma, AIDS-related,
58, 59
Conjunctival choristoma, 178
Conjunctival cysts, 177
Conjunctival intraepithelial neoplasia
(Conj.IN), 141, **178–9**
Conjunctival melanosis, secondary, 260
Conjunctival xerosis, vitamin A
deficiency, 13
Conjunctivitis, 49, 50–1
acute allergic, 61
artefacta, 3
bacterial, 50, 51, 92–3
chronic infection, 93
investigations, 93
chlamydial, 86
discharge, 50
follicular, 48, **50–1**, 77
giant papillary *see* Giant papillary
conjunctivitis
graft-versus host reactions, 76
ligneous, 50, **51**
lymphadenopathy, 51
membranes/pseudomembranes, 50
neonatal (ophthalmia neonatorum),
86, 93
oedema (chemosis), 50
papillae, **51**
sequelae, 49

toxic, 22
vasodilatation, 50
vernal *see* Vernal keratoconjunctivitis
viral, 50, 51
Connective tissue disorders, autosomal
dominant, 122–3
Consanguineous marriage, 123
Constant region, 40
Contact allergy, 60–1
Contact dermatoconjunctivitis/keratitis,
63
Contact lens disinfecting solutions, 22
Contact lens wear-related disorders,
21–3
allergic/toxic responses, 21
bacterial conjunctivitis, 93
conjunctiva, 22–3
cornea, 21–2
giant papillary conjunctivitis *see* Giant
papillary conjunctivitis
hypoxia/hypercapnia, 21, 22
infective keratitis, 22, 93
lids, 23
mechanical injury, 21
osmotic effects, 21
sterile infiltrates, 22
tear film, 23
Contagious pustular dermatitis (orf), 83
Contracture phase of wound healing, 16
sclera, 18
Contre coup injury, 3
Contusion, 3
Conus (congenital crescent), 161
Copper, 19
deposits, 257–8
ocular damage, 129
Coppock cataract, 156
Cornea
allergic disease, 61–4
blood staining, **259**
contact lens wear-related injury, 21–2
deformation, 22
deposits, 255–6, 258, 259, 263–4
developmental anomalies, 152
diabetic complications, 287
diffuse calcification, 256
electromagnetic radiation protection,
8
histological sections examination,
325
immune privilege
avascularity, 42–3
corneal allograft survival, 75
incisions, complications, 25
microbiological specimens
biopsy, 327
scrapings, 326–7
normal development, 151
tattoo pigment, **259**
ultraviolet light absorption, 10
ultraviolet light-related damage, 10
wound healing, 16–18
surgical wounds, 23
Cornea guttata, **216**, 241
Cornea plana, 152

Cornea verticillata (vortex keratopathy), 17, 264
Corneal allograft, 75–6
  corneal immune privilege, 75
  rejection, 26, 75–6
    endothelial, 75–6
    epithelial, 75
    stromal, 75
    Type IV hypersensitivity, 60-1
Corneal arcus, 263
Corneal degenerations
  pellucid marginal, 217
  spheroidal, *see* Climatic droplet
    keratopathy
  Salzmann's nodular, **215–16**
  Terrien's marginal degeneration, 215
Corneal discs, 319
Corneal dystrophies, 235–42
  anterior, 236–7
  Avellino, 238
  Cogan's microcystic (epithelial
    basement membrane dystrophy;
    map-dot-fingerprint dystrophy),
    236
  congenital hereditary endothelial, **242**
    dominant variant, 242
  endothelial, 241–2
  epithelial basement membrane
    dystrophy (Cogan's microcystic
    corneal dystrophy; map-dot-
    fingerprint dystrophy), **236**
  Fuchs' endothelial, **241**
  gelatinous drop-like, 239, **240**
  granular, **237–8**
  lattice, **238–9**
  map-dot-fingerprint (epithelial
    basement membrane dystrophy;
    Cogan's microcystic dystrophy),
    236
  Meesmann's juvenile epithelial, 236,
    237
  polymorphic stromal, 239
  posterior polymorphous, 241, **242**
  Reis–Bückler's, **236–7**
  Schnyder's central crystalline, 240,
    263
  stromal, 237–41
  Waardenburg Jonker's (superficial
    granular), 238
Corneal endothelium
  contact lens wear-related injury, 22
  surgery-related damage, 24
  surgical incisions, 25
  wound healing, 17–18
Corneal epithelium
  contact lens wear-related injury, 22
  iron lines, **256**
  microbial barrier function, 42
  surgical incisions, 25
  wound healing, 17
Corneal erosions
  punctate epithelial erosions (PEE), 51
  recurrent, 17
Corneal filaments, 51, 263
Corneal keloid, 216

Corneal neovascularization, 20–1
  pannus, 20, **21**
  stromal, 20, **21**
Corneal oedema, 51, 52
  glaucoma, 305
Corneal scarring, mustard gas, 12
Corneal siderosis, 3, **256**
Corneal stroma
  contact lens wear-related injury, 22
  neovascularization, 20, **21**, 22
  wound healing, 17
Corneal stromal oedema
  corneal allograft rejection, 75
  glaucoma, 305
  intraocular surgery-related, 24
  keratitis, 52
Corneal xerosis/ulceration, vitamin A
  deficiency, 13
Corneolimbal incisions, complications,
  25
Corneorefractive procedures,
  complications, 26
Corneoscleral coat
  autoimmune disorders, 66–7
  degenerations, 214–18
  developmental anomalies, 152-3
  ectasias, 216–18
  glaucomatous damage, 305
  inflammation, 49, 51–2
    sequelae, 49
  mechanical trauma, **3–4**
    perforation, **5–6**
  normal development, 151
  staphyloma, 216–18
Cortical cataract, 222
Corticosteroids
  endothelial cell proliferation
    inhibition, 19
  fungal endophthalmitis susceptibility,
    104
  glaucoma induction, **311–12**
  immunodeficiency, 55
  postoperative intraocular pressure
    elevation, 24
  trabeculectomy support, 28
  wound healing impairment, 16
Cortisol-binding globulin, 43
Corynebacterium, 91
Corynebacterium diphtheriae, 42, 50, 91
  conjunctivitis, 93
  keratitis, 93
Corynebacterium xerosis, 13, 91
Cotton-wool spots, 58, **278**, 281, 285,
  289, 297
Cowden's disease, 210
Cowdry type A inclusions, 79, 80, 81
Coxsackieviruses, 84, 317
Cranial neuropathies, 287, 313–14
Craniofacial dysostoses, 159
Crescent, congenital (conus), 161
Creutzfeldt–Jakob disease (CJD), 76
Crohn's disease, 68, 261
CRYBB2, 156
Cryotherapy, 7
Cryptococcus neoformans, 102, 103

AIDS opportunistic infection, 57, 59
Cryptosporidium, 104
Crystalline keratopathy, **263–4**
Crystallins, 219, 221
  age-related changes, 219, 220
  gene mutations, 156
Cutaneous leishmaniasis, 104
Cyanocobalamin (vitamin B_{12})
  deficiency, 13, 291, 302
Cyclectomy specimens, 319
Cyclitis, 52
Cyclocongestive glaucoma, 311
Cyclocryotherapy, 27
Cyclodestruction, 27
Cyclodialysis, 4, 27
  battered child, 5
Cyclophotocoagulation *see* Laser
  cyclophotocoagulation
Cyclopia, 148, 149
  del 18p, 119
Cylindroma, 173
Cystadenoma, apocrine, 173, **174**
Cystic eye, congenital (del 12p), 119
Cystic naevus, 179, **180**
Cystine deposits, 263–4
Cystinosis, 127, 264
Cystoid degeneration of peripheral
  retina, **229**
Cystoid macular oedema, **24–5**, 53
Cysts
  aneurysmal bone, 190
  Blessig–Iwanoff, 229
  conjunctiva, 177
  dermoid, **164**
  epidermoid (keratinous), **164**
  epithelial, 178
  hyaloid, 157
  inclusion, 16
  intraocular, 190
  iris, **190**
  leaking, **164–5**
  lids, 164–5
  microphthalmos with cyst, 184
  Moll, 165
  orbit, 183–4
  sweat gland (sudoriferous), **165**
Cystic eye, congenital, 148, 149
Cytokines, 38–9
  acute inflammation, 44
  acute phase response, 45
  cell-mediated immunity, 40
Cytology, 321
Cytomegalovirus, 73, 79, 81–2, 292
  AIDS opportunistic infection, 57, 59
  cytopathic effect, 81
  fetal infection, 81–2
  immunocompromised host, 82
  retinitis, 59, 71, **82–3**
Cytopathic effect, 77
Cytotoxic reactions *see* Hypersensitivity
  Type II reactions
Cytotoxic/suppressor T cells
  ($T_{C/S}CD8+$), 36, 37, 39, 40
  corneal allograft rejection, 75
Cytotoxicity, complement system, 39

D

Dacryocystitis, bacterial, 93
DAG-PKC pathway, 283, 287
Dalén–Fuchs' nodules, 70, **71**
Degenerations, 214–35
  age-related of macula/posterior pole,
    230–4
  conjunctiva, 214–18
  corneoscleral coat, 214–18
  lens, 218–22
  peripheral retina, 229–30
  retinal pigment epithelium (RPE),
    234–5
  vitreoretinal interface, 223–9
  vitreous, 223
  zonule, 223
Degenerative retinoschisis, 229–30
Degenerative vascular disease, 267–8
Delayed-type hypersensitivity *see*
    Hypersensitivity Type IV reactions
Deletions, 117, 118
  syndromic associations, 119
Demodex folliculorum, **112**
Demyelination
  primary, 296–7
  secondary, 297
  segmental, 313
Dendritic cells, 35, 40
  interdigitating, 35
  lids, 163
Denervation
  muscle atrophy, 314
  wound healing impairment, 16
Dental caries, 90
Deposits, 254–64
  amyloid, 261–3
  aromatic amino-acid derivatives,
    260–1
  blood pigment, 259, 270
  calcium salts, **254–6**
  cholesterol, 263–4
  copper, 257–8
  cystine, 263–4
  drugs, 264
  ferritin, 259
  gold (chrysiasis), 258–9
  haemosiderin, 270
  hexosylceramides, 264
  iron, 256–7
  leukaemic, 207
  lipid, 263
  mercury, 259
  metastatic, 144–5, 148, 210–11
  metals/metal compounds, 254–9
  paraproteins, 264
  silver (argyrosis), 258
  sub-retinal pigment epithelium (RPE),
    230–1
  uric acid, 263–4
Dermal melanocyte proliferations, 176
Dermatoconjunctivitis/keratitis, contact
  63
Dermatomyositis, 317
Dermoid cyst, **164**

orbit, 183
Dermoids, **178**
Dermolipoma, 177-8
Descemet's membrane
  folds, 52
  surgical incision injury, 25
  wound healing, 17
Desmosomes, 144
Determination, 139–40
Deuteranopia, 247
Development, 148
  anterior segment, 151–2
  cornea, 151
  corneoscleral coat, 151
  drainage angle, 151–2
  iris, 152
  lens, 154
  ocular adnexae, 161–2
  optic disc/optic nerve, 159
  retina, 157
  retinal circulation, 276
  sclera, 152
  trabecular meshwork, 151–2
  vasculature, 156
  vitreous, 156
Developmental anomalies, 148–62
  anterior segment, 151–4
  corneoscleral coat, 151–4
  lens, 154–6
  ocular adnexae, 162
  ocular vasculature, 156–7
  optic disc/optic nerve, 159–61
  organogenesis, 149–51
  retina, 157–9
  size of eye, 161
  vitreous, 156–7
Devic's disease (neuromyelitis optica),
  301
Di George syndrome, 55
Diabetes mellitus, 268, 273, 278, 282–7,
  301
  angiogenic growth factors, 283
  arteriolosclerosis, 283
  capillaropathy, 282, 283
  cataract, 222, 282, 287
  corneal complications, 287
  cranial neuropathies, 287, 313–14
  DAG–PKC pathway, 283
  ectropion uveae, 287
  genetic factors, 135, 282
  glycaemic control, 283
  haematological abnormalities, 282
  iridopathy, **287**
  macroangiopathy, 283
  microangiopathy, 283
  neovascular glaucoma, 287, 308
  optic nerve lesions, 287
  papillopathy, 287
  polyol pathway, 282
  protein glycosylation, 282
  retinopathy *see* Diabetic retinopathy
  rubeosis iridis, 287
  Type I (insulin-dependent), 282, 283
    HLA associations, 282

Type II (non-insulin-dependent), 282,
  283
Diabetic retinopathy, 19, 282–7
  angiogenic growth factors, 287
  DAG–PKC pathway, 287
  non-proliferative, 284–5
  background, **284–5**
  maculopathy, 285
  preproliferative, **285–6**
    intraretinal microvascular
      abnormalities(IRMAs), 286
  preretinopathy, 283–4
  proliferative, **286–7**
    neovascularization, 286–7
Diacylglyceral (DAG), 283
Diathermy, 7, 8
Dichromatism, 247
Differentiation, 139–40
  abnormalities in mature tissue, 141–8
  malignant cells, 144
Diffuse atrophy of choriocapillaris
    (diffuse choroidal sclerosis), 253
Diffuse choroidal atrophy, 245
Diffuse corneal calcification, 256
Diffuse melanosis of skin, 260
Diphtheroids, 42
  keratitis, 93
Diptera (flies), 112
Disciform keratopathy, 80
Disorganization of intraocular
    architecture, 5, **6**
Distal axonopathy, 313
DNA, 115, 116
  damage, 11
  mitochondrial, 116
  mutations, 116–17
  neoplasia-related changes, 143, 144,
    146, 147
  non-chromosomal, 116
  synthesis, 139
DNA repair disorders, 125, 132
  gene mutations, 147
DNA viruses, 77–84
Dominant drusen (Doyne's honeycomb
    choroiditis; Malattia-levantinese),
    232, 243, **252**
Dot-blot retinal haemorrhages, 270
Down's syndrome (trisomy 21), 118–19,
    154, 217, 218
Doyne's honeycomb choroiditis
    (dominant drusen; Malattia-
    levantinese), 232, 243, **252**
Drainage angle development, 151–2
Drug deposits, 264
Drug reactions
  contact dermatoconjunctivitis/
    keratitis, 63
  Stevens–Johnson syndrome (erythema
    multiforme), 65
Drug-related wound healing impairment,
  16
Drusen, **230–1**, 272
  age-related macular degeneration,
    231, 232, 233, 234
  calcification, **231**, 255

dominant, 232, 243, **252**
optic disc (hyaline bodies), 160–1
peripheral, 235
Dry eye, 49, 141
contact lens wear-related, 23
radiation exposure related, 11
Duplications, 117, 118
Dyschromatopsias, 244, 246–8
Dysgenesis, 140
Dyskeratosis, 141, **142**
Dysplasia, 2, 141, **142**
Dysplastic naevus (atypical mole) and
syndrome, 170–1
Dysthyroid orbitopathy, **73–4**
HLA associations, 73, 74
Dystrophic calcification, 254–5
Dystrophies, 235–54
choroidoretinal, 253–4
corneal, 235–42
macular, 239–40
muscular, 316
retina/choroid, 242–54
sclera, 242

E

E-selectin, 38
Eales' disease, 288
Eaton–Lambert syndrome *see*
Lambert–Eaton syndrome
Eccrine poroma, 174
Echinococcus granulosus, 112
Eclipse blindness, 10
Ectasias, corneoscleral coat, 216–18
Ectopia, 140
Ectopia lentis, 310
congenital, 155
Ectropion, lid, 49
Ectropion uveae, **20**
diabetes mellitus, 287
Eczema, 59
EDTA contact sensitivity, 63
Edward's syndrome (trisomy 18), 119
EFEMP1, 252
Ehlers–Danlos syndrome, 123, 217, 234,
235
Electrical injury, 8
Electrolysis, 8
Electromagnetic radiation, 8–11
ionizing, 8, 10–11
non-ionizing, 9
ocular protective mechanisms, 8–9
properties, 8
tissue effects, 9
tissue injury susceptibility, 8
tissue transmission/absorption, 8
Electromagnetic spectrum, 8
Electron microscopy, 320
Elschnig's pearls, 5
Elschnig's spots, 279, 282
Embolism, **275**
Embryonal sarcoma (embryonal
rhabdomyosarcoma), **189**
Embryonic fissure closure, 148, 149
failure, 150–1

Embryonic period, 148
Embryopathy
LSD, 150, 161
rubella (congenital rubella syndrome),
85, 161, 222
Embryotoxon, posterior, 153
Encephalopathy
bovine spongiform (BSE), 76
transmissible mink, 76
Wernicke's, 302
Encephalotrigeminal angiomatosis
(Sturge–Weber syndrome), 176,
201, 208
Endocarditis, bacterial, 90
Endocrine exophthalmos (dysthyroid
orbitopathy), **73–4**
Endophthalmitis, 52
bacterial, **94**
corneoscleral perforation, 5
fungal, 104
investigations, 94
lens-induced (phacoantigenic
endophthalmitis), 4, 5, 18, 60, **72**
Endothelium-derived inflammatory
mediators, 44
Endothelial cell angiogenesis factor
(ECAF), 15
Endothelial cell blebs, 22
Endothelial cells
corneal wound healing, 17–18
loss, 278, 284-5
migration, 19
proliferation, 19
Endothelins, 44
Endotoxins, 89
Enterobacter aerogenes, 92
Enterobacter cloacae, 92
Enterobacteriaceae, 91–2
exogenous endophthalmitis, 94
Enteroviruses, 84
Entropion, 49
cicatricial, 16
Enucleation specimens, 319–20
injection techniques, 321
museum specimen examination,
323–4
Enucleations, complications, 28
Enzyme deficiency, genetic aspects, 125
Enzyme immunoassay (enzyme linked
immunosorbent assay; ELISA), 328
Eosinophilic cationic protein, 33
Eosinophilic chemotactic factor of
anaphylaxis (ECF-A), 33, 59
Eosinophilic granuloma, 206
Eosinophilic major basic protein
(EMBP), 33, 34, 62
Eosinophilic peroxidase, 33
Eosinophils, **33–4**
degranulation, 33
inflammatory mediators, 44
non-granulomatous chronic
inflammation, 46
Type I hypersensitivity reactions, 59
Ephelis (freckle), 260
axillary, 209

Epibulbar osseous choristoma, 178
Epicapsular stars, 157
Epidemic keratoconjunctivitis, 78
Epidermal-associated structures, 163–4
Epidermal growth factor (EGF), 14
Epidermal melanocytes, 163
proliferations
benign, 168–71
intraepidermal, 171
malignant, 171–2
Epidermidalization, 13
Epidermis, 163
ultraviolet light absorption, 10
Epidermoid (keratinous) cyst, **164**
orbit, 183
Epinephrine, 260
Epiretinal membrane, 228
Episcleral fibrosis, 16
Episcleral wound healing, 16
Epithelial basement membrane corneal
dystrophy (Cogan's microcystic
dystrophy; map-dot-fingerprint
dystrophy), **236**
Epithelial cell proliferations, 178–9
benign, 178
intraepithelial, 178–9
malignant, 179
see also Epithelial melanocyte
proliferations
Epithelial cysts, 178
Epithelial displacement, **5**
Epithelial implantation
cysts, 5
surgical incision complications, 25
Epithelial keratitis, 79–80
Epithelial melanocyte proliferations,
179–81
benign, 179–80
intraepithelial, 180
malignant, 180–1
Epithelial oedema
glaucoma, 305
keratitis, 51
Epithelialization of anterior segment, 5
Epithelioid histiocytes (epithelioid cells),
granulomatous chronic
inflammation, **46**
Epithelium, conjunctiva, 177
Epstein–Barr virus, 58, 73, 79, 81
oncogenesis, 146–7
ophthalmic manifestations, 81
serological diagnosis, 81
Erdheim–Chester disease, 205
Erythema migrans, 100
Erythema multiforme *see*
Stevens–Johnson syndrome
Erythrocytosis *see* Polycythaemia
Escherichia coli, 64, 92
conjunctivitis, 93
keratitis, 93
Essential iris atrophy, 308
Eukaryotes, 76
Evisceration
complications, 28
specimens, 319

Excimer laser, 10
  mechanism of tissue damage, 9
  photorefractive keratectomy
    complications, **26**
Exenteration, complications, 28
Exenteration specimens, 320
  museum specimen examination,
    323–4
Exons, 116
Exophthalmos, endocrine (dysthyroid
    orbitopathy), **73–4**
Exotoxins, 89
Expulsive haemorrhage, **271**
Extracellular matrix
  corneal wound healing, 17
  scar tissue formation, 15
Extraocular inflammation, 49–51
  sequelae, 49
Extraocular muscles, 314
  complications of surgery, 28
Exudates, 269
Eyeworm, African (*Loa loa*), **111**

F

Fab fragments, 40
Fabry's disease (angiokeratoma
    diffusum; galactosidase deficiency),
    17, 133–4, 264
Familial exudative vitreoretinopathy,
    273
Farinaceous epithelial keratopathy of
    Tobgy, 62
Fas, 43
Fas ligand (Fas L)-mediated apoptosis,
    43
Fat necrosis, 2, 18
Fatty acids, 42
Fatty change, cell injury, 2
Fc fragment, 40
Fc receptors, 33, 41
Ferritin deposits, 259
Ferry's line, 256
Fetal period, 148
Fever, 45, 145
Fibre folds, lens substance, 221
Fibrillin, 122, 223
Fibrinoid necrosis, 2
Fibrinolysis, 44
Fibroblast growth factors (FGFs),
    14–15, 19
Fibroblasts
  cytokines, 38, 39
  proliferative lesions, 205–7
Fibroepithelial polyp (squamous cell
    papilloma; skin tag), **166**
Fibrosarcoma, 189
Fibrosis, 54
  anterior subcapsular of lens, 4
Fibrotic vasoproliferation, **19**
Fibrous dysplasia, 190
Fibrous histiocytoma (fibrous
    xanthoma), **205**
Fibrous ingrowth, surgical incision
    complications, 25

Fibrous xanthoma (fibrous
    histiocytoma), **205**
Filariasis, Bancroftian, 111
Filtering (fistulizing) procedures *see*
    Glaucoma surgery
Filtration bleb, 28
Fimbriae, 88, 91
Fine needle biopsy, 321
First (primary) intention healing, 16, 23
Fixation for histology, 319
Flagellae, 88
Flame-shaped haemorrhages, 270, 297
Fleischer's ring, 217, **256**
Fleurettes, 199, **200**
Flexner–Wintersteiner rosettes, 199, **200**
Flies (Diptera), **112**
Flukes (trematodes), 108, 111
5-Fluorouracil, 16, 28
Flynn Aird syndrome, 249
Follicular conjunctivitis, **50–1**
  adenoviruses, 77
  sarcoidosis, 48
Follicular dendritic cells, 35
Foreign bodies
  granulomatous reactions, 3, 46
  intraocular, 5–6, **7**
  mechanical trauma
    corneoscleral coat, **3–4**
    lids/conjunctiva, 3
Foreign body giant cells, 46, **47**
Foveal schisis, 243
Foveolar detachment, 228
Foveomacular dystrophy, adult-onset
    with choroidal neovascularization,
    245
Fowl pest (Newcastle disease), 85
Frameshift mutations, 117
Francisella, 92
Francisella tularensis, 92
Freckle (ephelis), 260
  axillary, 209
Free radical-mediated damage
  acute inflammation, 44
  carcinogenesis, 146
  radiation injury, 9, 11
  reperfusion injury, 12
  visible light, 10
  vitamin E/vitamin A protective effect,
    13
Freezing injury, slow/fast, 7
Friedreich's ataxia, 249, 298
Frozen orbit, 49
Frozen sections, 320
Fuchs' 'adenoma', **190**
Fuchs' endothelial corneal dystrophy,
    241
Fuchs' uveitis syndrome (Fuchs'
    heterochromic iridocyclitis), 70
Fundus albipunctatus, 246
Fundus coloboma, 150–1
Fundus flavimaculatus, 245, 251
  see also Stargardt's disease
Fungi, 22, 76, 100–4, 292
  classification, 101
  conidial, 102

endophthalmitis, 104
  granulomatous inflammation, 46, 60
  growth/culture, 101
  higher, 102–3
  keratitis, 103, **104**
  lower, 101–2
  microbiological specimens, 326–7
  ophthalmic infections, 101
  orbital cellulitis, 104
  reproductive processes, 100
  staining, 101
  structural aspects, 100
Fusarium, 102
  keratitis, 103
Fusarium solani, 102

G

Galactokinase deficiency, 128
Galactosaemia, 125, 127–8
  cataract formation, **128**
  galactokinase deficiency, 128
  galactose-1-phosphate uridyl
    transferase deficiency, 128
Galactose-1-phosphate uridyl transferase
    deficiency, 128
Galactosidase deficiency (Fabry's
    disease; angiokeratoma diffusum),
    17, 133–4, 264
Gamma-rays, 8, 11
Gangliosidoses, 130
Gangrene, 2
Gardner's syndrome, 158, 210
Gas gangrene, 94
Gelatinous drop-like corneal dystrophy,
    239, **240**, 263
Genes, 115–16
Genetic aspects, 115–35
  autoimmunity, 65
  differentiation, 139–40
  glaucoma, 135, **305**
  myopia, 135
  neoplasia, 143, 146
  oncogenesis, 147
  uveal melanoma, 147, 193
Genetic code, 116
Genetic counselling, 121
Genetic disorders, 115, 117–35
  chromosomal abnormalities, 117–19
  mitochondrial inheritance, 134–5
  multifactorial, 135
  radiation damage, 9
  single gene defects, 119–32
  see also Dystrophies
Genetic heterogeneity, 117, 243, 245
Genotype, 116
German measles *see* Rubella
Gerstmann–Straussler–Streinker
    syndrome, 76
Ghost cell glaucoma, 309
Giant cell arteritis/polymyalgia
    rheumatica, **290–1**
Giant cells, 46, **47**
Giant papillary conjunctivitis, 51, 59,
    62–3

contact lens wear-related, 22, 62, 63
  Type IV hypersensitivity, 61
Giant retinal tears, 225
Glands
  apocrine, 163
  eccrine, 163
  Meibomian, 163
  Moll, 164
  sebaceous, 163
  sweat (sudoriferous), 163
  Zeiss, 42
Glandular fever (infectious
    mononucleosis), 81, 146
Glassblowers' cataract, 9, 220
Glaucoma, 303–13
  acellular material and, 308–9
  alpha chymotrypsin-induced, 311
  cellular proliferation and, 308
  chemical injury-related, 12, 311
  classification, 303
  congenital, **312–13**
    buphthalmos, **312**, 313
    primary infantile, 312–13
  corneoscleral coat damage, 305
  cyclocongestive, 311
  genetic aspects, 135, **305–6**
  ghost cell, 309
  haemolytic, 309
  haemorrhage-related, **309**
  inflammation sequelae, 53, **307–8**, 310
  lens associated, 4, 5, 18, 222, **310**
  lens damage, 305
  malignant, 311
  mechanical trauma-related, 310–11
  medication-related, 311–12
    corticosteroids, **312**
  neoplasia-related, 310, **311**
  neovascular, 308
    diabetes mellitus, 287
  optic neuropathy, **304–5**
    optic disc cupping, 304
  phacolytic, 5, **310**
    lens trauma, 4, 18
  phacomorphic, 222, 310
  primary angle-closure, 306–7
  primary open-angle, 306
  secondary, 307–12
  silicone oil-induced, **311–12**
  surgical trauma complication, 24, 25,
    311
  thrombotic, 308
  tissue damage, 303–5
  uveal damage, 305
Glaucoma surgery
  ciliary body procedures, 27
  closed angle glaucoma, 27
  complications, 16, 27–8
  filtering (fistulizing) procedures, 16,
    27, 28
  implant devices, 28
  open-angle glaucoma, 27, 28
  trabecular meshwork procedures,
    27–8
Glaukomflecken, 221, 305
GLC1B, 306

Glioma, optic nerve, juvenile, 139, 187,
  188
Gliosis, 227, **296**, 303
  inflammation sequelae, **54**
  premacular (macular pucker), 228
Globular retinal haemorrhages, 271
Glomerulonephritis, 60
Glycocalyx, 88, 89
Glycogen storage diseases, 127
Glycosylated proteins, 282
GM$_1$ galactosidoses, 130, 131
  Type I (infantile), 131
  Type II (juvenile), 131
  Type III (adult), 131
GM$_2$ Type I (Tay–Sachs disease), **130**
GM$_2$ Type II (Sandhoff's disease), 130
Gold deposits (chrysiasis), 258–9
Goldenhar's syndrome, 162, 210
Goniodysgenesis, 312
Gonococcus see Neisseria gonorrhoeae
Goodpasture's syndrome, 60
Gorlin–Goltz syndrome, 159, 167,
  209–10
Gout, 264
Graft-versus host reactions, 76
Gram reaction, 88–9
Gram-negative bacilli, **91–2**
  autoimmune uveitis/arthritis
    association, 94
  keratitis, 93
Gram-negative cocci, **90**
  keratitis, 93
Gram-negative organisms, 89
Gram-positive bacilli, **91**
  keratitis, 93
Gram-positive cocci, **89–90**
  keratitis, 93
Gram-positive filamentous bacteria,
  keratitis, 93
Gram-positive organisms, 89
Granular cell layer, 163
Granular cell myoblastoma, 189
Granular corneal dystrophy, **237–8**
  Avellino dystrophy variant, 238
  molecular genetics, 239
  superficial variant (Waardenburg
    Jonker's dystrophy), 238
Granulation tissue, **15**, 23
  drug effects, 16
Granulocyte colony stimulating factor
  (G-CSF), 39
Granulocyte/macrophage colony
  stimulating factor (GM-CSF), 39
Granulocytes, **32–4**
  inflammatory mediators, 44
  Type I hypersensitivity reactions, 59
Granulocytic sarcoma ('chloroma'), 207
Granuloma, 46
  eosinophilic, 206
Granulomatous inflammation, **46**, **47**
  foreign bodies, 3, 6, **7**
  Type III hypersensitivity reactions, 60
  Type IV hypersensitivity reactions,
    60-1
Graves' disease, 60, 65

autoantibodies, 74
orbitopathy (dysthyroid orbitopathy),
  73, 74
HLA associations, 73
Growth, 139
  abnormalities in mature tissue, 141–8
  malignant cells, 144
  oncogenic process, 148
  tissue stress responses, 2
  see also Proliferative lesions
Growth factors
  angiogenesis, 19
  endothelial cell proliferation, 19
  neoplasia, 143
  receptors, 14
  wound healing, 14–15, 17
Growth hormone, 283
GUN syndrome, 204
Gyrate atrophy, 135
  choroid/retina with
    hyperornithinaemia, 253–4

H

Haab's striae, 305, 313
Haemangioma
  capillary (strawberry naevus), **175–6**
    orbit, 185
  cavernous, 176
    orbit, 185, **186**
    retina, 202
  choroidal, 201–2
  racemose
    orbit, 186
    retina, 202
Haemangioblastoma, retinal, **202**
Haemangiopericytoma, 186
Haematoma, 3
Haemochromatosis, 257, 259
Haemoglobin, 292
  structural variants, 292–4
Haemoglobinopathies, 234, 235, 292–4
Haemolytic glaucoma, 309
Haemolytic transfusion reactions, 60
Haemophilus, 92
  neonatal conjunctivitis (ophthalmia
    neonatorum), 93
Haemophilus aegyptius, 42, 64
Haemophilus ducreyi, 92
Haemophilus influenzae, 92
  conjunctivitis, 93
  orbital cellulitis, 94
Haemophilus influenzae aegyptius, 92
Haemorrhage, 270–1
  battered child, 5
  expulsive, **271**
  ophthalmic surgery complication, 24
  optic nerve, 271
  primary, 24
  reactionary, 24
  secondary, 24
  secondary glaucoma and, **309**
  shaken baby, 5
  subconjunctival, 270
  subhyaloid (preretinal), 4, 270

Haemorrhage (*cont.*)
  subretinal/sub-RPE, 271
  see also Retinal haemorrhage
Haemorrhagic glaucoma, **309**
Haemosiderin deposits, 270
Haemosiderosis bulbi, 259
Hair, 164
Hair follicle, 163–64
  proliferations, 175
Halo naevus, 170
Hamartoma, 141
Hand–Schüller–Christian disease, 206
Hansen's disease *see* Leprosy
Haptens, 32
  contact sensitising agents, 63
Hashimoto's thyroiditis, 73
Head louse (*Phthirus capitis*), 112
Healing *see* Wound healing
Heavy chains, 40
Helminths (worms), 76, 108–12
  cellular defences, 33, 34
  immune response, 41
  non-granulomatous chronic
    inflammation, 46
Helper T cells (T$_H$CD4 +), 36, 38, 39,
    40
  autoimmune disorders, 65
  corneal allograft rejection, 75
  cytokines, 38, 39
  HIV infection, 56, 57
  IL-1-mediated activation, 38
  immune response initiation, 40, 41
  T$_{H1}$/T$_{H2}$ subsets, 36, 39
Hemidesmosomes, 17
Hemispheric retinal vein occlusion, 280
Henoch–Schönlein purpura, 289
Heparin, 19, 34
Hepatolenticular degeneration *see*
    Wilson's disease
Herbert's pits, **87**
Hereditary endothelial dystrophy,
    congenital, **242**
  dominant variant, 242
Hereditary haemorrhagic telangiectasia
    (Rendu–Osler–Weber disease), 181,
    272
Hermansky–Pudlak syndrome, 126
Herpes simplex virus, 63, 64, 65, 79–80,
    292
  acute/acute bilateral retinal necrosis
    (ARN/BARN), **82**
  AIDS opportunistic infection, 57,
    59
  disciform keratopathy, 80
  epithelial keratitis, 79–80
  HSV-1, 79
  HSV-2, 79
  investigations, 80
  neonatal conjunctivitis (ophthalmia
    neonatorum), 79, 93
  post-herpetic (metaherpetic)
    keratopathy, 80
  reactivation of latent infection, 79
  retinitis, 71
  stromal keratitis, **80**

teratogenesis, 140
Herpes zoster ophthalmicus, 81
  corneal filaments, 51
Herpes zoster (shingles), 81
Herpesvirus retinitis, **82–3**
Herpesviruses, **78–83**
Heterolysis, 2
Heterotopia, 140
Heterozygous state, 116
Hexosylceramide deposits, 264
Hidradenoma, clear cell, 174
High endothelial venules, 40
Histamine, 34, 39, 44, 59, 62
Histiocytes *see* Macrophages
Histiocytic giant cells, 46
Histiocytic proliferations, 205–7
Histiocytosis, Langerhans cell, 206–7
Histological stains, 321
  pathogens, **322**
  specific structures, **321**
  specific substances, **322**
Histology, 319–20
  artefacts/irrelevant features, 325
  eye sections examination, 324–6
  tissue sections examination, 326
Histoplasma capsulatum, 102
  AIDS opportunistic infection, 59
  histoplasmosis, 102
  presumed ocular histoplasmosis
    syndrome (POHS), **102–3**
HIV infection/AIDS, 56–9, 85
  AIDS-indicator conditions, **58**
  anogenital carcinoma, 58
  CD4 T$_H$ cell effects, 56, 57
  CDC classification, **58**
  clinicopathological features, 57–9
  conjunctival carcinoma, 58, 59
  conjunctival squamous cell carcinoma,
    179
  cotton-wool spots, 278
  investigations, 59
  Kaposi sarcoma, 57, 58, 59
    conjunctiva, 181
  lymphoma, 57–8
  neoplasms, 146
  opportunistic infection, 57, 58, 59
    cytomegalovirus/cytomegalovirus
      retinitis, **82–3**
    fungal (oculomycosis), 101, 104
    Pneumocystis carinii, 101
    progressive outer retinal necrosis
      (PORN), **82**
    toxoplasmosis, 105
  retinal microangiopathy (HIV
    retinopathy), **58–9**
  transmission, 57
  virology, 56–7
HIV retinopathy, **58–9**
HIV-1, 56
HIV-2, 56
HLA (human leukocyte antigens), 37
  corneal allograft rejection, 75
  transplanted tissue compatibility, 74
HLA haplotype associations
  ankylosing spondylitis, 65

anterior uveitis, 68
  acute (AAU), 68–9, 94
  Behçet's disease, 65, 289
  birdshot retinochoroidopathy, 71
  diabetes mellitus, Type I (insulin-
    dependent), 282
  dysthyroid orbitopathy, 73, 74
  Graves' disease, 65
  juvenile chronic arthritis, 69
  multiple sclerosis, 301
  ocular cicatricial pemphigoid, 66
  posterior uveitis, 68
  presumed ocular histoplasmosis
    syndrome (POHS), 103
  reactive arthritis, 94
  sarcoidosis, 49
  seronegative spondyloarthropathies,
    68
  Sjögren's syndrome, 73
  Stevens–Johnson syndrome (erythema
    multiforme), 65
  sympathetic ophthalmitis, 71
  vasculitis, 288
  Vogt–Koyanagi–Harada syndrome,
    71
Hodgkin lymphoma, 203, 204
Homeobox-containing genes, 140
Homer Wright rosettes, 199
Homocystinuria, 123, 125, **127**, 223
Homozygous state, 116
Horner–Trantas' dots, **62**
Hudson–Stähli line, 256
Human herpesvirus serotypes, 79
Human papilloma virus (HPV), 77, 179
  oncogenesis, 146
Human T cell lymphotropic viruses
    (HTLV-1/HTLV-2), 85, 147
Humoral immunity *see* Antibody-
    mediated immunity
Hunter syndrome, 131
Hurler syndrome, 131, 249
Hutchinson's melanotic freckle
    (malignant lentigo), **171**
Hyaline bodies (optic disc drusen),
    160–1
Hyaloid cysts, 157
Hyaloid vascular system, 156
  persistent remnants, 156–7
Hydatid disease, 112
Hydrogel contact lenses, 63
Hydrogel intraocular lenses, 27
Hydropic change (acute cellular oedema;
    cloudy swelling), 2
Hydroquinones, 261
Hyperaemia *see* Vasocongestion
Hypercalcaemia, 255, 256
  vitamin D (calciferol) excess, 13
Hypercapnia, contact lens wear-related
    injury, 21, 22
Hyperchromatism, **144**
Hyperhomocysteinaemia, 268
Hyperornithinaemia, gyrate atrophy of
    choroid/retina, 253–4
Hyperplasia, 2, 139
  intraocular lesions, 190–1

pseudoadenomatous (of ciliary epithelium), **190**
pseudocarcinomatous, 168
reactive lymphoid, **203–4**
sebaceous, **172**
Hypersensitivity reactions, 54, 59–65
bacterial pathogenicity, 89
Gell and Coombs classification, 59
Hypersensitivity Type I reactions (anaphylaxis), 59
acute allergic conjunctivitis, 61
allergic microbial blepharoconjunctivitis, 64
effector cells, 34
giant papillary conjunctivitis, 63
non-granulomatous chronic inflammation, 46
surface IgE cross-linkage, 41, 59
vernal keratoconjunctivitis, 62
Hypersensitivity Type II reactions (cytotoxic), 59–60
Mooren's ulcer, 67
ocular cicatricial pemphigoid, 66
Hypersensitivity Type III reactions (immune complex-mediated), 33, 60
allergic granulomatous nodule, **61**
granulomatous inflammation, 46
marginal keratitis (catarrhal infiltrates/keratitis), 64
Mooren's ulcer, 67
phacoantigenic endophthalmitis, 72
scleritis, 67
sterile peripheral ulcerative keratitis, 66
Stevens–Johnson syndrome (erythema multiforme), 65
vasculitis, 289
Hypersensitivity Type IV reactions (cell-mediated; delayed-type hypersensitivity), 60–1
contact dermatoconjunctivitis/ keratitis, 63
corneal allograft rejection, 75
giant papillary conjunctivitis, 63
granulomatous inflammation, 46
Mooren's ulcer, 67
scleritis, 67
Sjögren's syndrome, 73
Stevens–Johnson syndrome (erythema multiforme), 65
sympathetic ophthalmitis, 70
vernal keratoconjunctivitis, 62
Hypersensitivity Type V reactions, 60
Hypersensitivity vasculitis, 289
Hypertension
intracranial, benign (idiopathic), 298
ocular, 303
systemic 268, 272, 278, 280–2
accelerated, 2
choroidopathy, **281**, 282
genetic factors, 135
optic neuropathy, 281–2
primary, 281
retinopathy, **281**
Hyperthermia, focal, 7

Hyperthyroidism, 73
Hypertrophy, 2, 139
Hypervariable regions, 40
Hyperviscosity states, 275
Hyphaema, 4
haemorrhagic glaucoma, 309
Hypoderma bovis, 112
Hypoperfusion retinopathy, 277
Hypophosphatasia, 242
Hypoplasia, 3, 140
optic nerve, 159
retinal, 140
Hypopyon, 52, **94**, 104
Hypothermia, focal, 7
Hypotony
inflammation sequelae, 53
ophthalmic surgery complication, 24
Hypoxic injury, 12
contact lens wear-related, 21, 22

I

ICAM-1/2/3 (intercellular adhesion molecule-1/2/3), 38
Idiopathic (benign) intracranial hypertension, 298
Idiopathic calcification, 255
Idiopathic juxtafoveal retinal telangiectasia, 272
Idiopathic retinal vasculitis, 273, **288**
Idiotype, 40
IgA, 33, 40, 41
tears, 42
IgD, 40, 41
IgE, 33, 34, 40, 41
acute allergic conjunctivitis, 61
receptors, 34
vernal keratoconjunctivitis, 62
IgG, 33, 39, 40, 41
vernal keratoconjunctivitis, 62
IgM, 40, 41
Immune complex formation, 33, 41
bacterial pathogenicity, 89
see also Hypersensitivity Type III reactions
Immune cross-reactions, bacterial pathogenicity, 89
Immune privilege, 42–3
corneal allograft survival, 75
Immune system, 32–9
adaptive, 32, 39–41, 42–3
cellular constituents, 32–7
disorders, 54–76
eyes/associated structures, 42–3
innate, 32, 42
malignant neoplasm responses, 145
molecular constituents, 37–9
regulation, 41–2
tissue transplantation responses, 74–6
Immune tolerance, 41–2, 65
Immunity
antibody-mediated (humoral), 40–1
cell-mediated, 40
bacterial pathogenicity, 89

response to malignant neoplasms, 145
Immunochemistry, 327–8
Immunocompromised host
bacterial keratitis, 93
cytomegalovirus retinitis, **82–3**
fungal infections (oculomycosis), 101
leukaemias, 292
progressive outer retinal necrosis (PORN), **82**
toxoplasmosis, 105
varicella zoster virus retinitis, 82
Immunodeficiency, 54–9
infection susceptibility, 55
neoplasms, 55
primary, 55–6
secondary, 56–9
Immunoenzymatic staining, 327, **328**
Immunofluorescence, 327–8
Immunoglobulin *see* Antibody
Immunoglobulin deficiency, 56
Immunoglobulin superfamily, 38
Immunosuppressive ocular fluids/factors, 43
Implant devices, 28
In-situ hybridization, 328
Incisions, 3
complications, 25
faulty technique, 24
wound healing, 16
Inclusion bodies, 77
chlamydial infection, 86, **87**
Inclusion body myositis, 317
Inclusion cyst, 16
Incontinentia pigmenti, 132–3
Infection, 76–113
corneoscleral perforation, 5
immunodeficiency-related susceptibility, 55
terminology, 76
Infectious mononucleosis (glandular fever), 81, 146
Infectious parotitis (mumps), 84
Infective keratitis, 22, 60
Inflammation, 43–54
acute, 43–5
cardinal signs, 43
chemical mediators, 44
leukocyte activation, 44, 45
organization, 45
phagocytosis, 45
resolution, 45
systemic response, 45
vascular changes, 44
chronic, 45–9
granulomatous, **46, 47**
non-granulomatous, 46
complement system activation, 39
corneoscleral coat, 5, 49, 51–2
extraocular, 49–51
histological sections examination, 325
intraocular, 52–4
lid, 162
ophthalmic surgery-related, 24–5
wound healing, 16

Inflammatory bowel disease, 68
Inflammatory glaucoma, **307–8**, 310
Inflammatory mediators, 44
  acute phase response, 45
  endothelial cell proliferation, 19
Inflammatory myopathies, 317
Inflammatory optic neuropathies (optic neuritis), 299–301
Influenza, 85, 317
Infrared radiation, 9–10
  injury, 8
  lasers, 9, 10, 27
  ocular protective mechanisms, 8
Inherited abnormalities see Genetic disorders
Injury, 2–14
  chemical, 11–12
  contact lens wear, 21–3
  electrical, 8
  electromagnetic spectrum, 8–11
  hypoxia, 12
  irreversible, 2–3
  mechanical, 3–6
  microwave, 8, 9
  non-accidental, children,, 4–5
  reversible, 2
  thermal, 6–7
  ultrasound, 7
    see also Ophthalmic surgery
Innate immune system, 32
  eyes/associated structures, 42
Inner blood–retinal barrier, 267
Insecta, **112**
Insertions, 117
Insulin-like growth factors (IGFs), 14, 19, 283
Integrins, 38, 144
Intercellular adhesion molecules (ICAMs), 38
Interdigitating dendritic cells, 35
Interferons (IFNs), 38–9
  acute inflammation, 44
Interleukins (TLs), 19, 36, 38
  acute inflammation, 44
  acute phase response, 45
  intraocular inflammatory response, 38
Interphotoreceptor retinoid binding protein (IRBP), 43
Intracranial pressure elevation, 297–8
  idiopathic (benign intracranial hypertension), 298
Intradermal naevus, 168, **170**
Intraepidermal carcinoma (carcinoma in situ; Bowen's disease), 141, **167**
Intraocular adhesions, 12
Intraocular aspirates, 321
Intraocular foreign bodies, 5–6, **7**
  copper, 257–8
  iron, 256–7
Intraocular gas injection, raised intraocular pressure, 312
Intraocular haemorrhages
  secondary glaucoma, **309**
  shaken baby, 5

Intraocular inflammation, 52–4
  anterior, 52
  interleukins, 38
  lens-associated secondary glaucoma, 310
  posterior, 53
  sequelae, 53–4
Intraocular lenses, 27
  complications of implantation, 27
  materials, 27
Intraocular pressure, 303
  ophthalmic surgery complications, 24
Intraocular proliferative lesions, 190–203
  choristoma, 191
  cysts, 190
  hyperplasias, 190–1
  melanocytic, 191–6
  neural, 202–3
  neuroepithelial, 197–201
  secondary glaucoma, 310, **311**
  smooth muscle, 203
  vascular, 201–2
Intraretinal microvascular abnormality (IRMA), 20
  diabetic retinopathy, 286
Intraretinal neovascularization, 19, 20
Intrascleral nerve loop, **178**
Introns, 116
Inversion, 118
Inverted follicular keratosis (irritated seborrhoeic keratosis), 165
Ionizing radiation see Radiation
Iridectomy specimens, 319
Iridocorneal adhesions, 53
Iridocorneal endothelial (ICE) syndrome, 308
Iridocyclectomy specimens, 319
Iridocyclitis, 52
Iridodialysis, 4
  battered child, 5
Iridolenticular adhesions, **53**
Iridopathy, diabetes mellitus, **287**
Iridotomy, 27
Iris
  atrophy, 308
  developmental anomalies, 153–4
  histological sections examination, 325
  ischaemia, 278
  mechanical trauma, 4
  normal development, 152
  response to injury, 18
  tissue incarceration, 5, **6**
  vasoproliferation, **20**
Iris bombé, **307**
Iris coloboma, **150**
Iris cysts, **190**
Iris melanoma, 193, **194**, 196
Iris naevi, , **191, 192**
Iris naevus (Cogan–Rees) syndrome, 308
Iritis, 52
Iron deposits, 256–7
  blood pigments, 259

Irritated seborrhoeic keratosis (inverted follicular keratosis), 165
Ischaemia, 274–9
  extravascular causes, 275
  intramural causes, 275
  intravascular causes, 274–5
  wound healing impairment, 16
Isografts, 74
Isospora belli, 104
Isotype switching, 41
Ixodidiae (ticks), **85, 113**

J

J chain, 41
Junctional naevus, 168, 169, **170**
  conjunctiva, 179, 180
Juvenile chronic arthritis, 69
Juvenile idiopathic arthritis, 69
Juvenile melanoma (Spitz naevus), 170
Juvenile optic nerve glioma, 139, 187, **188**
Juvenile xanthogranuloma, 205, **206**, 309

K

Kallikreins, 44
Kaposi sarcoma, 57, 58, 59
  conjunctiva, **181**
Kaposi sarcoma virus, 79, 82
Karyolysis, 2
  hypoxic damage, 12
Karyorrhexis, 2
Kawasaki disease, 65
Kayser–Fleischer ring, 129, **258**
Kearns–Sayre syndrome (chronic progressive ophthalmoplegia), 134–5, 249, 316
Keloid
  corneal, 216
  nodule, 16
Keratic precipitates, **52**
Keratin layer, 163
Keratinocyte growth factor (KGF), 14, 15
Keratinocytes, 163
  proliferations, 165–8
    benign, 165–6
    intraepidermal, 166–7
    malignant, 167–8
Keratinous cyst see Epidermoid cyst
Keratitis, 49, 51–2
  acanthamoebic, **107–8**
  bacterial, 93–4
  corneal filaments, 51
  epithelial, 79–80
  epithelial oedema, 51
  fungal, 103, **104**
  investigations, 93–4
  marginal, 64
  peripheral corneal melt, 66
  punctate epithelial, 51
  sequelae, 49
  stromal oedema, 52

ulcerative, 51, **52**, 60, 66
viral, 51
Keratoacanthoma (molluscum
sebaceum), **166**
Keratoconjunctivitis
atopic, 64–5
contact lens wear-related, 22–3
epidemic, 78
phlyctenular *see* Phlyctenular
keratoconjunctivitis
superior limbic, 22–3
vernal *see* Vernal keratoconjunctivitis
Keratoconjunctivitis sicca
corneal filaments, 51
graft-versus host reactions, 76
sarcoidosis, 48
Sjögren's syndrome, 72
Keratoconus, **216–17**, **218**, 242
associated disorders, 217
posterior, 153
Keratoepithelin gene mutations, 239
Keratoglobus, 217, 242
Keratomalacia, 12, 13
Keratopathy
band, **255**
glaucoma, 305
sarcoidosis, 48
vitamin D (calciferol) excess, 13
bullous, 305
climatic droplet (spheroidal
degeneration; Labrador
keratopathy), **215**
crystalline, **263–4**
disciform, 80
farinaceous epithelial (of Tobgy), 62
Labrador (spheroidal degeneration;
climatic droplet keratopathy),
215
lipid, 263, **264**
metaherpetic (post-herpetic), 80
Thygeson's superficial punctate, 67
vortex (cornea verticillata), 17,
264
Keratoplasty
normal wound healing, 25–6
see also Corneal allografts
Keratotomy, 26
Khodadoust line, 75
KID syndrome, 56
Kinin system, 44
Klebsiella, 68, 69
autoimmune uveitis/arthritis
association, 94
conjunctivitis, 93
Klebsiella pneumoniae, 92
keratitis, 93
Koch–Weeks bacillus *see Haemophilus
influenzae aegyptius*
Koeppe nodules, 52
Krypton laser
cyclophotocoagulation, 27
therapeutic burns, 10
Kupffer cells, 34
Kuru, 76
Kveim test, 48–9

L

L-selectin, 38
Labile cell populations, 15, 139
Labrador keratopathy (spheroidal
degeneration; climatic droplet
keratopathy), **215**
Lacerations, 3
Lacrimal gland proliferations, 184–5
Lacrimal sac, 162
carcinoma, 183
melanoma, 183
microbiological specimens, 327
papilloma, **183**
Lactic acid, 42
Lactoferrin, 32, 42
Lagophthalmos, 7, 16
Lambert–Eaton myasthenic syndrome,
145, 314–15
Lamellar cataract, congenital, 155
Langerhans cell histiocytosis, 206–7
Langerhans cells, **35**, 42
conjunctival epithelium, 177
lids, 163
Langhans' giant cells, 46, **47**
Lanolin sensitivity, 63
Large granular lymphocytes, 37
Laser-assisted *in situ* keratomileusis
(LASIK), 26
Laser, 7, 9
argon, 10
cyclophotocoagulation, 27
diode (infrared), 10, 27
excimer, 10
krypton, 10, 27
Nd:YAG (neodymium:yttrium
aluminium garnet), 10
tissue injury mechanisms, 10
trabeculoplasty, 27
Lashes, 42, 164
Latent viral infection, 77
Lattice retinal degeneration, 225
Lattice corneal dystrophy, **238–9**
amyloid deposits, 239, 263
Type 1, 238, 263
molecular genetics, 239
Type 2 (Meretoja's syndrome), 238,
263
Type 3, 238–9, 263
Lax ligament syndrome, 242
Leaking cyst, **164–5**
Leber's congenital amaurosis, 248
Leber's hereditary optic neuropathy,
134, 298, **299**
Leber's miliary aneurysms, 272
Leiomyoma, 189
intraocular, 203
Leiomyosarcoma, 189, 203
Leishmania, 104
Lens
ageing changes, 219–20
autoimmune disorders, 72
degenerations, 218–22
developmental anomalies, 154–6
electrical injury, 8

electromagnetic radiation protective
mechanisms, 8
glaucomatous damage, 305
histological sections examination, 325
inflammation sequelae, 53
infrared radiation damage, 9
intraocular surgery-related damage,
24
manipulation, cataract surgery, 27
mechanical trauma, 4
battered child, 5
corneoscleral perforation, 5
microwave-related damage, 9
normal development, 154
transparency, 220, 221
ultraviolet light-related damage, 10
wound healing, 18
Lens capsule, 218–19
degenerative abnormalities, 220–1
exfoliation, 220
manipulation, cataract surgery, 27
Lens coloboma, 155
Lens dislocation, 4, 223
Lens displacement, 4
secondary glaucoma, 309–10
Lens epithelium, 219
degenerative abnormalities, 221
Lens substance, 219
degenerative abnormalities, 221–2
fibre folds, 221
vacuoles, 221
water clefts, 221
Lens-induced endophthalmitis
(phacoantigenic endophthalmitis),
4, 5, 18, 60, **72**
corneoscleral perforation, 5
Type IV hypersensitivity, 60-1
Lenticonus, 155
Lenticular oxalosis, 256
Lentiglobus, 155
Lentigo, 171
conjunctiva, 180
malignant (Hutchinson's melanotic
freckle), **171**
Leprosy, 95, 96–8
borderline, 97
classification, 96, **97**
granulomatous inflammation, 46, 60
lepromatous, 96–7
ophthalmic, 97–8
reactions/reactional states, 97
tuberculoid, 97
Leptospira interrogans, 98
Leptospirosis, 98
Letterer–Siwe disease, 206
Leukaemias, 292
Leukaemic deposits, 207
Leukocyte activation, 44
Leukocyte migration, 44
Leukocyte-derived mediators, acute
inflammation, 44
Leukotrienes, 44, 59
LFA-1 (lymphocyte function-associated
antigen-1), 38
Lice, **85, 112**

Lid coloboma, 162
Lid margin specimens, 319
Lids
    allergic disease, 61–5
    bacterial flora, 42
    benign neoplasms, 162
    burns, 7
        alkali, 12
    contact lens wear-related injury, 23
    cysts, 164–5
    distortion, 49
    growth disorders/lid lumps, 162–76
    hair follicle proliferations, 175
    inflammatory lesions, 162
    innate immunity, 42
    keratinocyte proliferations, 165–8
    lymphatics, 35
    malignant neoplasms, 162
    mechanical trauma, 3
    melanocyte proliferations
        dermal, 176
        epidermal, 168–72
    metastatic deposits, 210
    microbiological specimens, 326
    neural proliferations, 176
    sebaceous gland proliferations, 172–3
    skin, 162–4
        epidermal-associated structures,
            163–4
        epidermis, 163
    sweat gland proliferations, 173–5
    vascular proliferations, 175–6
    wound contraction, 16
Light chains, 40
Light transduction, 244, 245
Lightning cataract, 8
Ligneous conjunctivitis, 50, **51**
Limbus, 177
    epithelium regeneration processes, 17
Lipid deposits, 263
Lipid keratopathy, 263, **264**
Lipid metabolism disorders, 125
Lipoma, 189
Lipopolysaccharide, 88, 89
Liposarcoma, pleomorphic, 189
Liquefaction (colliquative necrosis), 2
Lisch nodules, 209
Listeria, 91
Listeria monocytogenes, 42, 91
Loa loa (African eyeworm), **111**
Local invasion, 144, 148, 210
Louis–Bar syndrome (ataxia
    telangiectasia), 55, 56, 125, **132**,
    147, 272, 273
Low molecular weight angiogenic
    factors, 19
Low-density-lipoprotein (LDL)
    cholesterol, 268
LSD embryopathy, 150, 161
Lupus vulgaris, 96
Lyme disease, 98, 100, 113
Lymph nodes, 35
    antigen processing, 40
Lymphadenopathy, 51
    persistent generalized, 57

Lymphangiectasia, 181–2
Lymphangioma
    conjunctiva, 181–2
    orbit, 183–4
Lymphatic leukaemia, chronic, 264
Lymphatic proliferations, conjunctiva,
    181–2
Lymphatics, 35
    ocular immune privilege, 43
Lymphocytes, **35–7**
    activation, 40
    cytokines (lymphokines), 38
    inflammatory mediators, 44
    large granular, 37
    non-granulomatous chronic
        inflammation, 46
Lymphogranuloma venereum, 86
Lymphoid organs, 35
Lymphoid system
    cellular constituents, 32, 35–7
    lymphoid organs, 35
Lymphoid tissue, 35, 40
    conjunctival subepithelial connective
        tissue, 177
    mucosa-associated (MALT), 35, 40,
        42, 177, 184
Lymphokines, 60
Lymphoma, 203, 264
    AIDS-related, 57–8
    B cell, 261
    Burkitt's, 81, 146, 204
    central nervous system, 204
    conjunctiva, 204
    Hodgkin, 203, 204
    immunodeficiency-related, 55
    non-Hodgkin, 203, **204**
    orbit, 204
    Sjögren's syndrome-related, 73
Lymphoproliferative lesions, 203–4
    conjunctiva, **204**
    orbit, 204
    retina, 204
    uvea, 204
Lysosomal storage disorders, 125,
    129–32
Lysozyme, 32, 34
    tears, 42

M

Macrophage colony stimulating factor
    (M-CSF), 39
Macrophages (histiocytes), **34–5**
    acute inflammation, 44, 45
    antigen presentation, 40
    cell-mediated immunity, 40
    cytokines (monokines), 38, 39
    granulomatous chronic inflammation,
        46
    inflammatory mediators, 44
    non-granulomatous chronic
        inflammation, 46
    phagocytosis, 41
    surface receptors, 41
Macrophotographs, 326

Macrophthalmos, 161
Macular burn, 10
Macular coloboma, 151
Macular cyst, 228
Macular degeneration *see* Age-related
    macular degeneration
Macular dystrophy, **239–40**
    adult vitelliform, 245
    Best's vitelliform, 243, **251–2**
    North Carolina, 253
    pattern, 245
    pigment pattern, 232, 243, 252
Macular hole, 228
    staging, 228–9
Macular pucker (premacular gliosis),
    228
Macular xanthophyll, electromagnetic
    radiation protection, 8
Maculopathy
    cellophane, 228
    diabetic retinopathy, 285
MAd CAM-1, 38
Madarosis, 16, 49, 97
Major histocompatibility complex
    (MHC), 37–8
    T cell function, 36, 37, 38
Malaria, 104, 147
Malattia-levantinese (dominant drusen;
    Doyne's honeycomb choroiditis),
    232, 243, **252**
Malignant glaucoma, 311
Malignant lentigo (Hutchinson's
    melanotic freckle), **171**
Malignant neoplasms, **143, 144–5**
    local invasion, 144, 148, 210
    metastasis, 144–5, 148, 210–11
    radiation-induced, 11
Malnutrition, 302
    bacterial keratitis, 93
    wound healing impairment, 16
MALT *see* Mucosa-associated lymphoid
    tissue
Map-dot-fingerprint corneal dystrophy
    (epithelial basement membrane
    dystrophy; Cogan's microcystic
    dystrophy), **236**
Marfan's syndrome, **122**, 155, 217, 223
Marginal keratitis (catarrhal infiltrates/
    keratitis), 64
Marshall's syndrome, 249
Massive intraretinal haemorrhage, 271
Mast cells, 34
    cytokines, 38
    degranulation, 34, 39, 59
    inflammatory mediators, 44
MC1R, 193
MCDR1, 253
Measles (rubeola), 84, 300
Mechanical injury, 3–6
    contact lens wear-related, 21
    electromagnetic radiation, 9
    non-accidental injury in children, 4–5
    penetrating/perforating wounds, **5–6**
    secondary glaucoma, 310–11
Medulloepithelioma, **201**

Meesmann's juvenile epithelial corneal dystrophy, 236, **237**
Megalocornea, 152
'Meibomian cyst' (chalazion), 46–7, **48**, 165
Meibomian glands, 163
  antibacterial secretions, 42
  contact lens wear-related dysfunction, 23
Meiosis, 116
Melanin, 260
  deposition, 260
  dispersion, 4
  ocular protective functions, 8, 9
Melanocytes
  conjunctival epithelium, 177
  dermis, 176
  epidermis, 163
  lid skin, 163
Melanocytic naevus (mole), 142, **168–71**, 260
  classification, 168
  conjunctiva, **179–80**
Melanocytic proliferations
  conjunctival epithelium, 179–81
    benign, 179–80
    intraepithelial, 180
    malignant, 180–1
  conjunctival non-epithelial, 182–3
  dermis, 176
  epidermis, 168–72
    benign, 168–71
    intraepidermal, 171
    malignant, 171–2
  intraocular, 191–6
    malignant potential, 192
    pathology, **192**
Melanocytoma
  ciliary body, **192**
  malignant potential, 192
  optic nerve head, **191–2**
Melanocytosis
  ocular (melanosis oculi), **182**
  oculodermal (naevus of Ota), 182–3
Melanoma, 260
  conjunctiva, **180–1**
  iris, 193, **194**, 196
  juvenile (Spitz naevus), 170
  lacrimal sac, 183
  lids, **171–2**
  Pagetoid, 171
  uvea, **193–6**
    classification, 194–5
    clinical features, **193–4**
    extraocular extension, 194, 196
    genetic aspects, 147, 193
    metastases, 196
    pathology, **194–5**
    prognosis, 195–6
    secondary glaucoma, 310, **311**
Melanoma *in situ* (intraepidermal melanoma), **171**
  conjunctiva, 180
Melanoma-associated retinopathy, 146
Melanosis

diffuse of skin, 260
  ocular melanocytosis, **182**
  secondary conjunctival, 260
Membrane formation, 50
Memory cells, 39
Meninges, 296
  hyperplasia, 139
Meningioma, **186–7**
Meningocele, 184
Meningococcus *see Neisseria meningitidis*
Meningoencephalocele, 184
Mercury deposits, 259
Meretoja's syndrome (Type 2 lattice dystrophy), 238, 263
Merkel cell carcinoma, **172**
Merkel cells, 163
Metabolic disorders
  autosomal recessive disorders, 123, 125
  neoplastic cells, 143
Metaherpetic (post-herpetic) keratopathy, 80
Metalloproteinases, 18
Metals/metal compound deposits, 254–9
Metaplasia, 2, 18, 141
Metastasis/metastatic deposits, 144–5, 148, 210–11
Metastatic calcification, 255
Methanol toxicity, 302
MHC class I molecules, 37
  antigen processing, 40
MHC class II molecules, 38
  antigen processing, 40
  delayed-type hypersensitivity (Type IV reactions), 60-1
  ocular immune privilege, 43
MHC class restriction, 37, 38, 40
Microaerophilic micro-organisms, 88
Microbiological specimens, 326–7
Microcornea, 152
Microglia, 34, 297
Microphthalmos, 140, 161
  chromosomal abnormalities, 118
  colobomatous, 161
  with cyst, 184
  pure (nanophthalmos), 161
Microscopy
  electron, 320
  polarizing, 320–1
Microspherophakia (spherophakia), 155
Microwave injury, 8, 9
Mid-line differentiation abnormalities, 149
Migraine, 301
Mineral metabolism disorders, 125, 129
Mites, **85**
Mitochondrial DNA, 116
Mitochondrial gene disorders, 134–5, **299**
Mitochondrial ocular myopathy, 316, **317**
Mitomycin C, 16, 28
Mitosis, 116, 139
  neoplastic cells, 143
    malignant, 144

Mittendorf dot, 157
Mizuo–Nakamura phenomenon, 246
Mohs' technique, 168, 320
Mole *see* Melanocytic naevus
Molecular methods, 328
Moll
  cyst, 165
  glands, 164
Mollusca fibrosa, 209
Molluscum contagiosum, **83–4**, 166
  AIDS opportunistic infection, 59
Molluscum sebaceum (keratoacanthoma), **166**
Molteno implant, 28
Monochromatism, 246, 247
  atypical/incomplete, 247
  blue cone, 247
Monocytes, **34**
  cytokines (monokines), 38
  inflammatory mediators, 44
Monomorphic adenoma, 184
Mononuclear phagocytic cells, **34–5**
Monosomy, 117, 118
Mooren's ulcer, 60, 66–7
Moraxella, 91, **92**
  keratitis, 93
Moraxella lacunata, 64, 91
  conjunctivitis, 93
Morgagnian cataract, 222, **223**, 256
Morning glory syndrome, **160**
Morphogenesis, 140
Morquio syndrome, 131
Mosaicism, 118
Motor unit, 314
Mucin-like vascular addressins (MAd CAMs), 38
Mucocele, 184
Mucoepidermoid carcinoma
  conjunctiva, 179
  lacrimal gland, 185
Mucolipidoses, 125, 129, 132
Mucopolysaccharidoses, 125, 129, 131–2, 240
Mucor, 101
Mucormycosis, 101
  orbital cellulitis, 104
Mucosa-associated lymphoid tissue (MALT), 35, 42
  antigen processing, 40
  conjunctival subepithelial connective tissue, 177
  lacrimal gland, 184
Muir–Torre syndrome, 210
Müller cell dystrophy, 243–4
Multifactorial (polygenic) inherited disorders, 135
Multiple evanescent white dot syndrome (MEWDS), 71
Multiple sclerosis, 297, **300–1**
Mumps (infectious parotitis), 84, 300
  dacryoadenitis, 84, **85**
Muscle
  biopsies, 319
  disorders, 314–17
  wound healing, 18

Muscular dystrophies, 316
Museum specimen examination, 323–4
Mustard gas, 12
Mutagens, 117
Mutation, 116–17
  length, 117
  oncogenesis, 148
  point, 117
  somatic, 135
Mutton-fat keratic precipitates, **52**
Mutualism, 76
Myasthenia gravis, 60, 72, 145, 315–16
Mycobacteria, **95–8**
  AIDS opportunistic infection, 57
Mycobacterium avium, 95
Mycobacterium chelonae, 95
Mycobacterium fortuitum, 95
Mycobacterium intracellulare, 95
Mycobacterium leprae, 95, 96, 97, 98
Mycobacterium tuberculosis, **95**, 96
Mycoplasma pneumoniae, 65, 87
Mycoplasmas, 87
Mycotoxins, 101
Myelin, 296, 313
Myeloid cells, 32–5
Myeloid leukaemia, chronic, 147
Myeloma, 207, 261, 262, 264
Myeloperoxidase, 32, 207
Myoblastoma, granular cell, 189
Myofibrils, 314
Myofilaments, 314
Myopathies, 316–17
  inflammatory, 317
Myopia, 217–18
  genetic factors, 135
Myositis, ocular (orbital), **317**
Myotonic disorders, 316–17
Myotonic dystrophy, 317
Myxoliposarcoma, 189

N

Naevus
  balloon cell, **170**
  blue naevus, **176**
    conjunctiva, 182
  choroidal, **191**, 192
  compound, 168, **169–70**
    conjunctiva, 179, **180**
  cystic, 179, **180**
  halo, 170
  intradermal, 168, **170**
  iris, 191
  junctional, 168, 169, **170**
  melanocytic (mole), **168–71**, 260
  of Ota (oculodermal melanocytosis),
    182–3
Spitz (juvenile melanoma), 170
Naevus flammeus (port wine stain), 176,
  208
Nanophthalmos (pure microphthalmos),
  161
Nasolacrimal duct, 162
Nasolacrimal groove, 162

Nasolacrimal stenosis, congenital, 140,
  148, 162
Nasopharyngeal carcinoma, 146
Natural killer (NK) cells, 37, 40
  corneal allograft rejection, 75
Nd:YAG (neodymium:yttrium
    aluminium garnet) laser, 10
  cyclophotocoagulation, 27
  mechanism of tissue damage, 9
NDP, 272
Necrosis, 2
Necrotizing scleritis, 60
Neisseria, 90
Neisseria gonorrhoeae, 42, 64, **90**
  conjunctivitis, 93
    neonatal (ophthalmia neonatorum),
      93
  keratitis, 93
Neisseria meningitidis, 90
  keratitis, 93
Nematodes (roundworms), 108, 109-11
Neomycin, 63
Neonatal conjunctivitis (ophthalmia
    neonatorum)
  chemical irritants, 93
  chlamydial oculogenital disease, 86,
    87
  cocci/bacilli, 93
  Neisseria gonorrhoeae, 90
Neoplasms, 141–6
  behaviour, **143–5**
  benign, **143**
  classification, **141–2**
  definition, 141
  genetic aspects, 143, 146
  immunodeficiency-related, 55
  local effects, 145
  malignant, **143**, **144–5**
  nomenclature, **141–2**
  secondary, 210–11
  systemic effects, 145–6
Neoplastic cells, 143
  genetic abnormalities, 143, 147
Neovascular glaucoma, 287, 308
Neovascularization, 18–20
  basement membrane lysis, 18
  choroidal, 20
    age-related macular degeneration,
      232, **233–4**
  cornea, 20–1
  diabetic retinopathy, 286–7
  endothelial cell migration, 19
  endothelial cell proliferation, 19
  inflammation sequelae, 53, 54
  retinal, 19–20
    intraretinal, 19, 20
    preretinal, **19–20**
  retinopathy of prematurity *see*
    Retinopathy of prematurity
  sickle cell retinopathy, 293
  stromal, contact lens wear-related, 22
  uveal, **20**
Nephroblastoma (Wilms' tumour), 119
Nerve supply, wound healing influence,
  16

Nettleship–Falls albinism, 126
Neural proliferations
  intraocular, 202–3
  lids, 176
  orbit, 186–8
Neurilemmoma *see* Schwannoma
Neuroepithelial proliferative lesions,
  197–201
Neurofibroma, 176
  orbit, **188**
  plexiform, 188
  uvea, 202, **203**
Neurofibromatosis 1 (von
    Recklinghausen's disease), 176,
    187, 188, 202, 208–9
Neurofibromatosis 2, 209
Neurogenic muscle disorders, 314
Neuroma, amputation, 18
Neuromuscular syndromes, 145
Neuromuscular transmission disorders,
  314–16
Neuromyelitis optica (Devic's disease),
  301
Neuronal ceroid lipofuscinosis (Batten's
    disease), 125, 128
  infantile form, 128, **129**
  juvenile form, 128
Neuronopathy, 313
Neurons, 296
Neuro-ophthalmic lesions, AIDS-related,
  59
Neuropeptides, 44
Neuroretinal dysfunctions/dystrophies,
  243–4
Neutralization, 41
Neutrophils, **32–3**
  acute inflammation, 44, 45
  cytokines, 38
  phagocytosis, 41
  respiratory burst, 44
  surface receptors, 41
Newcastle disease (fowl pest), 84
Nezelof's syndrome, 55
NF1 gene, 208
NF2 gene, 209
Nickel sensitivity, 63
Niemann–Pick lipidoses, 130, 131
  group I, 131
  group II, 131
Night blindness
  choroideremia, 254
  gyrate atrophy of choroid/retina with
    hyperornithinaemia, 253
  retinitis pigmentosa, 248
  vitamin A deficiency, 12
  see also Stationary night blindness,
    congenital
Nissl substance, 296
Nitric oxide, 44
Nocardia, 91
Nocardia asteroides, 91
  keratitis, 93
Nodular fasciitis (pseudosarcomatous
    fasciitis), **205**
Nodules

Busacca, 47, 52
Dalén–Fuchs', 70, **71**
Koeppe, 47, 52
Lisch, 209
Non-accidental injury, 4–5
  battered child, 5
  shaken baby, 5
Non-antibody-dependent complement-
  mediated cell lysis, 45
Non-epithelial melanocyte proliferations,
  182–3
Non-granulomatous chronic
  inflammation, 46
Non-Hodgkin lymphoma, 203, **204**
Nondisjunction, 117
Norrie's disease, **133**, 158, 273
North Carolina macular dystrophy, 253
Nosema, 104–5
Nuclear cataract, 222
  congenital, 155
Nucleic acids, 115
Nucleocapsid, 77
Nutritional amblyopia, 13
Nutritional optic neuropathy
  (tobacco–alcohol amblyopia),
  301–2
Nutritional state, wound healing
  influence, 16

O

Obesity, 268
Ochronosis
  alkaptonuria, 125, 127, 260–1
  exogenous, 261
  ocular, **261**
Ochronotic pigment deposits, 260–1
Ocular albinism, 126
  myopia association, 218
Ocular cicatricial pemphigoid (ocular
  pemphigoid; benign mucous
  membrane pemphigoid) *see*
  Pemphigoid, ocular cicatricial
Ocular ischaemic syndrome, 279
Ocular melanocytosis (melanosis oculi),
  182
Ocular myopathy with progressive
  external ophthalmoplegia, 316
Ocular (orbital) myositis, **317**
Ocular pemphigoid *see* Pemphigoid,
  ocular cicatricial
Ocular thermal injury, 7
Oculocutaneous albinism, **126**
  Chédiak–Higashi syndrome, 55
  Type I, 126
  Type II, 126
  Type III (rufous), 126
Oculo–dental–digital syndrome, 161
Oculodermal melanocytosis (naevus of
  Ota), 182–3
Oculopharyngeal muscular dystrophy,
  316
Oedema, 269–70
  Berlin's (commotio retinae), 4

cellular, acute (hydropic change;
  cloudy swelling), 2
choroidal/suprachoroidal, 53
conjunctivitis, 50
corneal, 51, 52
cystoid macular, **24–5**, 53
keratitis, 51, 52
optic disc, 297–8
scleritis, 52
Oestrus ovis, **112**
Oguchi's disease, 246
Oligodendrocytes, 296–7
Onchocerca volvulus, **110**
Onchocerciasis, 110
  investigations, 111
  ocular, 110
Oncocytoma (oxyphil adenoma), **182**
  lacrimal gland, 184
Oncodevelopmental antigens, 145
Oncogenes, 147
Oncogenesis, 146–8
  genetic basis, 147
  stages, 147–8
Oncogenic mutagens, 117
Oncogenic viruses, 77, 146
Ophthalmia neonatorum *see* Neonatal
  conjunctivitis
Ophthalmic artery, 266
Ophthalmic surgery, 23–9
  complications, 24–9
    cataract surgery, 26–7
    corneal/corneolimbal incisions, 25
    corneorefractive procedures, 26
    eviscerations/enucleations/
      exenterations, 28
    extraocular surgery, 28
    glaucoma surgery, 27–8
    intraocular manipulation, 24
    keratoplasty, 25–6
    vitreoretinal surgery, 28–9
  wound healing, 23
Ophthalmomyasis, 112
Opsonization, 41, 60
  complement system, 39
Optic atrophy (optic nerve atrophy), 18,
  298, 300
  Schnabel's cavernous optic atrophy,
    304–5
Optic disc
  congenital excavated, 161
  crowded, 161
  development, 159
  developmental anomalies, 159–61
    minor anomalies appearance, 161
  tilted, 161
Optic disc coloboma, **151**
Optic disc drusen (hyaline bodies),
  160–1
Optic disc oedema, 297–8
  prelaminar causes, 297
  retrolaminar causes, 297
Optic disc pits, 160
Optic nerve
  aplasia, 159
  development, 159

developmental anomalies, 159–61
histological sections examination, 325
hypoplasia, 159
mechanical trauma, 4
myelination, 159
response to injury, 18
Optic nerve coloboma, 151
Optic nerve glioma
  adult, 188
  juvenile, 187, **188**
Optic nerve haemorrhage, 271
Optic nerve hypoplasia, 140
Optic nerve lesions, 297–313
  diabetes mellitus, 287
Optic nerve sheath haemorrhage, shaken
  baby, 5
Optic neuritis (inflammatory optic
  neuropathy), 299–301
  Type IV hypersensitivity, 60-1
Optic neuropathy
  acquired, 299–313
  anterior ischaemic, 287, 288, 301, **302**
  compressive, 303
  glaucomatous, **304–5**
  hypertensive, 281–2
  inflammatory (optic neuritis), 60,
    299–301
  inherited, **298–9**
  irradiation, 303
  Leber's hereditary, 134, 298, **299**
  nutritional, 301–2
  toxic, **302**
  traumatic, 303
  vascular, 301
Optic sulci, 148
Optic vesicles, 148
  inner layer developmental anomalies,
    158
  invagination abnormalities, 149–50
  outer layer developmental anomalies,
    158
  regression, 149
Oral streptococci, 90
Orbit
  autoimmune disorders, 72–4
  cartilaginous proliferations, 190
  cysts, 183–4
  growth disorders, 183–90
  inflammation, 60
  lacrimal gland proliferations, 184–5
  leukaemic deposits, 207
  lymphoproliferative lesions, 204
  mechanical trauma, 3
  metastatic deposits, 210
  neural proliferations, 186–8
  osseous proliferations, 190
  soft tissue proliferations, 188–9
  vascular proliferations, 185–6
  wound healing, 18
Orbital cellulitis, 49, 51
  bacterial, 94
  fungal, 104
  sequelae, 49
Orbital haemangiopericytoma, 186
Orbital (ocular) myositis, **317**

Orf (contagious pustular dermatitis), 83
Organic solvents, tissue damage, 12
Organization
    acute inflammation outcome, 45
    thrombus, 274
    tissue repair processes, 15
Organogenesis, 148–9
    anomalies, 149–51
Ornithine aminotransferase (OAT)
    deficiency, 253
Orthomyxoviruses, 85
Osmotic effects, contact lens wear-
    related injury, 21
Osseous choristoma
    choroidal, 191
    epibulbar, 178
Osseous metaplasia, 141
Osseous proliferations, orbit, 190
Ossification, intraocular, **54**
Osteoblastoma, 190
Osteoclasts, 34
Osteogenesis imperfecta, 242
Osteoma, 190
Osteomyelitis, 261
Osteopetrosis (Albers–Schönberg
    disease), 249
Osteosarcoma, 190
Outer blood–retinal barrier, 267
Oxalosis
    lenticular, 256
    retinal, **255**, 256
Oxyphil adenoma (oncocytoma), **182**

P

    p16 (CDKN2A) mutations, 193
    p53 mutations, 147
    p-phenylenediamine sensitivity, 63
P-selectin, 38
Pagetoid melanoma, 171
Pagetoid spread, 144
    sebaceous carcinoma, 172, **173**
Paget's disease, 234, 235
Panhypogammaglobulinaemia, 56
Pannus, 20, **21**
    degenerative, 20
    inflammatory, 20
Panophthalmitis, 52
    bacterial, **94**
        investigations, 94
    corneoscleral perforation, 5
Panuveitis, 70–1
    autoimmunity, 68
Papillary conjunctivitis, **51**
Papillary syringocystadenoma, 173–4
Papillitis, 299
Papilloedema, 297
Papilloma
    basal cell (seborrhoeic wart;
        seborrhoeic keratosis), 165, **166**
    lacrimal sac, **183**
    squamous cell, **166, 178**
Papilloma viruses, 77
Papovaviruses, 77
Parabens sensitivity, 63

Parakeratosis, 66, 141, **142**
Paramyxoviruses, 84
Paraneoplastic syndromes, 145
Paraprotein deposits, **263–4**
Parasitism, 76
Paratope, 40
Patau's syndrome (trisomy 13), 119,
    150, 156, 158, 161
Pathogens, 76
    histological stains, **322**
Paton's concentric lines, 297
Pattern macular dystrophy, 245
Pauciarticular juvenile chronic arthritis,
    69
Paving-stone degeneration of retinal
    pigment epithelium, 235
PAX6 mutations, 153, 154
Pellucid marginal corneal degeneration,
    217
Pemphigoid, ocular cicatricial (ocular
    pemphigoid; benign mucous
    membrane pemphigoid), 50, 60, **66**
Pemphigus, 60
Penetrating/perforating wounds, **5–6**
Perfluoropropane, 311
Pericytes, **266,** 273, 278, **284,** 285
Peripheral corneal melt (sterile
    peripheral ulcerative keratitis), 66
Peripheral iridotomy, laser, 27
Peripheral nerves, 313
    wound healing, 18
Peripheral neuropathies, 313
Peripheral retinal degenerations, 229–30
Peripheral retinoschisis, 243
Peripheral ulcerative keratitis, 60
Peripherin/RDS, molecular genetics/
    mutations, 245, 248, 252, 253
Permanent cell populations, 15, 139
Pernicious anaemia, 13, 291, 302
Persistent generalized lymphadenopathy,
    57
Persistent hyaloid artery, **156–7**
Persistent hyperplastic primary vitreous,
    148, 156
    anterior, 156
    posterior, 156
Persistent pupillary membrane, 154, **157**
Peter's anomaly, 153
Peyer's patches, 35
Phacoantigenic endophthalmitis see
    Lens-induced endophthalmitis
Phacoemulsification cataract surgery, 7
Phacolytic glaucoma, 5, **310**
    lens trauma, 4, 18
Phacomorphic glaucoma, 222, 310
Phagocytic deficiencies, 55
Phagocytosis, 33, 34, 45
Phakomatoses, 207–9
Pharyngoconjunctival fever, 78
Phenotype, 116
Philadelphia chromosome, 147
Phlyctenular keratoconjunctivitis
    (phlyctenulosis), 63
    Type IV hypersensitivity, 60-1
Phlyctenules (phlyctens), **63**

Phlyctenulosis see phlyctenular
    keratoconjunctivitis, Type IV
Photoablation, 9
Photocoagulation, 10
Photodisruption, 9, 10
Photomicrographs, 326
Photoreceptors
    age-related macular degeneration,
        231, 232
    ageing changes, 230
    dysfunctions, 244, 245–8
    dystrophies, 244, 248–50
        associated disorders, 217
    light transduction, 244, 245
    mechanisms of degeneration/death,
        245
    molecular genetics, 245
    pathophysiology, 245
        retinal detachment, 227
    structural aspects, 244
Photorefractive keratectomy (PRK), 26
Phototherapeutic keratectomy, 26
PHTC, 309
Phthirus capitis (head louse), 112
Phthirus pubis (pubic louse), **112**
Phthisis bulbi, 5, **54**
Physical carcinogens, 146
Picornaviruses, 84
Pigment deposits
    bilirubin, 259
    blood, 259, 270
Pigment dispersion syndrome, 309
Pigment pattern macular dystrophies,
    232, 243, 252
Pilomatricoma (benign calcifying
    epithelioma of Malherbe), **175**
Pilosebaceous units, 163–4
Pinealoblastoma, 201
Pinguecula, 10, 214–15
Plasma cells, **37**
    non-granulomatous chronic
        inflammation, 46
Plasmacytoma, **207**
Plasmids, 88
Plasmodium, 104
Platelet factor IV, 19
Platelet-activating factor (PAF), 33, 44,
    59
Platelet-derived growth factor (PDGF),
    14
Pleomorphic adenoma, 141, 175, 184,
    185
Pleomorphic carcinoma, 184–5
Pleomorphic liposarcoma, 189
Pleomorphism, corneal endothelium,
    22
Plexiform neurofibroma, 188
Pneumococcus see *Streptococcus
    pneumoniae*
Pneumocystis carinii, 101
    AIDS opportunistic infection, 57, 59
    choroidal pneumocystosis, 101
Point mutations, 117
Polar cataract, 155
Polarizing microscopy, 320–1

Polioviruses, 84
Polyarteritis nodosa, 66, 67, 73, 289, 301, 317
Polyarticular juvenile chronic arthritis, 69
Polycythaemia (erythrocytosis), 291
Polycythaemia rubra vera, 301
Polymegathism, corneal endothelium, 22
Polymerase chain reaction, 328
Polymethylmethacrylate (PMMA)
 contact lenses, 63
 intraocular lenses, 27
Polymorphic macular degeneration of Braley, 252
Polymorphic stromal corneal dystrophy, 239
Polymyalgia rheumatica see Giant cell arteritis/polymyalgia rheumatica
Polymyositis, 73, 317
Polyol pathway, 282
Polyoma viruses, 77
Polyp, fibroepithelial (squamous cell papilloma; skin tag), **166**
Polyploidy, 117, 143
Polypropylene intraocular lenses, 27
Pork tapeworm (Taenia solium), 111
Port wine stain (naevus flammeus), 176, 208
Posner–Schlossman syndrome, 308
Post-herpetic (metaherpetic) keratopathy, 80
Posterior chamber, histological sections examination, 325
Posterior ciliary artery, 266
Posterior embryotoxon, 153
Posterior intraocular inflammation, 53
 sequelae, 54
Posterior keratoconus, 153
Posterior multifocal placoid pigment epitheliopathy, acute (APMPPE), 71
Posterior polymorphous corneal dystrophy, 241, **242**
Posterior uveitis, 52, 53, 70–1
 autoimmunity, 68
Posterior vitreous detachment, 53, 224–5, 226, 229
Pott's disease, 96
Poxviruses, 83–4
Practolol-induced ocular toxicity syndrome, 66
Pre-embryonic period, 148
Pre-papillary veils, 157
Preauricular lymph nodes, 35
Preauricular lymphadenopathy, 51
Premacular gliosis (macular pucker), 228
Prematurity
 acquired retinal telangiectasia, 273
 retinopathy see Retinopathy of prematurity
Preretinal haemorrhage see Subhyaloid haemorrhage
Preretinal neovascularization, **19**

Preservatives, contact sensitivity, 63
Presumed ocular histoplasmosis syndrome (POHS), **102–3**
Primary (first) intention healing, 16, 23
Prions, 76–7
Progressive multifocal leukoencephalopathy, 77
Progressive ophthalmoplegia, chronic (Kearns–Sayre syndrome), 134–5, 249, 316
Progressive outer retinal necrosis (PORN), **82**
Prokaryotes, 76
Proliferation, neoplastic cells, 143
 malignant, 144
Proliferative lesions, 162–211
 bone, 190
 cartilage, 190
 conjunctiva, 176–83
 epithelial cell, 178–9
 epithelial melanocyte, 179–81
 histiocytic and fibroblastic, 205–7
 intraocular, 190–203
 lacrimal gland, 184–5
 lacrimal sac, 183
 lids, 162–76
 lymphatic, conjunctiva, 181–2
 lymphoproliferative, 203–4
 melanocytic
  conjunctival epithelium, 179–83
  dermis, 176
  epidermis, 168–72
  intraocular, 191–6
  non-epithelial, 182–3
 neural, 176, 186-8, 202-3
 neurilemmal, 18
 neuroepithelial, 197–201
 orbit, 183–90
 sebaceous glands, 172-3
 smooth muscle, 203
 soft tissue, 188-9
 sweat gland, 173–5
 vascular, 185-6
Proliferative vitreoretinopathy, 29, **227–8**
Propionibacterium, 91
Propionibacterium acnes, 42, 91
 exogenous endophthalmitis, 94
Prostacyclin, 44
Prostaglandins, 44, 59, 308
Protanopia, 247
Protein glycosylation, 282
Protein kinase C (PKC), 283, 287
Protein synthesis, 116
Proteus, 92
 keratitis, 93
Proteus mirabilis, 92
Proteus morgagni, 92
Proto-oncogenes, 147
Protozoa, 76, 104-8
Psammoma bodies, **187**
Pseudoadenomatous hyperplasia of ciliary epithelium, **190**
Pseudocarcinomatous hyperplasia, 168
Pseudoexfoliation syndrome, **220–1**, 309

Pseudomembranes, 50
Pseudomonas, 91
Pseudomonas aeruginosa, 22, 91, **92**
 conjunctivitis, 93
 keratitis, 93
Pseudophakie keratopathy, 25
Pseudopterygium, 215
Pseudosarcomatous fasciitis (nodular fasciitis), **205**
Pseudovitelliform lesions, 252
Pseudoxanthoma elasticum, **123**, 234, 235
Psoriatic arthritis, 68
Pterygium, 10, **214–15**
Pubic louse (Phthirus pubis), **112**
Punctate epithelial erosions (PEE), 51
Punctate epithelial keratitis (PEK), 51
Punctate inner choroidopathy (PIC), 71
Pupillary disorders, 4
Pupillary membrane, persistent, 154, **157**
Pus formation, 45
Pyknosis, 2
Pyogenic granuloma, 181

R
Rab escort protein-1 (REP-1), 254
Racemose haemangioma
 orbit, 186
 retina, 202
Radiation, 8–11
 carcinogenesis, 11, 146
 cataract, 11
 optic neuropathy, 303
 retinopathy, 11
 tissue damage, 8, 11
 vasculopathy, 11
 see also Gamma-rays, Infrared radiation, Ultraviolet radiation, Visible light, X-rays
Radiotherapy, 11
Rb1 (retinoblastoma gene), 147, 189, 197, 201
RDS locus see Peripherin/RDS
Reactive arthritis
 acute anterior uveitis (AAU) association, 68, 69
 Gram-negative bacilli in aetiology, 94
Reactive lymphoid hyperplasia, **203–4**
 conjunctiva, **204**
Refsum's disease, 249
Regeneration
 axons, 313
 cell potential, 15
 wound healing process, 15
Reis–Bückler's corneal dystrophy, **236–7**
 molecular genetics, 239
Reiter's syndrome, 68, 69, 87
 HLA associations, 68, 69
Relapsing polychondritis, 67
Rendu–Osler–Weber disease (hereditary haemorrhagic telangiectasia), 181, 272

Renin–angiotensin system, 280
Reperfusion injury, 12
Respiratory burst, 44
Rete mirabile, **19**
Reticular cystoid degeneration of
    peripheral retina, 229
Reticular degenerative retinoschisis, 230
Reticular dysgenesis, 56
Retina
    development, 157
    developmental anomalies, 157–9
    electromagnetic radiation protective
        mechanisms, 8
    glial proliferation, 54
    histological sections examination, 325
    infrared radiation damage, 9–10
    leukaemic deposits, 207
    lymphoproliferative lesions, 204
    mechanical trauma, 4
        battered child, 5
    posterior intraocular inflammation, 53
    vasoproliferation, 19–20
    wound healing, 18
Retinal aneurysms, 273–4
    macroaneurysms, **273–4**
    microaneurysms, **273**
Retinal artery, central, 266
    occlusion, **275–6**
Retinal arterioles, 266
    occlusion, branch 276
    sclerotic changes, 272
    sickle cell retinopathy, 293, 294
Retinal astrocytoma, **203**, 209
Retinal breaks, 225, 226
    classification, 225
Retinal capillaries, **266**
Retinal cavernous haemangioma, 202
Retinal circulation, **266**
    anomalous branching, 272
    development, 276
    embolism, **275**
    thrombosis, 274–5
    vessel calibre abnormalities, 272–4
Retinal degeneration
    lattice, 225
    peripheral, 229–30
    reticular cystoid, 229
Retinal detachment, 226–8
    battered child, 5
    choroid trauma, 4
    complications of surgery, 28
    exudation, 226
    intraretinal changes, **226–7**
    non-rhegmatogenous, 226
    preretinal changes (proliferative
        vitreoretinopathy), **227–8**
    retinopathy of prematurity, **277**
    rhegmatogenous, 226
    sickle cell retinopathy, 293
    subretinal changes, 227
    traction, 226
    vitreous trauma, 4
Retinal dialysis (disinsertion), 4, 225
Retinal digest preparations, 321
Retinal dysplasia, **158**

Retinal dystrophies, 242–54
    classification, 243
    genetic aspects, 243
    Müller cell, 243–4
    neurosensory retinal dysfunctions/
        dystrophies, 243–4
    photoreceptor dysfunctions/
        dystrophies, 244-52
    photoreceptor/RPE dystrophies,
        250–2
Retinal exudates, **269–70**, 297
Retinal folds, 297
    congenital, **159**
Retinal haemangioblastoma, **202**
Retinal haemorrhage, **270–1**
    battered child, 5
    dot-blot, 270
    flame-shaped, 270
    globular, 271
    massive, 271
    Roth's spots, 271
    shaken baby, 5
    sickle cell retinopathy, 294
Retinal holes, 225
    sickle cell retinopathy, 293
Retinal hypoplasia, 140
Retinal ischaemia, 274, 275–8
Retinal microangiopathy (HIV
    retinopathy), 58–9
Retinal necrosis, acute/acute bilateral
    (ARN/BARN), **82**
Retinal nerve fibre myelination, 159,
    160
Retinal non-attachment, congenital,
    148, 149–50, 158–9
Retinal outer segment membrane protein
    1 (ROM-1), molecular genetics/
    mutations, 245, 248
Retinal oxalosis, **255**, 256
Retinal pigment epitheliitis, acute, 71
Retinal pigment epithelium (RPE)
    age-related macular degeneration,
        231, 232
        detachment, 234
        tear, 234
    ageing changes, 230
    congenital hypertrophy (CHRPE),
        158, 191
        atypical multifocal bilateral lesions,
            158
        congenital grouped pigmentation
            (bear-track pigmentation), 158
    degenerations
        age-related, 235
        non-age-related, 234–5
    development, 157
    dystrophies
        photoreceptor/RPE, 250–2
        RPE/Bruch's membrane, 252–3
    focal proliferation, 227
    IL-6 production, 38
    wound healing/response to injury, 18
Retinal racemose haemangioma, 202
Retinal S-antigen, 43
Retinal tears

full-thickness, 225, 228
    giant, 225
    partial-thickness, 225
Retinal telangiectasia
    acquired, 273
    congenital, 272–3
Retinal vasculature
    anomalies, 157
    normal development, 156
Retinal vasculitis, 53
    idiopathic, **288**
Retinal vein occlusion, 273
    branch retinal vein occlusion, 19, 280
    central retinal vein occlusion, 278,
        279–80
    ischaemic, 279–80
    neovascular (thrombotic) glaucoma,
        308
    non-ischaemic, 279
        pathogenesis, 280
    hemispheric, 280
Retinal veins, 266
Retinal venules, 266
    dilatation, 272
Retinitis, 53
Retinitis pigmentosa, 243, 248–50
    clinical features, **248–9**
    molecular genetics, 245, 246, 248
    pathology, **249–50**
    systemic associations, 249
Retinitis punctata albescens, 245
Retinoblastoma, 146, 190, 197–201
    calcification, **255**
    chromosomal abnormalities, 147
    clinical features, **198**
    extraocular dissemination, 200
    familial/sporadic pattern, 197
    genetic aspects, 147, 197
    local invasion, 144
    pathology, **198–9**, **200**
    prognosis, 200
    secondary glaucoma, 308
    trilateral, 201
Retinoblastoma gene see Rb1
Retinocytoma (retinoma), 201
Retinopathy
    cancer-associated, 145–6
    diabetic see Diabetic retinopathy
    HIV (retinal microangiopathy), **58–9**
    hypertensive, **281**
    hypoperfusion, 277–8
    leukaemias, 292
    melanoma-associated, 146
    radiation, 11
    sickle cell, 293–4
    solar, 10
Retinopathy of prematurity (ROP),
    276–7
    angiogenic growth factors and, 276
    clinicopathological features, 277
    pathogenesis, 276–7
    preretinal neovascularization, 19
    vitamin E protective effect, 13
Retinoschisis
    degenerative, 229–30

peripheral, 243
  reticular degenerative, 230
X-linked juvenile, 243
Retrobulbar neuritis, 299
Retrocorneal fibrous membrane, **25**
Retrograde axonal changes, 313
Retrolental membrane, 53
Retroviruses, 85
  oncogenesis, 146, 147
Rhabdomyoma, 189
Rhabdomyosarcoma, 189
Rheumatoid arthritis, 60, 66, 67, 72–3,
  261, 289
Rhinosporidium seeberi, **101**, 102
Rhinoviruses, 84
Rhizopus, 101
Rhodopsin, 43, 244
  activation/deactivation, 245
  molecular genetics/mutations, 245
Riboflavin (vitamin B$_2$) deficiency, 13
Rickettsiae, **85**, 113
Rieger's anomaly (del 4q; del 4p;
  dup3p), 119, 153
Rieger's syndrome, 153, 305
RIEG1, 153
Rigg's type congenital stationary night
  blindness (CSNB 1), 246
Ring chromosomes, 118
Ringschwiele, 139, 190, **191**, 227
RNA, 116
RNA viruses, 84–5
Rods, 244
  light transduction, 244, 245
  stationary dysfunctions, 245–6
Rosai–Dorfman syndrome (sinus
  histiocytosis with massive
  lymphadenopathy), **205–6**
Roundworms (nematodes), 108
Rubella (German measles), 84–5, 300
  embryopathy (congenital rubella
    syndrome), 85, 161, 222
Rubeola (measles), 84, 300
Rubeosis iridis, **20**
  diabetes mellitus, 287
  inflammation sequelae, 53
  neovascular glaucoma, 308
Russell bodies, **37**

S

Salmonella, 68, 69, 92
  autoimmune uveitis/arthritis
    association, 94
Salzmann's nodular corneal
  degeneration, **215–16**
Sandhoff's disease (GM$_2$ Type II), 130
Sanfilippo syndrome, 131
Saprophytes, 76
Sarcoidosis, **47–9**
  causes, 49
  chronic anterior uveitis, 69
  genetic factors, 49
  granulomatous inflammation, 46
Sarcoma, 142

embryonal (embryonal
  rhabdomyosarcoma), **189**
Kaposi, 57, 58, 59
  conjunctiva, **181**
Scar tissue
  formation, 15–16, 45
  remodelling, 16
Scheie syndrome, 131
Schistosoma haematobium, 111
Schistosoma japonicum, 111
Schistosoma mansoni, 111
Schistosomiasis, 111
Schnabel's cavernous optic atrophy,
  304–5
Schnyder's central crystalline corneal
  dystrophy, 240, 263–4
Schubert–Bornschein type congenital
  stationary night blindness (CSNB
  2), 246
Schwann cells, 313
  proliferation, 18
Schwannoma (neurilemmoma), 176
  Antoni type A/type B, 188, **189**
  orbit, 188, **189**
  uveal, 203
Schwartz–Matsuo syndrome, 309
Sclera
  blue, 242
  histological sections examination, 325
  normal development, 152
  wound healing, 18
Scleral dystrophies, 242
Scleritis, 49, **52**, **67**
  necrotizing, 60
  sequelae, 49
Sclerocornea, 152
Scleroderma, 73
Sclerosing orbital inflammation, **74**
Scrapie, 76
Scurvy, 13
Sebaceous adenoma, 172
Sebaceous carcinoma, **172–3**
  pagetoid spread, 144, 172, **173**
Sebaceous glands, 163
  proliferations, 172–3
Sebaceous hyperplasia, **172**
Seborrhoeic dermatitis, 50
Seborrhoeic keratosis, 165, **166**
  irritated (inverted follicular keratosis),
    165
Seborrhoeic wart (basal cell papilloma;
  seborrhoeic keratosis), 165, **166**
Second intention healing, 16
  ophthalmic surgical wounds, 23
Secondary neoplasms, 210–11
Secretory IgA, 41
Segmental demyelination, 313
Selectins, 38
Selective IgA deficiency, 56
Selenium, 19
Senile keratosis (actinic keratosis; solar
  keratosis), 141, **167**
Senile lentigo, 171
Senile reticular hyperpigmentation, 235
Senile scleral plaque, 216

Seronegative spondyloarthropathies,
  acute anterior uveitis (AAU)
    association, 68
Serotonin, 34, 44, 59
Serratia marcescens, 92
  keratitis, 93
Serum amyloid A, 45
Serum amyloid P, 45
Serum sickness, 60
Severe combined immunodeficiency
  (SCID), 56
Sex chromosomes, 115
Shagreen patches, 209
Shaken baby, 5
Shigella, 68, 69, 92
  autoimmune uveitis/arthritis
    association, 94
Shingles (herpes zoster), 81
Sickle cell haemoglobinopathies, 273,
  278, 292–4, 301
  AS disease (sickle cell trait), 293
  preretinal neovascularization, 19
  retinopathy, 293–4
    black sunbursts, 294
    non-proliferative, 294
    proliferative, 293
    retinal haemorrhages, 294
    retinal vascular changes, 294
  SC disease (sickle cell C disease), 293,
    294
  secondary glaucoma, 309
  SS disease (sickle cell disease; sickle
    cell anaemia), 292–3, 294
  SThal disease (sickle cell ß-
    thalassaemia), 293
Siderosis, 6, **256**
  corneal, 3, **256**
Siderosis bulbi, **256–7**
Siegrist's streaks, 279, 282
Silicone intraocular lenses, 27
Silicone oil-induced glaucoma, **311**
Silver deposits (argyrosis), 258
Silver nitrate, 93
Simian vacuolating virus, 77
Single gene defects, 119–32
  autosomal dominant disorders, **120–3**
  autosomal recessive disorders, 121,
    123–32
  congenital malformations, 140 *see also*
    Developmental anomalies
  optic neuropathies, 298, **299**
  retinal dystrophies, 243
  X-linked disorders, 132–4
Sinus histiocytosis with massive
  lymphadenopathy (Rosai–Dorfman
  syndrome), **205–6**
Size of eye, developmental anomalies,
  161
Sjögren's syndrome, 72–3, 289
  autoantibodies, 73
  HLA associations, 73
  keratoconjunctivitis sicca, 72
  ophthalmic manifestations, 72
  oral manifestations, 72
  primary (sicca syndrome), 72

Sjögren's syndrome, (*Cont.*)
  secondary, 72
  Type IV hypersensitivity, 60-1
Skin
  allergic disorders, 64–5
  bacterial flora, 42
  diffuse melanosis, 260
  lids, 162–4
  wound healing, 16, 23
Skin tag (squamous cell papilloma;
    fibroepithelial polyp), **166**
Smallpox, 83
Smoking, 268
Smooth muscle proliferations, 203
Snow blindness, 10
Soemmering's ring cataract, 5, **6**
Soft tissue proliferations, orbit, 188–9
Solar keratosis (actinic keratosis; senile
    keratosis), 141, **167**
Solar retinopathy, 10
Solvent abuse, 302
Somatic mutation, 135
Sorsby's fundus dystrophy, 232, 253
Spheroidal corneal degeneration
    (climatic droplet keratopathy;
    Labrador keratopathy), 10, **215**
Spheroliths, 222
Spherophakia (microspherophakia), 155
Sphingolipidoses, 125, 129–31
Spiral bacteria (spirochaetes), **98–100**
Spitz naevus (juvenile melanoma), 170
Spleen, 35
  antigen processing, 40
Splendore–Hoeppli phenomenon, 61
Spores
  fungi, 100
  Gram-positive organisms, 88
Spotted fevers, **85**
Spring catarrh *see* Vernal
    keratoconjunctivitis
Squamous cell carcinoma
  conjunctiva, **179**
    AIDS-related, 59
  lacrimal gland, 185
  lids, 168, **169**
Squamous cell layer, 163
Squamous cell papilloma
  conjunctiva, **178**
  skin tag (fibroepithelial polyp), **166**
Squint surgery, complications, 28
Stable cell populations, 15, 139
Stains *see* Histological stains
Staphylococcus, 64, 65, **89**, 317
  allergic disorders, 63, 64
  neonatal conjunctivitis (ophthalmia
    neonatorum), 93
Staphylococcus aureus, 42, 89, **90**
  anterior blepharitis, 50
  canaliculitis/dacryocystitis, 93
  conjunctivitis, 93
  exogenous endophthalmitis, 94
  keratitis, 93
  orbital cellulitis, 94
Staphylococcus epidermidis, 42, 89
  conjunctivitis, 93

exogenous endophthalmitis, 94
  keratitis, 93
Staphyloma, 49, **50**, 216–18
Stargardt's disease/fundus
    flavimaculatus, 232, 243, 250–1
  maculopathy (Stargardt's disease), **251**
  peripheral retinopathy (fundus
    flavimaculatus), 251
Stationary night blindness, congenital
    see Congenital stationary night
    blindness
Sterile infiltrates, 22
Sterile peripheral ulcerative keratitis
    (peripheral corneal melt), 66
Stevens–Johnson syndrome (erythema
    multiforme), 50, 60, 65, 87
Stickler's syndrome, 122–3
Still's disease (systemic juvenile chronic
    arthritis), 69
Stocker's line, 214, 256
Strawberry naevus *see* Capillary
    haemangioma
Streptococcus, **89–90**, 317
  canaliculitis/dacryocystitis, 93
  exogenous endophthalmitis, 94
  neonatal conjunctivitis (ophthalmia
    neonatorum), 93
Streptococcus pneumoniae, 64, **90**
  conjunctivitis, 93
  exogenous endophthalmitis, 94
  keratitis, 93
  orbital cellulitis, 94
Streptococcus pyogenes, 50, **90**
  conjunctivitis, 93
  exogenous endophthalmitis, 94
  keratitis, 93
  orbital cellulitis, 94
Streptococcus viridans, 90, 93
Striated muscle, 314
Stroma *see* Corneal stroma
Stromal keratitis, **80**
Stromal oedema *see* Corneal stromal
    oedema
Sturge–Weber syndrome
    (encephalotrigeminal angiomatosis),
    176, 201, 208
Subconjunctival haemorrhage, 270
Subepithelial connective tissue, of
    conjunctiva, 177
Subepithelial fibrosis, of lens, 141
Subhyaloid (preretinal) haemorrhage, 4,
    270
  battered child, 5
  shaken baby, 5
Submandibular lymph nodes, 35
Submandibular lymphadenopathy, 51
Subretinal fluid, retinal detachment, 227
Subretinal haemorrhage, 271
  battered child, 5
  shaken baby, 5
Sub-retinal pigment epithelium (RPE)
    deposits, **230–1**
Sub-retinal pigment epithelium (RPE)
    haemorrhage, 271
Substance P, 44

Sudoriferous glands *see* Sweat glands
Sulphonamides, 65
Sulphur hexafluoride, 311
Sunflower cataract, 258
Sunlamps, 10
Sunlight, 10
Superior limbic keratoconjunctivitis,
    22–3
Surgical trauma, secondary glaucoma,
    311
Suspensory ligament *see* Zonule
Sutural cataract, congenital, 155
Sutures, 23
  faulty technique, 24
Sweat gland carcinoma, 175
Sweat gland proliferations, 173–5
Sweat gland (sudoriferous) cyst, **165**
Sweat glands (sudoriferous glands), 163
Symbiosis, 76
Symblepharon, 49, **49**
Sympathetic ophthalmitis, 68, **70–1**
  corneoscleral perforation, 5
  evisceration complication, 28
  granulomatous inflammation, 60
  HLA associations, 71
  Type IV hypersensitivity, 60-1
Synchisis scintillans, 223
Syneresis, 223
Synophthalmos, 149, **150**
Syphilis, 98–100, 301
  clinical stages, 98–9
  congenital, 99–100, 140
  granulomatous inflammation, 46
  investigations, 100
  ophthalmic, 99–100
Syringocystadenoma, papillary, 173–4
Syringoma, **174**
Systemic juvenile chronic arthritis (Still's
    disease), 69
Systemic lupus erythematosus, 60, 66,
    67, 73, 289, 317

T

T cell deficiencies, primary, 55–6
  combined B cell deficiencies, 56
T cell receptors (TCRs), 36, 38
T cells, 36
  activation, 36, 39, 40
  adhesion molecules, 38
  clonal deletion/inactivation, 41–2
  cytokines, 38, 39
  delayed-type hypersensitivity (Type IV
    reactions), 60
  differentiation, 35
  lymphoid organs, 35
  memory cells, 39
  MHC molecule interactions/
    restriction, 37, 38
  subsets, 36
  see also Cytotoxic/suppressor T cells
    ($T_{C/S}$CD8 +); Helper T cells
    (T_HCD4 +)
Taenia solium (pork tapeworm), 111,
    317

Takayasu's disease, 291
Tamoxifen, 264
Tapeworms (cestodes), 108, 111–12
Tay–Sachs disease (GM$_2$ Type I), **130**
T$_{C/S}$CD8 + cells *see* Cytotoxic/
    suppressor T cells
Tear film
    contact lens wear-related injury, 23
    leukocytes, 42
Tear gas, 12
Tears
    IgA, 41, 42
    innate immune function, 42
Telangiectasia, 181
    hereditary haemorrhagic
        (Rendu–Osler–Weber disease),
        181, 272
    retinal, 272-3
Temporal arteritis *see* Giant cell
    arteritis/polymyalgia rheumatica
Temporal artery biopsies, 319
Teratogens, 117, 140
Teratoma, 184
Terrien's marginal corneal degeneration,
    215
TGFB1, 239
T$_H$/CD4 + cells *see* Helper T cells
Thalassaemias, 292
Thalidomide, 150, 161
Thermal injury, 6–7
    electrical current, 8
    electromagnetic radiation, 9
    laser mechanisms of action, 9
Thermocoagulation, 7, 8
Thiamine (vitamin B$_1$) deficiency, 13,
    302
Thrombolysis, 274
Thrombosis, 274–5
    ophthalmic surgery complication, 24
Thrombotic glaucoma, 308
Thromboxane, 44, 59
Thygeson's superficial punctate
    keratopathy, 67
Thymus, 35
    developmental failure, 55
    T cell clonal deletion/inactivation,
        41–2
Thyroid carcinoma, 73
Thyroid eye disease (dysthyroid
    orbitopathy), **73–4**
Ticks (*Ixodidiae*), **85, 113**
TIMP3, 253
Tissue injury, 2–14
Tobacco–alcohol amblyopia (nutritional
    optic neuropathy), 301–2
Tocopherols (vitamin E family), 13
Togaviruses, 84–5
Tolerance, 41–2
    autoimmunity-related impairment, 65
Tolosa–Hunt syndrome, 74
Total cataract, congenital, 155
Touton giant cells, 46, **47**
Toxic conjunctivitis, 22
Toxic optic neuropathies, **302**
Toxins, 89

contact lens wear-related injury, 21,
    22
Toxocara, 109–10
    granulomatous inflammation, 46
    investigations, 109–10
    ocular toxocariasis, **109**
Toxocara canis, **109**
Toxocara cati, 109
Toxoplasma gondii, 59, 104, **105**, 106,
    140, 292, 317
Toxoplasmosis, 105–7
    AIDS opportunistic infection, 57, 59
    congenital, 105
    investigations, 106–7
    ocular, **105**, 106
Trabecular meshwork
    glaucoma procedures, 27–8
    normal development, 151–2
Trabeculectomy, 28
    failure/complications, 28
    specimens, 319
Trabeculitis, 308
Trachoma, 86–7
    Chlamydia trachomatis serovars,
        86, 87
    Herbert's pits, **87**
Transcription, 116, 139
Transducin, 245
Transforming growth factors (TGFs),
    14, 39, 43
    acute inflammation, 44
Translation, 116
Translocation, 117–18
    balanced, 118
Transmissible mink encephalopathy, 76
Transplantation, 74
    cytomegalovirus opportunistic
        infection, 82
    graft-versus host reactions, 76
    see also Corneal allografts
Transthyretin, 261
Transudates, 269
Traumatic optic neuropathy, 303
Treacher–Collins syndrome, 162
Trematodes (flukes), 108, 111
Treponema pallidum, **98**, 100, 140
Trichilemmoma, **175**
Trichinella spiralis, 110, 317
Trichoepithelioma, 175
Trichofolliculoma, 175
Trichromatism, anomalous, 247–8
Trisomies, 117, 118
Trisomy 13 (Patau's syndrome), 119,
    150, 156, 158, 161
Trisomy 18 (Edward's syndrome), 119
Trisomy 21 (Down's syndrome),
    118–19, 154, 217, 218
Tritanopia, 247
Tropheryoma whippeli, 91
Trypanosoma, 104
Tuberculosis, 2, 95–6, 261
    granulomatous inflammation, 46, 60
    investigations, 96
    ophthalmic, 96
    phlyctenular keratoconjunctivitis, 63

Tuberous sclerosis, 209
Tumour necrosis factors (TNFs), 36, 39,
    44, 145
Tumour-suppressor genes (anti-
    oncogenes), 147
Tumours
    definition, 141
    histological sections examination, 325
    museum specimen examination, 324
Turcot's syndrome, 158, 210
Turner's syndrome, 118, 217
Typhus, **85**
Tyrosinase pathway, 260
    defects, 126

U

Ulcerative colitis, 68
Ulcerative keratitis, 51, **52**
    peripheral, 60, 66
Ultrasound, 7
Ultraviolet radiation, 10
    carcinogenesis, 146
    chronic exposure, 10
    cornea/lens selective absorption, 8
    lasers, 9, 10
    ocular protective mechanisms, 8
    tissue damage, 8, 9, 10
Ureaplasma urealyticum, 87
Uric acid deposits, 264
Usher's syndrome, 249
UV-A, 10
UV-B, 10
UV-C, 10
Uvea
    autoimmune disorders, 67–71
    circulation, 267
    glaucomatous damage, 305
    ischaemia, 278–9
    leukaemic deposits, 207
    lymphoproliferative lesions, 204
    metastatic deposits, 211
    vasoproliferation, 20
    wound healing, 18
Uveal melanoma *see* Melanoma
Uveal neurofibroma, 202, **203**
Uveal schwannoma, 203
Uveitis, 4, 52
    autoimmune, 67–71
        Gram-negative bacilli in aetiology,
            94
        uveitogenic antigens, 43, 69
    graft-versus host reactions, 76
    intermediate (pars plana
        inflammation), 53
    secondary glaucoma, 308
    see also Anterior uveitis; Posterior
        uveitis

V

Vaccinia, 83
Vacuoles, lens, 155, 221
Variable region, 40
Varicella (chickenpox), 80, 81

Varicella zoster virus, 79, 80–1
  acute/acute bilateral retinal necrosis
    (ARN/BARN), 82
  AIDS opportunistic infection, 59
  herpes zoster ophthalmicus, 81
  progressive outer retinal necrosis
    (PORN), **82**
Varices, 186
Vascular disease, 267–80
  degenerative changes, 267–8
Vascular endothelial growth factor
    (VEGF), 14, 19, 202, 207, 280, 283,
    287
  retinopathy of prematurity, 276
Vascular optic neuropathies, 301
Vascular proliferations
  conjunctiva, 181
  intraocular, 201–2
  lids, 175–6
  orbit, 185–6
Vascular supply, wound healing
    influence, 16
Vascular system, ocular, 266–7
  blood–ocular barriers, 267
  development, 156
  developmental anomalies, 156–7
  retinal circulation, **266**
  uveal circulation, 267
Vascular tortuosity, 272
Vasculitis, 275, 288–91
  HLA associations, 288
  hypersensitivity, 289
  retinal, 53, 273, **288**
  Type III hypersensitivity, 60, 289
Vasculopathy, radiation, 11
Vasoactive amines, 44
Vasoactive intestinal peptide (VIP), 43,
    44
Vasocongestion (hyperaemia), 279–80
  scleritis, 52
Vasodilatation
  acute inflammation, 44
  conjunctivitis, 50
Vasospasm, 275
Venules, high endothelial, 40
Vernal keratoconjunctivitis (spring
    catarrh), 50, 51, 59, **61–2**
  Type IV hypersensitivity, 61
VHL, 207
Virokines, 77
Virulence factors, 89
Viruses, 76, 77–85
  cytopathic effect, 77
  DNA, 77–84
  inclusion bodies, 77
  latent infection, 77
  microbiological specimens, 326
  replication cycle, 77
  RNA, 84–5
  structural aspects, 77
  Type IV hypersensitivity reactions, 60
Visceral leishmaniasis, 104
Visible light, 10
  lasers, 9

ocular protective mechanisms, 8
  tissue injury, 8, 10
Vitamin A deficiency, 12–13, 93
Vitamin B complex deficiencies, 13,
    302
Vitamin B$_1$ (thiamine) deficiency, 13,
    302
Vitamin B$_2$ (riboflavin) deficiency, 13
Vitamin B$_{12}$ (cyanocobalamin)
    deficiency, 13, 291, 302
Vitamin C (ascorbic acid) deficiency, 13
  wound healing impairment, 16
Vitamin D (calciferol) excess, 13
Vitamin deficiencies, 12–14
Vitamin E family (tocopherols), 13
Vitamin K, 14
Vitelliform macular dystrophy,
  adult, 245
  Best's, 243, **251–2**
Vitreomacular traction, 224
Vitreoretinal interface degenerations,
    223–9
Vitreoretinal surgery, complications,
    28–9
Vitreoretinal traction, 223–4, 226
  blood vessel involvement, 224
  peripheral, 224
  sickle cell retinopathy, 293
Vitreoschisis, 224
Vitreous
  amyloid deposits, 263
  aspirates for microbiology, 327
  degenerations, 223
  detachment, 4
    posterior, 224–5, 226, 229
  development, 156
  developmental anomalies, 156–7
  haemorrhage, 270
    sickle cell retinopathy, 293
  histological sections examination,
    325
  immune function, 42
  mechanical trauma, 4
  posterior intraocular inflammation, 53
  posterior vitreous detachment, 53,
    224–5, 226, 229
Vitritis, 53
VMD2, 252
Vogt–Koyanagi–Harada syndrome, 68,
    71
  granulomatous inflammation, 60
  HLA associations, 71
  Type IV hypersensitivity, 60-1
Vogt's striae, 217
Vogt's white limbal girdle, 215
von Hippel–Lindau disease, 202, 207,
    272
  chromosomal abnormalities, 147
von Recklinghausen's disease *see*
    Neurofibromatosis 1
Vortex keratopathy (cornea verticillata),
    17, 264
Vortex veins, 266
Vossius' ring, 4, 260

W

Waardenburg Jonker's (superficial
    granular) corneal dystrophy, 238
Waardenburg's syndrome, 249
WAGR syndrome, 119, 154
Waldenström's macroglobulinaemia,
    264
Wallerian (axonal) degeneration, 18,
    304, 313
Water clefts, lens substance, 221
Wedl cells, 221
Wegener's granulomatosis, 66, 67, 72,
    289
Weight loss in neoplastic disease, 145
Weill–Marchesani syndrome, 155, 223,
    310
Weil's disease, 98
Weiss' ring, 225, 229
Welding arcs, tissue injury, 10
Wernicke–Korsakoff syndrome, 302
Wernicke's encephalopathy, 302
Wernicke's syndrome, 13
White dot syndromes, 68, 71
Wilms' tumour (nephroblastoma), 119
Wilson's disease (hepatolenticular
    degeneration), 125, 129, 258
  Kayser–Fleischer ring, 129
Wiskott–Aldrich syndrome, 56
Worms (helminths), 76, 108-12
Wound contraction, 15
Wound healing, 14–20
  adipose tissue, 18
  bone, 18
  Bowman's layer, 17
  cell regeneration capacity, 15
  cellular phase, 16
  contracture phase, 16
  corneal epithelium, 17
  episcleral, 16
  growth factors, 14–15
  keratoplasty, 25–6
  keratotomy, 26
  modifying influences, 16
  ophthalmic surgery, 23
  ophthalmic tissues, 16–18
  photorefractive/phototherapeutic
    keratectomy, 26
  primary (first) intention, 16, 23
  regeneration process, 15
  repair processes, 15–16
  second intention, 16, 23
Wuchereria bancrofti, 111
Wyburn–Mason syndrome, 185, 202,
    208, 272

X

X chromosome, 115
X-linked congenital stationary night
    blindness, 246
X-linked disorders, 132–4
  dominant, 132–3
  recessive, **133–4**

X-linked juvenile retinoschisis, 243
X-rays, 8, 11
Xanthelasma, 205, **206**
Xanthogranuloma, juvenile, 205, **206**, 309
Xanthophyll, 8
Xenografts, 74
Xeroderma pigmentosum, 125, 132, 146, 147

Xerophthalmia, vitamin A deficiency, 12–13
  conjunctival xerosis, 13
  corneal ulceration/keratomalacia, 13
  corneal xerosis, 13

Y

Y chromosome, 115
Yersinia, 68, 69

autoimmune uveitis/arthritis association, 94

Z

Zeiss glands, 42, 164
Zonule (suspensory ligament), 218
  degenerations, 223
  mechanical trauma, 4
Zygomycetes, 101–2